ENDOCRINE DISORDERS

BASIC AND CLINICAL ENDOCRINOLOGY

Editors

P. Reed Larsen
Brigham and Women's Hospital
Harvard Medical School
Boston, Massachusetts

David R. London
Queen Elizabeth Hospital
Edgbaston, Birmingham,
England

Peter Sönksen
St. Thomas's Hospital
Medical School
London, England

1. Radioassay Systems in Clinical Endocrinology, *edited by Guy E. Abraham*
2. Congenital Hypothyroidism, *edited by Jean H. Dussault and Peter Walker*
3. Cytochemical Bioassays: Techniques and Clinical Applications, *edited by J. Chayen and Lucille Bitensky*
4. Endocrine Disorders: A Guide to Diagnosis, *edited by Richard A. Donald*

Other Volumes in Preparation

ENDOCRINE DISORDERS
A Guide to Diagnosis

edited by

Richard A. Donald

Christchurch Clinical School of Medicine
The Princess Margaret Hospital
Christchurch, New Zealand

Marcel Dekker, Inc. New York • Basel

Butterworths London

Library of Congress Cataloging in Publication Data

Main entry under title:

Endocrine disorders.

(Basic and clinical endocrinology ; 4)
Includes indexes.
1. Endocrine glands–Diseases–Diagnosis–Addresses, essays, lectures. I. Donald, Richard A., [date] II. Series. [DNLM: 1. Endocrine diseases–Diagnosis. W1 BA813T v.4 / WK 100 E516]
RC649.E514 1983 616.4 83-18807
ISBN 0-8247-1913-1

MARCEL DEKKER, INC.
270 Madison Avenue, New York, New York 10016

Current printing (last digit):
10 9 8 7 6 5 4 3 2 1

PRINTED IN THE UNITED STATES OF AMERICA

Preface

This book is part of the "Basic and Clinical Endocrinology" series. It is intended to be a practical guide to diagnosis and to provide readily accessible information on the applications, interpretation and limitations of the various diagnostic tests and testing procedures used in endocrinology. It should be of interest not only to endocrinologists, but other clinicians who have patients with suspected endocrine disorders, undergraduate and postgraduate students in internal medicine, and nursing and technical staff who carry out endocrine tests. The temptation to cover other aspects of endocrinology has been resisted and exhaustive technical details of the various laboratory tests have been omitted. However, references to the relevant literature and other books in the "Basic and Clinical Endocrinology" series will provide further scientific and theoretical background. The practical emphasis and concise presentation should make this book suitable for use in the clinic rather than confining it to the library.

It is perhaps only to be expected that the approach to diagnosis will vary in different centers and in different parts of the world, depending on local expertise, equipment and financial considerations. It is hoped that the cosmopolitan authorship of this book (contributors from the United States, the United Kingdom, Switzerland, Scandinavia, and Australasia) will help to avoid a parochial approach to diagnosis. Inevitably there will be some highly valued technique which has been overlooked. Many centers would include endocrine gland biopsy as part of their diagnostic routine. However, there is still considerable lack of agreement regarding the indications for thyroid and testicular biopsies, and biopsies taken during endocrine gland surgery, such as parathyroid biopsies, were judged to be beyond the scope of this book. The immunology of endocrine disorders has made considerable progress recently and is likely to have an important effect on endocrine diagnosis in the future. These topics will be covered in further volumes on endocrine pathology and endocrine immunology in the "Basic and Clinical Endocrinology" series.

This book has been divided into three major categories. Chapters 1-18 give an overview of the methodology with emphasis on any factors which may affect clinical understanding and interpretation. It is hoped that these chapters will stimulate better liaison between the clinician and laboratory to the mutual benefit of both. Chapters 19-35 outline the background pathophysiology of the appropriate endocrine disorders and provide detailed analysis of the relevance and relative importance of the investigational procedures used. "Diagnostic summaries" provide a diagrammatic logical and sequential approach to diagnosis. In Chapters 36-47, detailed protocols of commonly used dynamic testing procedures are given, followed by comments on the application of the tests and interpretation of the results. This is a "how to do it" section which should reduce the need for telephoned advice and may encourage more standardized procedures. It is hoped that a satisfactory balance between theory and practice has been achieved. The ever-increasing size and specialization of endocrine texts has highlighted the need for a book which provides a practical guide to the diagnosis of endocrine disorders. At the same time, the widely acknowledged professional competence of the contributors will reassure the reader that he is being brought up to date with the current state of diagnosis in this rapidly advancing specialty.

I am indebted to the Series Editors for their advice and encouragement, all the authors for their cooperation and excellent contributions, and Mrs. Yvonne Skilton, Mrs. Shirley Gunnell, and Mrs. Paula Gilson for their expert secretarial assistance.

Richard A. Donald

Contributors

A. Brian Ayers, D.M.R.D., M.D., F.R.C.R. Consultant Radiologist, Radiology Department, St. Thomas' Hospital, London, England

Derek R. Bangham, M.B., F.R.C.P. Head, Division of Hormones, National Institute for Biological Standards and Control, London, England

Peter H. Baylis, B.Sc., M.D., F.R.C.P. Consultant Physician and Senior Lecturer, Department of Medicine, Royal Victoria Infirmary, Newcastle-Upon-Tyne, England

A. Caroline Berry, M.B., B.S., Ph.D. Consultant Clinical Geneticist, Pediatric Research Unit, Guy's Hospital, London, England

S. R. Bloom, M.A., D.Sc., M.D., F.R.C.P. Professor of Endocrinology, Department of Medicine, Royal Postgraduate Medical School, Hammersmith Hospital, London, England

Keith E. Britton, M.A., M.B., B.Chir., M.Sc., M.D., F.R.C.P. Consultant Physician and Physician in Charge, Department of Nuclear Medicine, St. Bartholomew's Hospital Medical College, London, England

R. V. Brooks, Ph.D., D.Sc., F.R.C.Path. Professor of Chemical Endocrinology, Department of Chemical Pathology, St. Thomas' Hospital Medical School, London, England

Stafford E. Brooks, FNZIMBI Chief Medical Photographer, Medical Illustration Department, North Canterbury Hospital Board, Christchurch, New Zealand

Henry G. Burger, M.D., F.R.A.C.P. Director, Medical Research Centre and Department of Endocrinology, Prince Henry's Hospital, Melbourne, Australia

Wilfrid R. Butt, D.Sc., F.R.S.C. Professor, Department of Clinical Endocrinology, Birmingham and Midland Hospital for Women, Birmingham, England

Tim Chard, M.D., F.R.C.O.G. Professor, Department of Reproductive Physiology, St. Bartholomew's Hospital Medical College, and the London Hospital Medical College, London, England

Richard A. Donald, M.D., Ph.D., F.R.A.C.P. Professor, Department of Medicine, Christchurch Clinical School of Medicine and Endocrinologist, Princess Margaret Hospital, Christchurch, New Zealand

Eric A. Espiner, M.B., B.Chir., M.D., F.R.A.C.P. Professor, Department of Medicine, Christchurch Clinical School of Medicine and Head, Department of Endocrinology, Princess Margaret Hospital, Christchurch, New Zealand

Stephen Franks, M.D., M.R.C.P. Senior Lecturer in Reproductive Endocrinology, Department of Obstetrics and Gynecology, St. Mary's Hospital Medical School, University of London, London, England

Bengt Fredricsson, M.D. Associate Professor, Department of Obstetrics and Gynecology, Karolinska Institute, Huddinge University Hospital, Stockholm, Sweden

David M. Hurley, M.B., F.R.A.C.P., N.H., M.R.C. Medical Postgraduate Scholar, Medical Research Centre, Prince Henry's Hospital, Melbourne, Australia

H. K. Ibbertson, M.B., F.R.C.P., F.R.A.C.P. Professor of Endocrinology, Department of Medicine, University of Auckland School of Medicine, Auckland, New Zealand

Stephen L. Jeffcoate, Ph.D., M.R.C.Path. Professor, Department of Biochemical Endocrinology, Chelsea Hospital for Women, London, England

Michael M. Kaplan, M.D., F.A.C.P. Assistant Professor, Department of Medicine, Brigham and Women's Hospital and Assistant Professor, Department of Medicine, Harvard Medical School, Boston, Massachusetts

P. G. Kopelman, M.D., M.R.C.P. Lecturer, Department of Metabolism and Endocrinology, London Hospital, London, England

Gabor Thomas Kovacs, M.R.C.O.G., F.R.A.C.O.G. Gynecologist, Reproductive Medicine Clinic, Medical Research Centre, Prince Henry's Hospital, Melbourne, Australia

Leslie Lazarus, M.B., B.S., F.R.A.C.P., F.R.C.P.A., F.A.A.C.B. Director, Garvan Institute of Medical Research, St. Vincent's Hospital, Sydney, Australia

John H. Livesey, Ph.D. Scientific Officer, Department of Endocrinology, Princess Margaret Hospital, Christchurch, New Zealand

A. Wayne Meikle, M.D. Professor, Division of Endocrinology and Metabolism, University of Utah School of Medicine, Salt Lake City, Utah

Don H. Nelson, M.D. Professor of Medicine and Physiology, and Chief, Division of Endocrinology and Metabolism, Department of Internal Medicine, University of Utah School of Medicine, Salt Lake City, Utah

M. Gary Nicholls, M.D., F.R.A.C.P. Physician, Departments of Endocrinology and Cardiology, Princess Margaret Hospital, Christchurch, New Zealand

Roger J. Pepperell, M.D., M.G.O., F.R.C.O.G., F.R.A.C.O.G., F.R.A.C.P. Professor, Department of Obstetrics and Gynecology, University of Melbourne, Melbourne, Australia

Solomon Posen, M.D., F.R.C.P., F.R.A.C.P. Associate Professor, Department of Medicine, University of Sydney, Sydney, Australia

Andrea Prader, M.D. Professor, Department of Pediatrics, University of Zurich, Zurich, Switzerland

Lesley H. Rees, M.Sc., M.D., M.R.C.Path., F.R.C.P. Professor, and Honorary Consultant Physician, Department of Chemical Endocrinology, St. Bartholomew's Hospital Medical College, London, England

Peter H. Sönksen, M.D., F.R.C.P. Professor of Endocrinology, Department of Medicine, St. Thomas' Hospital Medical School, London, England

Roderick D. Suckling, M.B.Ch.B., D.O., F.R.C.S., F.R.A.C.S. Visiting Ophthalmologist, Department of Ophthalmology, Christchurch Hospital, Christchurch, New Zealand

James M. Tanner, M.D., Ph.D., D.Sc., F.R.C.P. Professor, Department of Growth and Development, Institute of Child Health, University of London, London, England

Susan M. Wood, B.Sc., M.B.B.S. R. D. Lawrence Research Fellow and Registrar in Endocrinology and Diabetes, Department of Medicine, Royal Postgraduate Medical School, Hammersmith Hospital, London, England

Contents

Diagnostic Summaries

ENDOCRINE DISORDERS

CLINICAL MEASUREMENTS

1
Weight and Endocrine Function

P. G. Kopelman
London Hospital, London, England

Stephen L. Jeffcoate
Chelsea Hospital for Women, London, England

The definitions of overweight and underweight conditions are necessarily arbitrary since body weight (or alternatively the quantity of body fat) is, like many biological variables, continuously distributed in populations with no clear dividing line between individuals of "normal" weight and those who are obese or thin. The popular conception of ideal body weight varies from society to society and also over time, but an excessive amount of fat or excessive thinness are recognized as having serious consequences on health (1, 2). There is, however, no well-defined weight at which a clear influence of obesity or excessive thinness on morbidity or mortality begins. Nevertheless, there must be an optimal amount of body fat and this optimum must be determined by the environmental situation.

I. IDEAL WEIGHT TABLES

The commonest method of assessment of fat stores is to weigh an individual and compare this weight against published tables. There are two types of weight tables available: those based on average weights and those based on ideal weights. The former have the disadvantage that the average weight in one population may not be ideal for optimal health. Furthermore, it is not a static parameter. As the number of obese people increase in a society the average figure itself tends to be "overweight." Thus it is important to establish that obesity or thinness is being measured, not just the deviation from a mean weight.

One set of ideal weight tables is derived from the experience of insuring 4.5 million lives over the period 1935 to 1954 (3) and it shows that the desirable range of weight for men and women which is associated with greatest longevity. These tables have limitations because weight must be related to the individual, together with age, sex, and size of frame. The Metropolitan Life Insurance Company tables have to some extent overcome this problem (Table 1). These tables list desirable weight for height, established on the basis of weights associated with lowest mortality and related to frame size and age. Unfortunately, no criteria are given for what constitutes a small, medium, or large frame and the measurements were made with subjects dressed and wearing shoes.

There are other methods of assessing "fatness" or "thinness." Measurements of body fat can be made from underwater weighing, by determining total body water, or calculated indirectly by estimating lean body mass, but such procedures are too complicated for routine clinical practice. An alternative method is to measure skinfold thickness with calipers. Nevertheless, this may not be very accurate, as measurements are difficult or impossible in very obese subjects and the distribution of fat between subcutaneous and deep sites varies among ethnic groups and among sites.

A simple expression of body mass is W/H^2 (where W is the individual's weight in kilograms and H is height in meters) and this correlates sufficiently with body density and skinfold thickness (4) to allow it to be applied to the original insurance data for the limits of the desirable weight range. A nomogram has been published (5) and is given in Figure 1. From this the value of W/H^2 can easily be read; for men the boundaries of the desirable range are 20-25 and for women, 19-24.

The use of any of these techniques of measurement of weight or fatness may be associated with errors that limit their usefulness. In many respects the errors are analogous to those that may be encountered in hormone assay laboratories and it is ironic that one of us has used the analogy of the weighing machine to illustrate such errors (6, 7). The potential errors are of three types. Systematic errors in the calibration of the machine (in a hospital or clinic) or in the weighing technique will lead to a consistent bias associated with that clinic. Random errors leading to a poor reproducibility of weighing on different occasions may result from a poorly maintained machine or the use of different observers on different days. Finally, there may be errors of interpretation if the weighings, however accurate, are compared with inappropriate norms.

II. ENDOCRINE CORRELATES OF BODY WEIGHT

Although the importance for the individual of establishing body size is obvious, what is the importance and relevance to an endocrinologist? As discussed in later chapters, excessive weight or excessive thinness may be associated with alterations in hypothalamic, pituitary, thyroid, adrenal, pancreatic, and gonadal function (8-14). The changes that have been reported in association with simple obesity or excessive thinness are listed in Table 2. The extent of these changes in endocrine function do suggest that the attainment of a specific body weight or body composition constitutes a signal to the hypothalamus, which "switches" on or off specific neuroendocrine mechanisms. An example of this may be the timing of puberty.

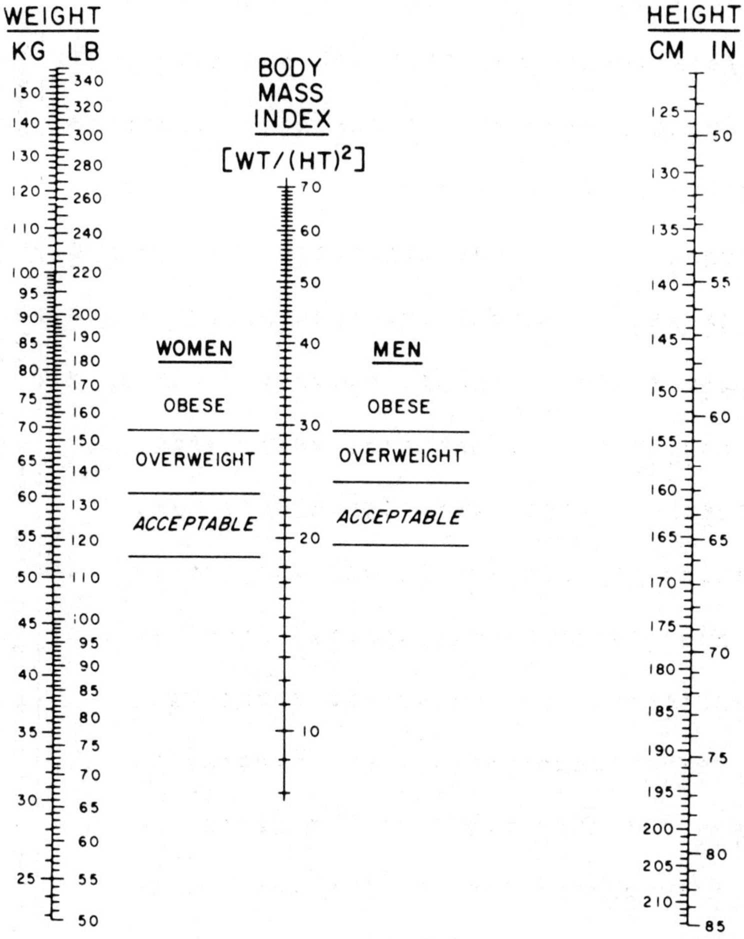

Figure 1 Nomogram for body mass. A straight edge is placed joining the body weight and the height of the subject. The body mass index is read from the middle scale. The limits of normal, overweight, and obese subjects are shown for each sex. (From Ref. 5.)

The decreasing age of menarche in successive generations of American women and the attainment of puberty at a certain ratio of body weight to height in girls were among the many epidemiological observations that Frisch has used to support the thesis that a critical body weight or, more precisely, a critical degree of fatness triggers the neuroendocrine initiation of puberty in girls (15). This original hypothesis has been criticized on the grounds that the method of calculating total body water for each girl (using a regression equation derived from

Table 1a Women: Percent Over or Under Ideal Weight

WEIGHT		HEIGHT cm	158	160	163	165	168	170	173	175	178	180	183	185	188	190	193
Pounds	Kilograms	in	62	63	64	65	66	67	68	69	70	71	72	73	74	75	76
100-104	45.5-47.0		-17	-20	-22	-23	-25	-27	-30	-32	-33	-35	-37	-39	-40	-42	-44
105-109	47.5-49.5		-13	-16	-18	-20	-22	-24	-26	-28	-30	-32	-34	-36	-37	-39	-41
110-114	50.0-52.0		- 9	-12	-14	-16	-18	-20	-23	-25	-27	-29	-31	-33	-35	-36	-38
115-119	52.5-54.0		- 5	- 8	-10	-12	-14	-17	-19	-21	-24	-26	-28	-30	-32	-34	-35
120-124	54.5-56.0		0	- 4	- 6	- 8	-11	-13	-16	-18	-20	-23	-25	-27	-29	-31	-33
125-129	56.5-58.5		3	0	- 2	- 5	- 7	-10	-12	-15	-17	-19	-22	-24	-26	-28	-30
130-134	59.0-60.5		7	4	0	0	- 3	- 6	- 9	-11	-14	-16	-19	-21	-23	-25	-27
135-139	61.0-63.0		11	8	5	3	0	- 2	- 6	- 8	-10	-13	-15	-18	-20	-22	-24
140-144	63.5-65.0		15	12	9	7	4	0	- 2	- 5	- 7	-10	-12	-15	-17	-19	-22
145-149	65.5-67.5		19	16	13	11	8	5	0	0	- 4	- 7	- 9	-12	-14	-16	-19
159-154	68.0-70.0		23	20	17	14	11	8	5	2	0	- 4	- 6	- 9	-11	-14	-16
155-159	70.5-72.0		27	24	21	18	15	12	8	5	3	0	- 3	- 6	- 8	-11	-13
160-164	72.5-74.5		31	28	25	22	19	15	12	9	6	3	0	- 3	- 5	- 8	-10
165-169	75.0-76.5		35	31	28	26	22	19	15	12	9	6	3	0	- 2	- 5	- 8
170-174	77.0-79.0		39	35	32	29	26	22	19	15	12	9	6	3	0	- 2	- 5
175-179	79.5-81.0		43	39	36	33	30	26	22	19	16	12	9	6	4	0	- 2
180-184	81.5-83.5		47	43	40	37	33	30	26	22	19	16	12	9	6	3	0
185-189	84.0-85.5		51	47	44	41	37	33	29	26	22	19	15	12	9	6	3
190-194	86.0-88.0		55	51	48	44	41	37	32	29	25	22	19	15	12	9	6
195-199	88.5-90.0		60	55	52	48	44	40	36	32	29	25	22	18	15	12	9
200-204	90.5-92.5		64	59	55	52	48	44	39	36	32	28	25	21	18	15	12
205-209	93.0-95.0		68	63	59	56	52	47	43	39	35	31	28	24	21	18	14
210-214	95.5-97.0		72	67	63	59	55	51	46	42	39	35	31	[illegible]	24	20	17
215-219	97.5-99.0		76	71	67	63	59	54	50	46	42	38	34	[illegible]	27	23	20
220-224	99.5-101.5		80	75	71	67	63	58	53	49	45	41	37	[illegible]	30	26	23
225-229	102.0-103.5		84	79	75	71	66	62	57	52	48	44	40	[illegible]	33	29	25
230-234	104.0-106.0		88	83	78	74	70	65	60	56	52	47	43	[illegible]	36	32	28
235-239	106.5-108.5		92	87	82	78	74	69	63	59	55	50	46	[illegible]	39	35	31
240-244	109.0-110.5		96	91	86	82	77	72	67	62	58	54	49	[illegible]	42	37	34
245-249	111.0-113.0		100	94	90	86	81	76	70	66	61	57	52	[illegible]	44	40	36
250-254	113.5-115.0		-	98	94	89	85	79	74	69	65	60	56	[illegible]	47	43	39
255-259	115.5-117.5		-	100	98	93	88	83	77	72	68	63	59	[illegible]	50	46	42
260-264	118.0-119.5		-	-	100	97	92	86	81	76	71	66	62	[illegible]	53	49	45
265-269	120.0-122.0		-	-	-	100	96	90	84	79	75	70	65	[illegible]	56	52	48
270-274	122.5-124.0		Blanks signify		-	-	99	94	88	83	78	73	68	[illegible]	59	55	50
275-279	124.5-126.5		more than 100%		-	-	100	97	91	86	81	76	71	[illegible]	62	57	53
280-284	127.0-129.0		overweight		-	-	-	100	94	89	84	79	74	[illegible]	65	60	56
285-289	129.5-131.0		-	-	-	-	-	-	98	93	88	82	77	[illegible]	68	63	59
290-294	131.5-133.5		-	-	-	-	-	-	100	96	91	85	80	75	71	66	61
295-299	134.0-135.5		-	-	-	-	-	-	-	99	94	89	83	78	74	69	64

Source: Based on desirable weights (in ordinary clothing) for women of medium frame, at ages 25 and over, according to height (with shoes). Derived from tables in: New weight standards for men and women. *Statistical Bulletin, Metropolitan Life Insurance Company*, 1959; 40:3, which were derived primarily from data of the Build and Blood Pressure Study, 1959, Society of Actuaries. Courtesy of Metropolitan Life Insurance Company, New York.

Table 1b Men: Percent Over or Under Ideal Weight

WEIGHT Pounds	Kilograms	HEIGHT cm / in	147 / 58	150 / 59	152 / 60	155 / 61	158 / 62	160 / 63	163 / 64	165 / 65	168 / 66	170 / 67	173 / 68	175 / 69	178 / 70	180 / 71	183 / 72
80-84	36.0-38.0		-19	-21	-23	-25	-27	-29	-31	-33	-36	-38	-39	-41	-43	-44	-46
85-89	38.5-40.0		-14	-16	-19	-21	-23	-25	-27	-29	-32	-34	-36	-38	-39	-41	-43
90-94	40.5-42.5		- 9	-12	-14	-16	-19	-21	-23	-25	-28	-30	-32	-34	-36	-38	-39
95-99	43.0-45.0		- 4	- 7	- 9	-12	-14	-16	-19	-21	-24	-26	-28	-30	-32	-34	-36
100-104	45.5-47.0		0	0	- 5	- 7	-10	-12	-15	-17	-20	-22	-25	-27	-29	-31	-33
105-109	47.5-49.5		5	3	0	- 3	- 5	- 8	-10	-13	-16	-19	-21	-23	-25	-27	-29
110-114	50.0-52.0		10	8	5	0	0	- 3	- 6	- 9	-12	-15	-17	-20	-22	-24	-26
115-119	52.5-54.0		15	12	9	6	4	0	- 2	- 5	- 8	-11	-14	-16	-18	-21	-23
120-124	54.5-56.0		20	17	14	11	8	5	2	0	- 4	- 7	-10	-13	-15	-17	-19
125-129	56.5-58.5		25	22	19	15	12	9	6	3	0	- 3	- 6	- 9	-11	-14	-16
130-134	59.0-60.5		30	27	23	20	17	14	10	7	4	0	- 3	- 5	- 8	-11	-13
135-139	61.0-63.0		35	32	28	25	21	18	15	11	7	4	0	- 2	- 5	- 7	-10
140-144	63.5-65.0		40	37	33	29	26	22	19	15	11	8	5	2	0	- 4	- 6
145-149	65.5-67.5		45	41	37	34	30	27	23	20	15	12	8	5	2	0	3
150-154	68.0-70.0		50	46	42	38	35	31	27	24	19	16	12	9	6	3	0
155-159	70.5-72.0		55	51	47	43	39	35	31	28	23	19	16	13	9	6	4
160-164	72.5-74.5		60	56	51	47	43	40	36	32	27	23	20	16	13	10	7
165-169	75.0-76.5		65	61	56	52	48	44	40	36	31	27	23	20	16	13	10
170-174	77.0-79.0		69	65	61	56	52	48	44	40	35	31	27	23	20	17	14
175-179	79.5-81.0		74	70	65	61	57	53	48	44	39	35	31	27	23	20	17
180-184	81.5-83.5		79	75	70	65	61	57	52	48	43	38	34	30	27	23	20
185-189	84.0-85.5		84	80	75	70	65	61	56	52	47	42	38	34	30	27	23
190-194	86.0-88.0		89	85	79	75	70	66	61	56	51	46	42	38	34	30	27
195-199	88.5-90.0		94	89	84	79	74	70	65	60	55	50	45	41	37	34	30
200-204	90.5-92.5		100	94	89	84	79	74	69	64	58	54	49	45	41	37	33
205-209	93.0-95.0		-	100	93	88	83	78	73	68	62	57	53	48	44	40	37
210-214	95.5-97.0		-	-	98	93	88	83	77	72	66	61	56	52	48	44	40
215-219	97.5-99.0		-	-	100	97	92	87	82	76	70	65	60	56	51	47	43
220-224	99.5-101.5		-	-	-	100	96	91	86	80	74	69	64	59	55	51	47
225-229	102.0-103.5		-	-	-	-	100	96	90	85	78	73	68	63	58	54	50
230-234	104.0-106.0		-	-	-	-	-	100	94	89	82	76	71	66	62	57	53
235-239	106.5-108.5		-	-	-	-	-	-	98	93	86	80	75	70	65	61	56
240-244	109.0-110.5		-	-	-	-	-	-	100	97	90	84	79	73	69	64	60
245-249	111.0-113.0		-	-	-	-	-	-	-	100	94	88	82	77	72	67	63

Blanks signify more than 100% overweight

Source: Based on desirable weights (in ordinary clothing) for men of medium frame, at ages 25 and over, according to height (with shoes). Derived from tables in New weight standards for men and women. *Statistical Bulletin, Metropolitan Life Insurance Company*, 1959; 40:3, which were derived primarily from data of the Build and Blood Pressure Study, 1959, Society of Actuaries. Courtesy of Metropolitan Life Insurance Company, New York.

Table 2 Changes in Endocrine Function Associated with Excessive Weight Gain or Loss[a]

	Weight gain	Weight loss
Adrenal		
Plasma cortisol		
Fasting concentration	N	N or ↑
Diurnal rhythm	Generally N	Generally N
Response to insulin hypoglycemia	N or ↓	N or ↓
Cortisol production rate	↓	N
24-hr urine steroid excretion		
17-oxosteroids	N or ↑	N or ↓
17-oxogenic steroids	N or ↑	N or ↓
Urinary free cortisol	Generally N	N
Sex steroids (plasma concentration)		
Sex hormone binding globulin (SHBG)	↓	↓
Androstenedione	↑	↑
Testosterone	↑	↑
Dihydrotestosterone	N	N
Esterone (E_1)	N	↓
Estradiol (E_2)	N	↓
E_1/E_2 ratio	↑	N
Gonadotropins		
Plasma luteinizing hormone (LH) concentration	N	↓
Plasma follicle stimulating hormone (FSH)	N	↓
LH and FSH response to LHRH	N	N or ↓
Nocturnal episodic release of LH	↓	↓
Thyroid (plasma concentration)		
Thyroxine	N	N or ↓
Triiodothyronine (T_3)	N or ↑	N or ↓
Reverse T_3	N or ↑	N or ↑
Thyroid stimulating hormone (TSH)	N	N
TSH response to thyroid releasing hormone (TRH)	N	N or ↑
Insulin		
Fasting plasma concentration	↑	↑
Response to oral glucose	↑	↑
Response to i.v. glucose	↑	↑
Growth hormone		
Fasting plasma concentration	↓	↑
Response to insulin hypoglycemia	↓	N or ↓
Nocturnal release	↓	↓
Prolactin		
Fasting plasma concentration	N	N
Response to insulin hypoglycemia	N or absent	–
Response to TRH	N or ↓	N

[a]N, normal; ↑ increased; ↓ decreased.

height and weight) was too inaccurate for statistical purposes (16). Nevertheless, support for the hypothesis comes from the clinical observation that secondary amenorrhea in patients with anorexia nervosa is reversed when patients regain a normal body weight and fat content.

Furthermore, excessive weight may also influence the endocrine mechanisms responsible for reproductive function; menarche tends to occur at a younger age in obese girls and menstrual abnormalities are more common (17). Abnormal menstrual cycles in obese women appear to be associated with alterations in plasma sex steroid secretion and binding (12). Such changes may result from the effect of body weight on adrenal function and the effect of fat on steroid interconversions and metabolism (18, 19). The reversal of these hormonal abnormalities by substantial weight loss is associated with more normal function (13).

It is of interest that a similar pattern of changes of sex steroid concentrations and binding to those found in obese women are also found in women with the polycystic ovary syndrome (20). The original description of this syndrome by Stein and Leventhal (21) included obesity as one of its clinical features but, in contrast to obese women, women with this syndrome have an abnormal luteinizing hormone (LH) response to pituitary stimulation with luteinizing hormone releasing hormone (LHRH). The polycystic ovary syndrome is thus an example of obesity in association with a primary disorder of endocrine function.

In most instances the more common primary disorders of endocrine function (e.g., of the adrenal or thyroid glands) presenting as excessive weight gain or loss are easily recognized, but there are occasions when this may be difficult. For example, if obese patients have fasted before being investigated, they may be found to have lost their diurnal plasma cortisol variation and to have an abnormally high excretion of urinary free cortisol (22); these patients may be distinguished from patients with Cushing's disease by showing that they have a normal suppression of plasma cortisol following a low dose of dexamethasone (23).

III. CONCLUSIONS

Ideal body weight tables are useful as a method for assessing body size and the expression W/H^2 is probably the most convenient clinical method of assessment. Nevertheless, because of their limitations, these tables should be used merely for guidance by clinicians and patients alike. They may help the clinicians to record the degree of excess weight or thinness and may provide an explanation for an apparent abnormality of endocrine function in patients in whom a primary disorder of function has been excluded. For the patient such tables may offer a means of monitoring the person's success or failure to gain or lose weight when medically advised or to quantify whether the person is "disgustingly fat" (or disgustingly thin) or "merely a little bit broad in the beam with a tendency to be barrel-shaped" (George Orwell, *Coming Up for Air*).

REFERENCES

1. James WPI (Ed). *Research on Obesity*. A report of the DHSS/MRC group. Her Majesty's Stationery Office, London, 1976.
2. Anonymous. The dangers of thinness. Editorial. Br Med J 1980; 281:894.
3. *Build and Blood Pressure Study*. Society of Actuaries, Chicago, 1959.
4. Keys A, Fidanza F, Karvonen MM, Kimura N, Taylor HZ. Indices of relative weight and obesity. J Chronic Dis 1972; 25:329–343.
5. Bray GA. Definition, measurement and classification of the syndrome of obesity. Int J Obes 1978; 2:99–112.
6. Jeffcoate SL. Who shall control the controllers? Ann Clin Biochem 1981;18:1–5.
7. Jeffcoate SL. *Efficiency and Effectiveness in the Endocrine Laboratory*. Academic, London, 1981.
8. Boyar RM. Endocrine changes in anorexia nervosa. Med Clin North Am 1978; 62:297–303.
9. Kalucy RS, Crisp AH, Chard T, McNeilly A, Chen CN, Lacey JH. Nocturnal hormonal profile in massive obesity, anorexia nervosa and normal females. J Psychosom Res 1976; 20:595–604.
10. Vigersky RA, Loriaux DL, Anderson AE, Lipsett MB. Anorexia nervosa: behavioral and hypothalamic aspects. Clin Endocrinol Metab 1976; 5:517–535.
11. Leslie RDG, Isaacs AJ, Gomez J, Raggatt PR, Bayliss R. Hypothalamo-pituitary-thyroid function in anorexia nervosa: influence of weight gain. Br Med J 1978; 2:526–528.
12. Kopelman PG, Pilkington TRE, White N, Jeffcoate SL. Abnormal sex steroid secretion and binding in massively obese women. Clin Endocrinol 1980; 12:363–369.
13. Kopelman PG, Pilkington IRE, Jeffcoate SL, White N. Persistence of defective hypothalamic control of prolactin secretion in some obese women after weight reduction. Br Med J 1980; 28:358–359.
14. Glass AR, Burman KD, Dahms WT, Boehm TM. Endocrine function in human obesity. Metabolism 1981; 30:89–104.
15. Frisch RE, McArthur JW. Menstrual cycle: fatness as a determinent of maximum weight for height necessary for maintenance or onset. Science 1974; 185:949–951.
16. Reeves J. Estimating fatness. Science 1969; 204:881.
17. Hartz AJ, Barboriak PN, Wong A, Katayama KP, Rimm AA. The association of obesity with infertility and related menstrual abnormalities in women. Int J Obes 1979; 3:57–73.
18. Migeon CJ, Green OC, Eckert JP. Study of adrenocorticol function in obesity. Metabolism 1963; 12:718–739.
19. Perel E, Killinger DW. The interconversion and aromatization of androgens by human adipose tissue. J Steroid Biochem 1979; 10:623–627.
20. Baird DT. Polycystic ovary syndrome. In *Advances in Gynaecological Endocrinology*, Jacobs HS (ed). Proceedings of the Sixth Group of the Royal College of Obstetricians and Gynaecologists, London, 1978, pp. 289–300.
21. Stein IF, Leventhal ML. Amenorrhoea associated with bilateral polycystic ovaries. Am J Obstet Gynecol 1935; 29:181–189.

22. Galvao-Teles A, Graves L, Burke CW, Fotherby K, Fraser R. Free cortisol in obesity: effect of fasting. Acta Endocrinol (Copenh) 1976; 81: 321–329.
23. Hankin ME, Theile HM, Steinbeck AW. Adreno-cortical function in obesity and Cushing's syndrome. Clin Sci Mol Med 1974; 47:119–129.

2
Growth Charts and Pubertal Staging

James M. Tanner
Institute of Child Health, University of London, London, England

I. GROWTH CHARTS

There are two sorts of growth charts: one which is suitable for making comparisons between populations or subpopulations—rich and poor, urban and rural, for instance—and the other which is suitable for following the growth of individuals. In clinical medicine it is usually the latter which is necessary; in community medicine, very often the former. There is still widespread confusion on this issue among pediatricians, endocrinologists, and chart makers, with the result that in many clinics population (i.e., cross-sectional) charts [such as, e.g., the recent U.S. National Center for Health Statistics charts (1)] are used where individual (i.e., longitudinal) charts are required.

Until about age nine, the cross-sectional and longitudinal standards for height and weight are essentially the same; but when puberty starts, the two sorts of standards part company. The reason for this is the variation in *tempo* of growth among children, coupled with the change in growth velocity which occurs at puberty. Some children have their growth spurts early, some late, and this distorts cross-sectionally derived standards in the way shown in Figure 1. A longitudinally followed child will plot along one of the sharper curves, not the flattened and lengthened one. Thus at puberty a child who is actually average in growth and tempo of growth will not follow the 50th percentile for height attained on cross-sectional charts; he or she will first fall below it, and then later catch up to it again; and these deviations are simply an artifact of the method of charting used.

The difficulty in constructing longitudinal standards is that in no longitudinal study are the numbers of children sufficient for the accurate location of the outside percentiles, the 97th and 3rd, which are the most important ones in clinical standards. This difficulty can be circumvented by using curves whose *shape* is based on longitudinal data, but whose *amplitude* (in the sense of distance between the percentiles) is based on large-scale cross-sectional surveys. In 1966, my colleagues and I introduced a new type of standard based on this tactic (3). When we published these standards, we left the old cross-sectional percentiles in and showed the new longitudinal percentiles shaded in gray. But increasing familiarity with the use of the longitudinal standards and with the misunderstandings engendered in the minds of auxologically unsophisticated pediatricians induced us to reissue the standards in the format shown in Figure 2. Here, the percentiles are longitudinal; thus the boy of average height who has his growth spurt at the average age does actually follow the 50th percentile throughout. We added shaded areas above the 97th and below the 3rd percentiles, however, to accommodate the whole 3rd to 97th percentile spectrum of cross-sectional data. Thus, in the initial screening, only children

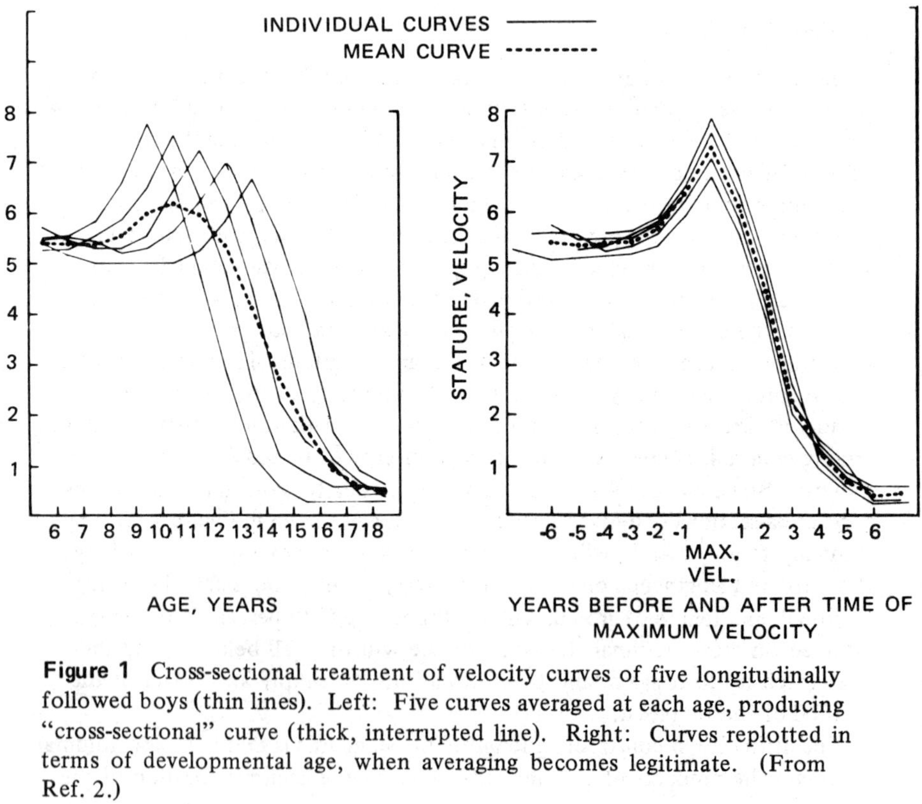

Figure 1 Cross-sectional treatment of velocity curves of five longitudinally followed boys (thin lines). Left: Five curves averaged at each age, producing "cross-sectional" curve (thick, interrupted line). Right: Curves replotted in terms of developmental age, when averaging becomes legitimate. (From Ref. 2.)

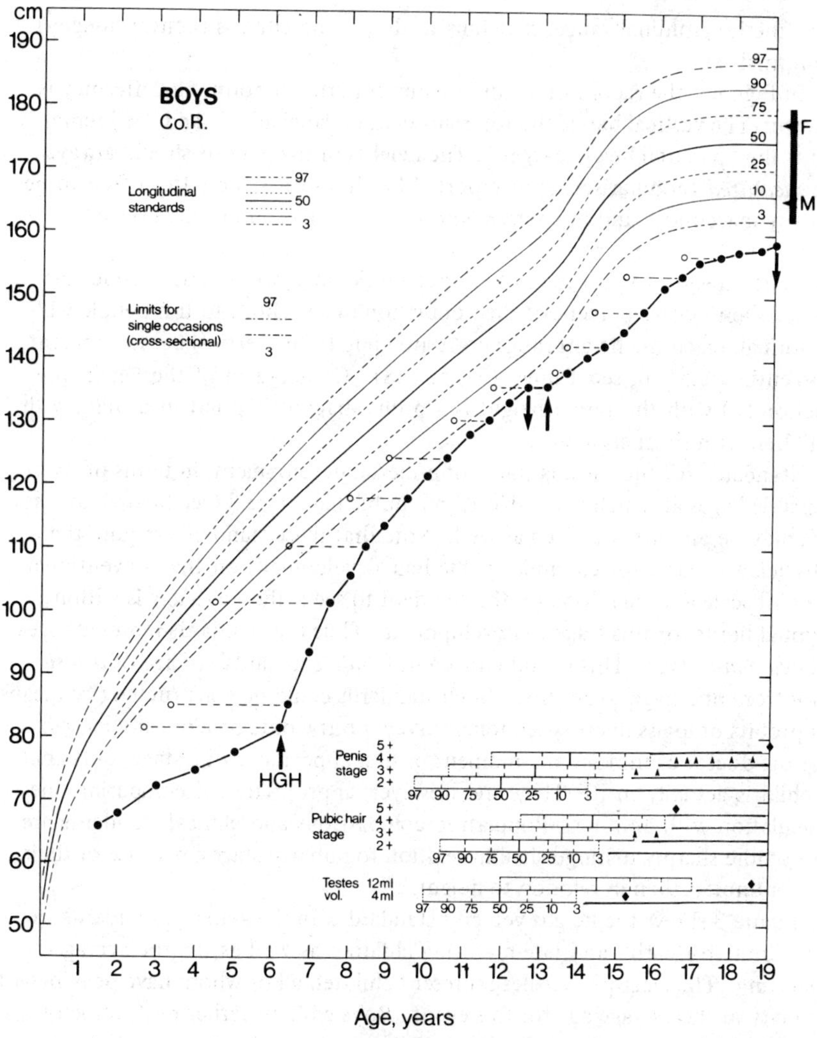

Figure 2 Standards of height attained at given age, boys. Plot is of growth hormone-deficient boy treated with hGH. Closed circles are height for chronological age, open circles height for bone age. (From Ref. 4.)

outside the shaded area should be considered "perhaps abnormal" (an arbitrary classification, of course, but the one conventionally used for probabilistic reasons). If a child lies within the shaded area, he or she is (conventionally) normal, but on subsequent visits the child's growth curve should move into the longitudinal range; if it fails to do so, the child is (conventionally) abnormal.

In Figure 2 the record of a child treated for growth hormone deficiency is shown. The vertical bar at the top right margin, labeled "F" and "M" represents the "parental height target." The heights of the parents should always be *measured* (comparison with reported heights shows the latter often to be grossly inaccurate) and the *percentiles* for father (F) and mother (M) are plotted. (To plot the mother's percentile on a boy's chart, add 13 cm or 5 in. to her measured height; to plot the father's percentile on a girl's chart, subtract the same.) Ninety-five percent of the population of sons born to this couple will, if normal, reach the height range corresponding to the vertical bar (midparent percentile ±8.5 cm; see Tanner (5), p. 168). Comparison of the height prediction (6) with the target height is a prime diagnostic point in dealing with children with short stature.

Standards for the various stages of pubertal development, in terms of "permissible" ages at which testis size 12 ml, pubic hair stage 3 (see below), and so on, may be present, are given as well. Note that these standards require the physician to rate, for example, pubic hair development on the conventional 5-point scale and then look up the standard to see if the boy's *age* is within normal limits for this stage of development. Thus the standards represent ages of *being-in-a-stage*. This is quite different from "standards" of age of *transition* from one stage to another. Such standards could be constructed (by means of probits or logits in cross-sectional surveys) but would be clinically useless, for the doctor cannot see the moment of first appearance of a stage, only that a child is actually in it. They are, however, appropriate for comparing one population with another. Population comparisons and clinical standards are even more sharply distinguished in relation to puberty stages, because of their discontinuity, than in relation to height.

Figure 3 shows the height velocity standards. In the velocity standards we give limits for early- and late-maturing children as well as for the average-maturing. The clear percentiles represent children all of whom have peak height velocity at the average age for this event. Boys with an earlier peak velocity have a higher peak. The 2 SD limit of "normal" earliness is approximately 2 years, and the left-hand edge of the shaded area encloses the velocity curve of such a boy. The upper arrow, diamond, and the lower arrow represent the 97th, 50th, and 3rd percentile peak velocities for boys with peaks 2 years early. Similarly, the right-hand edge of the shaded area represents boys with peaks 2 years late. Thus all boys with (conventionally) normal peaks at (conventionally) normal ages will have velocity curves lying within the shaded area. Those outside are abnormal. The example in Figure 3 shows the striking catch-up on treatment with human growth hormone (hGH). Note that velocities are calculated and plotted like annual rates of inflation announced at 3- or

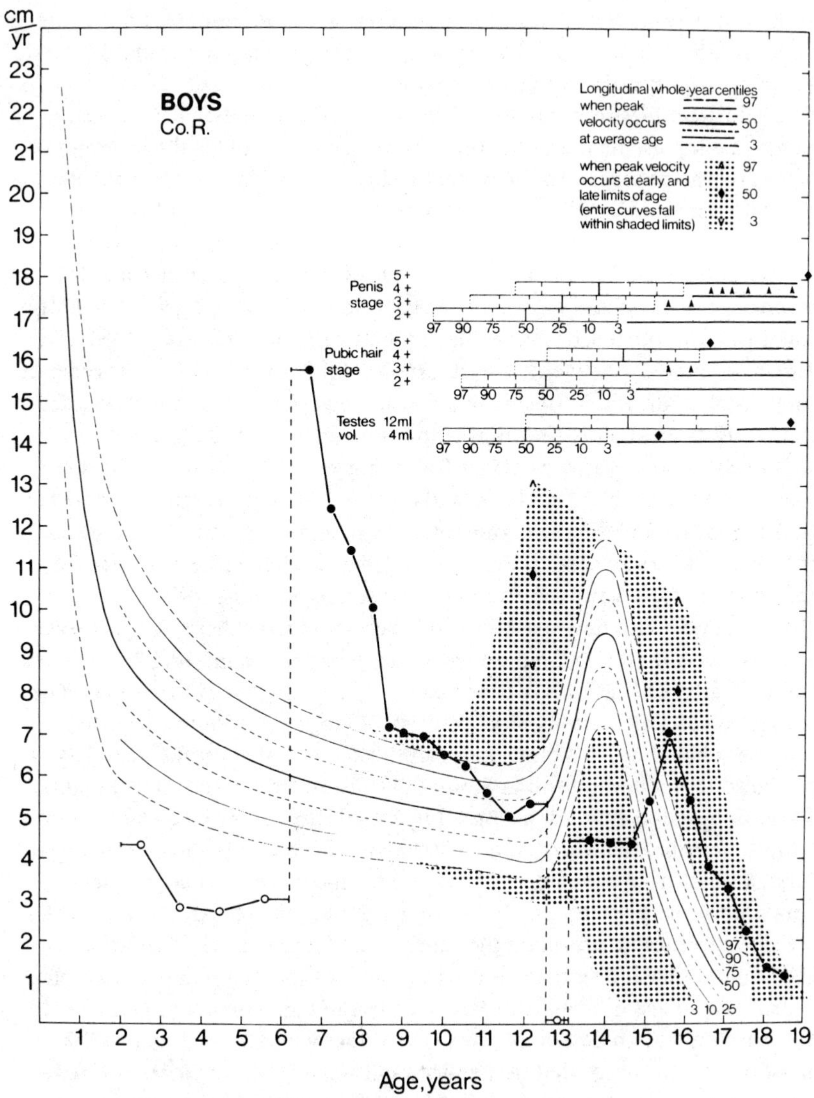

Figure 3 Standards of whole-year height velocity, boys. Plot is of growth hormone deficient boy treated with hGH. Each successive whole-year value of height velocity is plotted. Percentiles represent boys having peak velocity at average age of peak. Left shaded area represents percentiles for boys with peak occurring 2 SD of age before mean age (approximately 2 years early). Right shaded area represents percentiles for boys with peak occurring 2 SD after mean age (approximately 2 years late). (From Ref. 4.)

6-monthly intervals. Velocities over a whole year are represented, not those over a shorter period, multiplied up. Owing to seasonal variations, the shorter-period velocities have higher ranges of normality (7).

We used percentiles rather than standard deviations in these charts because the percentile represents the direct probability statement and is the interpretation given by the physician to the patient or his parents ("5% of normal children are shorter than your child"). Few pediatricians carry the tables of the normal deviate in their heads, and without this facility what exactly *do* they say when a child has a height of −1.65 SD? Formally, of course, percentiles and SD scores are equivalent if and only if the distribution of the variate, like height, is Gaussian [indeed, the height percentiles are best calculated via the SD (8)]. If the variate is skewed, like weight, or still more, skinfolds, then SD scores cannot be interpreted at all, and in this sense are erroneous. Percentiles then are calculated directly from the distribution, without assuming a distributional form. The use of SD scores as a convenience for saying *how* small a small child is is different from their use as standards, and entirely justifiable (even in a sense for weight) as a rather arbitrary way of expressing smallness (leading to the statement "He is not now so small in relation to other children as he was when he started treatment"). A full discussion will be found in Tanner (9).

Figures 4 and 5 give height attained and height velocity charts for girls, and Figures 6-9 weight attained and weight velocity charts for girls and boys. These and other charts (of skinfolds, sitting height and leg length, etc.) are obtainable from Castlemead Publications, 40 Greyfriars Wave, Herts, United Kingdom. A convenient handbook which includes all the charts is that by Buckler (10); they are also reproduced in full in Smith (11). These height and weight charts are based on London children measured in the 1950s; but recent surveys show that the percentiles represent very adequately the present population of England, at least from ages 5 to 11 (12). Where the mean heights or weights of a population are known to be above those given in the charts, the percentiles can be simply adjusted, assuming the variances to be the same. Such an adjustment presumes that the average tempo of growth of the two populations is the same: surveys of age of menarche [see, e.g., Eveleth and Tanner (13), p. 214] are the simplest way to determine this. The velocity charts are directly usable for most populations provided that adjustment is made for any mean difference in age of peak velocity (a year earlier in Japan, for example, than in England at present). Even for populations (such as the present Japanese) which end up (some 6 cm) below the English, the differences in *yearly* mean increments are so small as to be negligible. The simplest way to allow for differing tempo is to alter the age scale on the chart.

The charts are calibrated in years and tenths ("decimal age") rather than in years and months because when it comes to calculating a velocity in the clinic

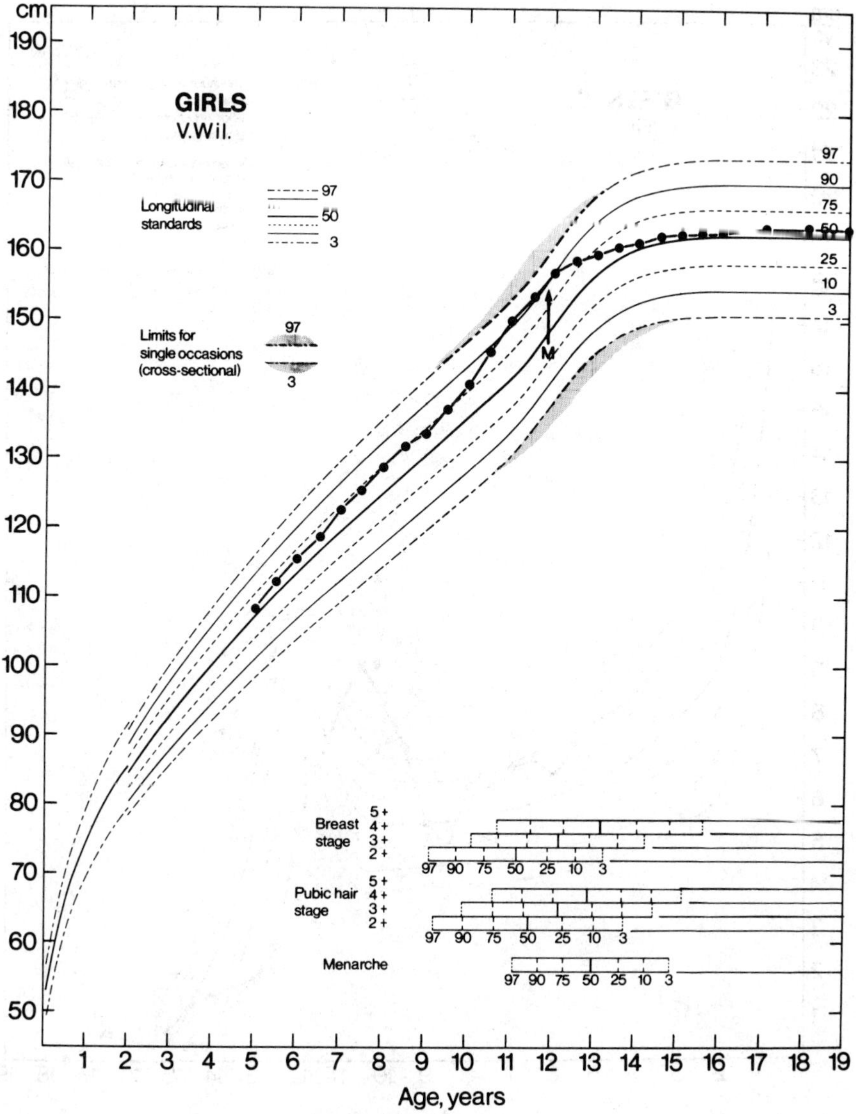

Figure 4 Standards of height attained at given age, girls. Plot is of a normal girl of average height, but maturity about 1½ years earlier than mean. (From Ref. 4.)

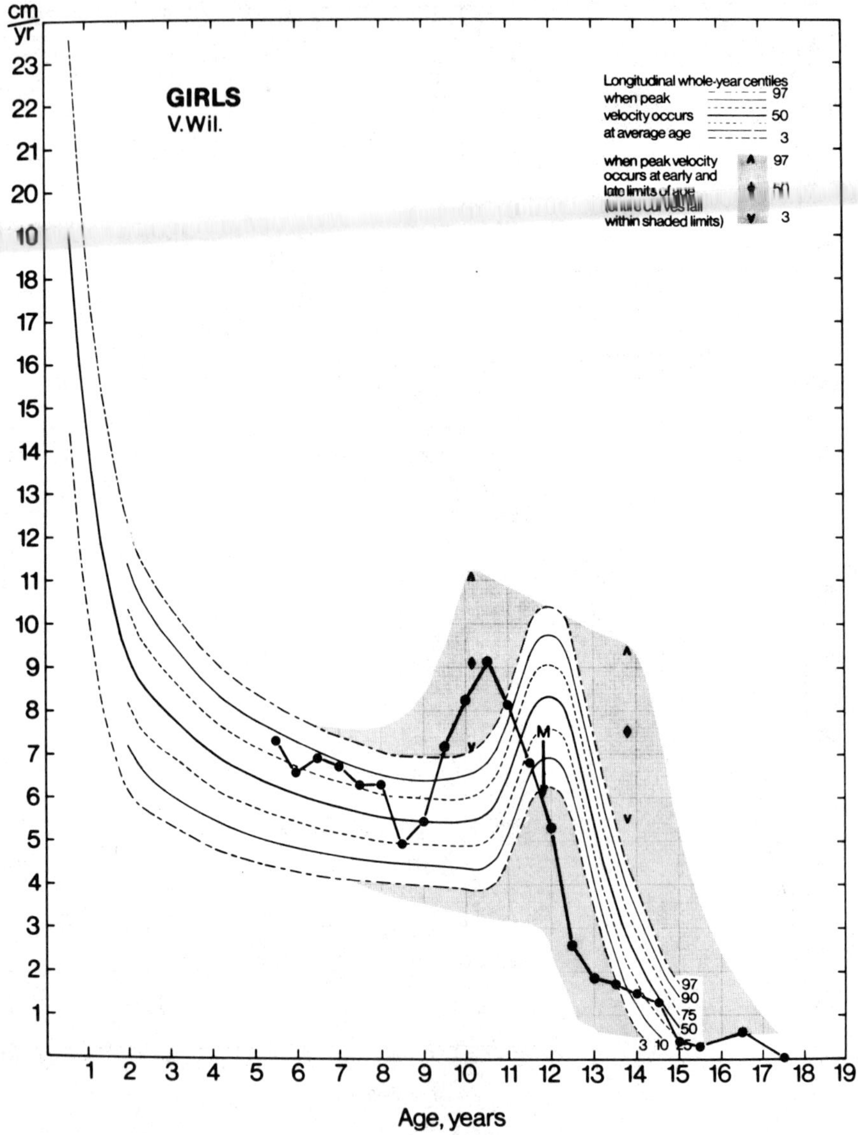

Figure 5 Standards of whole-year height velocity, girls. Plot is of a normal girl of average height, but maturity about 1½ years earlier than mean. Whole-year "rolling" velocities are plotted. (From Ref. 4.)

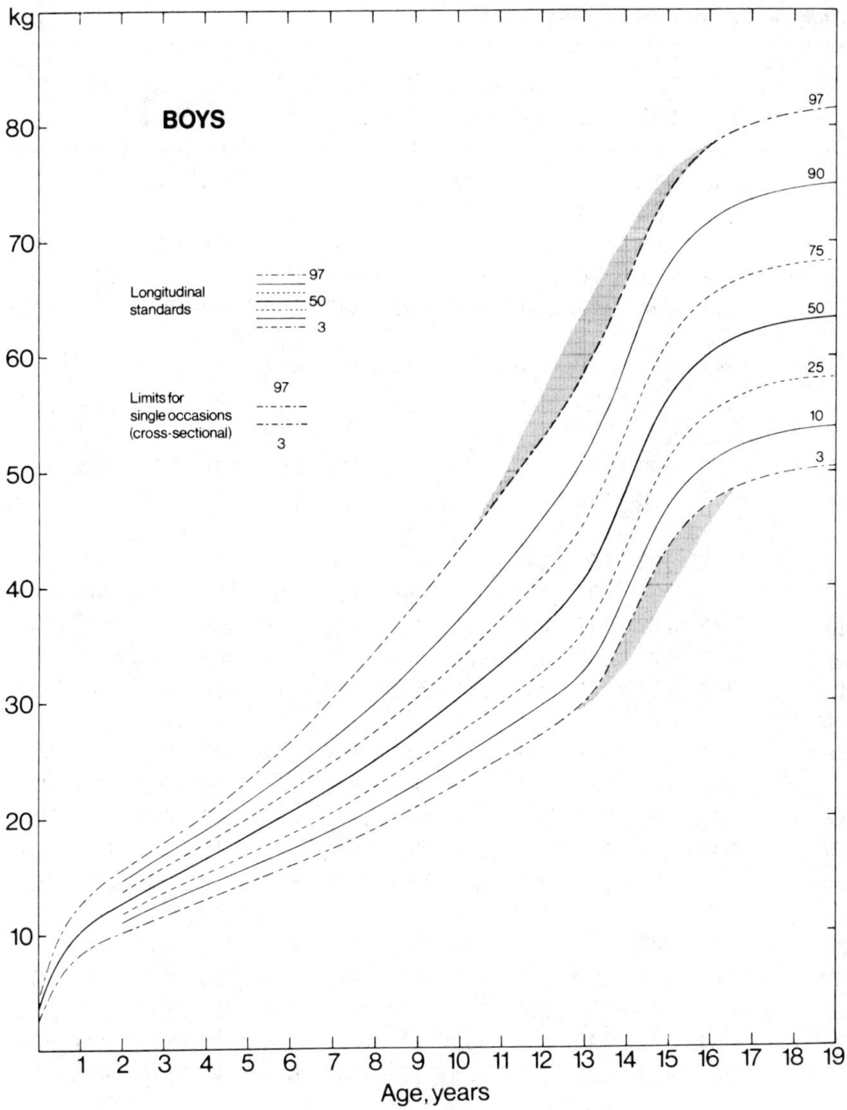

Figure 6 Weight standards for clinical use, boys. (From Ref. 4.)

it is enormously easier to do so if decimal age is used. For those who find decimals disturbing, however, Castlemead publishes versions overprinted with a 2-month scale. Decimals of the year are given in Table 1: June 1, 1980, reads 80.414. The child's birthdate in decimals is simply subtracted from the present date to get the child's decimal age; the interval between two examinations

Table 1 Table of Decimals of Year

	1 Jan.	2 Feb.	3 Mar.	4 Apr.	5 May	6 June	7 July	8 Aug.	9 Sept.	10 Oct.	11 Nov.	12 Dec.
1	000	085	162	247	329	414	496	581	666	748	833	915
2	003	088	164	249	332	416	499	584	668	751	836	918
3	005	090	167	252	334	419	501	586	671	753	838	921
4	008	093	170	255	337	422	504	589	674	756	841	923
5	011	096	173	258	340	425	507	592	677	759	844	926
6	014	099	175	260	342	427	510	595	679	762	847	929
7	016	101	178	263	345	430	512	597	682	764	849	932
8	019	104	181	266	348	433	515	600	685	767	852	934
9	022	107	184	268	351	436	518	603	688	770	855	937
10	025	110	186	271	353	438	521	605	690	773	858	940
11	027	112	189	274	356	441	523	608	693	775	860	942
12	030	225	192	277	359	444	526	611	696	778	863	945
13	033	118	195	279	362	447	529	614	699	781	866	948
14	036	121	197	282	364	449	532	616	701	784	868	951
15	038	123	200	285	367	452	534	619	704	786	871	953
16	041	126	203	288	370	455	537	622	707	789	874	956
17	044	129	205	290	373	458	540	625	710	792	877	959
18	047	132	208	293	375	460	542	627	712	795	879	962
19	049	134	211	296	378	463	545	630	715	797	882	964
20	052	137	214	299	381	466	548	633	718	800	885	967
21	055	240	216	301	384	468	551	636	721	803	888	970
22	058	142	219	304	386	471	553	638	723	805	890	973
23	060	145	222	307	389	474	556	641	726	808	893	975
24	063	148	225	310	392	477	559	644	729	811	896	978
25	066	151	227	312	395	479	562	647	731	814	899	981
26	068	153	230	315	397	482	564	649	734	816	901	984
27	071	145	233	318	400	485	567	652	737	819	904	986
28	074	159	236	321	403	488	570	655	740	822	907	989
29	077	–	238	323	405	490	573	658	742	825	910	992
30	079	–	241	326	408	493	575	660	745	827	912	995
31	082	–	244	–	411	–	578	663	–	830	–	997

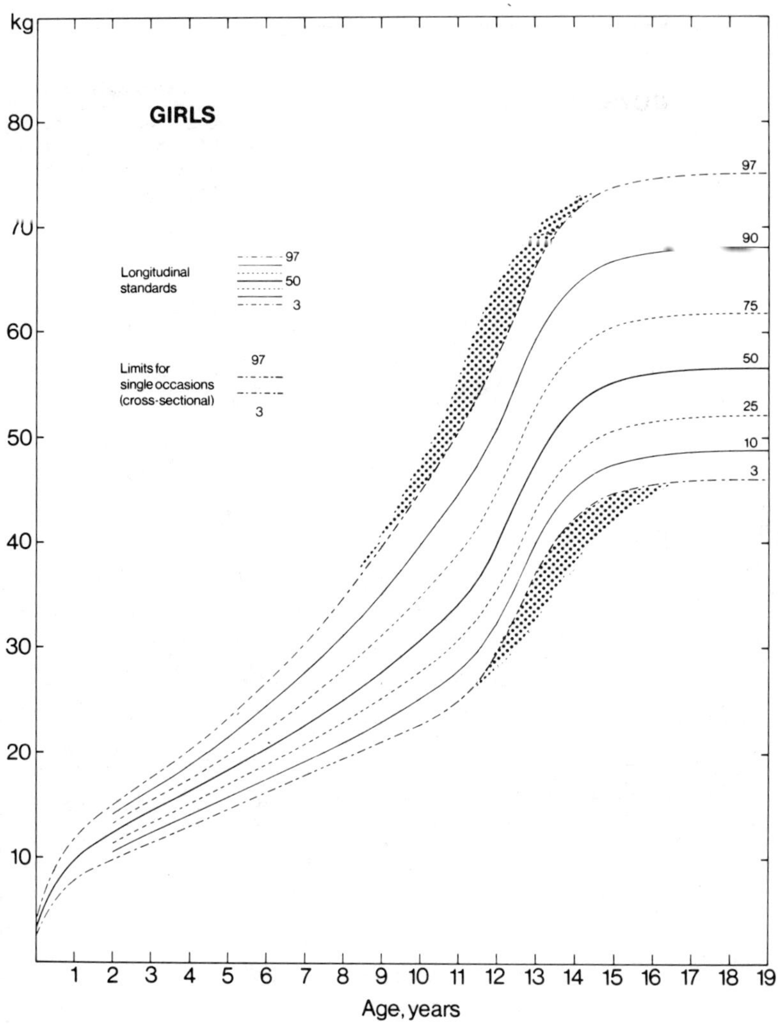

Figure 7 Weight standards for clinical use, girls. (From Ref. 4.)

becomes a simple decimal proportion of the year and from it velocity is readily calculated. Examples of the use of these charts are given in Tanner (5).

In weight-for-height (as opposed to weight-for-age) standards, a further problem arises. The distribution of weight of children of a given height interval may be different in six-year-olds than in seven-year-olds, say. Thus the average 7-year-old boy of height 110 cm may not have the same weight as the average 6-year-old boy of 110 cm. And even if these *average* children do have the same weights, then the *range* of weights of the 110 cm six- and seven-year-olds may

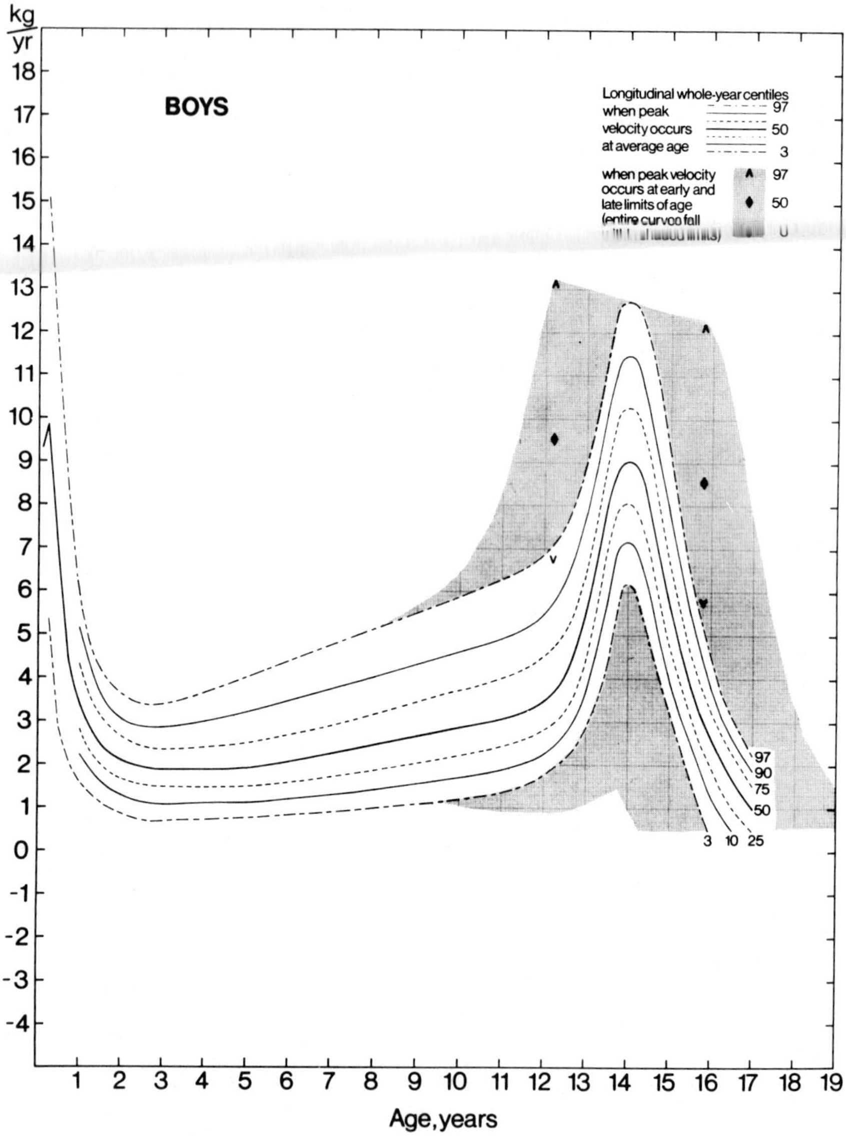

Figure 8 Weight velocity standards for clinical use, boys. (From Ref. 4.)

not be the same. This problem, recently reinvestigated by Waterlow et al. (14) and Chinn and Morris (15), is a difficult one. Between the ages of one and nine the error in using a single chart with all ages pooled is not very great, and the U.S. National Center for Health Statistics has published a chart of weight per-

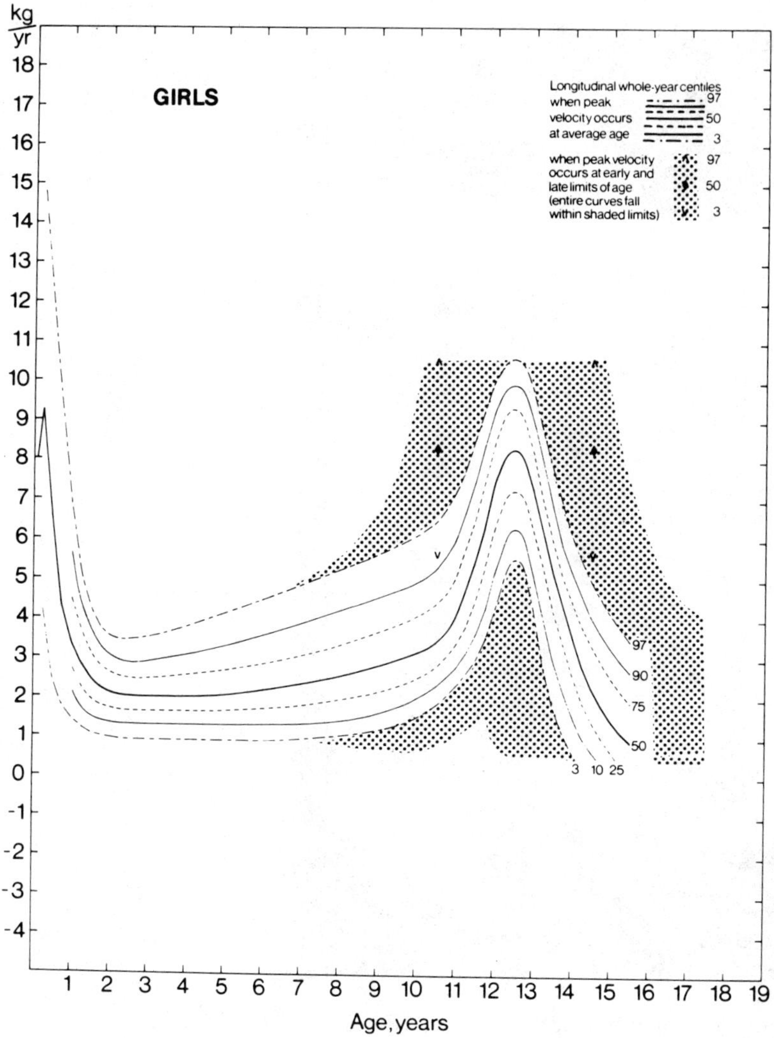

Figure 9 Weight velocity standards for clinical use, girls. (From Ref. 4.)

centiles for given height, covering age one to puberty (at whatever age) (1). Chinn and Morris (15) have published more accurate charts, for each year singly, from 5+ through 10+. Both sets of charts, are, of course, cross-sectional, but this is unimportant in the range of ages dealt with. There are no satisfactory weight-for-height standards for pubertal ages.

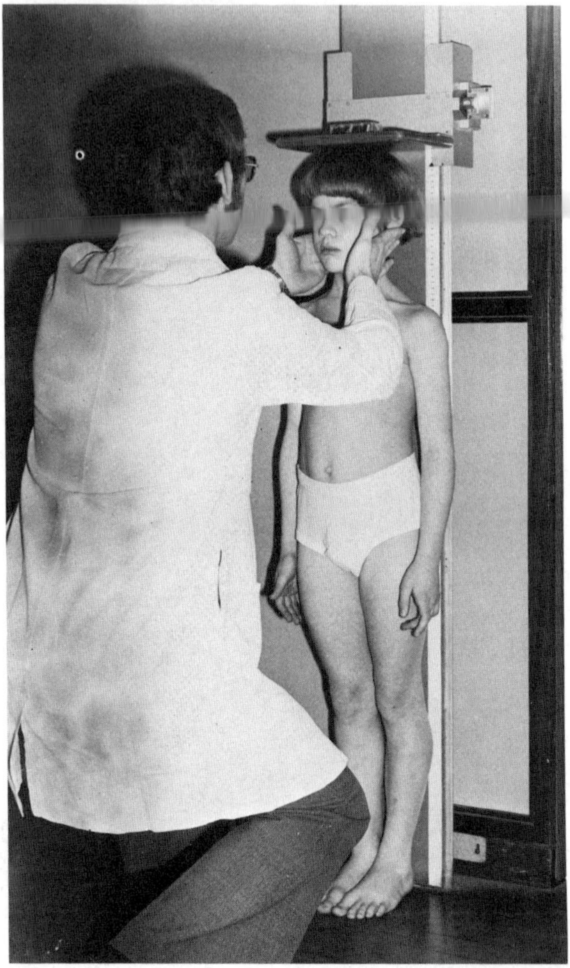

Figure 10 Method of measuring stature. (From Ref. 16.)

II. MEASUREMENT TECHNIQUE

No standards of growth are better than the measurements of the children from which they are derived and of the child who is being compared with them. "Garbage in, garbage out" is the motto of the auxologist no less than the biometrician. Measurements of growth, exactly like measurements of growth hormone, begin with modern well-maintained equipment and a trained technician using it. The apparatus for measuring stature and the method of doing it are shown in Figure 10 (stadiometer obtainable from Holtain Limited, Crosswell, Crymmych, Pembrokeshire, Wales). In the figure, the headboard is counter-

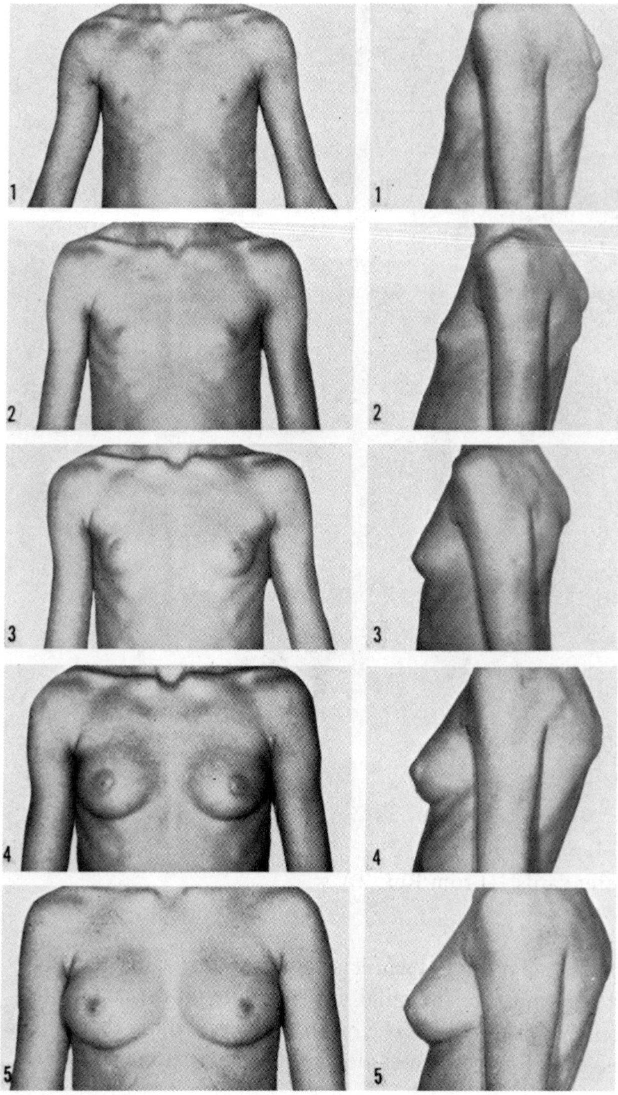

Figure 11 Breast standards. (From Ref. 2.)

balanced and the height read from a rack-and-pinion digital counter. More sophisticated apparatus uses an electronic scale to read on-line to a small computer in which the measurement is checked against previous ones and other body measurements, the velocities computed and displayed, and a warning given if sets of limits are passed so that a check may be made at once. In less sophisticated clinics the same checks can be made by a trained recordist. In

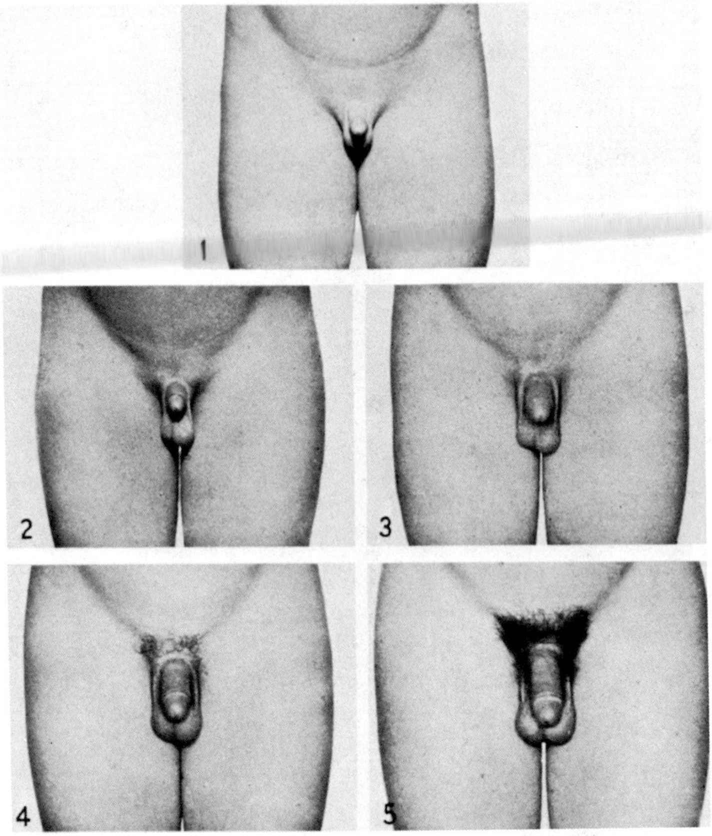

Figure 12 Genitalia standards. (From Ref. 2.)

any clinic there should be one or more technicians who are specially trained as anthropometrists and who measure the child each time he or she comes, to minimize errors, especially in velocities. The heights "measured" in the average casual clinic are useless even for accurate clinical purposes, let alone research.

III. PUBERTAL STAGES

Figures 11-13 illustrate the conventional rating scales used for giving semi-quantitative assessments of the development of breasts, male genitalia, and pubic hair. Verbal descriptions of each stage are given in Tables 2-4. The relationship between the different sequences is described in Marshall and Tanner (18, 19) and in Taranger et al. (20). Scales that confound genitalia and pubic hair in boys, or breasts and pubic hair in girls, are not recommended for use by endocrinologists, who have to deal with extreme normal variants and actual ab-

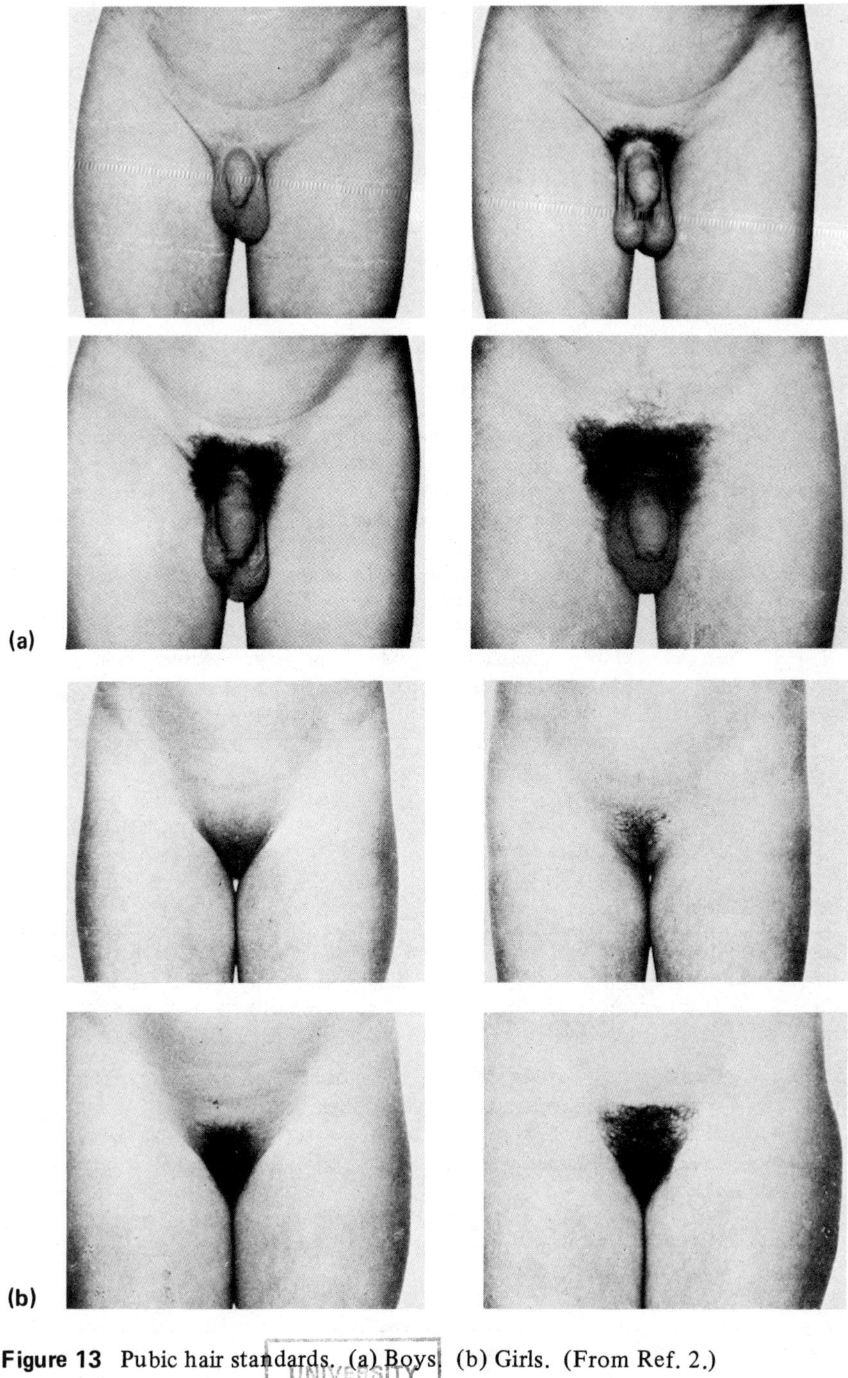

Figure 13 Pubic hair standards. (a) Boys. (b) Girls. (From Ref. 2.)

Table 2 Breast Development Stages

Stage 1:	Preadolescent: elevation of papilla only.
Stage 2:	Breast bud stage: elevation of breast and papilla as small mound. Areola diameter enlarged over stage 1.
Stage 3:	Breast and areola both enlarged and elevated more than in stage 2 but with no separation of their contours.
Stage 4:	The areola and papilla form a secondary mound, projecting above the countours of the breast.
Stage 5:	Mature stage: papilla only projects, with areola recessed to the general contour of the breast.

Source: Ref. 17.

Table 3 Genital Development Stages

Stage 1:	Preadolescent. Testes, scrotum, and penis are of about the same size and proportion as in early childhood. Testes 1 or 2 ml.
Stage 2:	Enlargement of scrotum and of testes. The skin of the scrotum reddens and changes in texture. Little or no enlargement of penis at this stage. Testes 3, 4, or 6 ml.
Stage 3:	Penis slighly enlarged, at first mainly in length. Scrotum further enlarged than in stage 2. Testes usually 6 or 8 ml.
Stage 4:	Penis further enlarged with growth in breadth and development of glands. Scrotum further enlarged than in stage 3; scrotal skin darker than in earlier stages. Testes usually 10 or 12 ml.
Stage 5:	Genitalia adult in size and shape. Testes usually 15, 20, or 25 ml.

Source: Ref. 17.

Table 4 Pubic Hair Stages

Stage 1:	Preadolescent. The vallus over the pubes is not further developed than with that over the abdominal wall (i.e., no pubic hair).
Stage 2:	Sparse growth of long, slightly pigmented downy hair, straight or only slightly curled, chiefly at the base of the penis or along the labia.
Stage 3:	Considerably darker, coarser, and more curled. The hair spreads sparsely over the junction of the pubes.
Stage 4:	Hair now adult in type, but the area covered by it is still considerably smaller than in the adult. No spread to the medial surface of the thighs.
Stage 5:	Adult in quantity and type with distribution of the horizontal (or classically "feminine") pattern. Spread to medial surface of thighs but not up linea alba or elsewhere above the base of the inverse triangle.

Source: Ref. 17.

normalities of pubertal sequence. The information obtained from staging may be plotted in the height-attained charts (see above) or on separate, larger charts. Frequently, plotting against bone age (6) is more important than plotting against chronological age [see Marshall (21)].

REFERENCES

1. National Center for Health Statistics. NCHS growth curves for children, birth to 18 years, United States. National Center for Health Statistics, Hyatsville, Md., 1977. (Vital and health statistics. Series 11: Data from the National Health Survey, No. 164.) DHEW Publ. (PHS) 78-1650.
2. Tanner JM. *Growth at Adolescence*, 2nd ed. Blackwell, Oxford, 1962.
3. Tanner JM, Whitehouse RH, Takaishi M. Standards from birth to maturity for height, weight, height velocity and weight velocity: British children 1965. Arch Dis Child 1966;41:454–471, 613–635.
4. Tanner JM, Whitehouse RH. Clinical longitudinal standards for height, weight, height velocity and weight velocity and the stages of puberty. Arch Dis Child 1976;51:170–179.
5. Tanner JM. *Foetus into Man*. Open Books, London/Harvard University Press, Cambridge, Mass, 1978.
6. Tanner JM, Whitehouse RH, Marshall WA, Healy MJR, Goldstein H. *Assessment of Skeletal Maturity and Prediction of Adult Height*. Academic, London, 1975.
7. Marshall WA. Evaluation of growth rate in height over periods of less than a year. Arch Dis Child 1971;46:414–420.
8. Healy MJR. Notes on the statistics of growth standards. Ann Hum Biol 1974;1:41–46.
9. Tanner JM. The assessment of growth and development in children. Arch Dis Child 1952;27:10–33.
10. Buckler JMH. *A Reference Manual of Growth and Development*. Blackwell, Oxford, 1979.
11. Smith DW. *Growth and Its Disorders*. Saunders, Philadelphia, 1977.
12. Rona RJ, Altman DG. National Study of Health and Growth: standards of attained height, weight and triceps skinfold in English children 5 to 11 years old. Ann Hum Biol 1977;4:501–524.
13. Eveleth PB, Tanner JM. *Worldwide Variation in Human Growth*. Cambridge University Press, Cambridge, 1976.
14. Waterlow JC, Buzina R, Keller W, Lane JM, Nichaman MZ, Tanner JM. The presentation and use of height and weight data for comparing the nutritional status of groups of children under the age of 10 years. Bull WHO 55:489–498.
15. Chinn S, Morris RW. Standards of weight-for-height in English children from age 5.0 to 11.0 years. Ann Hum Biol 1980:7:457–472.
16. Cameron N. Methods of auxological anthropometry, Vol. 2. In *Human Growth*, Falkner F, Tanner JM (eds). Plenum, New York, 1978.
17. Tanner JM. Physical growth and development. In *Textbook of Paediatrics*, Forfar JO, Arneil GC (eds). Churchill Livingstone, Edinburgh, 1973.

18. Marshall WA, Tanner JM. Variation in the pattern of pubertal changes in girls. Arch Dis Child 1969;44:291-303.
19. Marshall WA, Tanner JM. Variation in the pattern of pubertal changes in boys. Arch Dis Child 1970;45:13-23.
20. Taranger J, Engström I, Lichenstein H, Svennberg-Redgren I. The somatic development of children in a Swedish urban community. VI. Somatic pubertal development. Acta Paediatr Scand 1976;258:121-135.
21. Marshall WA. Inter-relationships of skeletal maturation, sexual development and somatic growth in man. Ann Hum Biol 1974;1:29-40.

3
Orchiometry

Andrea Prader
University of Zurich, Zurich, Switzerland

Testicular volume is determined primarily by the mass of the seminiferous tubules. The Leydig cells occupy only a small part of the testis. The size of the testicles therefore gives clinical information only about tubular function and not about testosterone secretion, which can be evaluated by the degree of sexual maturation and sexuality. Abnormally small testicles indicate deficient spermatogenesis, while the production of testosterone may be more or less normal. Abnormally large testicles are found in several special conditions.

I. METHOD

The most precise method to estimate testicular volume is to measure the maximum length and breadth with the help of calipers and to calculate the volume mathematically (1). Such methods are tedious and require considerable handling of the genitalia, which should be avoided for psychological reasons. The estimation by comparable palpation with the help of an orchiometer is simpler, quicker, and of sufficient precision for clinical use. It needs some experience, however. The most widely used orchiometer is probably the one designed by the author (Fig. 1). With this instrument the inexperienced examiner will rather overestimate than underestimate testicular volume. One should try to estimate only the testicle, without the surrounding skin. The results of different examiners should not differ by more than one size. In normal males there is no difference or at most a one-size difference between the left and the right side.

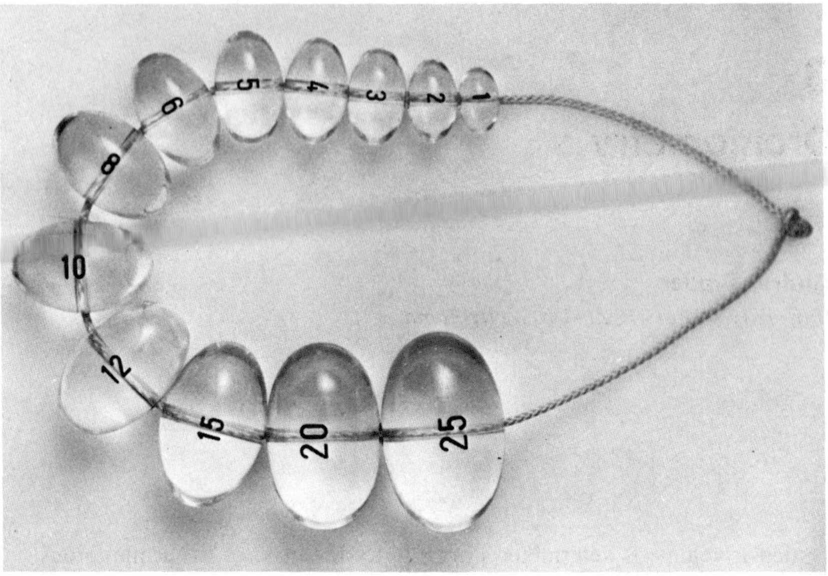

Figure 1 Orchiometer; each model (size) carries a number which indicates its volume in milliliters. (From Ref. 2.)

II. NORMAL VALUES

The variability of testicular volume is large (3) (see Fig. 2). Normal testicles of adult men have a volume of 10-25 ml. Values slightly outside this range may still be normal but require investigation. The smallest volume in a fertile man seen by the author was 6 ml. In children before puberty the normal values are 1-2 ml. Usually, the volume increases to 3-6 ml in the year before the appearance of pubic hair and the pubertal increase in penile size. Sometimes the testicles begin to grow later, simultaneously with the appearance of the other pubertal signs.

III. DECREASED TESTICULAR VOLUME

Small testicles are found in patients with hypothalamopituitary gonadotropin deficiency and in patients with primary hypogonadism. In the second group there is a negative correlation between testicular volume and follicle stimulating hormone (FSH) values (4). There exist borderline situations with relatively small testicles (6-8 ml) and slightly increased FSH values with normal spermatogenesis, which may be considered as compensated primary

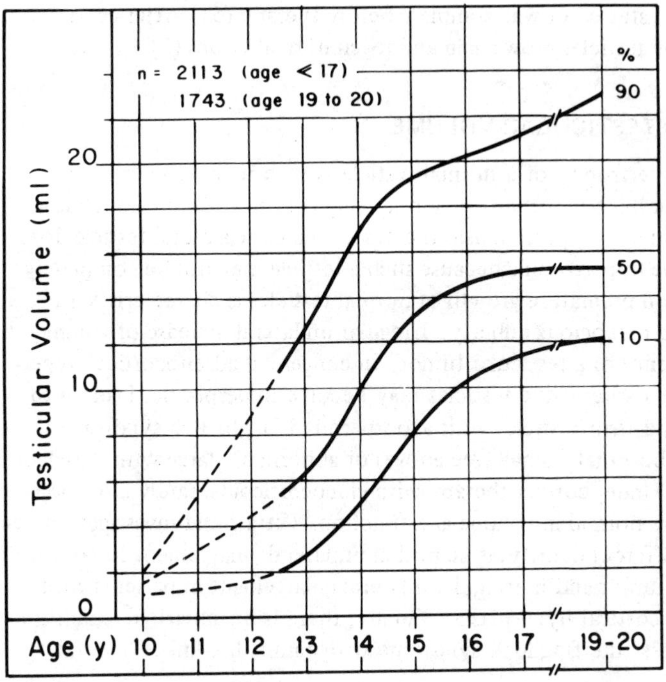

Figure 2 Testicular volume (10th, 50th, and 90th percentiles) in boys and young men. (From Ref. 2.)

hypogonadism. Many patients with cryptorchidism who have been treated successfully as far as the position of the testicles is concerned have small testes, high FSH values, normal or high lutenizing hormone (LH) values, and deficient spermatogenesis. Patients with Klinefelter's syndrome usually show some testicular growth during puberty up to a volume of 4-6 ml, with subsequent shrinkage and a final volume of 1-4 ml. They have high FSH values and azoospermia.

Abnormally high levels of androgenic or estrogenic steroids inhibit gonadotropin secretion, with consequent lack of testicular growth in puberty or testicular atrophy after puberty. This situation is found in sex steroid-producing tumors, untreated congenital adrenocortical hyperplasia, and treatment with high doses of sex steroids. Small doses of testosterone, such as 100 mg monthly of a long-acting preparation, as may be used to stimulate growth and physical maturation in patients with constitutional delay of growth and puberty, do not prevent normal testicular growth at puberty. Larger doses, however, prevent growth or are followed by decrease of testicular volume if pubertal growth of of the testicles had started or was complete before therapy (5). After cessation of therapy the testicles grow again and reach normal values (5).

IV. INCREASED TESTICULAR VOLUME

Compensatory hypertrophy of a normal testicle is seen if the contralateral testicle is absent or has become atrophic following torsion or trauma in childhood (6). In unilateral cryptorchidism the descended contralateral testicle does not always become hypertrophic because such a testicle may not be completely normal. In children premature growth of normal testicles is characteristic of true hypothalamic precocious puberty. Irregular unilateral increase of volume indicates the presence of a testicular tumor. In congenital adrenocortical hyperplasia adrenal rest tissue in the testicles may become hyperplastic, leading to large, irregular, and firm testicles with azoospermia (7). In this syndrome testicles may be abnormally small (see above) or abnormally large with deficient spermatogenesis. Under correct therapy with glucocorticoids, rarely also spontaneously, they are normal in volume and function. Ultrasound investigation, revealing areas of different density, is helpful in unilateral enlargement to confirm the presence of a tumor and in irregular bilateral enlargement in patients with congenital adrenocortical hyperplasia. Finally, there is an inherited condition with large testicles: the fragile X syndrome with familial X-linked mental deficiency (8).

REFERENCES

1. Hansen PF, With TK. Clinical measurements of the testes in boys and men. Acta Med Scand 1952; 142 (Suppl 266):457.
2. Zachmann, M, Prader A, Kind HP, Häfliger H, Budliger H. Testicular volume during adolescence. Cross-sectional and longitudinal studies. Helv Paediatr Acta 1974; 29:61.
3. Largo RH, Prader A. Pubertal development in Swiss children. (A longitudinal study.) Helv Paediatr Acta 1983; in press.
4. Prader A. Testicular growth in puberty. In *Puberty: Biologic and Psychosocial Components*, Berenberg SR (ed). Stenfert Kroese, Leiden, 1975.
5. Zachmann M, Ferrandez A, Mürset G, Gnehm HE, Prader A. Testosterone treatment of excessively tall boys. J Pediatr 1976; 88:116.
6. Laron Z, Zilka E. Compensatory hypertrophy of testicle in unilateral cryptorchidism. J Clin Endocrinol Metab 1969; 29:1409.
7. Zachmann M, Prader A, Illig R. Testicular maturation in congenital adrenal hyperplasia due to 21-hydroxylase deficiency. In *Pathophysiology of Puberty*, Cacciari E, Prader A (eds). Academic, London, 1980, p 213.
8. Gerald PS. X-linked mental retardation and an X-chromosome marker. N Engl J Med 1980; 303:696.

4
Visual Fields

Roderick D. Suckling
Christchurch Hospital, Christchurch, New Zealand

I. SYMPTOMS

The patient may complain of difficulty seeing to one side if there is a homonymous hemianopia, but bitemporal defects are usually silent.

II. ACUITY

Visual field testing must include testing the best central vision (i.e., the visual acuity). If, with distance glasses, the patient reads down the chart leaving off the first letters of each row with the left eye, and the last letters with the right eye, a bitemporal field loss should be suspected. If the same end of the line is omitted with each eye, suspect a homonymous hemianopia. If the patient cannot read down to 6/6 (20/20) a refractive error should be corrected if present. If the acuity is improved by looking through a 1¼-mm pinhole, a refractive error is confirmed and a refraction test is required. If, with the best glasses, the acuity is still below 6/9 (20/30), and no obvious ocular cause is found, it is likely that the field loss has crossed the midline. A truly hemianopic patient would see half of the 6/6 (20/20) line with each eye, not 6/12 (20/40) right and left. To detect this the chart should be a full one with lines of letters. When each half of the central field is depressed, suspect the lesion to be in the optic nerve, the chiasma, or rarely in both occipital cortices.

III. CONFRONTATION FIELD TESTING

The patient is next asked to cover one eye and look toward the doctor, who preferably faces the window or lighting. The doctor holds up one or two fingers of each hand in the two lower quadrants, asking the patient to add the fingers. The examiner then shifts to the upper quadrants, repeating the question. If there is a dense quadrant defect, the patient will only see the number of fingers in the other quadrant. If there is only a slight defect, it may only be detected by a color test. A red object, like a red-topped eye-drop bottle, is held up in each quadrant about 10° off fixation and the patient asked: "Can you see it as red out of the side of your vision while you keep looking at me? Is it a good red? Is it as bright a red here in this quadrant as it is in this one"? This is a suprathreshold test; the quality of the object is described, not its presence or absence. Most defects will be revealed with this test (1), provided that the background is even and the light is behind the patient, although measurement and followup comparisons require screen or perimeter testing.

IV. BJERRUM SCREEN TEST

This screen consists of a black cloth with a central fixation spot and fine stitch markings in circles at 5, 10, 15, 20, 25, and 30°. Many screens have an oval marked at 18° on each side to indicate the blind spots. This test is best used in dull illumination, the patient being seated 1 m away with one eye covered. The patient should keep fixing on the central mark while the examiner moves a 10-mm white circular disk near the blind spot area until the target disappears. The patient is reassured that it is normal for it to disappear in that area; then the same target is moved in from the periphery of the screen until seen, then continued in to the fixation spot. The examiner continuously inquires "Can you still see it?" while moving it in. This is quickly repeated in the quadrants, paying particular attention to each side of the midline at 12 and 6 o'clock, where a step defect often shows in early chiasmal or tract lesions (2, 3). A smaller target is then used (e.g., 2-mm diameter, white) and the process repeated, again paying particular attention to each side of the vertical line. Next a 20-mm-diameter red disk is used in each upper quadrant at 15° from fixation as a suprathreshold test. Rather than requesting "Tell me when you first see it," the examiner asks: "Tell me, is that as good a red on that side as it is on this side?" Then the examiner compares the lower quadrants, then the upper with the lower if the patient is not too tired. Red field defects appear as pink, yellow, or gray. If the difference is slight, it is better ignored. If the 10- and 2-mm white isopters show a wide gap, intermediate white sizes should be used to confirm and to give the gradient of the defect.

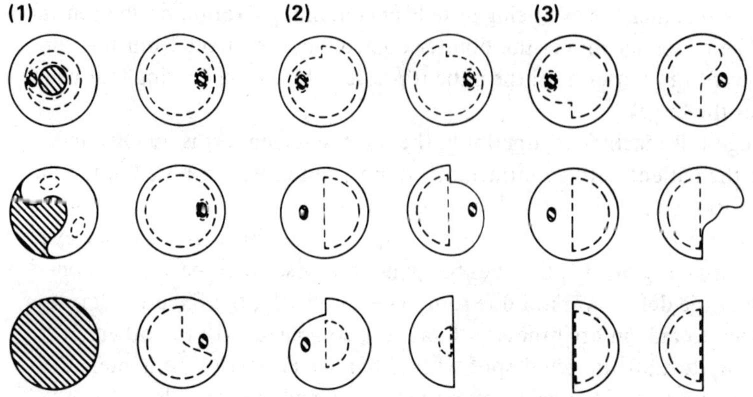

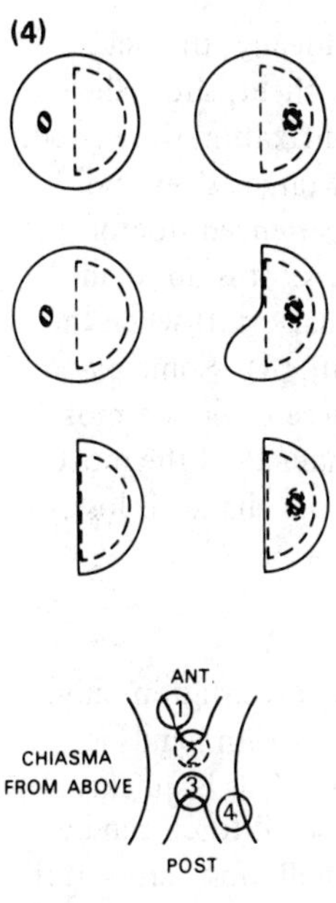

Figure 1 Expected field defects resulting from compression of the optic nerve within the skull. chiasma from above and below, and the left tract. (1) Optic nerve: The first stage of compression shows a central scotoma which with further compression extends to the periphery. If the lesion is in the presella region, the next defect is often the upper temporal field on the other side, a signal for semiurgent treatment before total blindness. (2) Chiasma from below: The first detectable field loss is often a step at the midline above when using small targets. Colored targets are most useful at this stage. (3) Chiasma from above: Similarly, careful attention to the juxta midline field below may show the earliest defect. (4) Tract: A progressive homonymous hemianopia *with optic atrophy* places the lesion in tract rather than radiation.

V. THE GOLDMANN PERIMETER

The Goldmann perimeter is a hemispherical shell with standardized illumination on its inner surface. Light-beam targets of varying size and intensity are directed onto the inner side by the operator via an amazing series of levers and mirrors from a manually controlled pointer on a chart on the outside. The patient sits with his chin on a rest and his head strapped into a forehead rest so that the eye being examined is at the center of the hemisphere, which has a radius of 0.33 m. Appropriate lenses for the patient for this distance are worn or inserted into a special holder. The examiner can watch the patient's eye through a small telescope to see whether the eye being tested is maintaining fixation on the central target. The examiner moves the pointer controlling the target from the periphery toward the center until the patient presses a buzzer indicating that he or she sees the target.

Although this machine is superior in theory, the screen test is quicker and easier for the patient with an intracranial tumor, and more magnified in the important central area. Also, with the screen test one can quickly compare one eye's field with the other's by leaving the target in a doubtful area for one eye, and by alternately covering the eyes the patient may see it come and go, confirming that the defect was not due to fatigue. Similarly, the fixed red target may be seen to fade in brightness with one eye compared with the other. If it is impossible to find the blind spot with either screen test or perimeter, the accuracy of the rest of the test must be suspected, and may even have to be abandoned.

If a chart is made it should be marked "poor fixation." Ideally, the field charts should include both left and right fields on the one sheet, show the acuity, whether glasses were worn, whether cooperation and fixation were good, both the examiner's and the patient's name, the date, and target sizes and colors. Fields should be done by the most senior and experienced doctor available, and preferably by the same examiner over the years. It is quite unfair to the patient to have fields done by temporary or ancillary staff when the result may strongly influence the decision whether to operate (4). Some patients are unable to maintain attention for long, and in these cases the most rapid test is the most accurate. The examiner must fully understand the most likely defect and test for that as quickly as possible, before the chance is lost.

VI. FIELD TESTING IN CHILDREN

From 3 years up to 6 or 7, field testing may have to be by confrontation only. Rather than asking the child to add fingers, a finger on one or both hands is wiggled, and the child asked to point to the one that wiggles. This is quickly repeated in the other two quadrants. With small children a small torch can be held in one of the hands and made to flash, when the child will look across at it if he sees it. It is then palmed into the other hand and the test repeated. Speed is essential with children, as attention is very limited. Adults who have suffered a stroke will look across to a moving hand if they see it; for example, a patient with homonymous hemianopia will consistently look across to one hand when both are moved.

VII. FOLLOW-UP

In acute cases it may be necessary to retest the fields the next day if the patient is too ill the first time. A suspected papilledema may need to be checked daily for the first small hemorrhage. In less acute cases (e.g., where a doubtful early field defect is found in someone with an enlarged pituitary fossa), a further check in 3 weeks would be appropriate. In postoperative cases fields should be checked at yearly intervals unless some additional symptoms are noted. Pregnant women with prolactinomas should have a field check every 2 months.

VIII. EYE CONDITIONS SOMETIMES ASSOCIATED WITH VISUAL FIELD DEFECTS

A. Pseudopapilledema and Papilledema

The question of papilledema may well arise in suspected hypothalamic or pineal tumors.

1. Pseudopapilledema

Pseudopapilledema is due to:

1. A congenitally small scleral opening in a small hypermetropic eye, so that the axons crowd at the disk, heaping up to pass through at right angles,
2. Drusen at the disk head, that is, small congenital buried glial cysts which tend to reach the surface as the child grows, and as they tend to present in other family members, an examination of the parents' disks may be rewarding in difficult cases.

In both of these types of pseudopapilledema the retinal vessels lie on the surface of the disks and the central retinal artery shows early and multiple branching; that is, five arteriole branches may be seen at once, instead of the usual two which branch again. There is no venous engorgement, hyperemia, edema, or obscuration of part of the vessels on or near the disk. The disk and vessels have a gleaming light reflex.

2. Papilledema

In true papilledema there is venous engorgement, disappearance of venous pulsation (present in 70% of people with normal intracranial pressures), some hyperemia, and blurring of the disk edge, while the physiological cup reduces in size as this swelling increases. The swelling is due to vascular engorgement edema and enlargement of axons due to obstruction to the flow of axoplasm. A small cup may remain to a late stage. The diagnosis is confirmed when the first small hemorrhage is seen near or on the disk.

Serial fundus photography can sometimes confirm a gradual change. In florid cases fluorescein angiography shows marked leakage around the disk, but in very early papilledema this test is often equivocal, and has not been as useful as had been initially hoped. However, fundus photography, in conjunction with fluorescein angiography, is of great use prior to applying laser treatment for diabetic retinopathy, a condition that can accompany some endocrine disorders (5).

B. Optic Atrophy

It is normal to have some temporal pallor, especially if the physiological cup is large. One should strongly suspect atrophy when the nasal side of the disk shows pallor, and at a later stage when few if any bands of ganglion cell axons are seen. Disk atrophy in chiasmal lesions tends to be horizontal, while in tract lesions it is horizontal on the opposite side, but vertical on the same side. This is because the axons of the ganglion cells in the temporal retina sweep around to reach the disk above and below (6).

C. Pupils

A useful comparison between the direct light reaction and the consensual light reaction can be made by the swinging light test. With the patient focusing in the distance, a strong light is directed at one eye for a few seconds, then quickly moved to the other. The first movement of this second pupil is noted. If it dilates a little, the retina or optic nerve on the second side is weaker than the first. This is a most useful test to show up optic nerve conduction defects, as in atrophy or neuritis. It tests whether the consensual reflex is better or worse than the direct light reflex (7). Both pupils tend to be semidilated in midbrain damage from a pinealoma.

D. Diplopia Due to Cranial Nerve Involvement

Horizontal diplopia, more marked to one side, indicates a sixth cranial nerve lesion; vertical diplopia, especially marked down to one side, indicates a probable fourth nerve lesion; while ptosis, enlarged pupil, and diplopia on lifting lid indicates a third nerve lesion. If on lifting the lid in a third nerve lesion the eye is found to be abducted, one can assume that the sixth nerve is intact, and if the patient is asked to look down and the affected eye is seen to rotate inward slightly, one can assume that the fourth nerve is intact.

REFERENCES

1. Frisén L. A versatile color confrontation test for the central visual field: a comparison with quantitative perimetry. Arch Ophthalmol 1973; 89:3–9.
2. Wilson P, Falconer MA. Patterns of visual failure with pituitary tumours: clinical and radiological correlations. Br J Ophthalmol 1968; 52:94–110.
3. Chamlin M, Davidoff LM, Feiring EH. Ophthalmologic changes produced by pituitary tumors. Am J Ophthalmol 1955; 40:3, 353–367.
4. Elkington SG. Pituitary adenoma: preoperative symptomatology in a series of 260 patients. Br J Ophthalmol 1968; 52:322–327.
5. Bresnick GH, Davis MD, Myers FL, De Venecia, G. Clinicopathological correlation in diabetic retinopathy. Arch Ophthalmol 1977; 95:1215–1220.
6. Hoyt WF, Kommerell G. Der Fundus oculi bei homonymer Hemianopie. Klin Monatsbl Augenheilkd 1973; 162:456–464.
7. Thompson HS. Afferent pupillary defects: pupillary findings associated with defects of the afferent arm of the pupillary light reflex arc. Am J Ophthalmol 1966; 62:860–873.

5
Cervical Mucus Assessment

Gabor Thomas Kovacs and Henry G. Burger
Prince Henry's Hospital, Melbourne, Australia

The physical properties of cervical mucus exhibit a changing pattern in response to the hormonal changes during the menstrual cycle. These changes provide a clinical index of ovarian function, which can be utilized by either the gynecologist or the patient.

Gynecological assessment is used in evaluation of the infertile couple, assessing the time of ovulation for treatments such as artificial insemination and in vitro fertilization, ascertaining that there is a response to ovulation induction, and in the study of the cervical factor in subfertility.

Patient self-assessment can be used both to enhance fertility by appropriate timing of intercourse, and for fertility regulation based on periodic abstinence from intercourse during the fertile phase of the cycle.

I. MOLECULAR BIOLOGY OF CERVICAL MUCUS

Mucus is a hydrogel, whose components change markedly in response to the circulating level of estrogen and progesterone. Estrogenic mucus (type E) is thin and watery (water content 95-98%) with a protein content of less than 1%, a mucin content of 0.5-1.5% and few cells present. The mucin is arranged in micelles which line up parallel with the cervical canal, with relatively few cross-links, thus providing channels for sperm migration. Progestogenic mucus (type G) has a decreased water content (85-92%), higher protein content (2-4%) and 2-10% mucin, with an abundance of cells. The mucin is arranged as a dense network with extensive cross-linkage, without micelle formation; thus sperm penetration is inhibited (1). The makeup of cervical mucus is heterogeneous, with one or other type of mucus predominating. At ovulation, 95% of mucus is of type E, and during the luteal phase up to 90% is type G.

These changes in the molecular biology of cervical mucus result in varying physical (rheological) properties. Of clinical interest are:

Viscosity. This is minimum at or just prior to ovulation and maximum during the luteal phase.

Spinnbarkeit. This is its ability to be drawn into threads, and gradually increases during the proliferative phase until ovulation, after which there is a rapid decline.

Crystallization (ferning). This is one of the most sensitive parameters of change in sex hormone concentration. The appearance of ferning is a result of the formation of four sets of crystals at right angles, in a solution containing proteins and electrolytes (NaCl). It is a result of the action of estrogen on viscosity and spinnbarkeit, appears during the early proliferative phase, and increases with the degree of estrogenic activity, to a maximum just before ovulation. It is replaced by a cellular pattern within 24-72 hr of ovulation.

II. METHODOLOGY

A. Gynecological Assessment

1. Cervical Score

The examination of the cervix and cervical mucus can be used as a semiquantitative index of estrogen secretion (2).

The cervix should be exposed with the speculum and the amount of mucus visible at the external os, as well as the degree of cervical opening is noted. A specimen of mucus is obtained either with a cotton wool swab or an inoculation loop. The mucus is placed on a microscope slide, and stretched so that the spinnbarkeit can be measured and graded. The mucus is then spread along the slide and allowed to dry. It is examined under a microscope on low power and the degree of ferning is quantitated. The scoring system is described in Table 1.

The cervical score after cessation of menstruation is very low, with closed cervix and scanty turbid mucus. As the cycle progresses, the quantity of mucus increases, as does its stretchiness. When dried mucus is inspected under the microscope the amount of ferning increases throughout the proliferative phase of the cycle. It is almost absent in the postmenstrual days and then the quality and degree of ferning steadily increase to reach a maximum just prior to ovulation. In the preovulatory phase the cervical score is usually 8-12. Following ovulation, it rapidly plunges to levels of less than 6 within 2 days or so. There is very little mucus produced and this is usually thick and tacky. It is not

Table 1 Definition of a Scoring System for Cervical Mucus

	Score			
	0	1	2	3
Quantity of mucus	None	Scant	Dribble	Cascade
Spinnbarkeit	None	Slight, 2–4 cm	Moderate, 4–8 cm	Copious, >8 cm
Ferning	None, cellular	Linear mucus	Partial	Complete
Cervix	Closed	–	Partly open	Gaping

Source: Ref. 2.

possible to stretch it and the ferning will have disappeared when inspected under the microscope.

The observed changes in the cervix and the cervical mucus are closely correlated with the periovulatory changes in gonadotrophins and gonadal steroids, and with ultrasonic evidence of follicular growth and rupture (3). In particular, a rising cervical score parallels the preovulatory rise in plasma estradiol, and the maximal score is seen at the time of the luteinizing hormone (LH) and follicle stimulating hormone (FSH) midcycle peaks. Ovulation, as observed ultrasonically, occurs on the day following the LH peak.

2. In Vivo Test of Sperm Mucus Interaction—The Postcoital Test (PCT)

Examination of cervical mucus after intercourse was first described by Sims in 1866 (4). He stated that this enabled the observation of spermatozoa in their natural environment, and that the presence of motile spermatozoa confirmed that the semen sample was satisfactory, the spermatozoa could enter the uterocervical canal, and the secretions were favorable for their vitality.

This test next received attention in 1913 from Huhner (5), who described it as the "assessment of the husband's semen in genitals of his own wife." He simplified the whole concept as follows:

> If living spermatozoa are present in the specimen, then the cervix is in the right position for that particular penis, and the couple's coital technique must be adequate. The concentration of spermatozoa in the semen must also be satisfactory.

If all the spermatozoa present appear dead, and a freshly examined semen specimen shows live spermatozoa, then "something about the female secretions is inimical to the vitality of the spermatozoa."

If no spermatozoa can be detected, a fresh semen specimen needs to be examined. If this is satisfactory, then mechanical problems such as inadequate coitus, premature ejaculation and penile abnormalities need to be excluded.

Surprisingly, our understanding of the Sim's-Huhner postcoital test has not improved during the last 68 years.

There is also debate about how long after intercourse the mucus should be examined. Sims suggested between 15 and 20 hr, and Huhner examined the specimen as soon after the coitus as the patient could get to the office. Others suggest performing intercourse in the office to enable examination of mucus within seconds of ejaculation (6).

It is important that if the postcoital test is performed, it should be carefully timed for the preovulatory phase when there is a good cervical score. The couple are asked to abstain from intercourse for 48-72 hr before having coitus for the test. Other advice that needs to be given is that the woman should remain supine for 20 min or so after intercourse and she should refrain from douching or bathing prior to attending the hospital. The timing between intercourse and the test being performed is not critical, and probably several hours is a reasonable range.

On attending the clinic, the woman should be examined in a dorsal position, cervix displayed with a bivalve speculum, and the cervical score ascertained. A specimen of mucus should be placed on a glass slide under a coverslip to keep it from drying out. Several fields should then be inspected under high-power microscopy (X400). Those areas with maximal spermatozoal activity should be selected. It is the practice in our laboratory to count up to about 300 spermatozoa. The average number of spermatozoa per high-power field, and percentages of purposefully progressing, progressing in circles, shaking, and non-motile spermatozoa, are recorded.

3. In Vitro Tests of Sperm Mucus Interaction

Two types of in vitro tests of sperm mucus interaction have been used, a microscope slide method (7) and a capillary tube testing system (8).

In the slide method, a small amount of fresh semen and preovulatory cervical mucus are placed on a microscope slide about 3 mm apart, and the specimens are then brought into contact by placing a coverslip over them. The interface between the semen and mucus is observed microscopically to see if spermatozoa could penetrate the mucus. If this takes place, the test is positive and hostility is thought to be excluded. However, if the sperms do not penetrate or if they appear to be shaking but not progressing in the mucus, "cervical hostility" has been postulated. This apparent cervical hostility may be caused by many factors, including the presence of antisperm antibodies in the female or in the male.

Other modifications of the slide technique include sealing it from air so that observation can take place without the mucus drying (9), and standardizing the area of sperm mucus interface by using a hemocytometer (10). However, slide tests have the shortcomings that the distance spermatozoa travel in the mucus cannot be quantitated, nor can their longevity be determined.

These disadvantages can be overcome by using a capillary method, which enables the observer to determine the penetration density, the qualitative motility, and the longevity of spermatozoa in cervical mucus. The first publication using this technique came from Lamar et al. in 1940 (11). They performed the tests by aspirating small quantities of cervical mucus and fresh semen into a capillary tube, being 0.1-0.4 mm in diameter, separating the two tissues by a small air bubble. They then observed sperm penetration into the mucus, the distance of spermatozoal travel, and the duration of motility of the spermatozoa which had penetrated the mucus. Capillary methods were modified by several other workers but were greatly refined by Kremer. He designed a simple apparatus—a sperm penetration meter (SPM)—which requires only 2 drops of semen and less than 0.05 cc of cervical mucus (8). Using this apparatus, he found that the results were sufficiently reproducible to employ as a routine part of the fertility workup.

The test can be refined further by performing it as a "crossover test" (12). This means testing the husband's semen in his wife's mucus as well as in fertile donor mucus; and testing the wife's mucus against fertile donor semen as well as her husband's semen. Thus, theoretically, it can be determined whether the spermatozoa or the mucus is at fault in a case of apparent cervical hostility.

B. Self-Assessment

The changes in cervical mucus can be recognized by the woman herself as a series of changes in the secretions observable at the vulva (13-15). Observations are best made at the end of the day, when cervical secretions have reached the vulva with the aid of gravity. They are facilitated by the use of toilet tissue wiped over the vulva prior to micturition, and are complemented by the sensations produced by the mucus. In healthy women, experiencing regular ovulatory menstrual cycles, 28-29 days in length, the following series of changes are usually observed. Following the cessation of menstrual bleeding (usually lasting about 5 days), no secretion or discharge may be noted for 2-5 days; these days may be termed "dry" days. The commencement of detectable mucus discharge is marked by the appearance of thick, sticky, tacky, or cloudy mucus,

Table 2 Sequential Self-Recognizable Changes in Cervical Mucus at the Vulva

1. Menstrual bleeding
2. Absence of secretion–"dry" days
3. Onset of thick, sticky, or cloudy mucus
4. Change to thin, clear, lubricative mucus resembling raw egg white
5. Change to sticky, tacky mucus

which may persist for 2-3 days, gradually increasing in quantity, and then changing in its characteristics, to become clear, wet, stretchy, lubricative, and resembling raw egg white. Such mucus is of "fertile" type, and the last day on which it is observable is termed the "peak" day. The mucus changes its characteristics relatively abruptly following the peak day, and becomes sticky and tacky. It may persist for one or more days, or may disappear until just prior to the next menses. The changes are summarized in Table 2. The changes can be used to define the fertile phase of the menstrual cycle. Several studies (13-15) have shown that the peak day is correlated closely with the estimated day of ovulation, and over 90% of women of widely differing social, cultural, educational, and economic characteristics are able to learn self-recognition of the fertile phase in the first cycle in which they are taught (16).

III. CLINICAL APPLICATION

A. Ovulation Timing

Ovulation timing is necessary in a number of clinical applications:

1. *The management of idiopathic infertility*. The teaching of self-recognition of the fertile phase is helpful in assessing optimal timing of coitus for couples wishing to achieve pregnancy.
2. *The timing of artificial insemination*. Both gynecological and self-assessment methods are useful in ensuring optimal timing of artificial insemination, using either husband's or donor semen. The combined use of the cervical score and basal temperature charting can lead to pregnancy rates with donor insemination which are not significantly lower than those using hormonal assessment or ultrasound for timing (17).
3. *Timing of in vitro fertilization*. Gynecological or self-assessment of cervical mucus is useful in the timing of hormone assays and ultrasound examinations prior to laparoscopy for ovum collection (18).

B. Assessment and Management of Clinical Factors in Infertility

The value of the postcoital test has been much debated. The controversy is associated with the fact that the role of the cervix in reproduction has not been defined. There are two schools of thought about this; the barrier theory and the reservoir theory. The barrier theory states that the cervix acts as a filter to prevent abnormal spermatozoa from reaching the upper reproductive tract. The evidence for this is that normal spermatozoa can be detected in the fallopian tubes within minutes of intercourse (19). If this is in fact true, then a postcoital test is looking only at the spermatozoa that failed to migrate and thus has little meaning.

The reservoir theory postulates that the cervical mucus acts as a reservoir from which spermatozoa are steadily released, and in this case sampling the mucus some hours after intercourse will give information about potentially fertile spermatozoa. It is probable that as in most other biological systems, the cervix plays a combined role of these two extremes, and as long as tests are performed at similar intervals (i.e., some hours after coitus) are compared with each other, it will still be meaningful.

What is a normal PCT? It has always been suggested that a normal PCT should have 10 motile spermatozoa per high-power field. However, a review of the literature showed that this mystical figure of 10 has never been substantiated. A study of 50 fertile women volunteers (20) suggested that if the mucus is examined several hours after coitus, the presence of *some* motile spermatozoa indicated normality.

Thus we postulate that if motile purposefully progressive spermatozoa are present on a PCT, then it is unlikely that there is cervical factor as a basis of the fertility problem, and that the couple's coital technique and anatomical normality are confirmed. However, if none or very few motile spermatozoa are detected in fertile preovulatory mucus in two separate cycles, the cervical factor should be investigated further. Our next test is a crossover Kremer test, and the screening of both partners for antisperm antibodies. A discussion on antisperm antibodies is beyond the scope of this chapter and readers are directed to recent reviews at a physiological level by Beer and Neaves (21), and at a clinical level by Jones (22).

The priority of the postcoital test among fertility investigations is also debated. Some workers claim that as the first requirement for fertilization is that a large number of motile spermatozoa should reach the cervix, the PCT should be the first test performed in investigating the subfertile couple.

It is the authors' practice to investigate the cervical factor once the three major fertility parameters (semen, ovulation, and tubal function) have been shown to be satisfactory.

C. Fertility Regulation

Self-recognition of the fertile phase is used as the basis of the natural methods of fertility regulation. In the ovulation method (23), couples are taught that the onset of detectable mucus secretion at the vulva marks the beginning of the fertile phase of the cycle. The end of the phase is the third day following the peak day, so that intercourse may be resumed on the fourth day after the peak. The method is readily taught, and has a low method failure rate of approximately one to three pregnancies per 100 women-years (24, 25). User failure rates are much higher, and result from intercourse during the fertile phase, with disregard by the couple for a variety of reasons, of the indications of fertility. The other major natural method, the sympto-thermal method, relies on a combination of calendar calculations, self-recognition of cervical mucus changes, and temperature measurements; pregnancy rates are comparable to those with the ovulation method. The so-called rhythm method is now obsolete.

REFERENCES

1. Elstein M. Functions and physical properties of mucus in the female genital tract. Br Med Bull 1978; 34:83–88.
2. Insler V, Melmed H, Eichenbrenner I, Serr D, Lunenfeld B. The cervical score. A simple semiqualitative method for monitoring of the menstrual cycle. Int J Gynaecol Obster 1972; 10:223–228.
3. Renaud RL, Maclear J, Dervan I, Ahret M, Aron Plas-Rosert S, Spida A, Pollack H. Echographic study of follicular maturation and ovulation during the normal menstrual cycle. Fertil Steril 1980; 33:272–276.
4. Sims JM. *Clinical Notes on Uterine Surgery with Special Reference to the Management of the Sterile Condition.* Robert Hardwicke, London, 1866.
5. Huhner M. *Sterility in the Male and Female and Its Treatment.* Rebman, New York, 1913.
6. Sobrero AJ, MacLeod J. The immediate post coital test. Fertil Steril 1962; 13:184–189.
7. Miller EG, Kurzrok R. Biochemical studies of human semen. III. Factors affecting migration of sperm through the cervix. Am J Obstet Gynecol 1932; 24:19–26.
8. Kremer J. A Simple sperm penetration test. Int J Fertil 1965; 10: 209–215.
9. Barton M, Wiesner BP. The receptivity of cervical mucus to spermatozoa. Br Med J 1946; 2:606–610.
10. Guard HR. New technic for sperm-mucus penetration tests, using a hemocytometer. Fertil Steril 1960; 11:392–398.
11. Lamar JK, Shettles LB, Delfs E. Cyclic penetrability of human cervical mucus to spermatozoa in vitro. Am J Physiol 1940; 129:234–241.

12. Morgan H, Hendry WF, Stedronska J, Chamberlain GVP, Dewhurst CJ. Sperm/cervical mucus cross hostility testing and antisperm antibodies in the husband. Lancet 1977; 1:1228–1230.
13. Billings EL, Billings JJ, Brown JB, Burger HG. Symptoms and hormonal changes accompanying ovulation. Lancet 1972; 1:282–284.
14. Flynn AM, Lynch SS. Cervical mucus and identification of the fertile phase of the menstrual cycle. Br J Obstet Gynaecol 1976; 83:656–659.
15. Hilgers TW, Abraham GE, Cavanagh D. Natural family planning. 1. The peak symptom and estimated time of ovulation. Obstet Gynaecol 1978; 52:575–582.
16. World Health Organization. Task force methods for the determination of the fertile period, special programme of research, development and research training in human reproduction. A prospective multicentre trial of the ovulation method of natural family planning. 1. The teaching phase. Fertil Steril 1981; in press.
17. Kovacs GT, Lording DL. Artificial insemination with donor semen—a review of 252 patients. Med J Aust 1980; 2:609–611.
18. Trounson AO, Leeton JF, Wood C, Webb J, Wood J. Fertilization in vitro and embryo transfer in the controlled ovulatory cycle. Science 1981; 212; 681–682.
19. Settlage D, Motoshima M, Tredway D. Sperm transport from the external cervical os to the follopian tubes in women. Fertil Steril 1973; 24: 655–661.
20. Kovacs GT, Norman GB, Henson GL. The post-coital test. What is normal? Br Med J 1978; 1:818.
21. Beer AE, Neaves WB. Antigenic status of semen from the viewpoint of the female and male. Fertil Steril 1978; 29:3–22.
22. Jones WR. The investigation of immunological fertility. Med J Aust 1979; 2:188–192.
23. Billings EL, Billings JJ, Catarinich, Rev M. *Atlas of the Ovulation Method: Mucus Patterns of Fertility and Infertility*, 3rd ed., Advocate Press, Melbourne, 1979.
24. Ball M. A prospective field trial of the "ovulation method" of avoiding conception. Eur J Obstet Gynaecol Reprod Biol 1976; 6:63–66.
25. Klaus H, Goebel JM, Muraski B, Egizio MT, Weitzel D, Taylor RS, Fagan MU, Ek K, Hobday K. Use-effectiveness and client satisfaction in six centers teaching the Billings ovulation method. Contraception 1979; 19:613–629.

HORMONE ASSAY METHODOLOGY

6

Peptide, Protein, and Glycoprotein Hormones

Wilfrid R. Butt
Birmingham and Midland Hospital for Women, Birmingham, England

Before binding-type assays such as radioreceptor and radioimmunoassays were available, the assay of peptide, protein, and glycoprotein hormones depended entirely on biological methods. Steroids and other hormones of low molecular weight, on the other hand, can be characterized so that physicochemical methods of measurement are applicable. Generally, bioassay methods are difficult to use routinely and lack sensitivity, have poor reproducibility, and are expensive. Major advances in our knowledge of the secretion of protein hormones and in the discovery of new ones have resulted since the new methods of assay were developed.

The molecular structure which is responsible for the biological activity of a hormone, however, may not be identical to that recognized by nonbiological methods. A hormone is defined by its biological actions and the first detection is therefore by bioassay. An assessment of the biological activity is also necessary when the hormone is to be used for therapy: for example, in treatment with insulin, growth hormone, or gonadotropins.

I. STANDARDS

Biological standards and reference materials available for use as standards to define units of biological activity or as reference materials in other assays have been listed (1) and discussed in detail in the regular Technical Report Series of the World Health Organization. There are a number of problems in setting up suitable standards: the material is usually extracted and purified from the gland of origin, and the chemical manipulations used may alter the chemical structure.

The assays in which they are to be used are usually for the hormone circulating in blood, where it may exist in different forms, which include precursors, metabolites, subunits, and variants such as are derived from tumors. Not all these forms may be biologically active, but clinically useful information may still be obtained by determination of their immunological activity (e.g., for proinsulin).

II. BIOASSAYS

It is important to validate any bioassay in terms of specificity, accuracy, precision, and parallelism of the dose-response lines for unknown and standard (2). The assays can be of the in vivo or in vitro varieties. Total hormone activity is measured by the in vivo methods since the transport mechanism to the target organ, the recognition of the receptor, and the binding and action at the receptor site are all involved. Only some of these properties are required for in vitro responses: the hormone is presented to the target organ so that any change in the molecule (e.g., loss of terminal sialic acid residues in glycoproteins) which affects the biological half-life in the circulation will not be detected. The end points may depend on binding to the target cells or on action at the receptor site as indicated by the production of another substance [e.g., corticosteroids from the adrenal in response to adrenocorticotropic hormone (ACTH), progesterone from the corpus luteum under the influence of luteinizing hormone (LH) or human chorionic gonadotropin (hCG), or glucose-6-phosphate dehydrogenase activity from the kidney in response to parathyroid hormone (PTH)].

A. Specificity

The development of specific assays may be difficult for closely related families of proteins: for example, the gonadotropins, which consist of common α subunits but distinctive β subunits; the peptide hormones related to pro-ACTH, such a lipotropin (LPH), ACTH, melanocyte stimulating hormone (MSH), and endorphin; and for growth hormone and prolactin. The development of relatively simple and specific bioassays for the gonadotropins helped to monitor the purification procedures and led to the eventual preparation of follicle stimulating hormone (FSH) separate from LH, from which specific reagents for immunoassay could be obtained. Evidence for the separate existence of growth hormone and prolactin in the human came from experiments with pituitary cell cultures from which prolactin activity measured by bioassay was maintained, whereas growth hormone activity measured immunologically decreased.

B. In Vitro Assays

1. Radioreceptor Assays

The requirements for this type of assay are a suitable tissue preparation and a labeled form of the hormone to be measured. The only difference from radioimmunoassays is that a natural binding protein is used instead of an artificially produced antibody. For clinical applications a series of assays is usually required and therefore a homogeneous preparation of binding tissue which is stable on storage is needed.

Labeling for this type of assay is usually by radioiodine and similar methods to those used for radioimmunoassay are applicable. It is even more important, however, to avoid damage to the protein molecule, and therefore the concentration of oxidant and of radioiodine is kept to a minimum and mild methods of iodination (e.g., using the enzyme lactoperoxidase) are used.

2. Assays Depending on a Metabolic End Point

As well as indicating a further biological property of the hormone, this type of assay does not require the use of a labeled hormone. The final product released and used as a measure of response may, however, be determined by radioimmunoassay, for instance, where a steroid is produced. Alternatively, a labeled intermediate may be included in the medium which under the influence of a hormone may be converted to another compound (e.g., 19-hydroxyandrostenedione converted to estradiol under the influence of FSH) (3).

3. Cytochemical Methods

Methods of assay depending on a cytochemical end point sometimes afford very high sensitivity hitherto obtainable only by radioimmunoassay (4). In principle the target tissue is exposed to the hormone and a suitable chemical change identified by a specific reaction. Quantitative measurement is obtained by microscopic inspection of a selected cell type and analysis of a chromogenic reaction by a microdensitometer. The reaction may be the same as that used in vivo (e.g., depletion of ascorbic acid in the cases of ACTH and LH). The assays are frequently sufficiently sensitive for the detection of circulating levels of the hormone, and since they depend on some biological function, they may not detect inactivated material recognized by radioimmunoassay.

III. IMMUNOASSAYS

A. Preparation of Antibodies

Protein and glycoprotein hormones are generally good immunogens, but peptides, because of their relatively low molecular weights, may be only weak immunogens and require coupling to a larger molecule before they become immunogenic. Alternatively, it may be possible to produce a derivative which is immunogenic, as for pancreatic glucagon, where the 27-S-methyl-glucagon has been found to be a good immunogen (5).

Fortunately, quantities of highly purified hormone required for raising antisera and for using as antigen in labeling procedures are quite small. Only microgram amounts are required for immunization by the multisite technique (6), and frequently antisera are obtained which may be used in very high dilutions.

1. Agglutination Inhibition Reactions

These methods are inexpensive and rapid for the determination of hormones which occur in fairly high concentrations in body fluids (e.g., for hCG in pregnancy diagnosis). This type of assay is subject to interference by nonspecific substances, however, and has seldom been applied successfully to the determination of hormones in blood. In the case of hCG, however, concentrations are so great in early pregnancy that the test has useful clinical applications. For this purpose the technique of complement fixation is also satisfactory (7).

2. Radioimmunoassay

This most commonly used method of hormone assay has several advantages over others: it is convenient, may be carried out in large numbers, can be automated, and can usually be developed with high sensitivity and specificity. Care is needed in the performance of the assay, however, and efficient quality control is essential. Factors contributing to the performance are the use not only of common reagents, but also common protocols. The large quantitative differences between results from different laboratories when these factors are not taken into account have been well illustrated by many examples [e.g., for LH (8), growth hormone (9,10), and PTH (11)].

The labeling procedure has frequently caused trouble. An oxidant is required for liberating iodine from the reagent, $Na^{125}I$, and this oxidant can cause chemical change to the protein. The minimum concentration of oxidant and the shortest exposure to its action compatible with satisfactory incorporation of iodine is therefore chosen. The most widely used of these oxidants is chloramine-T (12). Alternative techniques, including the use of the enzyme lactoperoxidase (13) and the generation of chlorine (14), both of which are mild methods, may be used to preserve biological as well as immunological activity. More recently the reagents Iodo-Gen (15) for glycoprotein hormones and N-bromosuccinimide (16) for prolactin, have been introduced and show great promise.

Another method is the conjugation labeling technique (17), in which direct contact of oxidant and antigen is avoided. Here it is not essential for the protein to contain tyrosine, as an iodinated reagent is linked covalently to the antigen. The rather tedious manipulations required probably account for the limited number of applications reported so far.

Another stage in the method where there are many alternatives is in the separation of free from bound labeled fractions. The use of the second antibody to afford an immunological separation of the bound fraction is commonly used, but solid phase methods have much to recommend them: they are rapid and the centrifuging is simple. For the best performance, however, several washing stages are required, offsetting some of the advantages. Magnetic particles offer an interesting alternative, as the magnetic separation of the bound fraction avoids centrifugation (18,19).

Serum may contain variable amounts of nonspecific material which may be mistaken for hormone. Response curves are generally, but not always, less steep than for standards or endogenous homologous hormone. The nonspecific material may obscure measurements at low concentrations. Hunter and Bennie (20) overcame the problem in gonadotropin assays by optimizing the assays, by purifying the labels before use, and by not accepting less than 15% inhibition. In earlier assays for TSH the nonspecific effects were overcome by adding TSH-free serum to the standards, but this has been avoided by raising antisera which are more specific.

Certain precautions are required when dealing with the assay of peptide hormones: this is because peptides may be degraded by proteolytic activity in blood. Plasma is therefore separated immediately after collection of the sample using a refrigerated centrifuge and it is stored at -70°C. Additives to inhibit proteolytic activity, such as Trasylol, may be used (21) or the plasma may be separated and extracted immediately after the blood has been collected, as described for glucagon (5).

3. Labeled Antibody Methods

The immunoradiometric assay (IRMA) was originally introduced for serum insulin (22). The technique is potentially more sensitive than the equivalent radioimmunoassay since sensitivity is limited by the avidity of the specific antibody which reacts with antigen in radioimmunoassay, while it is dependent on the specific activity of the label used (^{125}I) in the IRMA method.

Greater overall specificity may be achieved by using a so-called sandwich or two-site assay. An adsorbent such as an antibody attached to a solid phase is used to extract the antigen from the sample and the antibody hormone complex is then exposed to a labeled antibody to give a solid phase-antibody-antigen-labeled antibody complex. An example of this type of assay is the determination of proinsulin, where insulin and the C peptide need to be separately recognized. Plastic pipette tips coated with guinea pig anti-insulin antibodies are used to extract proinsulin together with insulin from the serum (23). The proinsulin is then identified by reaction with rabbit antibodies to the C peptide and the reaction is quantified by iodine-labeled sheep antibodies to rabbit gamma globulin.

This type of assay also overcomes the problem sometimes associated with labeling of hormone antigen, but there are problems to overcome in the setting up of these assays and a good deal of preliminary experimentation is needed. This is probably why many years have elapsed between the original description of the method and its widespread use.

4. Nonisotopic Labels

Nonisotopic labels are intrinsically more stable than radioisotopes, they carry no radiation hazard, and they may be used in countries where there are no facilities for handling and counting radioisotopes. Many types have been suggested and until now, enzymes have been the most studied (24). It has sometimes been difficult to attain the same sensitivity as in radioimmunoassay by this method; an ultrasensitive method described recently (25) is therefore of great interest as a potentially useful development, although as presently described it is somewhat unwieldy and requires a radioactive substrate ([^{3}H] adenosine monophosphate).

It is likely that other nonisotopic methods will become increasingly important in the future. These include laser immunonephelometry (26); chemiluminescence, where there are several excellent labels offering high sensitivity, stability, and theoretically zero background interference (27); and fluorescence, particularly with the rare earth fluorophores readily distinguishing the specific and background fluorescence by time resolution techniques (28).

5. Assay Performance

For many hormones commercial kits are available which give good performance. There are also separate reagents and when these are used in well-tried procedures there may be little to choose on the grounds of analytical performance between the kits and laboratory procedures. Both external and internal quality assessment is required so that results between and within laboratories may be related.

In view of the different mechanisms involved it is not surprising that differences are recognized between in vivo or in vitro bioassays compared with radioimmunoassays. Radioreceptor assays for the somatomedins (29) measure a variety of somatomedins, including growth hormone-dependent somatomedin A and C as well as the insulin-like growth factor 2, thought to be independent of growth hormone. Radioimmunoassays, on the other hand, can be designed to measure these individual components. In the radioreceptor assay for growth hormone using lymphocytes, growth hormone of various species will displace human growth hormone, whereas there is less cross-reaction between species in immunoassays. Hyperfunctioning human parathyroid glands secrete significant quantities of C-region immunoreactive PTH fragments. C-region immunoreactive PTH estimates therefore exceed the values obtained in radioimmunoassays for intact PTH (30).

IV. FUTURE TRENDS

There is a resurgence of interest in the IRMA method since it is particularly useful for the microdetermination of proteins and offers wide working ranges with shorter incubation and counting times and lower detection limits than some radioimmunoassays. The method will certainly be improved if monoclonal antibodies become available. These are produced by the hybrid myeloma technique (31). Continuous cultures of fused cells secreting antibody of predefined specificity have several potential advantages over conventional polyclonal antibodies. The monospecific antibodies may be produced in unlimited quantities with defined and constant characteristics even when the antigen is not available in pure form. The antibody may be readily purified from contaminating immunoglobulins in high yield, so that labeling in IRMA methods and the preparation of immunoadsorbents is much easier.

There are difficulties to overcome in this technique. Some antigens may produce only a low titer on immunization and a large number of antibodies has to be investigated to obtain one with the correct combination of specificity, affinity, and other properties required for immunoassay purposes. The method shows much promise, however, so that the considerable effort is justified.

REFERENCES

1. Bangham DR. Standards for hormones, 3rd ed. In *Hormones in Blood,* (Gray, C. H., and James, V. H. T., eds). Academic, London, 1979, vol. 1, pp IX-XIV.
2. Loraine JA, Bell ET. General principles in hormone assay. In *Hormone Assays and Their Clinical Application,* 4th ed. Churchill Livingstone, Edinburgh, 1976, pp 2-20.
3. Van Damme MP, Robertson DM, Marana R, Ritzen EM, Diczfalusy E. A sensitive and specific in vitro bioassay method for the measurement of follicle-stimulating hormone activity. Acta Endocrinol (Copenh) 1979, 91:224-237.
4. Chayen J. The cytochemical bioassay of polypeptide hormones. *Monographs on Endocrinology No. 17,* Springer-Verlag, Berlin, 1980.
5. Nooijen WJ, Koppert PM. Radioimmunoassay for pancreatic glucagon based on specific derivatisation of the hormone. Ann Clin Biochem 1981, 18:118-122.

6. Vaitukaitis J, Robbins JB, Nieschlag E, Ross GT. A method for producing specific antisera with small doses of immunogen. J Clin Endocrinol Metab 1971; 33:988-990.
7. Brody S. Immunoassay of gonadotrophins using complement fixation. Acta Endocrinol [Suppl] (Copehn) 1970; 142:113-130.
8. Taymor, MC. Discrepancies and similarities of serum FSH and LH patterns as evaluated by different assay methods. Acta Endocrinol [Suppl] (Copenh) 1970; 142:324-337.
9. Herington AC, Jacobs LS, Daughaday WH. Radioreceptor and radioimmunoassay quantitation of human growth hormone in acromegalic serum: overestimation by immunoassay and systematic differences between antiserum. J Clin Endocrinol Metab 1974; 39:257-262.
10. Root AW. Regulation of secretion of human growth hormone. In *Problems in Pediatric Endocrinology,* La Cauza, C, Root, AW (eds). Academic, London, 1980, vol 32, pp 3-20.
11. Berson SA, Yalow RS. Immunochemical heterogeneity of parathyroid hormone in plasma. J Clin Endocrinol Metab 1968; 28:1037-1047.
12. Greenwood FC, Hunter WM, Glover JS. The preparation of ^{131}I-labeled human growth hormone of high specific activity. Biochem J 1963; 89: 114-123.
13. Thorell JI, Johansson BG. Enzymatic iodination of polypeptides with ^{125}I to high specific activity. Biochim Biophys Acta 1971; 251:363-366.
14. Butt WR. The iodination of follicle-stimulating and other hormones for radioimmunoassay. J Endocrinol 1972; 55:453-454.
15. Fraker, PJ, Speck JC Jr. Protein and cell membrane iodinations with a sparingly soluble chloramine 1,3,4,6-tetrachloro-3α,6α-diphenyl glycoluril. Biochem Biophys Res Commun 1978; 86:849-857.
16. Reay P. The use of N-bromosuccinimide for the iodination of proteins for radioimmunoassay. Ann Clin Biochem 1981; in press.
17. Bolton AE and Hunter WM. The labelling of proteins to high specific activities by conjugation to an ^{125}I-containing acylating agent. Biochem J 1973; 133:529-539.
18. Nye L Forrest GC, Greenwood H, Gardner JS, Jay R, Roberts JR, Landon J. Solid-phase, magnetic particle radioimmunoassay. Clin Chim Acta 1976; 69:387-396.
19. Al-Dugaili EAS, Forrest GC, Edwards CRW, Landon J. Evaluation and application of magnetizable charcoal for separation in radioimmunoassays. Clin Chem 1979; 25:1402-1405.
20. Hunter, WM, Bennie JG. Reduction of non-specific serum responses in human pituitary gonadotrophin radioimmunoassays. J Endocrinol 1979; 80:59-68.
21. Zyznar E. A rationale for the application of Trasylol as a protease inhibitor. Life Sci 1981; 28:1861-1866.

22. Miles LE and Hales CN. The preparation and properties of purified ^{125}I-labelled antibodies to insulin. Biochem J 1968; 108:611-618.
23. Sopwith AM, Hales CN. Micromodification of an immunoradiometric assay for proinsulin. Ann Clin Biochem 1980; 17:185-187.
24. Schuurs AHWM, van Weeman BK. A powerful analytical tool. J Immunoassay 1980; 1:229-249.
25. Harris CC, Yolken RH, Krokan H, Hsu IC. Ultrasensitive enzymatic radioimmunoassay: application to detection of cholera toxin and rotavirus. Proc Nat Acad Sci USA 1979; 76:5336-5339.
26. Shulman G. Quality of commercially available controls in laser immunonephelometry. Ann Clin Biochem 1980; 17:178-182.
27. Simpson JSA, Campbell AK, Ryall MET, Woodhead JS. A stable chemiluminescent-labelled antibody for immunological assays. Nature 1979; 279:646-647.
28. Soini E, Hemmila. Fluoroimmunoassay: present status and key problems. Clin Chem 1979; 25:353-361.
29. Kemp SF, Rosenfeld RG, Liu F, Gaspich S, Hintz RL. Acute somatomedin response to growth hormone: radioreceptor assay versus radioimmunoassay. J Clin Endocrinol Metab 1981; 52:616-621.
30. Nissenson RA, Abbott SR, Teitelbaum AP, Clark OH, Arnaud CD. Endogenous biologically active human parathyroid hormone: measurement by a guanyl nucleotide-amplified renal adenylate cyclase assay. J Clin Endocrinol Metab 1981; 52:840-846.
31. Kohler G, Milstein C. Continuous cultures of fused cells secreting antibody of predefined specificity. Nature 1975; 256:495-497.

7

Steroid Hormones

R. V. Brooks
St. Thomas' Hospital Medical School, London, England

The application of radioimmunoassay during the course of the last 10 years has transformed steroid analysis and accelerated the trend toward measurement in blood rather than urine. However, there are still circumstances in which urine assays give more appropriate information and others where a dual approach is desirable.

Hormones are measured for one of the following reasons:

1. To explain a clinical condition in terms of increased or decreased hormonal stimulus to the tissues.
2. To assess the secretory activity of an endocrine gland. It may be that the rate of secretion of a hormone by an endocrine gland and the rate of excretion of its metabolites in the urine are within normal limits, but the concentration of hormone in the region of the target organ may be increased due to an abnormally low rate of inactivation of the hormone.
3. To test the system controlling the secretion of a hormone. Abnormalities in the control system can be detected by the use of dynamic stimulation and suppression tests. Specificity requirements of methods used for this purpose may be lower than those required for other purposes.
4. To evaluate treatment.

The test used and the most appropriate compartment in which to measure the hormone or its metabolites depends on the objective. The steroid hormone is secreted by the endocrine gland directly into the blood, but perhaps the best index of the hormonal stimulus to the tissues would be the concentration in the extracellular fluid (ECF). Because of the difficulty of sampling the ECF compartment the concentration of steroid in the blood is usually measured. The concentration of steroid in the blood is related to that in the ECF only indirectly through the nonprotein-bound fraction of the steroid (free steroid). All the steroid hormones are bound to albumin and some of them are bound also to specific binding proteins in the plasma: cortisol and corticosterone to cortisol binding globulin (CBG); testosterone and estradiol to sex hormone binding globulin (SHBG). For these steroids the total concentration in the plasma depends as much on the concentration of the specific binding protein as it does on the activity of the gland secreting the hormone. Furthermore, if the subject has a low concentration of specific binding protein the tissues can be subject to pathologically high concentrations of hormone even though the total concentration of hormone in the plasma is within normal limits.

The free steroid and part of the steroid bound to albumin is available for metabolism by the liver cells, where most of the inactivation takes place. In the case of the steroid hormones with the typical 4-en, 3-oxostructure (e.g., progesterone, testosterone, aldosterone, and cortisol) this inactivation is by forming a tetrahydro derivative in which the double bond betweens carbons 4 and 5 is saturated and the oxo group on carbon 3 is reduced to an hydroxy group. These reduced metabolites are then usually conjugated with glucuronic or sulfuric acids, returned to the blood, and rapidly excreted in the urine.

The unchanged free (i.e., nonprotein bound) steroid in the blood also passes into the glomerular filtrate and, although it is mainly passively reabsorbed in the renal tubule, some passes into the urine. In some ways the measurement of this small proportion of the hormone which is excreted unchanged into the urine approaches the ideal index for measuring the hormonal stimulus to the tissues. It is fairly directly related to the concentration of nonprotein-bound steroid in the blood and therefore to the concentration in the ECF. It has the further advantage, when a 24-hr urine collection is used, of giving an integral value for the whole day, whereas a blood value gives only the concentration at one instant. This may be of particular value in the hormones which exhibit a marked circadian rhythm or sharp fluctuations due to episodic secretion. Both of these phenomena occur with cortisol, the urinary excretion of which is a very useful test in Cushing's syndrome in spite of the fact that only about 0.5% of the cortisol secreted is eliminated in this way (1). In the case of testosterone an even smaller proportion (0.01%) is eliminated unchanged in the urine, but since this is accompanied by a very much larger quantity of the glucuronide conjugate, which may undergo a variable degree of hydrolysis, it is an unreliable index.

The concentrations of steroid hormones in saliva are also related to the biologically active nonprotein-bound fraction in the plasma. The collection of salivary samples is of course a noninvasive technique and would seem to be of particular value in infertility studies (e.g., to monitor the concentrations of estradiol and progesterone throughout the menstrual cycle).

In the past, estimations of steroids in urine have most often been of the reduced metabolites excreted in the form of sulfate and glucuronide conjugates. This may be estimation of a single major metabolite (e.g., pregnanediol), the reduced product from progesterone, or a group of related metabolites such as the 17-oxogenic steroids, which together represent 50-60% of secreted cortisol. If the proportion of the secreted hormone excreted in the form of these metabolites was the same at all times and for different subjects, then such estimations would give a reliable indication of the rate at which the hormone was being secreted. Unfortunately, this is not always the case. For example, some patients with Cushing's syndrome excrete less than 25% of the cortisol they secrete in the form of 17-oxogenic steroids. In such cases their rate of cortisol secretion may be considerably elevated, although the 17-oxogenic steroid excretion is within normal limits. Isotope methods are available for measuring the secretion rates of steroids.

I. TYPES OF TECHNIQUES AVAILABLE FOR STEROID ANALYSIS

Methods for steroids may be broadly divided into those for *individual steroids,* which depend on a very specific property or employ chromatographic purification stages, and *group methods,* which measure together substances possessing certain functional groups on the molecule.

Most methods of analyzing steroids in body fluids begin by extracting the steroid from the aqueous medium with an organic solvent. With the development of specific antisera of high affinity it is now sometimes possible to measure certain steroid hormones in the plasma without the need for extraction ("direct" methods). Since the major metabolites of the steroid hormones are excreted in the urine in the form of water-soluble glucuronide and sulfate conjugates, these conjugates must be split before the steroid can be extracted. In some group methods of analysis it may be sufficient to effect this hydrolysis by heating the urine with mineral acid. Since this violent method of hydrolysis causes some molecular rearrangement it is an unsuitable prelude to the measurement of specific analytes. In such cases mild enzymatic methods must be used.

A. Physical Methods of Measurement

Steroids with the 4-en, 3-oxo structure may be measured by virtue of a physical property, the absorption of ultraviolet light at 240 nm. However, extensive purification is necessary if this method is to be used for measuring the concentrations of steroids in blood and urine. In recent years the development of high-performance liquid chromatography (HPLC) with its high resolving power has provided an excellent complement to quantitation by ultraviolet absorption.

B. Chemical Methods

These may be of two types. In one type the analyte acts on a reagent to alter its physical properties (e.g., corticosteroids reducing tetrazolium salts to colored formazans). In the other type the steroid reacts with a reagent to form a derivative which may also be estimated spectrophotometrically. An example of the second type is the Zimmermann reaction for 17-oxosteroids. Such methods have limited sensitivity but were among the first available techniques with reasonable precision.

C. Fluorometric Methods

These are in general capable of much greater sensitivity but are of more restricted application and subject to interference and quenching.

D. Gas-Liquid Chromatography (GLC)

GLC using a flame ionization detector is an effective method of quantitating urinary steroids. The system is best suited to the less polar steroids, but even the corticosteroids can be measured after conversion to suitable derivatives. GLC methods are generally robust, capable of good precision and specificity, but fairly time consuming. The sensitivity of the flame ionization detector is not adequate for measuring plasma steroids, but the electron capture detector is if the steroids are first converted to halogen-containing derivatives. Electron capture methods are, however, less robust and therefore less suited to routine application.

The recent introduction of capillary columns for the GLC of steroids has made steroid profiling a possibility. These columns have much greater resolving power, so it is possible to separate all the urinary steroids from the nonpolar androgen metabolites to the polar corticosteroid metabolites in a single run. This approach has been particularly successful in the investigation of steroid enzyme defects in pregnancy and in the newborn (2).

In another application the gas chromatograph is coupled to a mass spectrometer to establish the "true" concentration of an analyte in a pool of reference plasma or urine. Such values can then be compared with the results obtained by routine methods (3).

E. Double Isotope Methods

Some of the earliest methods for measuring steroids other than cortisol in the plasma used the principle of double isotope dilution (4). These methods were research procedures, being too slow and complicated for routine application.

F. Displacement Analysis Methods

These methods depend on the existence of proteins with the property of binding certain steroids in a relatively specific way. The protein may be a naturally occurring one: either a steroid binding protein in the plasma or a steroid receptor protein in a target tissue. CBG in the plasma binds cortisol and corticosterone at high affinity; similarly, SHBG binds testosterone and estradiol. These plasma proteins can be used for assaying their particular steroids with no more preparation than an appropriate dilution of the plasma. The tissue receptor proteins must be isolated from the target tissue, a process that takes several hours. At one time routine methods both for estradiol and aldosterone used receptor proteins, but these have now been replaced by examples of the third group of assaying proteins; those produced by an immune process. This is a much more general method applicable to any steroid. The steroid is rendered immunogenic by attaching it to a pure protein and then injecting the steroid-protein conjugate into an animal of different species from that from which the protein was derived. Some of the antibodies produced are specific for the steroid part of the conjugate and can be used to estimate the steroid without separation from the antiserum.

With all these steroid binding proteins the percentage of steroid bound to the protein depends on the relative amounts of protein and steroid present. They can therefore be used as a means of assaying steroids provided that we have a technique for separating the protein-bound steroid from the free steroid and a method of labeling the steroid so that its distribution between the two fractions can be observed. Several different approaches to the labeling of steroids have been tried: labeling with a radioactive isotope, an enzyme, a fluorescent, or a chemiluminescent substance.

1. Radioactive Labels

These have been used exclusively in competitive protein binding assays with plasma and tissue-receptor proteins and have also been used in the majority of steroid immunoassay procedures. The maximum specific activity of ^{14}C labels is too low but ^{3}H, ^{125}I, and ^{75}Se have all been successfully employed. Because of its higher specific activity, ^{125}I can give a more sensitive assay, but this increase in sensitivity is not always realized because of the phenomenon of "bridge recognition" (5). Tritium labels can be used for many years if their radiochemical purity is checked periodically, but ^{125}I labels must be freshly prepared every few months. On the other hand, ^{125}I labels can be counted more easily, more cheaply, and if use is made of one of the 12- or 16-place counters, much more quickly. Even these multiplace gamma counters, although cheaper than autosample changer beta and gamma counters, are expensive. In an attempt to reduce costs and to avoid the health hazards inherent in isotopic methods, much effort has been expended in the development of nonisotopic immunoassays.

2. Enzyme Labels

The steroid covalently linked to enzyme competes with unlabeled steroid for binding to a limited quantity of antibody. The antibody-bound antigen is separated from the free antigen by the use of solid-phase antibody or a second antibody with specificity for the first. The enzyme activity in either the bound or free fraction is determined and related to the concentration of unlabeled steroid.

3. Fluorescent Labels

A steroid similarly linked to a fluorescent molecule such as fluorescein may also be used to indicate the distribution of the steroid between the bound and the free fraction. Indeed, it may be possible to carry out the assay without the need to separate bound and free fractions if binding of the steroid fluorescent label to antibody substantially decreases its fluorescence or increases its polarization.

4. Chemiluminescent Labels

Luminescent substances can be used as labels in immunoassays in various ways. One technique is to prepare a label in which the steroid is linked covalently to a luminescent substance such as isoluminol. The resultant steroid-isoluminol conjugate emits light when oxidized with peroxidase and hydrogen peroxide. When the steroid-isoluminol conjugate is bound to the specific antibody the production of light may be increased. This binding and consequently the production of light is reduced by the addition of free steroid which competes for sites on the antibody. This technique has the advantage that there is no need to separate the bound and free steroid.

II. METHODS FOR DIFFERENT STEROID TYPES

A. Estrogens

Unlike the other steroid hormones, the estrogens undergo an extensive enterohepatic circulation which results in a time lag of 24-48 hr between secretion by the ovary or placenta and excretion in the urine. This delay may make assays in plasma preferable for clinical management in some cases.

Except in pregnancy the secretions of estrogens are low, so that until sensitive methods became available, measurements had to be made in urine where concentrations are higher. Even in urine extensive purification was necessary, so that methods were tedious until the highly developed fluorometric method of Brown was introduced in 1968 (6). This method has a high throughput and good precision but demands a fairly high level of skill on the part of the analyst. The much higher concentrations of estrogens in pregnancy urine permits the use of colorimetry as an alternative to fluorometry (7), while fluorometry is sensitive enough to measure total estrogens in the plasma in late pregnancy (8). Nevertheless, plasma estrogens are most often estimated now by radioimmune or enzyme immunoassays, the most useful assays being estradiol for evaluating ovarian function and estriol for monitoring fetal well-being.

In spite of the very low concentration of estradiol in the plasma of nonpregnant subjects, methods have been devised to measure them without prior chromatography. This specificity is achieved by means of antisera raised to estradiol linked to protein through C-6 (9) or C-11 (10), in both cases leaving the functional groups on the A and D rings available for recognition by the antibody. The most abundant estrogen in peripheral plasma is estrone sulfate, which may be quantitated without hydrolysis or chromatography using an antiserum to estrone glucuronide linked to bovine thyroglobulin (11). Such antisera, derived from antigens in which the steroid glucuronide is coupled to the carrier protein via the carboxyl group in the glucuronic acid portion, lack specificity and, in particular, they cross-react with the corresponding free steroids. Nambara and his colleagues (12) have described three types of estradiol-17β-glucuronide-bovine serum albumin (BSA) conjugates in which the haptens are linked to the protein through C-2 or C-4. These have good specificity and do not cross-react with free estrogens.

The most usual steroid index of fetal well-being is the concentration of unconjugated estriol (13). Kerr (14) has claimed that because estriol-16α-glucuronide is cleared more quickly than estriol or any of its sulfated metabolites, its plasma concentration reflects more closely the current state of the fetus. Their assay has an exceptionally good interassay coefficient of variation of 3.4%. The plasma concentration of conjugated and unconjugated estetrol is also claimed to be a better indicator of fetal viability than estriol, but the reported precision of this assay is considerably lower (15).

Enzyme immunoassays using estriol covalently linked to horseradish peroxidase are available for monitoring pregnancy (16). The assay, using polyethylene glycol separation of bound and free fractions, is rapid and especially suitable for small clinical laboratories. However, enzyme immunoassays are not, in general, sufficiently sensitive for the measurement of plasma estrogens in nonpregnant subjects. An exception appears to be the method of Nicolas and his colleagues (17), which uses the transhydrogenase activity of the estradiol dehydrogenase of human placenta.

Gas-liquid chromatography is now used much less in the analysis of estrogens, but there may be occasions when the high resolutions of capillary columns may be useful in fractionating urinary estrogens (18).

B. Progesterone and Pregnanediol

The concentration of progesterone in plasma and of its metabolite pregnanediol in urine reaches a maximum in the middle of the luteal phase at about 10 times the follicular level. Single estimations are therefore of little value in the assessment of luteal function. On the other hand, an analytical procedure with a very high precision is perhaps unnecessary. In investigations of infertility it may be desirable to analyze samples every 2 or 3 days over a period of several weeks. For the convenience of the patient, pregnanediol (or its glucuronide conjugate) in urine or progesterone in saliva (19) may be preferable to plasma estimations.

For many years luteal function was monitored by methods which measured the yellow color produced by pregnanediol with concentrated sulfuric acid. The color reaction is not very specific, so that hydrolyzed urine extracts from nonpregnant subjects had to be purified by double chromatography on alumina columns (20). The colorimetric method was largely superseded by GLC methods (21). More rapid methods are available in which pregnanediol glucuronide is measured directly in the urine by radioimmunoassay (22). These have a somewhat lower precision.

Progesterone in blood may be measured by competitive protein binding (23) or radioimmunoassay (24) methods. Corrie and his colleagues have produced a particularly sensitive radioimmunoassay by using an ^{125}I label. They have avoided the difficulty usually caused by "bridge recognition" by linking the steroid to bovine serum albumin in the antigen and to iodinated tyramine in the radioligand using in each case glucuronic acid on an 11α-hydroxy group attached to the progesterone molecule (25). A sensitivity only a little lower than this has been achieved in an enzyme immunoassay, in which progesterone is linked to horseradish peroxidase, again through an 11α-hydroxy group (26). The method is rapid and the enzyme label is reported to be stable for at least 18 months. Other nonisotopic immunoassays for progesterone in plasma have also been reported using chemiluminescent labels (27).

C. Androgens

For many years the only routine measurement of androgenic steroids available was the excretion of 17-oxosteroids in the urine. The 17-oxosteroids are a very heterogeneous group of steroids derived in the main from weak androgens secreted by the adrenal cortex. Even in the male only about 25% of the 17-oxosteroid precursors are of testicular origin. The 17-oxosteroids are measured using the Zimmermann color reaction (28) and may be greatly elevated in some cases of androgen-secreting tumors. In adrenal carcinoma the excretion of one particular 17-oxosteroid, dehydroepianderosterone, is especially increased. It may therefore be worth measuring urinary 17-oxosteroids or dehydroepiandrosterone in hirsutism and virilism of sudden onset.

About 1% of testosterone secreted is excreted in the urine in the form of the glucuronide conjugate. In men this may be used as an indicator of testosterone production and may be conveniently measured by gas chromatography or radioimmunoassay. In women, however, the testosterone excretion does not faithfully represent the biologically active testosterone available to the tissues (29).

At present the most important index of androgenicity is the concentration of testosterone in the plasma and it is usually measured by radioimmunoassay (30). Testosterone antisera cross-react 10-20% with 5-dihydrotestosterone and positive interference with radioimmunoassay of plasma testosterone has been found in women treated with large doses of danazol (31). Enzyme immunoassays have been devised in which the testosterone is linked to glucoamylase (32), penicillinase (33), and peroxidase (34). The latter procedure has been applied to the estimation of testosterone in both plasma and saliva.

In congenital adrenal hyperplasia due to a 21-hydroxylase or 11β-hydroxylase block, the androgen whose concentration in the blood is most increased is not testosterone but androstenedione. The measurement of androstenedione (35) in plasma has been reported to be the best way of monitoring the treatment of these patients (36).

D. Cortisol and Its Metabolites

1. Plasma Cortisol

Because of its relatively high concentration in plasma, cortisol was the first steroid hormone for which routine methods were available. First in the field was the colorimetric-phenylhydrazine method of Porter and Silber, which was replaced by the more sensitive, precise, rapid, but less specific fluorometric technique of Mattingly (37). Despite its lack of specificity this method yields useful clinical information when used in conjunction with adrenal stimulation and suppression tests. Currently, the most widely used techniques are competitive protein binding using CBG in diluted plasma (38,39) and radioimmunoassay using either a ^{3}H (40) or an ^{125}I label (41). Enzyme labels have also been used in which cortisol is linked to β-galactosidase (42) or alkaline phosphatase (43). One advantage of the competitive binding methods is that the specificity of the binding protein is constant within the species. Thus the CBG in human plasma from one individual has the same ratio of affinities for 17-hydroxyprogesterone relative to that for cortisol as would be found in any other individual. The relative specificity of antibodies varies not only from animal to animal but even in the same animal from time to time (44). Problems of specificity are likely to be of greater importance in the plasma of subjects with congenital adrenal hyperplasia, patients being treated with synthetic corticosteroids, and in the newborn.

2. Free Cortisol in Urine

The clinical usefulness of this measurement, especially in the diagnosis of Cushing's syndrome, has been noted already. Fluorometric techniques have insufficient specificity for the measurement of cortisol in urine and a chromatographic stage is often included to increase the specificity of methods based on competitive protein binding (44) and radioimmunoassay (45). Alternative approaches for assessing the biologically active level of cortisol are to measure the nonprotein-bound fraction in the plasma by steady-state gel filtration (46) or by equilibrium dialysis (47) or measure the concentration in saliva (48).

3. Cortisol Metabolites

For many years the assessment of cortisol secretion was based on the excretion of the major metabolites of cortisol in the urine. These were group methods which measured either the tetrahydro metabolites (49) or the sum of the tetrahydro and the hexahydro metabolites (17-oxogenic steroids) (50). While these methods give a reliable indication of the response to adrenal stimulation and suppression tests, the basal values may be misleading either because of a departure from the normal proportion of cortisol being excreted in the form of these metabolites or because of the inclusion of metabolites of cortisol precursors.

4. Cortisol Secretion Rate

Two types of isotopic methods can be used. In one, isotopically labeled cortisol is infused at a constant rate until the concentration in the blood reaches a steady state. From this equilibrium concentration of radioactive cortisol the metabolic clearance rate can be calculated and the product of this with the mean plasma concentration of unlabeled hormone gives the secretion rate. In the alternative approach the urine is collected for 48 hr after the administration of a known amount of isotopically labeled cortisol. The specific activity of cortisol metabolites isolated from this urine enables the amount of cortisol secreted in this period to be calculated (51). Measurements of the rate of secretion of cortisol are particularly valuable in assessing the completeness of adrenalectomy and hypophysectomy.

5. Intermediates in Cortisol Biosynthesis

Measurement of the concentration of precursors of cortisol in the plasma or of their metabolites in the urine may be necessary in cases of suspected congenital adrenal hyperplasia.

17α-Hydroxyprogesterone. Measurement of the concentration of this steroid in plasma is probably the best diagnostic test of a defect in the 21-hydroxylating enzyme system (52). A method in which a drop of blood from a heel prick is taken onto filter paper is convenient for screening infants (53). Urinary measurements of the metabolite pregnanetriol (54) or of the 11-oxygenation index (55) are less reliable indices in the newborn.

11-Desoxycortisol. The concentration in the plasma of this steroid is raised when there is impairment of the 11β-hydroxylating enzyme system. It may be determined by radioimmunoassay (56) or HPLC (57). The latter technique has the advantage of giving a simultaneous estimation of cortisol and is also of value in quantitating the levels of synthetic corticosteroids during treatment (58).

E. Aldosterone

The concentration of aldosterone in plasma is very low, partly because of the low rate of secretion and partly because it is bound to plasma proteins to a much smaller extent than other corticosteroids. In spite of the low concentration it is possible to measure aldosterone directly in plasma without either solvent extraction or chromatography (59). This is due to the preparation of very good antibodies to aldosterone-3-carboxymethyloxime conjugated to bovine serum albumin.

18-Hydroxycorticosterone. This steroid does not have mineralocorticoid properties of its own, but it appears to be a useful marker of the later stages of aldosterone biosynthesis. Its measurement is helpful in the diagnosis of primary aldosteronism (60).

References

1. Cope CL, Black EG. The reliability of some adrenal function tests. Br Med J 1959; 2:1117-1122.
2. Taylor NF, Shackleton CHL. Gas chromatographic steroid analysis for diagnosis of placental sulfatase deficiency: a study of nine patients. J Clin Endocrinol Metab 1979; 49:78-86.
3. Bjorkheim I, Blomstrand R, Lantto O, Svenson L, Ohman G. Toward absolute methods in clinical chemistry: application of mass fragmentography to high accuracy analysis. Clin Chem 1976; 22:1789-1801.

4. Burger HG, Kent JR, Kellie AE. Determination of testosterone in human peripheral and adrenal venous plasma. J Clin Endocrinol Metab 1964; 24: 432-441.
5. Cameron EHD, Scarisbrick JJ, Morris SE, Read G. ^{125}I-Iodohistamine derivatives as tracers for the radioimmunoassay of progestagens. In *Steroid Immunoassay,* Cameron EHD, Hillier SG, Griffiths K (eds). Cardiff Alpha Omega Publishing Ltd., 1975, pp 153-164.
6. Brown JB, Macleod SC, MacNaughton C, Smith MA, Smyth B. A rapid method for estimating estrogens in urine using a semiautomatic extractor. J Endocrinol 1968; 42:5-15.
7. Oakey RE, Bradshaw LRA, Eccles SS, Stitch SR, Heys RF. The rapid estimation of estrogens in pregnancy to monitor fetal risk. Clin Chim Acta 1967; 15:35-45.
8. Goutte-Coussien C, Sanchez D, Adessi G, Jayle MF. Semi-automated fluorometry of total estrogens in plasma during late pregnancy. Clin Chem 1980; 26:190-193.
9. Korenman SG, Stevens RH, Carpenter LA, Robb M, Niswender GD, Sherman BM. Estradiol radioimmunoassay without chromatography: procedure, validation and normal values. J Clin Endocrinol Metab 1974; 38:718-720.
10. England BG, Niswender GD, Midgley AR. Radioimmunoassay of estradiol 17β without chromatography. J Clin Endocrinol Metab 1974; 38:42-50.
11. Wright K, Collins DC, Masey PI, Preedy JRK. A specific radioimmunoassay for estrone sulfate in plasma and urine without hydrolysis. J Clin Endocrinol Metab 1978; 47:1092-1098.
12. Nambara T, Numazawa M, Tanaka T, Ohkubo T. Preparation of specific antisera to estradiol-17-glucuronide. J Steroid Biochem 1978; 9:785-790.
13. Liedtke RJ, Grieves JP Jr, Batjer JD, Busby B. ^{125}I-Radioimmunoassay for unconjugated estriol in serum of pregnant women. Clin Chem 1978; 24:1100-1104.
14. Kerr EJ, Park BK, Dean PDG. A specific direct radioimmunoassay for estriol-16α-glucuronide in pregnancy plasma. Clin Chim Acta 1977; 77: 77-82.
15. Den K, Matsumoto H, Fujii KT, Furaya K, Yoshida T, Takaji S. A radioimmunoassay of plasma unconjugated and conjugated estetrol. Steroids 1977; 30:521-529.
16. Osterman TM, Juntunen KO, Gothoni GD. Enzyme immunoassay of estrogen-like substances in plasma with polyethylene glycol as precipitant. Clin Chem 1979; 25:716-718.
17. Nicolas JC, Boussioux AM, Descomps B, Crastes de Paulet, A. Enzymatic determination of estradiol and estrone in plasma and urine. Clin Chim Acta 1979; 92:1-9.
18. Fels JP, Dehennin L, Grenier J, Scholler R. Quantitative estimation of urinary estrogens during the menstrual cycle by gas liquid chromatography with a glass capillary column. J Steroid Biochem 1979; 11:1303-1308.

19. Walker RF, Read GF, Riad-Fahmy D. Radioimmunoassay of progesterone in saliva: application to the assessment of ovarian function. Clin Chem 1979; 25:2030-2033.
20. Klopper A, Michie EA, Brown JB. A method for the determination of urinary pregnanediol. J Endocrinol 1955; 12:209-219.
21. Goldzieher JW, Matthijssen C, Gual C, Vela BA, De La Pena A. A simplified gas chromatographic method for large numbers of urinary pregnanediol determinations. Am J Obstet Gynecol 1967; 98:739-766.
22. Samarajeewa P, Cooley G, Kellie AE. The radioimmunoassay of pregnanediol-3α-glucuronide. J Steroid Biochem 1979; 11:1165-1171.
23. Yoshimi T, Lipsett MB. The measurement of plasma progesterone. Steroids 1968; 11:527-540.
24. Morgan CA, Cooke ID. A comparison of the competitive protein-binding assay and radioimmunoassay for plasma progesterone during the normal menstrual cycle. J Endocrinol 1972; 54:445-456.
25. Corrie JET, Hunter WM, Macpherson JS. A strategy for radioimmunoassay of plasma progesterone with use of a homologous site ^{125}I-labelled radioligand. Clin Chem 1981; 27:594-599.
26. Joyce BG, Wilson DW, Read GF, Riad-Fahmy D. An improved enzyme immunoassay for progesterone in human plasma. Clin Chem 1978; 24: 2099-2102.
27. Kohen F, Kim JB, Lindner HR, Collins WP. Development of a solid-phase chemiluminescence immunoassay for plasma progesterone. Steroids 1981; 38:73-88.
28. Gray CH, Baron DN, Brooks RV, James VHT. A critical appraisal of a method of estimating urinary 17-oxosteroids and total 17-oxogenic steroids. Lancet 1969; 1:124-127.
29. Korenman SG, Lipsett MB. Is testosterone glucuronide uniquely derived from plasma testosterone? J Clin Invest 1964; 43:2125-2131.
30. Anderson PH, Fukushima K, Schiller HS. Radioimmunoassay of plasma testosterone with use of polyethylene glycol to separate antibody bound and free hormone. Clin Chem 1975; 21:708-714.
31. Sharp AM, Fraser IS, Robertson S, Turtle JR. Positive interference by danazol in a testosterone radioimmunoassay kit procedure. Clin Chem 1981; 27:603-604.
32. Tateishi K, Yamamoto H, Ogihara T, Hayashi C. Enzyme immunoassay of serum testosterone. Steroids 1977; 30:25-32.
33. Yoshi UM, Shah HP, Sudhama SP. A sensitive and specific enzyme immunoassay for serum testosterone. Steroids 1979; 34:35-46.
34. Turkes A, Turkes O, Joyce BG, Read GF. A sensitive solid-phase enzyme immunoassay for testosterone in plasma and saliva. Steroids 1979; 33:347-359.
35. Lejeune-Lenain C, Wolter R, Franckson JRM. A direct radioimmunoassay for plasma Δ^4-androstenedione: application to children. Clin Chim Acta 1979; 94:327-329.

36. Korth-Schutz S, Virdio R, Saenger P, Chow DM, Levine LS, New MI. Serum androgens as a continuing index of adequacy of treatment of congenital adrenal hyperplasia. J Clin Endocrinol Metab 46:452-458.
37. Mattingly DA. A simple fluorimetric method for the estimation of free 11-hydroxycorticoids in human plasma. J Clin Pathol 1962; 15:374-379.
38. Murphy BEP, Engleburg W, Pattee CJ. Simple method for the determination of plasma corticoids. J Clin Endocrinol Metab 1963; 28:293-300.
39. Nugent CA, Mayes DM. Plasma corticosteroids determined by use of corticosteroid-binding globulin and dextran-coated charcoal. J Clin Endocrinol Metab 1966; 26:1116-1122.
40. Morris R. A simple and economical method for the radioimmunoassay of cortisol in serum. Ann Clin Biochem 1978; 15:178-183.
41. Riad-Fahmy D, Read GF, Gaskell SJ, Dyas J, Hindawi R. A simple direct radioimmunoassay for plasma cortisol featuring a ^{125}I radioligand and solid phase separation technique. Clin Chem 1979; 25:665-668.
42. Comoglio S, Celada F. An immuno-enzymatic assay of cortisol using *E. coli* β-galactosidase as label. J Immunol Methods 1976; 10:161-170.
43. Ogihara T, Miyai K, Nishi K, Ishibashi K, Kumahara Y. Enzyme-labelled immunoassay for plasma cortisol. J Clin Endocrinol Metab 1977; 44:91-95.
44. Murphy BEP. Pitfalls in the assay of cortisol. J Immunoassay 1980; 1:413-434.
45. Chattoraj SC, Turner AK, Pincus JL, Charles D. The significance of urinary free cortisol and progesterone in normal and anencephalic pregnancy. Am J Obstet Gynecol 1976; 124:848-854.
46. Fisher RA, Anderson DC, Burke CW. Simultaneous measurement of unbound testosterone and estradiol fractions in undiluted plasma at 37°C by steady state gel filtration. Steroids 1974; 24:809-824.
47. Clerico A, Del Chicca MG, Ghione S, Matterazzi F, Zuchelli GC. Radioimmunoassay determination of apparent free cortisol concentration: some physiological and clinical applications. Clin Chim Acta 1979; 91:227-231.
48. Walker RF, Riad-Fahmy D, Read GF. Adrenal status assessed by direct radioimmunoassay of cortisol in whole saliva or parotid saliva. Clin Chem 1978; 24:1460-1463.
49. Glenn EM, Nelson DH. Chemical method for the determination of 17-hydroxycorticosteroids and 17-ketosteroids in urine following hydrolysis with β-glucuronidase. J Clin Endocrinol Metab 1953; 13:911-921.
50. Few JD. A method for the analysis of urinary 17-hydroxycorticosteroids. J Endocrinol 1961; 22:31-46.
51. Kelly WG. Questions concerning the validity of one of the assumptions underlying the determination of the secretory rate of cortisol. Steroids 1970; 16:579-602.

52. Abraham GE, Swerdloff R, Tulchinsky D, Odell WD. Radioimmunoassay of plasma progesterone. J Clin Endocrinol Metab 1971; 32:619-624.
53. Pang S, Hotchkiss J, Drash AL, Levine LS, New MI. Micro filter paper method for 17α-hydroxyprogesterone radioimmunoassay; its application for rapid screening for CAH. J Clin Endocrinol Metab 1977; 45:1003-1008.
54. Ros A, Sommerville IF. Gas-liquid chromatography with high resolution glass capillary columns for simultaneous determination of urinary steroids J Obstet Gynaecol 1971; 78:1096-1107.
55. Edwards RWH, Makin HLJ, Barratt TM. The steroid 11-oxygenation index: a rapid method for use in the diagnosis of congenital adrenal hyperplasia. J Endocrinol 1964; 30:181-194.
56. Fukushima DK, Nishina T, Wu RHK, Hellmann L, Finkelstein JW. Rapid assay of plasma 21-deoxycortisol and 11-deoxycortisol in CAH. Clin Endocrinol 1979; 10:367-375.
57. Canalis E, Caldarella AM, Reardon GE. Serum cortisol and 11-deoxycortisol by liquid chromatography: clinical studies and comparison with radioimmunoassay. Clin Chem 1979; 25:1700-1703.
58. Frey FJ, Frey BM, Benet LZ. Liquid chromatographic measurement of endogenous and exogenous glucocorticoids in plasma. Clin Chem 1979; 25:1944-1947.
59. Al-Dujaili EAS, Edwards CRW. The development and application of a direct radioimmunoassay for plasma aldosterone using ^{125}I labelled ligand-comparison of 3 methods. J Clin Endocrinol Metab 1978; 46:105-113.
60. Biglieri EG, Schambelan M. The significance of elevated levels of plasma 18-hydroxycorticosterone in patients with primary aldosteronism. J Clin Endocrinol Metab 1979; 49:87-91.

8
Thyroid Hormones

Michael M. Kaplan
Brigham and Women's Hospital and Harvard Medical School, Boston, Massachusetts

Thyroxine (T_4), the main secretory product of the thyroid gland, is by far the most abundant thyroid hormone in blood. T_4 circulates in plasma largely bound to proteins, principally thyroxine binding globulin (TBG), but the unbound, or free, T_4 is the portion thought to be available to tissues. 3,5,3′-Triiodothyronine (T_3) is, of course, a very potent thyroid hormone, and also circulates tightly bound to the same plasma proteins. As with T_4, it is the unbound, or free, T_3 that is generally considered to be biologically active. In contrast, 3,3′,5′-triiodothyronine (reverse-T_3 or rT_3) has no identified metabolic effects at concentrations observed in vivo. Seventy-five to eighty percent of the circulating T_3 and about 95% of the circulating rT_3 are produced by extrathyroidal deiodination of T_4 (1-4), the remainder being secreted directly by the thyroid. Measurements of serum concentrations of T_4 and T_3 and assessment of the extent of protein binding of these hormones are fundamental tools for the evaluation of patients' thyroid status. Measurements of rT_3 may have some utility in separating primary derangements of thyroid function from abnormalities of thyroid function tests due to systemic illnesses. This chapter deals with techniques for assaying iodothyronines and protein binding and with the complexities in the interpretation of these tests caused by interactions of pathophysiological abnormalities and test methodology.

I. GENERAL PRINCIPLES OF THYROID HORMONE MEASUREMENTS

A. Measurements of Total Serum Hormone Concentrations

Competitive protein binding (CPB) analysis (5), used for T_4 measurements, and radioimmunoassay (RIA), used for T_4 (6-9), T_3 (9-13), and rT_3 (14-22) measurements, are based on the same principles. Competition for a constant number of high-affinity protein binding sites is set up between the radioactive iodothyronine (tracer) and either known amounts of iodothyronine standards or the endogenous iodothyronine in patients' sera. TBG is used in the CPB technique and a specific antiserum is used in RIA. To measure total iodothyronine concentrations, binding of the iodothyronine to endogenous serum proteins must be eliminated; in CPB this is achieved by extracting T_4 from serum with ethanol, whereas in RIA a blocking compound, which inhibits binding of iodothyronines to serum proteins, but not to the antibody, is generally used. Both CPB and RIA eliminate the problem of cross-reaction of iodinated drugs, which plagued older iodimetric T_4 assays. T_4, T_3, and rT_3 values by CPB or RIA are rather free of artifactual errors, with the few exceptions discussed below.

B. Assessment of T_4 and T_3 Binding to Endogenous Serum Proteins

There are two direct techniques for assessing serum protein binding: dialysis (or ultrafiltration) of serum to which radioactive T_4 or T_3 has been added (23-27), and RIA of T_4 or T_3 in ultrafiltrates of dialysates of serum (28,29). These direct techniques suffer from the disadvantages of being technically demanding and costly. For this reason, indirect measurements of serum protein binding of T_4 and T_3 are more commonly employed. Most are based on the principle of competition for tracer T_4 or T_3 between serum proteins and fixed amounts of an adsorbent substance such as anion exchange resin, charcoal, dextran beads, talc, and immobilized antibodies (30-33). The percent of tracer bound to adsorbent can be used as an index of the percent free hormone in serum or can be used to derive a function more linearly related to the percent free hormone (30-32) by the equation

$$\text{binding index} = \frac{[b \div (100 - b)]_{\text{unknown serum}}}{[b \div (100 - b)]_{\text{normal serum pool}}}$$

where b is the percent tracer bound to adsorbent. The binding index is multiplied by the total serum T_4 or T_3 concentration to obtain an index of the free T_4 or free T_3 concentration in serum. When abnormalities exist in protein binding, they are almost always similar in degree for T_4 and for T_3. Therefore, the indirect assessment of protein binding obtained with either tracer T_4 or tracer T_3 may be used to calculate both a free T_4 index and a free T_3 index (34).

Another indirect method for estimating the free T_4 in serum is to calculate the ratio of the serum T_4 and TBG concentrations. This ratio is proportional to the free T_4 concentration except in patients with marked TBG deficiency. The serum TBG concentration can be measured by immunodiffusion, rocket immuno-electrophoresis, or RIA (35-40). We have found the T_4/TBG ratio to be about as closely related to the serum free T_4 concentration (by dialysis) as the conventional free T_4 index (using a T_3-charcoal uptake binding index), but no more so (41). It may therefore be considered an alternative, rather than a supplementary, method for estimating the serum free T_4.

C. Other Methods

Several chromatographic methods have been used to measure iodothyronines: gas-liquid (9), gas (42), and high-performance liquid chromatography (43). These methods at present are too demanding to be clinically useful. Enzyme-linked and enzyme-multiplied immunoassays for T_4 have been developed (44, 45); these are variants of the RIA which avoid the use of radioactive material and eliminate the necessity to separate bound and free tracer.

II. RADIOIMMUNOASSAY METHODOLOGY

In this section the methodology of iodothyronine RIAs is discussed. Additional specific details will be found in the references cited. The CPB method will not be detailed here.

A. Antibody Production

Iodothyronines must be bound to proteins to be effective antigens. Bovine and human thyroglobulin contain much more T_4 than T_3 or rT_3, and either thyroglobulin can be used for production of a T_4 antibody (6, 8). For T_3 and rT_3, conjugation to bovine serum albumin or other peptides using a carbodiimide (9, 11-13, 46, 47) yields a satisfactory immunizing agent. Because there is much more T_4 in serum than T_3 or rT_3, cross-reactivity of T_4 with anti-T_3 or anti-rT_3 antibodies must be suitably low.

B. Iodothyronine Standards

Standards made up in human serum and stored frozen in small aliquots are stable for months to years. Pooled normal human serum, tested to be free of hepatitis B antigen, is stripped of endogenous iodothyronines by treatment with anion exchange resins or with charcoal (9). The stripped serum must have the same nonspecific binding as several individual normal sera and the same zero binding as a previous, satisfactory, batch of stripped serum. Synthetic T_4, T_3, and rT_3 are dissolved and diluted in the stripped serum to give the desired concentrations for the standard curve.

C. Blocking Agents

Sodium salicylate, 8-anilino-1-naphthalenesulfonic acid (ANS), and merthiolate have been used in T_4, T_3, and rT_3 assays, and phenytoin has been used in T_3 assays [(6, 8, 14-22), and for a comparative study of blockers, see Ref. 48]. These substances all inhibit iodothyronine binding to serum proteins at concentrations which do not interfere with the binding of iodothyronines to antibodies.

D. Tracers

T_4, T_3, and rT_3 labeled with ^{125}I can be purchased commercially. For very high volume laboratories or for those in which radioiodinations are carried out routinely, it may be economical to prepare tracer iodothyronines by the chloramine-T method (22, 49-51). Protein is required in the assay buffer to prevent adsorption of tracers to the glass or plastic of incubation tubes. Bovine serum albumin, ovalbumin, and gelatin are often used, typically in concentrations of 0.02-0.25% (w/v).

E. Separation of Free from Antibody-Bound Ligand

The easiest methods of separating bound from free ligand are the use of a second antibody, dextran-coated charcoal, or polyethylene glycol. The double antibody technique (6, 11, 14, 19) can be used readily for large-scale assays, because once the insoluble immune complex is formed, the time needed for centrifugation and removal of supernatant is not critical. The disadvantages of the double antibody technique are that it prolongs the time required to complete the assay and that it obscures both the nonspecific binding of tracer to serum proteins and contamination of tracer by iodide. Polyethylene glycol, which precipitates immunoglobulins, is used in some thyroid hormone assays (52), and *Staphlococcus aureus* protein A, which has the same effect, has been used as well (53). Both of these agents provide a rapid separation of bound from free tracer, but neither discloses the true nonspecific binding of tracer to serum proteins or iodide contamination of tracer in the assay system.

The principle of the dextran-charcoal separation (7-9, 12) is that small organic molecules adsorb to charcoal which is readily pelleted, whereas proteins, both antibodies and serum proteins, and iodide do not. Thus dextran-coated charcoal separation does disclose the true nonspecific binding of tracer to serum proteins and the iodide in the tracers. It provides rapid separation, but because it is not a steady-state system, both temperature and timing are important variables which must be attended to carefully.

Another method of separating bound from free ligand, often employed in commercial kits, utilizes an antibody immobilized by covalent linkage to glass beads, the walls of assay vessels, and so on (54, 55). Because this technique uses large quantities of antibody and requires the extra step of linking the antibody to a solid matrix, it is not practical to establish de novo in a clinical laboratory.

F. Normal Serum Concentrations and Requirements for Assay Sensitivity

Normal serum T_4 concentrations in man fall in the range 65-140 nmol/liter [5-11 μg/dl (5-8)]. It is preferable to quantitate accurately both low and high values; therefore, a good T_4 assay should span a range of 25-250 nmol/liter (2-20 μg/dl). Defining the normal range for serum T_3 is difficult. The normal upper limit for serum T_3 appears to fall with age (30, 56), and serum T_3 concentrations regularly decrease in patients with nonthyroidal illness. We have found a "normal range" (mean ± 2 SD) for serum T_3 in adults seeking medical attention, but not acutely ill, of 1.0-2.6 nmol/liter (65-170 ng/dl) (unpublished data) and another "normal range" for completely healthy adults 22-55 years old of 1.2-3.7 nmol/liter (75-220 ng/dl). Moreover, we have encountered a few elderly hyperthyroid patients whose serum T_3 concentrations and free T_3 indices fall in the upper part of the normal range for young adults but above the normal range for older patients. Because the primary use of the serum T_3 assay is in diagnosing hyperthyroidism and monitoring its treatment, an appropriate range for a serum T_3 assay is 0.75-7.5 nmol/liter (50-500 ng/dl).

Defining a normal concentration range for rT_3 in human serum is also difficult in light of current disagreement among laboratories. Reported normal mean serum concentrations vary from 0.3 to 0.9 nmol/liter (20-60 ng/dl (14-22), although most workers report mean values of 0.3-0.6 nmol/liter (20). A practical range for measurements in clinical samples, if the normal mean is 0.3-0.4 nmol/liter is 0.15-1.5 nmol/liter (10-100 ng/dl). It is desirable to use a rT_3 antiserum sufficiently specific that T_4 cross-reactivity is low ($\leqslant$0.06%, w/w). In this case, correction for T_4 cross-reactivity is probably unnecessary. With less specific antisera, T_4 cross-reactivity must be accounted for in calculating rT_3 values, and this is not always a straightforward correction (19, 20).

III. CLINICAL APPLICATIONS

A. Thyrotoxicosis

In thyrotoxicosis from thyroidal hypersecretion, both the serum T_4 and T_3 (and free T_4 and T_3)* concentration are usually elevated, with the serum T_3

*In the rest of this section and in Section III.B, statements about serum T_4 and T_3 concentrations also apply to free T_4 and free T_3 concentrations.

generally more markedly elevated than the serum T_4 (57, 58). In an occasional individual with mild or early hyperthyroidism, the serum T_4 may remain in the mid- or high-normal range, while the serum T_3 concentration rises unequivocally above the normal range, a pattern termed "T_3-thyrotoxicosis." This combination of serum T_4 and T_3 levels may also be seen in the early phases of treatment of hyperthyroidism with thionamide drugs, in those relapsing from remitted Graves' disease, and in patients taking slightly excessive doses of desiccated thyroid, thyroglobulin, or synthetic T_4 and T_3 combinations (57, 58). A more extreme disparity of serum T_4 and serum T_3 is found in thyrotoxicosis induced by ingestion of excessive amounts of T_3: the serum T_4 falls to a subnormal level while the serum T_3 concentration is elevated. In thyrotoxicosis caused by exogenous T_4, serum T_4 and T_3 concentrations are proportionately elevated (19). Elevation of the serum T_4 concentration with a normal serum T_3 is seen rarely, and represents hyperthyroidism ("T_4-thyrotoxicosis") in some but not all patients (59-61). Even in hyperthyroidism, much of the T_3 produced daily originates from extrathyroidal deiodination of T_4. If this process is strongly inhibited by concomitant, severe, nonthyroidal illness, or by administration of drugs such as the cholecystographic dyes iopanoate and ipodate, or the antiarrythmic agent amiodarone, the serum T_3 in a hyperthyroid person may fall into the normal range, while the serum T_4 remains elevated (62-64).

B. Hypothyroidism

Hypothyroidism is characterized by a subnormal serum free T_4 concentration, with the total serum T_4 usually being low, also. The ratio of T_3 to T_4 in the serum is increased in hypothyroidism, as in hyperthyroidism. As the thyroid gland fails, therefore, the serum T_3 concentration remains normal much longer than the serum T_4, falling to a subnormal level only in severe thyroid failure (57, 58). Thus serum T_3 measurements are not useful in the diagnosis of hypothyroidism, while serum T_4 and protein binding measurements are essential.

C. High and Low TBG States

The causes of high and low TBG states are listed in Table 1. The effects of high and low TBG states on thyroid hormone measurements in euthyroid individuals are summarized in Table 2, together with examples of the interaction of abnormal TBG states, exemplified by pregnancy and congenital TBG deficiency, with true thyroid disease. As seen, this interaction is an additive one.

D. Nonthyroidal Illness

Severe or prolonged illness of almost any variety can alter the body's thyroid hormone economy in the absence of any intrinsic thyroid or pituitary disease.

Table 1 Causes of Abnormal Serum TBG Concentrations

Increased serum TBG	Decreased serum TBG
Pregnancy	Very severe systemic illness
Newborn period	Protein-calorie malnutrition
Chronic active or acute hepatitis	Cushing's syndrome
Porphyria	Acromegaly
Familial	Nephrotic syndrome
Drugs	Severe hepatic failure
Estrogen	Familial
Methadone	Drugs
Heroin	Glucocorticoids
Perphenazine	Androgens
Clofibrate	Danazol
	L-Asparaginase

Commonly seen abnormalities include (1) a low total serum T_4 with a normal free T_4, (2) both low and high serum free T_4, and (3) low total and free serum T_3 concentrations (30, 33, 41, 65). Some, but not all, indirect methods of assessing percent free T_4 and T_3 (including some T_3-uptake tests and the T_4/immunoreactive TBG ratio) underestimate the free fractions in sera of very sick patients when values are compared to equilibrium dialysis results (33, 41, 65).

Inasmuch as most of the abnormal thyroid function tests consequent to nonthyroidal illness suggest hypothyroidism, the clinician is often faced with the difficult question of whether a severely ill patient has coincidental hypothyroidism complicating another illness. As a group, patients with systemic illness have elevated serum rT_3 concentrations (41, 65), because rT_3 is degraded by the same enzymes that convert T_4 to T_3, and, in illness, activity of these enzymes are lowered, resulting in a slowing of rT_3 degradation (4, 66). There is no direct kinetic evidence supporting the concept of a major shift of T_4 metabolism toward rT_3 in illness. Chopra and co-workers have proposed that serum rT_3 measurements can be used to separate patients with low serum T_4 and free T_4 index values due to systemic illness from those with hypothyroidism (65). We, on the other hand (41), have found a considerable overlap of serum rT_3 concentrations in hypothyroid patients with or without other illnesses and sick euthyroid patients with low free T_4 levels. While our study confirmed that serum rT_3 concentrations are elevated in most acutely ill patients, it indicated that serum TSH measurements are superior to rT_3 determinations in establishing or excluding

Table 2 Effect of Altered Thyroid Hormone Binding to Serum Proteins on Thyroid Function Tests[a]

	Serum T_4 and T_3 concentrations	×	Free hormone fractions (or protein binding index)	=	Free T_4 and free T_3 concentrations (or free hormone indices)
A. High TBG[b]	↑	x	↓	=	N
Low TBG	↓	x	↑	=	N
B. Hyperthyroidism	↑	x	↑	=	↑
Pregnancy	↑	x	↓	=	N
Hyperthyroidism in pregnancy[c]	↑↑	x	↓	=	N
C. Hypothyroidism	↓	x	↓	=	↓
Pregnancy	↑	x	↓	=	N
Hyperthyroidism in pregnancy[c]	N or ↓	x	↓↓	=	↓
D. Hyperthyroidism	↑	x	↑	=	↑
Familial TBG deficiency	↓↓	x	↑↑	=	N
Hyperthyroidism with TBG deficiency[c]	Low or N	x	↑↑↑	=	↑

[a]N, normal; ↑, increased; ↓, decreased.
[b]Effects of primary alterations in TBG on thyroid function tests in normal individuals.
[c]Examples of the additive interaction of changes in thyroid function tests induced by coincident abnormalities in binding proteins and thyroid status.

hypothyroidism. These differing conclusions about the utility of rT_3 measurements may stem both from differences in the assays and differences in selection criteria used for hypothyroid and sick-euthyroid patients. It seems fair to say that, at present, the precise patient group for whom rT_3 measurements are a cost-effective means of excluding hypothyroidism requires better definition.

E. Abnormal Tests Caused by Drugs that Compete for TBG Binding Sites

Commonly used drugs which compete with T_4 and T_3 for TBG binding sites are listed in Table 3. When sufficiently high blood levels are attained for more than a few days, a steady state is reached with a decreased serum T_4, increased free fraction, and normal free T_4 concentration. Phenytoin has an additional effect of accelerating the intracellular metabolism of T_4, thereby causing a genuine fall in the serum free T_4 concentration (26), without the expected increase in thyrotropin secretion (67), and without manifestations of thyroid hormone deficiency.

Two types of measurement artifacts are seen in patients treated with these drugs. First, in the CPB method of T_4 measurement, drugs, like fenclofenac, which are extracted into ethanol with T_4, will displace tracer T_4 from the TBG used in the assay (68), causing an anomalous, elevated serum T_4 measurement. T_4 RIAs reflect the true lowering of the total serum T_4 concentration. Second, these drugs may cause the free fraction of T_4 and T_3 to be underestimated. Their ability to displace iodothyronines from TBG is highly concentration dependent, and, when serum is diluted, either for the T_3-uptake test or for dialysis, the drug concentration falls below the threshold for displacement of T_4 and T_3 from TBG (69). This phenomenon is also seen if free T_4 is estimated by the T_4/TBG ratio (36). The only techniques that avoid this artifact are ultrafiltration or dialysis of undiluted serum (69). In our hospital, phenytoin is the drug which most commonly causes abnormal thyroid function tests (41).

F. Endogenous Anti-T_4 or Anti-T_3 Antibodies and Abnormal Binding Proteins

Occasional patients with thyroid disorders have endogenous antibodies which bind T_4 or T_3 (70-73). These are presumably formed against the individual's own thyroglobulin. In vivo, the result is the same as if the serum TBG were elevated: a low percent free hormone. In vitro, such endogenous antibodies can cause perplexing RIA results. If the technique for separating bound from free tracer does not discriminate between rabbit and human immunoglobulins (e.g., dextran-charcoal or polyethylene glycol), then the percent of tracer apparently bound to the assay antiserum will be artifactually elevated. This can cause a false-low value or can cause the percent of tracer apparently bound to the assay antibody to be off the standard curve entirely, giving an uninterpretable result. Occurrence of this phenomenon can be verified by assaying the sample without the assay antibody, in which case the percent tracer bound will be much higher than the nonspecific binding of normal serum. If an immobilized antibody is

Table 3 Drugs That Displace T_4 and T_3 from TBG

Anticonvulsant: phenytoin, carbamazepine
Anti-inflammatory agents: salicylates, phenylbutazone, fenclofenac
Hypolipidemic agent: halofenate
Antineoplastic agents: mitotane (o,p′-DDD), 5-fluorouracil

used, or a double antibody technique wherein the second antibody does not react with human immunoglobulins, the endogenous antibody will sequester some of the tracer, and the percent of tracer bound to the assay antibody will be artifactually lowered, yielding a falsely high iodothyronine concentration. In this case, suspicion should be raised by a discrepancy between the measurement and the patient's clinical status, or between the serum T_4 and T_3 concentrations, inasmuch as the antibodies tend to react more strongly with one or the other hormone. This suspicion can be most easily confirmed by measuring the binding of tracer in the presence and absence of assay antibody in a system using a charcoal or polyethylene glycol separation.

Supranormal serum T_4 concentrations have been reported due to the familial occurrence of raised serum levels of thyroxine binding prealbumin (73) and of an abnormal albumin with a high affinity for T_4 (74-77). The prevalences of these conditions are not precisely known, but they are probably uncommon. The estimated free T_4 is artifactually high if a T_3 uptake method is used to measure protein binding or if the T_4/TBG ratio is used (74-77), but, if the dialyzable fraction of tracer T_4 or a T_4 uptake method is used, the free T_4 concentration is found to be normal. The total serum T_3 concentrations in these patients are normal.

REFERENCES

1. Braverman LE, Ingbar SH, Sterling K. Conversion of thyroxine (T_4) to triiodothyronine in athyreotic subjects. J Clin Invest 1970; 49:855-864.
2. Pittman CS, Chambers JB Jr, Read VH. The extrathyroidal conversion of thyroxine to triiodothyronine in normal man. J Clin Invest 1971; 50:1187-1196.
3. Surks MI, Schadlow AR, Stock JM, Oppenheimer JH. Determination of iodothyronine absorption and conversion of L-thyroxine (T_4) to L-triiodothyronine (T_3) using turnover techniques. J Clin Invest 1973; 52:805-811.
4. Chopra IJ. An assessment of daily production and significance of thyroidal secretion of 3,3′,5′-triiodothyronine (reverse T_3) in man. J Clin Invest 1976; 58:32-40.
5. Murphy BEP, Pattee CJ. Determination of thyroxine utilizing the property of protein binding. J Clin Endocrinol Metab 1964; 24:187-196.
6. Chopra IJ. A radioimmunoassay for measuring of thyroxine in unextracted serum. J Clin Endocrinol Metab 1972; 34:938-947.
7. Mitsuma T, Colucci J, Shenkman L, Hollander CS. Rapid simultaneous radioimmunoassay for triiodothyronine and thyroxine in unextracted serum. Biochem Biophys Res Commun 1972; 46:2107-2113.
8. Larsen PR, Dockalova J, Sipula D, Wu M. Immunoassay of thyroxine in unextracted human serum. J Clin Endocrinol Metab 1973; 37:177-182.
9. Larsen PR. Radioimmunoassay of thyroxine, triiodothyronine and thyrotropin in human serum. In *Manual of Clinical Immunology*, Rose NR, Friedman H (eds). American Society for Microbiology, Washington, DC, 1976, pp 222-230.

10. Mitsuma R, Nehei N, Gershengorn M, Hollander CS. Serum triiodothyronine measurements in human serum by radioimmunoassay with corroboration by gas liquid chromatography. J Clin Invest 1971; 50:2679-2688.
11. Lieblich J, Utiger RD. Triiodothyronine radioimmunoassay. J Clin Invest 1972; 51:157-166.
12. Larsen PR. Direct immunoassay of triiodothyronine in human serum. J Clin Invest 1972; 51:1939-1949.
13. Chopra IJ, Ho RS, Lam R. An improved radioimmunoassay of triiodothyronine in serum: its application to clinical and physiological studies. J Lab Clin Med 1972; 80:729-739.
14. Chopra IJ. Radioimmunoassay for measurement of 3, 3′,5′-triiodothyronine (reverse T_3). J Clin Invest 1974; 54:583-592.
15. Hufner N, Grussendorf M. Radioimmunoassay for 3,3′,5′-triiodothyronine (reverse T_3, R-T_3) in unextracted human serum. Clin Chim Acta 1976; 69:497-504.
16. Nicod P, Burger AG, Staeheli V, Vallotton MB. A radioimmunoassay for 3,3′,5′-triiodo-L-thyronine in unextracted serum: method and clinical results. J Clin Endocrinol Metab 1976; 42:823-829.
17. Ratcliffe WA, Marshall J, Ratcliffe JG. The radioimmunoassay of 3,3′,5′-triiodothyronine (reverse T_3) in unextracted human serum. Clin Endocrinol 1976; 5:631-641.
18. Griffiths RS, Black EG, Hoffenberg R. Measurement of serum 3,3′,5′-(reverse) T_3, with comments on its derivation. Clin Endocrinol 1976; 5: 679-685.
19. Kaplan MM, Schimmel M, Utiger RD. Changes in serum 3, 3′,5′-triiodothyronine (reverse T_3) concentrations with altered thyroid hormone secretion and metabolism. J Clin Endocrinol Metab 1977; 45:447-456.
20. Mathur H, Ekins RP, Brown BL, Malan PG, Kurtz AB. Correction for the presence of cross-reactants in saturation assays: application to thyroxine cross-reactivity in 3,3′,5′-(reverse)-triiodothyronine radioimmunoassay. Clin Chim Acta 1979; 91:317-327.
21. Meinhold H, Wenzel KW, Schurnbrand P. Radioimmunoassay of 3,3′,5′-triiodo-L-thyronine (reverse-T_3) in human serum and its application in different clinical states. Z Klin Chem Klin Biochem 1975; 12:571-574.
22. Burman KD, Dimond RC, Wright FC, Earll JM, Bruton J, Wartofsky L. A radioimmunoassay for 3,3′,5′-L-triiodothyronine (reverse T3): assessment of thyroid gland content and serum measurements in conditions of normal and altered thyroidal economy and following administration of thyrotropin releasing hormone (TRH) and thyrotropin (TSH). J Clin Endocrinol Metab 1977; 44:660-672.
23. Oppenheimer JH, Squef R, Surks MI, Hauer H. Binding of thyroxine by serum proteins evaluated by equilibrium dialysis and electrophotetic contechniques. Alterations in non-thyroidal illness. J Clin Invest 1963; 42: 1769-1782.
24. Sterling K, Brenner MA. Free thyroxine in human serum: simplified mea-

surement with the aid of magnesium precipitation. J Clin Invest 1966; 45: 153-163.
25. Schussler GC, Plager JE. Effect of preliminary purification of ^{131}I-thyroxine on the determination of free thyroxine in serum. J Clin Endocrinol Metab 1967; 27:242-250.
26. Larsen PR, Atkinson AJ Jr, Wellman HN, Goldsmith RD. The effect of diphenylhydantoin on thyroxine metabolism in man. J Clin Invest 1970; 49:1266-1279.
27. Ingbar SH, Braverman LE, Dawber NA, Lee GY. A new method for measuring the free thyroid hormone in human serum and an analysis of the factors that influence its concentration. J Clin Invest 1965; 44:1679-1689.
28. Ellis SM, Ekins RP. Direct measurement by radioimmunoassay of the free thyroid hormone concentration in serum. Acta Endocrinol (Copenh) 1973; Suppl 177:106.
29. Yeo PPB, Lewis M, Evered DC. Radioimmunoassay of free thyroid hormone concentrations in the investigation of thyroid disease. Clin Endocrinol 1977; 6:159-165.
30. Bermudez F, Surks MI, Oppenheimer JH. High Incidence of decreased serum triiodothyronine concentration in patients with nonthyroidal disease. J Clin Endocrinol Metab 1975; 41:27-40.
31. Schussler GC, Schaffner F, Korn F. Increased serum thyroid hormone binding and decreased free hormone in chronic active liver disease. N Engl J Med 1978; 299:510-515.
32. Felicetta JV, Green WL, Haas LB, Kenny MA, Sherrard DJ, Brunzell JD. Thyroid function and lipids in patients with chronic renal disease treated by hemodialysis: with comments on the "free thyroxine index." Metabolism 1979; 28:756-763.
33. Kaptein EM, MacIntyre SS, Weiner JM, Spencer CA, Nicoloff JT. Free thyroxine estimates in nonthyroidal illness: comparison of eight methods. J Clin Endocrinol Metab 1981; 52:1073-1077.
34. Sawin CT, Chopra D, Albano J, Azizi F. The free triiodothyronine (T_3) index. Ann Intern Med 1978; 88:474-477.
35. Bradwell AR, Burnett D, Ramsden DB, Burr WA, Prince HP, Hoffenberg R. Preparation of a monospecific antiserum to thyroxine binding globulin for its quantitation by rocket immunoelectrophoresis. Clin Chim Acta 1976; 71:501-510.
36. Burr WA, Evans SE, Lee J, Prince JP, Ramsden DB. The ratio of thyroxine to thyroxine-binding globulin in the assessment of thyroid function. Clin Endocrinol 1979; 11:333-342.
37. Attwood EC, Probert DE. An assessment under routine conditions of an immunoelectrophoretic assay for thyroxine-binding globulin. Clin Biochem 1978; 11:226-229.

38. Kagedal B, Kallberg M. Determination of thyroxine-binding globulin in human serum by single radial immunodiffusion and radioimmunoassay. Clin Chem 1977; 23:1694-1699.
39. Haddow JE, Ritchie RF. Newer immunochemical techniques for the quantification of serum proteins. In *Recent Advances in Clinical Immunology,* Thompson RA (ed). Churchill-Livingstone, New York, 1980, pp. 293-301.
40. Gershengorn MC, Larsen PR, Robbins J. Radioimmunoassay for serum thyroxine-binding globulin: results in normal subjects and in patients with hepatocarcinoma. J Clin Endocrinol Metab 1976; 42:907-911.
41. Kaplan MM, Larsen PR, Crantz FR, Dzau VJ, Rossing TH, Haddow JE. Prevalence of abnormal thyroid function tests in patients with acute medical illnesses. Am J Med, 1982; 72:9-16.
42. Peterson BA, Giese RW, Larsen PR, Karger BL. Measurement of free thyroid hormones in serum by dialysis and gas chromatography. Clin Chem 1977; 23:1389-1396.
43. Alexander NM, Nishimoto M. Rapid analysis for iodotyrosines and iodothyronines in thyroglobulin by reversed-phase liquid chromatography. Clin Chem 1979; 25:1757-1760.
44. Schall RF Jr, Fraser AS, Hansen HW, Kern CW, Tenoso HJ. A sensitive manual enzyme immunoassay for thyroxine. Clin Chem 1978; 24:1801-1804.
45. Galen RS, Forman D. Enzyme immunoassay of serum thyroxine with the "autochemist" multichannel analyzer. Clin Chem 1977; 23:119-121.
46. Brown BL, Ekins RP, Ellis SM, Reith WS. Specific antibodies to triiodothyronine hormone. Nature 1980; 226:359.
47. Chopra IJ, Nelson JC, Solomon DH, Beall GN. Production of antibodies specifically binding triiodothyronine and thyroxine. J Clin Endocrinol 1971; 32:399-308.
48. Hufner M, Hesch RD. A comparison of different compounds for TBG-blocking used in radioimmunoassays for triiodothyronine. Clin Chim Acta 1973; 44:101-107.
49. Weeke, J, Orskov H. Synthesis of ^{125}I monolabelled 3,5,3′-triiodothyronine and thyroxine of maximum specific activity for radioimmunoassay. Scand J Clin Lab Med 1973; 32:357-360.
50. Kjeld JM, Kuku SF, Diamant L, Fraser TR, Joplin GF, Mashiter K. Production and storage of [^{125}I] thyroxine and [^{125}I] triiodothyronine of high specific activity. Clin Chim Acta 1975; 61:381-389.
51. Kochupilla N, Yalow RS. Preparation, purification, and stability of high specific activity ^{125}I-labeled thyroxines. Endocrinology 1978; 102:128-135.
52. Sourgens H, Winterhoff H, Kemper FH, Aenstoots F. The relative merits of polyethyleneglycol as a separating agent in the radioimmunoassay of thyroid hormones. Clin Chim Acta 1979; 97:179-190.

53. Mitchell ML, McKenna JJ, McIver J. Radioimmunoassay of thyrotropin and thyroxine in dried blood by use of *Staphylococcus aureus* containing "protein A." Clin Chem 1980; 26:1140-1142.
54. Wide L. Radioimmunoassays employing immunosorbents. Acta Endocrinol (Copenh) 1969; 63 (Suppl 142):207-218.
55. Catt KJ. Radioimmunoassay with antibody-coated discs and tubes. Acta Endocrinol (Copenh) 1969; 63 (Suppl 142):222-243.
56. Snyder PJ, Utiger RD. Response to thyrotropin releasing hormone (TRH) in normal man. J Clin Endocrinol Metab 1972; 34:380-385.
57. Larsen PR. Triiodothyronine: review of recent studies of its physiology and pathophysiology in man. Metabolism 1972; 21:1073-1092.
58. Utiger RD. Serum triiodothyronine in man. Annu Rev Med 1974; 25: 289-302.
59. Joasoo A. T_4 thyrotoxicosis with normal or low serum T_3 concentration. Aust NZ J Med 1975; 5:432-434.
60. Birkhauser M, Burer T, Busset R, Burger A. Diagnosis of hyperthyroidism when serum-thyroxine alone is raised. Lancet 1977; 2:53-56.
61. Gavin LA, Rosenthal M, Cavalieri RR. The diagnostic dilemma of isolated hyperthyroxinemia in acute illness. JAMA 1979; 242:251-253.
62. Burgi H, Wimpfheimer C, Burger A, Zaunbauer W, Rosler H, Lemarchand-Beraud T. Changes of circulating thyroxine, triiodothyronine and reverse triiodothyronine after radiographic contrast agents. J Clin Endocrinol Metab 1976; 43:1203-1210.
63. Wu S-Y, Chopra IJ, Solomon DH, Johnson DE. The effect of repeated administration of ipodate (Oragrafin) in hyperthyroidism. J Clin Endocrinol Metab 1978; 47:1358-1362.
64. Burger A, Dinichert D, Nicod P, Jenny M, Lemarchand-Beraud T, Vallotton MB. Effect of amiodarone on serum triiodothyronine, reverse triiodothyronine, thyroxin, and thyrotropin. J Clin Invest 1976; 58:255-259.
65. Chopra IJ, Solomon DH, Hepner GW, Morgenstein AA. Misleadingly low free thyroxine index and usefulness of reverse triiodothyronine measurement in nonthyroidal illnesses. Ann Intern Med 1979; 90:905-912.
66. Pittmann CS, Suda AK, Chambers JB Jr, McDaniel HG, Ray GY, Preston BK. Abnormalities of thyroid hormone turnover in patients with diabetes mellitus before and after insulin therapy. J Clin Endocrinol Metab 1979; 48:854-880.
67. Heyma P, Larkins RG, Perry-Keene D, Peter CT, Ross D, Sloman JG. Thyroid hormone levels and protein binding in patients on long-term diphenylhydantoin treatment. Clin Endocrinol 1977; 6:369-376.
68. Ratcliffe WA, Hazelton RA, Thomson JA, Ratcliffe JG. The effect of fenclofenac on thyroid function tests in vivo and in vitro. Clin Endocrinol 1980; 13:569-575.
69. Larsen PR. Salicylate-induced increases in free triiodothyronine in human serum. J Clin Invest 1972; 51:1125-1134.

70. Robbins J, Rall JE, Rawson RW. An unusual instance of thyroxine binding by human serum gamma globulin. J Clin Endocrinol Metab 1956; 16: 573-579.
71. Premachandra BN, Blumenthal HT. Abnormal binding of thyroid hormone in sera from patients with Hashimoto's disease. J Clin Endocrinol Metab 1967; 27:931-936.
72. Wu SY, Green WL. Triiodothyronine (T_3)-binding immunoglobulin in a euthyroid woman: effects on measurement of T_3 (RIA) and on T_3 turnover. J Clin Endocrinol Metab 1976; 42:642-652.
73. Moses AC, Lawlor J, Haddow J, Jackson IMD. Familial euthyroid hyperthyroxinemia resulting from increased thyroxine binding to thyroxine binding prealbumin. N Engl J Med 1982; 306:966-969.
74. Docter R, Bos G, Krenning EP, Fekkes D, Visser TJ, Hennemann G. Inherited thyroxine excess: a serum abnormality due to an increased affinity for modified albumin. Clin Endocrinol (Oxford) 1981; 15:363–371.
75. Ruiz M, Rajatanavin R, Young RA, Taylor C, Brown R, Braverman LE, Ingbar SH. Familial dysalbuminemic hyperthyroxinemia. A syndrome that can be confused with thyrotoxicosis. N Engl J Med 1982; 306: 635-639.
76. Barlow JW, Csicsmann JM, White EL, Funder JW, Stockigt JR. Familial euthyroid thyroxine excess: characterization of abnormal intermediate affinity thyroxine binding to albumin. J Clin Endocrinol Metab 1982; 55:244-250.
77. Silverberg JDH, Premachandra BN. Familial hyperthyroxinemia due to abnormal thyroid hormone binding. Ann Int Med 1982; 96:183-186.

9
Catecholamines

M. Gary Nicholls
Princess Margaret Hospital, Christchurch, New Zealand

The catecholamines (norepinephrine, epinephrine, and dopamine) may be measured in plasma or urine, either unchanged or in the form of major metabolites [usually, vanillylmandellic acid (VMA) or metanephrine and normetanephrine]. By far the commonest indication for catecholamine measurements in clinical medicine is the biochemical diagnosis of pheochromocytoma. In this case, urinary levels of catecholamines, VMA, and total metanephrines (metanephrine and normetanephrine) are commonly used, and will detect all but a tiny minority of catecholamine-secreting tumors. The recent introduction of sensitive radioenzymatic techniques for the measurement of catecholamines in plasma not only allows the detection of patients with pheochromocytoma, but also permits the accurate quantitation of the separate catecholamines in a variety of medical conditions, such as essential hypertension and autonomic insufficiency. This new advance has clarified the physiological functions of circulating catecholamines. Thus epinephrine is a hormone in the classic sense: it is secreted by the adrenal medulla and has numerous metabolic actions in many tissues at physiological concentrations (1). In contrast, norepinephrine in plasma represents a tiny percentage ("spillover") of the total amount released from sympathetic axon terminals, the principal routes of dissipation being axonal reuptake and local metabolism. Under normal circumstances the levels of circulating norepinephrine have little or no metabolic effects (2); the threshold at which observable metabolic changes occur is about 1800 μg/ml (2). Plasma concentrations of the neurotransmitter norepinephrine have been used as a guide to the activity of the sympathetic system, and many studies indicate that this might be rational (3,4). However, as with any circulating substance, its level reflects not only production rate but also its rate of removal (clearance). High circulating norepinephrine levels might therefore represent increased production (and thereby reflect augmented sympathetic activity) or decreased clearance. For example, the well-documented age-related increase in plasma norepinephrine (5) appears to reflect a decline in clearance rather than an increase in sympathetic activity (6). Also complicating the interpretation of norepinephrine levels is the fact that sympathetic outflow to the different organs or anatomical regions may not be uniform (7). Hence increases or decreases in plasma norepinephrine cannot be taken to imply a global activation or reduction of sympathetic activity.

I. METHODOLOGY

A. Urine Assays

When screening for pheochromocytoma, it is usual to obtain a 24-hr urine collection in 15 ml of 6 N hydrochloric acid. Alternatively, a urine collection over some hours may be made during and after a symptomatic episode, and the result expressed per unit creatinine excretion. Finally, some workers have claimed equal or improved diagnostic accuracy by analyzing catecholamines or metabolites in a 12-hr nocturnal period (8,9), since normal subjects (in contrast to patients with pheochromocytoma) exhibit a diurnal fall in catecholamine production in the sleep hours (9).

If one urine assay method is to be used, many authorities favor total metanephrines (10-12) in view of its reliability and relative ease of performance. However, VMA and urine catecholamine measurements will also detect almost all patients harboring a pheochromocytoma (10-12). Ideally, two or even three of these products should be measured in the same urine collection.

Although a variety of procedures have been reported, analysis of urinary VMA, metanephrines, and catecholamines in most laboratories is based on long-established spectrophotometric or fluorometric methods (13-15). Newer radioenzymatic methods for the measurement of urine catecholamines are being used in some centers, but whether diagnostic accuracy is improved remains to be seen. Since many drugs can interfere with the estimation of urine catecholamines and their metabolites (16-18), especially when fluorometric techniques are used, the laboratory must be aware of this potential for misdiagnosis, and the physician should endeavor to withdraw all but essential medications some days before the urine collection. Severe renal impairment may reduce excretion of catecholamines and metabolites; thus more reliance should be placed on the measurement of catecholamines in plasma under these circumstances.

B. Plasma Catecholamines

Early fluorometric methods have largely given way to more sensitive and specific radioenzymatic assays. The concept is based on the use of an enzyme, usually harvested from liver (19), to transfer a tritiated methyl group from a donor [S-adenosyl-L-methionine (SAM)] to norepinephrine and epinephrine (and dopamine) to form their respective derivatives, tritiated normetanephrine, and metanephrine (and methoxytyramine). These metabolites can be separated (e.g., by thin-layer chromatography) oxidized to vanillin, and the radioactivity counted. The original assays used two isotopes, the methyl donor being ^{14}C labeled, and trace quantities of tritiated catecholamines were added to plasma samples thus allowing correction for recovery (20). Recent techniques usually utilize a single isotope, [^3H] SAM. The much higher specific activity of [^3H] SAM compared to the ^{14}C-labeled methyl donor has produced a considerable increase in sensitivity. Although assessment of recovery is sacrificed, most workers using single isotope derivative assays report excellent sensitivity, high specificity, good reproducibility, a straight-line relationship of catecholamines added to final counts at the completion of the assay, and minimal cross-reactivity between the catecholamines (21-23). Small volumes of plasma (25-250 μl) are required. Very few drugs (isoproterenol, L-dopa, and α-methyldopa) interfere with the assay. Variations of this new technique are being reported with great frequency (24-27). The method may be used for measurements of catecholamines in cerebrospinal fluid, urine, and tissue extracts as well as in plasma. One drawback of the method is the high purchase cost of commercially available [^3H] SAM.

With this major advance in methodology, it has become evident that many factors can alter plasma catecholamine levels (28, 29), and these must be taken into account in their interpretation. For example, increasing age, body posture, exercise, dietary sodium intake, caffeine, smoking, fasting, mental stress, physical stress (surgery, cardiac failure, myocardial infarction, cerebrovascular accident), and hypoglycemia can affect norepinephrine and epinephrine levels. Arteriovenous differences have been documented (30, 31). Ideally, then, blood for catecholamine measurements should be drawn under standardized conditions. The patient should be resting supine in quiet surroundings, and a heparinized venous line inserted 30 min prior to withdrawal of the blood sample. Where impaired function of the sympathetic nervous system is suspected (e.g., in patients with postural hypotension), a stimulatory maneuver such as 10 min of upright posture, isometric exercise, or treadmill exercise should be performed prior to the withdrawal of a second blood sample (32). Although catecholamines in blood and plasma might be more stable than was previously thought (33), it is currently suggested that blood be taken into chilled containers, centrifuged without delay at 4°C, and the plasma stored at below −20°C. Samples should be analyzed as soon as possible since the long-term stability of catecholamines in plasma is not known.

Smoking, caffeine, severe exercise, or "stress" should be avoided for some hours before blood sampling. Medications which may interfere with the assay (especially α-methyldopa, isoproterenol, and L-dopa), or can augment (diuretics, beta blockers, vasodilators) or inhibit norepinephrine release (clonidine, ganglion blockers, adrenergic neurone blockers), should be noted to allow accurate interpretation of the results. The "normal range" of plasma catecholamines for each laboratory should, ideally, be derived using healthy subjects sampled under the same condition as the patients, preferably with a range of age decades represented to allow age matching with the patients.

II. CLINICAL APPLICATIONS

Catecholamine or metabolite measurements have been used almost exclusively in clinical medicine for the diagnosis of pheochromocytoma (Chap. 27). Radioenzymatic methods have sufficient sensitivity to define normal and even low levels of plasma catecholamines, and are increasingly used to document sympathetic activity in patients with suspected impairment of the autonomic nervous system. For example, postural hypotension in patients with diabetes mellitus is generally associated with impaired plasma norepinephrine increments during change in body posture or with exercise (34), although a small minority of patients exhibit an exaggerated postural norepinephrine response (35), presumably because of a subnormal blood volume.

The role of the sympathetic nervous system in the pathogensis and maintenance of essential hypertension has been extensively studied, but limitations in design or catecholamine assay technique ensure that questions remain to be answered (36). It is possible that disordered functioning of catecholaminergic neurones in the brain forms the basis of some endocrine disorders such as acromegaly (37) and prolactin-secreting tumors (38). In view of the potent effects of epinephrine on glucose homeostasis (1, 39), it is likely that destruction of the adrenal medulla removes one important defense mechanism against hypoglycemia. Circulating norepinephrine levels tend to be high in primary hypothyroidism and normal or low in hyperthyroidism (40-42).

In clinical practice, catecholamine measurements are essential to confirm or refute the presence of pheochromocytoma, and most other requirements relate to research into sympathetic nervous system or adrenal medullary involvement in various disorders.

REFERENCES

1. Clutter WE, Bier DM, Shah SD, Cryer PE. Epinephrine plasma metabolic clearance rates and physiologic thresholds for metabolic and hemodynamic actions in man. J Clin Invest 1980; 66:94-101.
2. Silverberg AB, Shah SD, Haymond MW, Cryer PE. Norepinephrine: hormone and neurotransmitter in man. Am J Physiol 1978; 234:E252-E256.
3. Esler M, Zweifler A, Randall O, Julius S, DeQuattro V. Agreement among three different indices of sympathetic nervous system activity in essential hypertension. Mayo Clin Proc 1977; 52:379-382.
4. Lake CR, Ziegler MG, Kopin IJ. Use of plasma norepinephrine for evaluation of sympathetic neuronal function in man. Life Sci 1976; 18:1315-1326.
5. Ziegler MG, Lake CR, Kopin IJ. Plasma noradrenaline increases with age. Nature 1976; 261:333-335.
6. Esler M, Skews G, Leonard P, Jackman G, Bobik A, Korner P. Age-dependence of noradrenaline kinetics in normal subjects. Clin Sci 1981; 60:217-219.
7. Vallbo AB, Hagbarth KE, Jorebjork HE, Wallin BG. Somatosensory, proprioceptive, and sympathetic activity in human peripheral nerves. Physiol Rev 1979; 59:919-957.
8. Sullivan JM, Solomon HS. The diagnosis of pheochromocytoma: overnight excretion of catecholamine metabolites. JAMA 1975; 231:618-619.
9. Ganguly A, Henry DP, Yune HY, et al. Diagnosis and localization of pheochromocytoma: detection by measurement of urinary norepinephrine excretion during sleep, plasma norepinephrine concentration and computerized axial tomography (CT-scan). Am J Med 1979; 67:21-26.
10. Crout JR, Pisano JJ, Sjoerdsma A. Urinary excretion of catecholamines and their metabolites in pheochromocytoma. Am Heart J 1961; 61:375-381.
11. Gitlow SE, Mendlowitz M, Bertani LM. The biochemical techniques for detecting and establishing the presence of a pheochromocytoma. Am J Cardiol 1970; 26:270-279.
12. Remine WH, Chong GC, VanHeerden JA, Sheps SG, Harrison EG. Current management of pheochromocytoma. Ann Surg 1974; 179:740-747.
13. Pisano JJ. A simple analysis for normetanephrine and metanephrine in urine. Clin Chim Acta 1960; 5:406-414.
14. Pisano JJ, Crout JR, Abraham D. Determination of 3-methoxy-4-hydroxymandelic acid in urine. Clin Chim Acta 1962; 7:285-291.
15. Crout JR. Catecholamines in urine. In *Standard Methods of Clinical Chemistry,* Seligson D (ed). Academic, New York, 1960, vol 3, p. 62.
16. Caraway WT, Kammeyer CW. Chemical interference by drugs and other substances with clinical laboratory tests. Clin Chim Acta 1972; 41:395-434.

17. Hamilton CA, Jones DH, Dargie HJ, Reid JL. Does labetalol increase excretion of urinary catecholamines? Br Med J 1978; 2:800.
18. Manger WM, Gifford RW. *Pheochromocytoma.* Springer-Verlag, New York, 1977, pp 214-215.
19. Axelrod J, Tomchick R. Enzymatic O-methylation of epinephrine and other catechols. J Biol Chem 1958; 233:702-705.
20. Engelman K, Portnoy B. Sensitive double-isotope derivative assay for norepinephrine and epinephrine: normal resting human plasma levels. Circ Res 1970; 26:53-57.
21. Cryer PE, Santiago JV, Shah S. Measurement of norepinephrine and epinephrine in small volumes of human plasma by a single isotope derivative method: response to the upright posture. J Clin Endocrinol Metab 1974; 39:1025-1029.
22. Da Prada M, Zurcher G. Simultaneous radio-enzymatic determination of plasma and tissue adrenaline, noradrenaline and dopamine within the femtomole range. Life Sci 1976; 19:1161-1174.
23. Peuler JD, Johnson GA. Simultaneous single isotope radioenzymatic assay of plasma norepinephrine, epinephrine, and dopamine. Life Sci 1977; 21: 625-636.
24. Ben-Jonathan N, Porter JC. A sensitive radioenzymatic assay for dopamine, norepinephrine, and epinephrine in plasma and tissue. Endocrinology 1976; 98:1497-1507.
25. Hortnagl H, Benedict CR, Grahame-Smith DG, McGrath B. A sensitive radioenzymatic assay for adrenaline and noradrenaline in plasma. Br J Clin Pharmacol 1977; 4:553-558.
26. Martin IL, Baker GB, Fleetwood-Walker SM. Modification of the radioenzymatic assay for the catecholamines. Biochem Pharmacol 1978; 27: 1519-1520.
27. Bauce L, Thornhill JA, Cooper KE, Veale WL. A radioenzymatic assay for femtomole determination of catecholamines using α-methyldopamine as an internal standard. Life Sci 1980; 27:1921-1928.
28. Cryer PE. Physiology and pathophysiology of the human sympathoadrenal neuroendocrine system. N Engl J Med 1980; 303:436-444.
29. Sever PS, Roberts JC, Snell ME. Phaeochromocytoma. Clin Endocrinol Metab 1980; 9:543-568.
30. Sole MJ, Drobac M, Schwartz L, Hussain MN, Vaughan-Neil EF. The extraction of circulating catecholamines by the lungs in normal man and in patients with pulmonary hypertension. Circulation 1979; 60:160-163.
31. Halter JB, Pflug AE, Tolas AG. Arterial-venous differences of plasma catecholamines in man. Metabolism 1980; 29:9-12.
32. Robertson D, Shand DG, Hollifield JW, Nies AS, Frolich JC, Oates JA. Alterations in the response of the sympathetic nervous system and renin in borderline hypertension. Hypertension 1979; 1:118-124.

33. Pettersson J, Hussi E, Janne J. Stability of human plasma catecholamines. Scand J Clin Lab Invest 1980; 40:297-303.
34. Hilsted J, Galbo H, Christensen NJ. Impaired responses of catecholamines, growth hormone, and cortisol to graded exercise in diabetic autonomic neuropathy. Diabetes 1980; 29:257-262.
35. Tohmeh JF, Shah SD, Cryer PE. The pathogenesis of hyperadrenergic postural hypotension in diabetic patients. Am J Med 1979; 67:772-778.
36. Goldstein DS. Plasma norepinephrine in essential hypertension. A study of the studies. Hypertension 1981; 3:48-52.
37. Van Loon GR. Abnormal plasma catecholamine responses in acromegalics. J Clin Endocrinol Metab 1979; 48:784-789.
38. Van Loon GR. A defect in catecholamine neurons in patients with prolactin-secreting pituitary adenoma. Lancet 1978; 2:868-871.
39. Santiago JV, Clarke WL, Shah SD, Cryer PE. Epinephrine, norepinephrine, glucagon, and growth hormone release in association with physiological decrements in the plasma glucose concentration in normal and diabetic man. J Clin Endocrinol Metab 1980; 51:877-885.
40. Christensen NJ. Increased levels of plasma noradrenaline in hypothyroidism. J Clin Endocrinol Metab 1972; 35:359-363.
41. Coulombe P, Dussault JH, Letarte J, Simard SJ. Catecholamine metabolism in thyroid disease. I. Epinephrine secretion rate in hyperthyroidism and hypothyroidism. J Clin Endocrinol Metab 1976; 42:125-131.
42. Coulombe P, Dussault JH, Walker P. Catecholamine metabolism in thyroid disease. II. Norepinephrine secretion rate in hyperthyroidism and hypothyroidism. J Clin Endocrinol Metab 1977; 44:1185-1189.

10
Standardization

Derek R. Bangham
National Institute for Biological Standards and Control, London, England

I. ESSENTIAL STANDARDIZATION: CONCEPT AND MISCONCEPT

The aim of standardization is to make results of assays valid and accurate and reliably reproducible; this makes it possible to compare the results from assays made with different reagents and personnel, in different laboratories, and at various times. In clinical endocrinology most assays are done to estimate the amount of a hormone in a specimen solution. All such assays to quantify an analyte require standardization, including those which test the change of an analyte in a body fluid in response to a stimulus, such as a rise in plasma thyroid stimulating hormone (TSH) in response to thyroid releasing hormone (TRH), and those which are intended simply to detect whether an analyte is present, such as human chorionic gonadotropin (hCG) in a pregnancy test. Standardization is needed for the former so that the change of response in successive tests carried out over a period of time can be compared; and for the latter so that the sensitivity of the test (the lowest concentration of analyte detectable) can be described with a stated probability.

Standardization in hormone assays consists of the application of a discipline which consists of good technical procedure and good biometry—the application of statistical design and tests to the results and their interpretation. Standardization does not mean the rigid imposition of a stipulated test procedure: on the contrary, if the principles are correctly applied, this discipline allows the development of indefinite improvement in assay methods. Standardization is like the discipline of good grammar: if a sentence is not correctly structured, its contents may be meaningless or vague, or inaccurate and dangerously misleading.

Principles of standardization in biological assays were first developed for the control of potency of drugs such as insulin (1). There is excellent succinct guidance in the design, conduct, and statistical analysis of results for a wide variety of assays given in pharmacopoeias (British, 1980, European, vol II, 1971, and United States, 1980). Pharmacopoeias also give descriptions of well-tried classical assay methods for several hormones, including insulin, glucagon, corticotrophins, hCG, luteinizing hormone (LH), follicle stimulating hormone (FSH), oxytocin, vasopressins, luteinizing hormone releasing hormone (LHRH), thyroid releasing hormone (TRH), and steroids. It is noteworthy that protein-binding assay methods have not yet been included as official tests, because of the difficulty in achieving reliable standardization.

This chapter will emphasize certain aspects of standardization. More detailed discussion of standardization, especially in relation to standards, is given in Bangham and Cotes (2), the 26th Report of the WHO ECBS (3), and successive reports of that committee. Detailed requirements for the manufacture and characterization of binding assay kits have been published by WHO (4). Anyone intending to assemble an immunoassay system should consult these requirements; indeed, the purchase of any assay kit could now be made conditional that it complies with them.

II. VALIDITY OF THE ASSAY SYSTEM: BIOMETRIC VALIDITY; BASIC ASSUMPTIONS FOR VALID ASSAYS; VARIABLES OF ASSAY SYSTEMS; RANDOMIZATION

The validity of an assay has two interrelated aspects (5). The validity of the assay system (reagents, conditions, and procedure) is its ability to measure the analyte. Specificity for the analyte should be suitable for the types of specimen (pharmaceutical preparation or body fluid) for which the assay would be used. *Biometric validity* is the numerical correctness of the assay result.

Assays for many hormones involve biological materials (animals, tissues, cells, extracts, or proteins such as antibodies) all of which are intrinsically variable. Hence most assays performed to quantify a hormone are comparison assays, in which the test specimen is compared with a reference standard. The validity of such a comparison assay depends on certain fundamental assumptions: (1) that the analyte in the test specimen is identical to the component in the standard with which it is compared, or at least similar to the extent that they behave identically in the assay system; and (2) that the test specimen and standard are compared under identical circumstances: with the same reagents, under the same conditions, and preferably at the same time. In certain types of assays, especially where identical reagents or conditions cannot be used it is essential that the variables be allocated to the test and standard in a strictly randomized way. The need for proper randomization in assays involving variables cannot be overstressed (6).

III. NUMERICAL VALIDITY OF ASSAY RESULTS

Statistical numerical procedures can assess the biometric validity and the precision of assay results. *Precision* means the consistency of agreement of repeated measurements, and *bias* is the extent to which results are consistently inaccurate. In the biometric sense the validity of an assay result can be assessed if the measured responses to at least two dose levels each of test specimen and of standard are compared. A statistical test for parallelism of the log dose-response relationship (e.g. Ref. 6) can be applied to assess whether the same increase in dose of specimen and analyte each gave rise to the same proportional increase in response. The test for parallelism should be applied to assess whether the requirement that "like is compared to like" has been satisfied. Parallelism is essential for a valid result; but by itself it is not a guarantee that the result is valid or that the test analyte and standard are identical.

The validity and precision of an assay result depend on both the design of the assay and on the way the results are analyzed. Pragmatic guidance on assay designs and analysis is given in pharmacopoeias.

Statistical tests also enable one to calculate the precision of the result of a single assay or of the combination of a series of results. Precision is commonly calculated as the range of values, confidence limits, within which results would be expected to occur if that assay was repeated. Generally, 95% confidence values are used, that is, the range within which a result would occur if that assay was repeated 20 times. This calculation documents the imprecision of bioassays. It explains why an experienced bioassayist calls an assay result an "estimate" and states the confidence limits of that estimate. Those with more conviction than insight call it a "determination." Another statistical test for validity can be applied to the results of repeated assays of the same specimens to assess if they are consistent (i.e., *homogeneous*). If results do not agree within a certain range of probability they are *heterogeneous*. This suggests either that there is a significant difference between the test analyte and standard—that like was not compared with like—or that there was something wrong with the assays, such as bias due to nonrandomization.

IV. STANDARDIZATION IN DIAGNOSTIC PROTEIN BINDING ASSAYS

Evaluation of numerical veracity is necessary for science and for the legal control of drugs and is not normally applied to the results of the multitude of specimens assayed in a busy clinical laboratory. In contrast, a clinician generally needs to know only if a result is too high, too low, or about normal, or if it was notably different from the result of a previous test.

In diagnostic laboratories specimens are generally tested at one dose level only. The validity of the assay system (reagents, conditions, and procedures) and its performance characteristics must then be assessed when the assay system is assembled and conditions optimized. These characteristics are then held to apply to each individual specimen in a whole series of estimations. But it is worth remembering that with only one dose level it is not possible to identify nonparallelism for the individual specimen, which might indicate an invalid result, perhaps due to an abnormal form of hormone analyte from a tumor.

V. COMPONENTS OF IN VITRO BINDING ASSAY SYSTEMS

Clinical diagnostic assays are now routinely done by one or another kind of in vitro protein binding assay, such as radioimmunoassay. The main components of such assays consist of the analyte in the specimen, a standard, a binding molecule (antibody, receptor protein, or the hormone itself for assays of hormone binding protein), and a signal and amplification system. The tracer label, which may be a radionuclide, fluophor, enzyme, or other tracer substance, provides a signal which enables the proportion of analyte bound to the binding molecule to be measured. A systematic classification of all such binding assay systems is being prepared for the International Federation of Clinical Chemistry (IFCC); but they fall into two basic categories: those assay systems which use a measured limited amount of binding component (e.g., antibody in a classical radioimmunoassay), and those in which there is an excess of the binding component (immunoradiometric assay). Certain performance characteristics (e.g., sensitivity) of each are different (7), but the criteria for standardization are similar.

VI. STANDARDS AND REFERENCE MATERIALS: IMPLICATIONS OF DISSIMILARITIES BETWEEN ANALYTE AND STANDARD

If biometry is the "grammar" of standardization, reference materials are the subject nouns of assays. Essentially all hormone assays depend on comparison with a reference material. Traditionally, hormones have been categorized into those which are "pure chemicals" such as steroids and those "biological substances" such as proteins of complex structure which cannot be characterized completely by chemical and physical methods alone. Any sample of an attested "pure chemical" should be the same as another and suitable for use as a standard. But standardization requires that each reference preparation of a peptide hormone be ultimately related—calibrated by assays—in terms of a single reference material. It is for this reason that a service of international reference materials (standards or reference preparations) is provided by the WHO (8). Ampules of these materials are available for calibration of national and manufacturers' standards. The essential properties of a reference material are that each sample is identical to another and that it is stable. The preparation and characterization of biological standards is described (9).

Standardization is made very complex because many hormone analytes are heterogeneous. Heterogeneity may be intrinsic, such as in the glycoprotein hormones hCG, LH, FSH, and TSH; brought about by alteration of molecules during their extraction; or be due to their instability. Thus in practice the fundamental requirement that the standard should be identical to the analyte probably occurs only rarely.

Furthermore, it is characteristic of immunoassay systems that each one has a slightly different spectrum of nonspecificity, which is rarely evaluated and documented in detail, and which may be altered by changes of reagents or procedure. In other words, the bias of each assay system may be influenced by unknown factors and leads to irregularities of results. Such irregularities are often due to dissimilarities between analyte and standard, which may be expressed as nonparallelism or as significant heterogeneity of results of repeated assays with one assay system or with different assay systems. In many instances the irregularities of results are minor and can be ignored. However, a change of standard is likely to give some discontinuity in the results (2, 3). Discontinuity is especially liable to occur with standards consisting of heterogeneous materials and also when there is a change from a standard of impure material to one which is highly purified. In such cases it may be necessary to recalibrate a working standard with the new primary (i.e., international) reference material when it is established (10). In practice it is particularly worthwhile having a common working standard for any substance which is scarce, heterogeneous, unstable, or difficult or costly to characterize and calibrate. It is thus essential that the record of an assay result include a statement of the assay method (and preferably the kit batch number) and the standard used and its assigned mass or unitage.

VII. STABILITY

WHO international biological standards are very stable. This is due primarily to the fastidious way in which they are prepared—free of bacteria and enzymes, desiccated, sealed in ampules with an inert gas, and kept in the dark at −20°C. Instability is due to chemical change, which is accelerated at higher temperatures. Stability is accurately and economically measured by accelerated degradation tests in which samples kept at higher temperatures (say 37°C and 46°C) for various periods of time are compared with samples kept at low temperatures. Calculation of the rate of change at given temperatures allow one to predict stability at other temperatures.

Table 1 List of Standards

Standard[a]	Ampule code no.	Defined activity[a]	Approximate composition of ampule contents	Other informatiuon (reference)
Angiotensin I (Asp-Isoleu[5])	71/328	9 μg/amp nominal	9 μg synthetic angiotensin I 2 mg mannitol	11
Angiotensin II (Asp-Ileu[5])	70/302	24 μg/amp nominal	24 μg synthetic angiotensin II 2 mg mannitol	11
First IS for arginine vasopressin	77/501	8.2 IU/amp	20 μg synthetic arginine vasopressin 5 mg human albumin Citric acid	12
First IRP of calcitonin, human, for bioassay	70/234	1.0 U/amp	8.5 μg synthetic calcitonin of sequence found in tumors 5 mg mannitol	13
First IRP of calcitonin, porcine, for bioassay	70/306	1.0 IU/amp	10 μg purified extract 5 mg mannitol	T_3 and T_4 trace amounts 14
First IRP of calcitonin, salmon, for bioassay	72/158	80 IU/amp	20 μg synthetic salmon calcitonin II 2 mg mannitol	14
First IRP of chorionic gonadotropin for immunoassay	75/537	650 IU/amp	70 μg chorionic gonadotropin 5 mg human albumin	15, 16
First IRP of α subunit of chorionic gonadotropin	75/569	70 IU/amp	70 μg chorionic gonadotropin α subunit 5 mg human albumin	15, 16

First IRP of β subunit of chorionic gonadotropin	75/551	70 IU/ amp	70 μg chorionic gonadotropin β subunit 5 mg human albumin	15, 16
Second IS for chorionic gonadotropin for bioassay	61/6	5300 IU/ amp	2 mg chorionic gonadotropin 5 mg lactose	17
Corticotropin, human	74/555		11.6 μg corticotropin 5 mg human albumin 2.5 mg mannitol	Bioassay vs. third IS: s.c. adrenal ascorbate depletion assay = 3.19 IU/ amp
Third IS for corticotropin (ACTH) porcine, for bioassay; International Working Standard	59/16 Various	5.0 IU/ amp 5.0 IU/ amp	50 μg pituitary extract 5 mg lactose	18, 19 Vasopressin <25 mu/ ampule by rat blood pressure assay terms of IS
First IS for desmopressin	78/573	27 IU/ amp	27 μg purified desmopressin 5 mg human albumin Citric acid	20
Second IRP of erythropoietin human, urinary, for bioassay	67/343	10 IU/ amp	2 mg urinary extract containing erythropoietin 3 mg sodium chloride	21
Second IRP of FSH/LH, human, pituitary for bioassay	78/549	FSH:10 IU/amp LH: 25 IU/ amp	0.5 mg FSH/LH 1.25 mg lactose	4, 22
First FSH/LH human, urinary, for bioassay	70/45	FSH: 54 IU/amp LH: 46 IU/ amp	1 mg human postmenopausal urine extract 5 mg lactose	23

Table 1 (Continued)

Standard[a]	Ampule code no.	Defined activity[a]	Approximate composition of ampule contents	Other information (reference)
Gastrin, human	68/439	12 U/amp	12.6 μg synthetic gastrin, as hexamonium salt 5 mg lactose Phosphate buffer	
Gastrin II, porcine	66/138	10 U/amp	10 μg gastrin II 5 mg sucrose Phosphate buffer	
First IRP of glucagon, porcine, for bioassay	69/194	1.49 IU/amp	1.5 mg glucagon 5 mg lactose 0.24 mg sodium chloride	24, 25
First IS for glucagon, porcine, for immunoassay	69/194	1.49 IU/amp	1.5 mg glucagon 5 mg lactose 0.24 mg sodium chloride	24, 25
First IRP for gonadorelin (LHRH) for bioassay	77/596	31 IU/amp	31 nmol synthetic gonadorelin 2.5 mg lactose 0.5 mg human albumin	Ovine/porcine sequence 4
First IRP of growth hormone, human, for immunoassay	66/217	0.35 IU/amp	175 μg growth hormone 5 mg sucrose Phosphate buffer	Prolactin activity: pigeon 1 IU/amp; rabbit; 7 IU/amp; decidual response (mice) 1 IU/amp
First IS for growth hormone, human, for bioassay	80/505	4.4 IU/amp	1.74 μg LGH with glycine, mannitol, $NaHCO_3$ and lactose	

First IS for human growth hormone for bioassay	80/505	4.4 IU/amp	1.74 mg human growth hormone with glycine, mannitol, $NaHCO_3$, and lactose	41
Insulin C peptide for immunoassay	76/561	~2.5 nmol/amp	10 μg synthetic human insulin C peptide analog 50 μg human albumin; 0.05 nmol phosphate buffer	Synthetic (64-formyllysine) human proinsulin 31-65 26
First IRP of insulin, human, for immunoassay	66/304	3.0 IU/amp	130 μg insulin 5 mg sucrose	27
Fourth IS for insulin, bovine and porcine, for bioassay	58/6	24.0 IU/mg	110-125 mg crystals 48% porcine insulin 52% bovine insulin	28, 29
First IS for kininogenase porcine pancreatic	78/543	22.5 IU/amp	20 μg porcine pancreatic kininogenase 5 mg human albumin	42
First IRP of LH, human pituitary, for immunoassay	68/40	77 IU/amp	11.6 μg LH 5 mg lactose 1 mg human albumin 1 mg sodium chloride	30
First IS for lysine vasopressin	77/512	7.7 IU/amp	30 μg synthetic lysine-vasopressin acetate 5 mg human albumin Citric acid	31
Fourth IS for oxytocin	76/575	12.5 IU/amp	24 μg synthetic oxytocin acetate 5 mg human albumin Citric acid	32

Table 1 (Continued)

Standard[a]	Ampule code no.	Defined activity[a]	Approximate composition of ampule contents	Other information (reference)
Parathyroid hormone, human, for immunoassay	75/549	0.025 U/ amp	250 ng extract of human adenomata 250 μg human albumin 1.25 mg lactose	Estimated to contain ~25 ng parathyroid hormone 33
First IRP of parathyroid hormone, human, for immunoassay	79/500	0.100 IU/ amp	100 ng purified extract of human adenomata 250 μg human albumin 1.25 mg lactose	
First IRP of parathyroid hormone bovine, for bioassay	67/342	200 IU/ amp	0.6 mg gland extract 5 mg lactose	34
First IRP of parathyroid hormone bovine, for immunoassay	71/324	2.0 IU/ amp	1 μg purified extract 200 μg human albumin 1 mg lactose	34
IRP of placental lactogen, human, for immunoassay	73/545	0.000850 IU/amp	850 μg placental lactogen 5 mg mannitol	35
First IRP of prolactin, human, for immunoassay	75/504	650 MU/ amp	20 μg extract 1 mg human albumin 5 mg lactose	36

Second IS for prolactin, ovine, for bioassay	57/8	22 IU/mg	10 mg extract	37
First IRP of renin, human, for bioassay	68/356	0.1 IU/amp	0.27 mg renal extract 5 mg lactose Phosphate buffer	11
Second IS for serum gonadotropin equine, for bioassay	62/1	1600 IU/amp	0.8 mg extract 5 mg lactose	38
First IRP of tetracosactrin, for bioassay	80/590	490 IU/amp	490 μg tetracosactrin 20 mg mannitol	
First IRP of TSH, human, for immunoassay	68/38	150 mU/amp	46.2 μg TSH extract 5 mg lactose 1 mg human albumin	39
First IS for thyrotropin, bovine, for bioassay	53/11	74 mU/mg	1 part pituitary extract 19 parts lactose	40

[a]IS, International Standard; IRP, International Reference Preparation.
[b]Amp, ampule.

A standard made up into solution should include a small amount of suitable bacteriocide (e.g., azide) and about 0.5% carrier protein [free from peptidase (9)] in a suitable buffer. This solution should be subdivided in small volumes into well-sealed containers and frozen to −20°C or less and stored at −40° or less (i.e., well below the eutectic freezing point of the solution) (9).

VIII. LIST OF STANDARDS

A list of standards is given in Table 1. Many of the preparations have been set up as a result of international collaborative effort by several laboratories contributing materials and work. They are available only in strictly limited quantities. International standards are intended primarily to calibrate national standards. Except for those designated, they are not for use as working standards. They are not intended for administration to humans.

Applications for ampules of these reference materials should be made as a written request by the scientist concerned, stating the purpose for which the material is needed, to the Hormones Division, the National Institute for Biological Standards and Control, Hampstead, London NW3 6RB, United Kingdom.

REFERENCES

1. Gaddum J. In *Reports on Biological Standards.* III. *Methods of Biological Assay Depending on a Quantal Response*. MRC Spec Rep Ser 183, 1933.
2. Bangham DR, Cotes PM. Standardization and standards. Br Med Bull 1974; 30:12-17.
3. WHO Expert Committee on Biological Standardization. 26th Report. WHO Tech Rep Ser 565, 1975.
4. WHO Expert Committee on Biological Standardization. 31st Report. WHO Tech Rep Ser 658, 1981.
5. Jerne NK, Wood EC. The validity and meaning of the results of biological assays. Biometrics 1949; 5:273.
6. Finney DJ. *Statistical Method in Biological Assay,* 3rd ed. Charles Griffin, London, 1978.
7. Ekins RP. General principles of hormone assay. In *Hormone Assays and Their Clinical Application,* Loraine JA, Bell ET (eds). Churchill Livingstone, London, 1976, pp 1-72.
8. *Biological Substances.* World Health Organization, Geneva, 1982.
9. WHO Expert Committee on Biological Standardization. Annex 4, 29th Report. WHO Tech Rep Ser 626, 1978.
10. WHO Expert Committee on Biological Standardization. 32nd Report. WHO Tech Rep Ser 673, 1982.

11. Bangham DR, Robertson I, Robertson JIS, Robinson CJ, Tree M. An international collaborative study of renin assay: establishment of the international reference preparation of human renin. Clin Sci Mol Med 1975; 48:135S.
12. World Health Organization. Unpublished working document WHO/BS/78. 1231.
13. Gaines Das RE, Zanelli JM. The IRP of calcitonin, human, for bioassay: assessment of material and definition of the international unit. Acta Endocrinol 1980; 93:37-42.
14. World Health Organization Unpublished working document WHO/BS/ 74.1077.
15. Canfield RE, Ross GT. A new reference preparation of human chorionic gonadotrophin and its subunits. Bull WHO 1976; 54:463-470.
16. Storring PL, Gaines Das RE, Bangham DR. International reference preparation of human chorionic gonadotrophin for immunoassay: potency estimates in various bioassay and protein binding assay systems, and international reference preparations of the alpha and beta subunits of HCG for immunoassay. J Endocrinol 1980; 84:295-310.
17. Bangham DR, Grab B. The 2nd international standard for chorionic gonadotrophin. Bull WHO 1964; 31:111-125.
18. Bangham DR, Mussett MV, Stack-Dunne MP. The 3rd international standard for corticotrophin. Bull WHO 1962; 27:395-408.
19. Storring PL, Gaines Das RE, Tiplady RJ, Stenning B, Mistry Y. Stability of the 3rd international standard for corticotrophin: accelerated degradation study using different bioassays and isoelectric focusing. J Endocrinol 1980; 85:533-539.
20. World Health Organization. Unpublished working document WHO/BS/ 80.1226.
21. Cotes PM, Annable L, Mussett MV. The 2nd international reference preparation of erythropoietin, human, urinary for bioassay. Bull WHO 1972; 47:99-122.
22. Bangham DR, Berryman I, Burger H, Cotes PM, Furnival BE, Hunter WM, Midgley AR, Mussett MV, Reichert LE, Rosemberg E, Ryan RJ, Wide L. An international collaborative study of 69/104: a reference preparation of human pituitary FSH/LH. J Clin Endocrinol Metab 1973; 36:647-660.
23. Storring PL, Dixon H, Bangham DR. The 1st international standard for human urinary FSH and human urinary LH (ICSH) for bioassay. Acta Endocrinol (Copenh) 1976; 83:700-710.
24. Bangham DR, Salokangas AA, Annable L, Storring PL. The 1st international standard for glucagon. Acta Endocrinol (Copenh) 1974; 77:705-714.
25. Calam DH, Storring PL. The heterogeneity and degradation of glucagon studied by polyacrylamide gel electrophoresis. J Biol Stand 1975; 3:263-265.

26. Caygill CPJ, Gaines Das RE, Bangham DR. Use of a common standard for comparison of insulin C-peptide. Diabetologia 1980; 18:197-204.
27. World Health Organization. Unpublished working document WHO/BS/74. 1084.
28. Bangham DR, Musset MV. The 4th international standard for insulin. Bull WHO 1959; 20:12.
29. Storring PL, Greaves PL, Mussett MV, Bangham DR. Stability of the 4th international standard for insulin. Diabetologia 1975; 11:581-584.
30. Storring PL, Bangham DR, Cotes PM, Gaines Das RE, Jeffcoate SL. The international reference preparation of human pituitary luteinizing hormone for immunoassay. Acta Endocrinol (Copenh) 1978; 88:250-259.
31. World Health Organization. Unpublished working document WHO/BS/78. 1230.
32. World Health Organization. Unpublished working document WHO/BS/78. 1227.
33. Zanelli JM, Gaines Das RE. International collaborative study of NIBSC Research Standard A for human PTH for immunoassay. J Endocrinol 1980; 86:291-304.
34. World Health Organization. Unpublished working document WHO/BS/74. 1078.
35. Cotes PM, Gaines Das RE. An international collaborative study of the assay of human placental lactogen: establishment of WHO IRP of human placental lactogen. Br J Obstet Gynaecol 1978; 85:451-459.
36. Gaines Das RE, Cotes PM. International reference preparation of human prolactin for immunoassay: definition of the international unit, report of a collaborative study and comparison of estimates of human prolactin made in various laboratories. J Endocrinol 1979; 80:157-168.
37. Bangham DR, Mussett MV, Stack-Dunne MP. The 2nd international standard for prolactin. Bull WHO 1963; 29:721.
38. Bangham DR, Woodward PM. The 2nd international standard for serum gonadotrophin. Bull WHO 1966; 35:761.
39. Cotes PM, Gaines Das RE, Kirkwood TBL, Bennie JG, Hunter WM. The stability of standards for radioimmunoassay of human TSH: Research Standard A and the IRP initially 68/38. Acta Endocrinol 1978; 88:291-297.
40. Mussett MV, Perry WLM. The international standard for thyrotrophin. Bull WHO 1955; 13:917-929.
41. World Health Organization. Unpublished working document WHO/BS/82. 1369.
42. World Health Organization. Unpublished working document WHO/BS/82. 1367.

11
Collection, Transport, and Storage of Samples

John H. Livesey
Princess Margaret Hospital, Christchurch, New Zealand

By comparison with the vast literature detailing methods of hormone assay, relatively little attention has been paid to the collection and treatment of the sample prior to assay. This is despite the obvious fact that suitable collection, transport, and storage techniques are essential if an accurate estimate of a hormone concentration in a biological fluid is to be obtained. Because of the importance of correct procedures, this chapter will cover some general considerations regarding the obtaining and handling of samples. Specific information regarding particular hormones may be available in the literature pertaining to that hormone. However, well-documented studies, performed under appropriate conditions, on the effects of methods of collection, transport, and storage of hormone on assayable levels are not available for many hormones.

The laboratory to which the specimens are to be sent should always be consulted as to their specific requirements for collection, storage, and transport of samples for particular tests. They will often also be able to supply requisition forms and special containers for transporting specimens.

I. COLLECTION

A. Plasma/Serum

1. Ascertain whether the laboratory requires serum or plasma. Where there is a choice, plasma is frequently preferable, since clotting releases proteolytic enzymes.
2. For plasma, use the recommended anticoagulant. Heparin, for instance, interferes in some radioimmunoassays.

3. Avoid hemolysis when taking the blood, as hemolysis may increase the rate of degradation of peptide hormones or interfere in the assay. For example, both effects have been reported for insulin (1, 2).
4. Minimize venous stasis during blood collection, as stasis will, at least in principle, raise the concentration of peptides, protein-bound hormones, and calcium.
5. Keep blood samples for plasma in iced water prior to separation (lowering the temperature minimizes degradation of the analyte).
6. Separate the cells from the plasma promptly at 4°C in a refrigerated centrifuge or a centrifuge in a cold room.
7. If serum is desired instead of plasma, allow blood to clot at room temperature for 30 min in a glass tube and press down the clot.
8. Aliquot a sufficient volume (usually 1.5-2 ml) of plasma or serum into one or preferably two plastic tubes with secure watertight caps. Do not fill more than three-fourths full.
9. Enter the details on sample tubes and requisition forms with care, paying particular attention to patient and hospital identification, time and conditions of sampling (e.g., fasting, stress, posture, etc.), clinical details, and current drug therapy. The latter is particularly important as drugs may entirely alter the interpretation of a hormone assay result [e.g., many drugs cause hyperprolactinemia, renin determination may be affected by diuretics, and hypotensive therapy and glucocorticoids will affect adrenocorticotropic hormone (ACTH) and adrenal steroid results].
10. Freeze samples.

B. Urine

An aliquot of a timed 24-hr sample is usually required, although for some tests a spot sample (usually first morning) is suitable if the urinary creatinine concentration is also measured (3).

1. Provide the patient with a plastic 2-liter bottle labeled with the patient's name and the sample collection times. Providing women with a funnel may facilitate their use of narrow-mouthed bottles.
2. Instruct the patient to empty the bladder and discard the urine at, say, 8 A.M., to collect all urine in the bottle until 8 A.M. the following morning, and then again to empty their bladder, collecting the urine in the bottle.
3. Measure and note on the requisition form the 24-hr volume of the specimen.

4. Mix the specimen well, take a sufficient aliquot for assay, and store the aliquot at 4°C or frozen.

Determination of the 24-hr urinary creatinine output can be a useful check on the completeness of the 24-hr collection.

II. STORAGE

A. Plasma/Serum

Plasma and serum are usually stored frozen at about -20°C prior to assay. Although this is frequently satisfactory, plasma is not frozen solid at this temperature. It has been shown experimentally that it is partially liquid at least down to -35°C (4) and as the eutectic temperature for the system $NaCl/CaCl_2/H_2O$ is -52.5°C, even lower temperatures may be necessary to solidify plasma completely and prevent all chemical changes.

The pH of plasma rises on storage to 8-9 because CO_2 is lost, and this may influence the stability of plasma hormones.

B. Urine

Many steroids in urine may be preserved by acidification. Where the required pH is 2-3, buffering with an equimolar mixture of Na_2SO_4 and $NaHSO_4 H_2O$ (1 g per 50 ml urine) is more convenient and safer than the use of HCl (5).

Storage at temperatures of 4°C or lower will generally assist preservation. However, we have found that immunoreactive follicle stimulating hormone in urine is less stable at -20°C than at 4°C (J. H. Livesey, M. G. Metcalf, unpublished observations, 1981).

II. TRANSPORT

Samples to be transported within a few hours to a local laboratory can usually be sent packed in ice, as most peptide and steroid hormones are stable at 0-4°C in plasma for many hours. Ideally, if transport of samples to a laboratory will take more than a few hours, they should generally be sent frozen in dry ice in an insulated container. However, this is expensive, often not easy to organize, and unreliable if delays occur in transit. Ice cubes or packs made from 27 parts by weight KCl and 100 parts by weight water melt at -11°C and can be useful for keeping samples in a well-insulated container frozen. Plain ice cubes or commercially available ice packs that melt at about 0°C will not keep samples as cold, although they will last longer before melting.

Transport at ambient temperatures is convenient and is certainly feasible for human plasma samples to be assayed for luteinizing hormone, follicle stimulating hormone, and thyroid stimulating hormone and is probably possible also for growth hormone and prolactin but is not for insulin (6). However, there are few published studies for other hormones.

In some cases transport at ambient temperatures may be possible with the addition of a preservative. For example, addition of 0.002 M N-phenylmaleimide or potassium tetrathionate stabilizes insulin immunoreactivity in plasma buffered with 0.05 M ammonium phosphate pH 7.4 (J. H. Livesey, unpublished observations, 1979). Alternatively, and especially where transport may be prolonged or conditions uncertain, samples can be freeze-dried and sent at ambient temperatures. The original volume must be stated on the sample.

IV. TESTING OF STABILITY

Several approaches to the testing of the stability of samples are possible. If the judgment can be made that a certain average loss of activity, say 10%, is the maximum acceptable, then a number of different samples may be incubated under the conditions of interest for varying lengths of time. From the regression of the analyte concentration on time, the time required to attain an average loss of 10% can be estimated [see, e.g., Livesey et al. (6)]. Alternatively, the acceptable change in the mean concentration with storage may be defined as a multiple of the error of the analytical method (7). However, with either definition, if some samples deteriorate much faster or slower than the average, a good estimate of the length of time that a sample can be considered stable may not be obtainable.

A shortcoming of stability studies in which the method of analysis is any form of immunoassay is that the results obtained may be valid only for the particular antiserum used. This is because different antisera may have differing binding affinities for fragments or modified forms of the original hormone.

REFERENCES

1. Nerukar SG, Gambhir KK. Insulin degradation by human erythrocyte lysates. Clin Chem 1981; 27:607-609.
2. Ziegler M, Michael R, Hommel H, Klatt D. The interference of hemolysis on radioimmunoassay of insulin and its prevention by pre-incubation with anti-insulin serum. J Clin Endocrinol Metab 1972; 35:317-318.
3. Metcalf MG. Are 24-hour urine collections necessary for the measurement of steroid excretion rates? NZ Med J 1976; 84:150-153.
4. Simatos D, Faure M, Bonjour E, Couach M. The physical state of water at low temperatures in plasma with different water contents as studied by

differential thermal analysis and differential scanning calorimetry. Cryobiology 1975; 12:202-208.

5. Metcalf MG. Use of a sulphate: hydrogen sulfate buffer to preserve urine for steroid analysis. Clin Biochem 1978; 11:101-102.
6. Livesey JH, Hodgkinson SC, Roud HR, Donald RA. Effect of time, temperature and freezing on the stability of immunoreactive LH, FSH, TSH, growth hormone, prolactin and insulin in plasma. Clin Biochem 1980; 13:151-155.
7. Thiers RE, Wu GT, Reed AH, Oliver LK. Sample stability: a suggested definition and method of determination. Clin Chem 1976; 22:176-183.

MICROSCOPIC DIAGNOSIS

12

Chromosome Analysis and Buccal Smear

A. Caroline Berry
Guy's Hospital, London, England

Since full chromosome analysis is so much the more useful investigation, this will be described first. Success depends on obtaining a good number of dividing cells, as the individual chromosomes are only visible at metaphase, one of the stages of cell division. Any dividing cells can be used but blood lymphocytes are easily obtained and multiply rapidly once they have been stimulated by phytohemagglutinin so that whole blood is the specimen usually requested for chromosome studies.

I. BLOOD CULTURE AND CHROMOSOME ANALYSIS

As living cells are essential, any factors promoting either cell death or infection must be avoided and the laboratory must receive the specimen as fresh and as clean as possible. Lithium heparin and certain rubber stoppers are toxic, so that the choice of container is important and some laboratories prefer to receive the specimen in their own sterile heparinized bottle. Where a specimen has to be sent by post, it is important to ensure that it is kept sterile and sent so that it does not languish at room temperature over the weekend. Overnight storage in a domestic refrigerator preserves the cells satisfactorily, but deep freezing is lethal.

The lymphocytes are cultured by taking small aliquots of whole blood and adding them to culture medium and incubating at 37°C for 2½-3 days. Laboratories vary in details, but an outline of basic techniques is given in standard laboratory manuals (1,2). After incubation, the cultures are terminated. Colcemid is added for about 1½ hr to arrest the cells at the stage of cell division in order to maximize the number of metaphases present. Later the cells are harvested by a series of centrifugations and washings and the final suspension is used to make slides. Making good cell preparations is essential for accurate cytogenetic results and requires skill and experience in getting the chromosomes to spread out clearly.

Simple orcein stain can be used where only a chromosome count is necessary, but now that so many chromosomal abnormalities are recognized, even where the actual number is normal, most laboratories use the Giemsa banding technique (G banding), which allows identification of individual chromosomes and the delineation of small deletions, insertions, and rearrangements. G bands may be produced in a number of ways, but the most widely used method is that developed by Seabright (3). This involves brief treatment with a solution of trypsin prior to staining with Giemsa. A light microscope giving magnification up to ×1000 is used and analysis is a skilled, time-consuming, and labor-intensive procedure since no automation procedures have been successfully developed to match the accuracy of the human eye. One graduate technician should not be expected to read more than 15-20 specimens per week, and a further individual would be required to make the cultures and prepare the slides.

A. Abnormalities Detected

Of chief concern to the endocrinologist are those involving the sex chromosomes. Monosomy X (45X or XO) is readily recognized in those with clinical features of Turner's syndrome or ovarian dysgenesis and the 47XXY constitution of those with Klinefelter's syndrome is also easy to detect. Less frequent are women with testicular feminization syndromes and normal male chromosome complement, and even rarer is the Klinefelter-like male with a normal female chromosome complement. Equally important, although rare, are the intersexes.

More skill is required in detecting the various structural abnormalities of the X chromosome which may occur in girls with features of ovarian dysgenesis; an isochromosome (Fig. 1a) is made up of two long arms of the X only so that these individuals have altogether three long arms and only one short arm. It is interesting that clinically their features are usually indistinguishable from those with chromosome complement 45X. Deletions (usually partial) of either long (q) or short (p) arm may occur (Fig. 1b,c) and are of interest in that girls with deletions of the long arm tend to be taller than girls with chromosome complement 45X but only rarely menstruate, whereas those with deletion of the short arm may go into spontaneous puberty and menstruate but are always short. Attempts to relate the cytogenetic findings to the clinical features were initially made by Ferguson-Smith (4) and, more recently, by Teyssier et al. (5) and Fryns et al. (6).

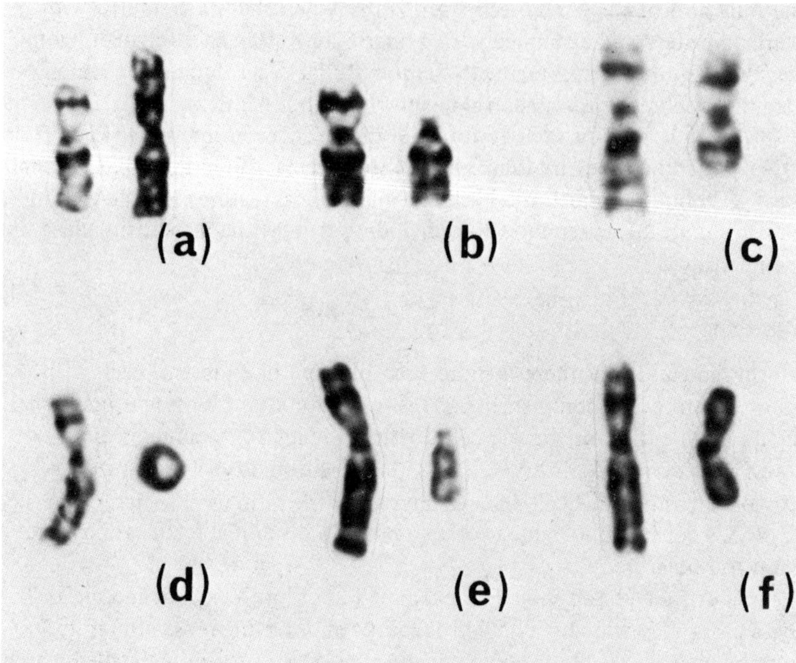

Figure 1 Normal X chromosome (left-hand member of pair) with (a) isochromosome of long arms of X; (b) X with deleted short arm; (c) X with deleted long arm; (d) ring X; (e) normal Y; (f) dicentric Y with the 2 Y chromosomes joined by their short arms. Note the varying size and shape of the normal X chromosome, which depends on the prevalent laboratory culture and staining conditions. The banding pattern remains consistent. (Courtesy of L. Kelberman.)

Occasionally, the X chromosome is present as a ring chromosome, the terminal portions having been deleted and the two ends joined (Fig. 1d). The larger the ring, the smaller the deletion and the less severe the clinical features. However, the ring tends to be unstable during cell division and many girls are mosaic with a second 45X cell line (see below).

Reciprocal translocations involving the X and an autosome must also be looked for as these too may present with features of ovarian dysgenesis since the normal X is preferentially inactivated (see below). Occasionally, only one X chromosome is present and a small fragment or marker chromosome is present instead. It is important to ascertain whether it represents a Y chromosome (Fig. 1e), since where ovarian dysgenesis occurs in the presence of a Y, gonadal malignancies arise in perhaps as many as 20% of cases (7).

The long arm of the Y fluoresces brilliantly when slides are stained with quinacrine mustard and examined with a microscope using an ultraviolet light source, but unfortunately, fragments frequently lack the fluorescent region. This staining technique is also useful in showing abnormalities of the Y chromosome such as deletions, or the two forms of dicentric Y chromosome (Fig. 1f); in one, two Y chromosomes are joined by the short arms, and in the other, by their long arms. In both, mosaicism is common and clinical features include varying degrees of failure of masculinization, including true hermaphroditism and a female phenotype.

B. Mosaicism

This term indicates that there is more than one cell line present, each with different chromosome complement. This will have arisen by nondisjunction occurring at an early postzygotic cell division, giving, for example, cell lines 45X/46XY or even 45X/46XX/47XXX. Iso X chromosome and ring X frequently occur with a 45X cell line. Chimerism is the term used to describe the 46XY/46XX constitution, which corresponds to a dispermic fertilization (e.g., of ovum and polar body).

How many metaphases should be examined in order to exclude mosaicism? Analysis of 11 cells will give a 95% probability of detecting mosaicism if 25% or more of the cells are chromosomally abnormal (8), but a more detailed search requiring the reading of 30, 50, or even 100 cells is necessary if one abnormal cell is detected. The discovery of one 45X cell among many normal ones can be difficult to interpret, as it may result from random cell breakage and be of no clinical significance.

C. Fibroblast Culture

This can be used for confirming the presence of mosaicism and has the advantage that such cells can be frozen down and stored in liquid nitrogen until required for research; but the cells are more difficult to culture and not all laboratories have this facility. These cells, which may be obtained from skin or gonad, require growth over several weeks before sufficient dividing cells are avilable for slide preparation. A small (2 mm) skin biopsy can be taken using curved scissors after freezing the skin with an ethyl chloride spray. It should be placed directly in culture medium such as Hams F10 and can be stored at 4°C or transported in this. Many solid tissue culture techniques have been described; summaries of methods in current use are given in standard laboratory manuals (1, 2).

II. USE OF THE ORAL SMEAR AND BLOOD SMEAR

The techniques described so far have all required cell culture and chromosome analysis which are time consuming and expensive. Two chromosomes can be distinguished in nondividing (interphase) cells and these are the Y and inactivated X chromosome(s).

A. Examination of Blood Smear for Y Dot

A blood smear is made on the microscope slide as would be done for hematological analysis. After fixing with methanol, the smear is stained with a fluorescent dye such as quinacrine mustard and examined using a microscope with ultraviolet light source. The fluorescent long arm of the Y appears as a fluorescent dot (Y chromatin mass) when present, so that this technique allows identification of this chromosome, if present, within a few hours of taking the sample. The most useful application is in cases of intersex at birth or in a survey for XYY males. Its reliability is limited by the fact that some (0.8%) (9) entirely normal men have a Y chromosome with only a very small fluorescent region, and occasionally parts of an autosome may fluoresce as brilliantly as the Y, so that both false positives and false negatives may occur and confirmatory chromosome analysis should be done if an abnormality is suspected.

B. Oral Smear

Where more than one X chromosome is present, one is inactivated and can be seen as a mass of heterochromatin (the Barr body or X chromatin mass) in interphase cells. Buccal squames are obtained by scraping the inside of the cheek with a metal spatula and smearing the material obtained over a microscope slide. It is fixed with methanol or a commercial spray fixative, stained with orcein, and the number of Barr bodies counted using a light microscope. They are not visible in every cell, so that about 100 cells must be examined and if the mass is found in about 25%, two X chromosomes can be assumed to be present, but there is individual variation in scoring. Two Barr bodies are seen in cells from triple X females and occasionally an experienced reader can distinguish that the Barr body is extra large in individuals with an Iso X chromosome. Although this technique might sound like a quick and cheap method for identifying those with Turner's and Klinefelter's syndromes, it is not accurate enough to be more than a screening test and confirmatory chromosome analysis is essential if abnormality is suggested by the oral smear. A further disadvantage is that those with structural abnormalities of the X chromosome may well have an entirely normal Barr body count, so that on the whole where the clinical picture is suggestive, full chromosome analysis is the better investigation.

REFERENCES

1. Yunis JJ (ed). *Human Chromosome Methodology*, 2nd ed. Academic, New York, 1974.

2. Schwarzacher HG, Wolf U, Passarge E (eds.). *Methods in Human Cytogenetics*. Springer-Verlag, Berlin, 1974.
3. Seabright M. A rapid banding technique for human chromosomes. Lancet 1971; 2:971-972.
4. Ferguson-Smith MA. Karyotype-phenotype correlations in gonadal dysgenesis and their bearing on the pathogenesis of malformations. J Med Genet 1965; 2:142–155.
5. [illegible] J-R, Bajolle F, Caron J. Complete deletion of long arm of X chromosome in woman without Turner syndrome. Lancet 1981; 1:1158-1159.
6. Fryns JP, Petit P, Van den Berghe H. The various phenotypes in Xp deletion. Observations in eleven patients. Hum Genet 1981; 57:385-387.
7. Simpson JL. Male pseudo hermaphroditism: genetics and clinical delineation. Hum Genet 1978; 44:1–49.
8. Bochkov NP, Kuleshov NP, Chebotarev AN, Alekhin VI, Midian SA. Population cytogenetic investigation of newborns in Moscow. Human Genet 1974; 22:139–152.
9. Lin CC, Gedeon MM, Griffith P, Smink, WK, Newton DR, Wilkie L, Sewell LM. Chromosome analysis on 930 consecutive newborn children using quinacrine fluorescent banding technique. Hum Genet. 1976; 31: 315-328.

13
Semen Analysis

Bengt Fredricsson
Karolinska Institute, Huddinge University Hospital, Stockholm, Sweden

The analysis of semen gives limited but useful information about the hormonal condition of the individual. Many steps are involved between the endocrine prerequisites and the end product, and these steps may be disturbed by several conditions (e.g., anatomical, developmental, infectious, and environmental). Nevertheless, patients with a normal sperm density seldom have disorders of the hypothalamic-pituitary-gonadal axis and a simple semen analysis is often easier to accomplish than more sophisticated endocrine tests.

This is not the place to give a detailed description of the endocrinology and hormonal regulation of the functions of the testes and the accessory genital organs. The reader is referred to the chapter on gonadal disorders and to appropriate surveys (e.g., Refs. 1,2). In summary, the Sertoli cell is stimulated by follicle stimulating hormone (FSH) and the Leydig cell by luteinizing hormone (LH). Inhibin and testosterone are responsible for the respective negative feedback control loops. Testicular steroidogenesis is not only quantitatively but also qualitatively under gonadotrophic regulation (3).

Although FSH stimulates the seminiferous tubules, the direct effect of this hormone seems to be restricted to the Sertoli cells. The germinative cells do not themselves produce any known substance exerting feedback on FSH production. High FSH levels characteristic of absence of germinative cells may be due to concurrent damage to the Sertoli cells. However, high intratesticular levels of testosterone are needed for spermatogenesis, in which prolactin also may play a role. Testosterone is transported to the seminiferous epithelium via the Sertoli cells. Damage to the blood-testis barrier seems to involve damage also to the Sertoli cells and hence results in disturbed testicular testosterone transport. A defective blood-testis barrier may also result in the formation of antispermatozoal antibodies.

The constituents of semen are for the major part derived from the accessory sex organs, mainly the seminal vesicles, which contribute about two-thirds. About one-fifth, in general the first part of the ejaculate, is derived from the epididymis. Hence the content of spermatozoa differs considerably between different portions of the ejaculate, in general being highest in the first. The process from the first meiotic division to the appearance of the resulting spermatozoa in the ejaculate may take 10 weeks or more, a period that includes morphologic and functional maturation and storage within the epididymis. An unsatisfactory semen sample may therefore be due to interference from disease or other events during this period. This must be considered by the clinician and multiple samples over a prolonged period may be required.

Semen analysis is most often requested because of infertility. Although self-evident, it should be stressed that the result pertains to the particular sample and does not implicate the retrospective or prospective fertility of the couple or the man and is not a diagnosis in itself. A poor result should be explained by further investigation if possible. A proper evaluation of the results needs sampling and analysis under standardized and well-defined conditions. A manual for the examination of human semen has recently been elaborated within the WHO (4). Some additional comments will be given here for the benefit of the clinician.

I. COLLECTION OF SAMPLE

A. Abstinence

The period of abstinence before sampling should correspond to the coital activity of the couple (i.e., in general 3-5 days). Long periods of abstinence may impose a higher degree of uncertainty to the evaluation than short periods.

B. Collection of the Semen Sample

The sample should preferably be produced by masturbation and the complete ejaculate collected. The different portions of the ejaculate differ in composition. Collection by coitus interruptus may be incomplete and is therefore inappropriate. The use of condoms is condemned as they may affect the spermatozoa, in particular their motility.

C. Transport to the Laboratory

For the study of sperm count, motility, and morphology the ejaculate may be produced at home and delivered to the laboratory within a few hours. For special studies the patient may have to produce the sample at the laboratory. The sample should be protected against cooling below room temperature at least before assessment of sperm motility. Patients living far away from the laboratory may deliver the sample to the nearby clinic, where motility and concentration is assessed and permanent preparations for the study of morphology and vitality can be made. The sample may be centrifuged and the seminal plasma frozen and transported when special tests are requested.

In a small number of cases the patient is not able or willing to produce a sample and a postcoital test will then give indirect information which may be of value.

In cases with aspermia (no semen), retrograde ejaculation may be the cause. The bladder contents should then be examined after orgasm has been achieved. Spermatozoa are as a rule immobilized in the urine unless this has been made alkaline (e.g., by previous oral intake of sodium bicarbonate).

II. ANALYSIS

A. Physical Characteristics

The volume of the sample is recorded. The presence of particulate material, inhomogeneity, abnormal color, incomplete liquefaction, or increased viscosity should be recorded. There are no simple methods to measure these variables objectively. Complete liquefaction should normally be achieved within 20 min from ejaculation.

B. Motility

The relative number of motile spermatozoa is evaluated in the microscope as is progressive motility. The evaluation is subjective and therefore often inaccurate (5, 6). The problem with the subjective evaluation can be overcome by employing photographic or other objective methods (7-9). The presence and type of spermatozoal agglutination (head to head, tail to tail, or mixed) should be recorded.

C. Sperm Concentration

Sperm concentration is determined in a hemocytometer after appropriate dilution in an immobilizing medium such as 0.4% formaldehyde (1 part 40% formalin in 100 parts distilled water), preferably brought to a neutral pH.

D. Morphology

Seminal smears are prepared. After fixation in ethanol, spray-cyte, or equivalent they can be stored and later stained using the method of Papanicolaou or similar staining technique. A differential morphologic count at high magnification (oil immersion lens) implies a subjective evaluation, and both normal range and clinical interpretation show local variation. The sperm head, midpiece, and tail should be examined. Different taxonomies are employed. In general practice, abnormalities of the head are allowed to "cover" abnormalities within midpieces and tails. The sum of the frequencies of the different abnormalities and normal spermatozoa is then 100%. It has been advocated, however, that the frequency of each type of abnormality is more of interest and therefore should be recorded irrespective of other abnormalities simultaneously present. In this way the sum of frequencies will exceed 100% (10).

E. Leukocytes

Leukocytes are frequently present. Their occurrence is best determined by counting their number per 100 spermatozoa in the stained smear. Knowing the sperm concentration, the number per cubic millimeter is easily calculated.

F. Vitality

Determination of sperm vitality may sometimes be of interest. This depends on the fact that all immotile spermatozoa may not be dead. Discrepancy between the figures of motility and vitality may have biochemical or immunological reasons. Vitality is easily determined after supravital staining with eosin in a buffered solution (11). Only dead spermatozoa take up the stain.

G. Biochemical Tests

Biochemical tests may be of value in selected cases. Fructose and prostaglandins are excreted from the seminal vesicles, acid phosphatase, citric acid, Mg and Zn from the prostate, glycerolphosphorylcholine, and carnitine from the epididymis. Although the secretory functions of these organs are hormonally controlled, interference from irregular emissions, infection, and benign prostatic hyperplasia renders their analysis of no value in the endocrine evaluation of the individual.

III. INTERPRETATION

A. General Comments

It should be remembered that the values of analysis relate to a particular sample and not necessarily to the individual's reproductive capability. The implication of normal or abnormal values in the strict sense may therefore be misleading. Normal does not mean fertile. The reference ranges given here (Table 1) are

Table 1 Evaluation of Semen Findings

	Normal	Abnormal
Volume (ml)	2-6	<1.5
Sperm concentration (millions/ml)	20-250	<10
Total sperm number (millions)	>80	<20
Motile spermatozoa exhibiting good progression	≥50	≤30
Morphology (spermatozoa of normal configuration, %)	>40	<30
Acid phosphatase[a] (mkat/liter)	>6.9	<4.2
Zinc[a] (mmol/liter)	1.2-3.8	<0.8
Magnesium[a] (mmol/liter)	2.9-10.3	<2.1
Fructose[a] (mmol/liter)	6.7-33	<4.4

[a]Biochemical borders are valid only if volume is normal.
Source: Modified from Ref. 10.

those generally employed. They are based on studies of samples delivered within a reasonable time of conception. However, the results in infertile males extend very much into the fertile reference range. This means that discrimination between fertile and infertile patients is often not possible by the variables of semen analysis. The reference ranges given indicate instead the cases in which further investigation or particular consideration may be worthwhile. Findings in the interval between the normal and abnormal values of the table are often difficult to explain clinically.

If a reproductive problem is present, in general more than one semen sample should be analyzed covering a period of at least 10 weeks, whereby proper consideration is given to the length of the spermatogenic cycle. Additional information of considerable clinical value is gained by penetration tests in vivo (the postcoital test) and in vitro (see below).

B. Volume

The major part of the ejaculate is derived from the seminal vesicles, and from the prostate gland to a lesser degree. Small volumes may indicate disorders of these glands but seldom have reproductive significance. However, in a few cases with retroflection of the uterus or a wide, voluminous vagina (e.g., after surgical removal of the rectum), a small volume may become crucial. A normal postcoital test will rule out this problem. If this test shows no penetration of spermatozoa into the cervical secretion, treatment by insemination with husband's semen is logical.

C. Sperm Concentration

There are indications of a decline of the sperm counts of fertile men during the past decades (12). However, sperm density shows very considerable intraindividual and interindividual variation (4, 13). Paternity has been proven in occasional cases with sperm counts persistently in the order of 1 million per milliliter.

D. Total Sperm Number

The total number of spermatozoa may be of greater clinical significance than the concentration, although proper documentation of this statement seems to be lacking.

E. Motility

Poor motility reduce the chances of conception significantly. The cause may be extrinsic or intrinsic. Varicocele, prostatovesiculitis, and environmental factors should be ruled out. Agglutinating or immobilizing antibodies may be present, particularly if progressive motility is poor or if vitality is much better than motility. No motile spermatozoa in spite of normal degree of vitality may indicate the presence of the immotile cilia syndrome (see below).

F. Morphology

The study of sperm morphology shows considerable local variation due to the subjective evaluation. Studies of sperm ultrastructure indicate that aberrations are more frequent than previously anticipated (14). If spermatozoa of normal appearance are few, the supravitally stained preparation can be used to assess the frequency of normal and abnormal spermatozoa within the live sperm population (15, 16). The photomicrographic technic of Makler may be used for the same purpose (17).

In general, the clinical significance of the different types of abnormality is not known. The presence of increased numbers of tapered sperm heads is considered to indicate stress to spermatogenesis (e.g., caused by infections, or associated with varicocele). Round sperm heads affecting all spermatozoa indicates a constitutional abnormality which imports sterility and cannot be treated (18). Increased numbers of coiled tails also reduces the fertilizing capacity of the semen (19).

If all spermatozoa are immotile although the cells are alive, this may indicate the presence of the immotile cilia syndrome. This condition cannot be treated.

It is due to absence of the dynein arms of the cilia and the diagnosis can only be settled by electron microscopy (20, 21). The condition also results in difficulties of clearing the bronchial tree, resulting in chronic bronchitis and bronchiectasis. About 50% of the cases also have situs inversus.

IV. COMMENTS

A. Aspermia

Failure to deliver a semen sample may indicate cohabitation difficulties but may also be due to side effects of medical treatment, or endocrine or metabolic abnormality (e.g., hyperprolactinemia may disturb male sexual potency).

Aspermia, no visible ejaculate in spite of orgasm, may indicate retrograde ejaculation, which in turn may have very different causes which merit thorough investigation. Motile spermatozoa may be recovered from the bladder as described above. These spermatozoa may then be used for insemination (22, 23).

B. Azoospermia

Azoospermia means complete absence of spermatozoa in the ejaculate. A congenital or acquired block of the excretory duct system is not uncommon. The endocrine balance is not disturbed and a testicular biopsy will reveal normal spermatogenesis. Defects within the pelvis affecting the ejaculatory duct and associated structures are as a rule characterized by the absence of fructose (derived from the seminal vesicles) in the seminal fluid.

High serum levels of FSH indicate the absence of seminiferous epithelium either due to secondary damage (e.g., previous mumps orchitis or congenital germ cell aplasia such as in Klinefelter's syndrome). This syndrome is frequently diagnosed first after the finding of azoospermia in the infertility investigation.

C. Low Sperm Counts (Oligozoospermia)

Patients with very low counts should be clinically examined and subjected to endocrine investigation. However, hormone estimations seem not to be helpful in patients with a sperm density exceeding 5 million per milliliter (24). The value of testicular biopsy remains to be proven, but it offers the possibility of studying the pattern of testicular steroidogenesis, which may be of interest not only in hypogonadal states (3, 25).

D. Normal Sperm Count

Moderate disturbances of thyroid and adrenal function, of glucose metabolism (diabetes), and of liver function may interfere with testicular function to a degree which may not be clinically overt or even indicated by commonly employed laboratory tests.

E. Functional Tests

There has been some concern about the significance of the apparently excessive numbers of spermatozoa in the ejaculate. No doubt, a significant number of spermatozoa are either immotile or dead, or anatomically or functionally defective. The crucial point is that no reliable criterion can be ascribed to the spermatozoon capable of fertilization. Functional tests have therefore been elaborated, of these the postcoital test and in vitro penetration tests are more or less indispensable in the infertility investigation.

No penetration of spermatozoa into a favorable cervical secretion suggests a poor prognosis for fertility and may be due to antispermatozoal antibodies within either man or woman. Good morphology of those spermatozoa which are found in the cervical secretion close to the external os speaks against a male cause of infertility (16, 26).

In vitro penetration into cervical mucus may be assessed quantitatively under standardized conditions (27). Cross-checking employing, in addition, donor semen and donor mucus will rule out if a poor result is due to a male or female factor. If bovine mucus (27, 28) or an artificial medium (30) is used, the test will be exclusively focused on spermatozoal function. However, these media are still under study and not yet recommended for general use.

Human spermatozoa are under certain conditions capable of penetrating zona-free hamster eggs, and it has been suggested that such a test can be used to characterize the fertilizing capacity of human spermatozoa (31-35). This test may be a valuable preliminary before attempting human in vitro fertilization.

REFERENCES

1. Burger HG, deKretser D, Hudson B. Spermatogenesis and its endocrine control. In *Human Semen and Fertility Regulation in Men,* Hafez ESE (ed). Mosby, St Louis, 1976, pp 3-16.
2. diZerega GS, Sherins RJ. Endocrine control of adult testicular function. In *Comprehensive Endocrinology, The Testis,* Burger H, deKretser D (eds). Raven, New York, 1981, pp 127-140.
3. Berg AA, Kjessler B. Effect of long term treatment with gonadotrophic hormones on in vitro metabolism of (^{3}H) progesterone in human testicular tissue. Int J Androl 1:53-60, 1978.
4. Belsey MA, Eliasson R, Gallegos AJ, Moghissi KS, Paulsen CA, Prasad MRN. Laboratory manual for the examination of human semen and semen-cervical mucus interaction. WHO, Geneva/Press Concern, Singapore, 1980.

5. Levin RM, Greenberg SH, Wein AJ. Clinical use of the turbidimetric analysis of sperm motility: comparison with visual techniques. Fertil Steril 1981; 35:332-336.
6. Amelar, RD, Dubin, L, Schoenfeld C. Sperm motility. Fertil Steril 1980; 34:197-215.
7. Jouannet P, Volochine B, Deguent P, Serres C, David G. Light scattering determination of various characteristics parameters of spermatozoa motility in a series of human sperm. Andrologia 1977; 9:36-49.
8. Makler A. A new multiple exposure photography method for objective human spermatozoal motility determination. Fertil Steril 1978; 30:192-199.
9. Katz DF, Overstreet JW. Sperm motility assessment by videomicrography. Fertil Steril 1981; 35:188-193.
10. Eliasson R. Analysis of semen. In *Comprehensive Endocrinology, The Testis,* Burger H, deKretser D (eds). Raven, New York, 1981, pp 381-399.
11. Eliasson R, Treichl L. Supravital staining of human spermatozoa. Fertil Steril 1971; 22:134-137.
12. James WH. Secular trend in reported sperm counts. Andrologia 1980; 12:381-388.
13. Schwartz D, Laplanche A, Jouannet P, David G. Within-subject variability of human semen in regard to sperm count, volume, total number of spermatozoa and length of abstinence. J Reprod Fertil 1979; 57:391-395.
14. Bartoov R, Eltes F, Weissenberg R, Lunenfeld B. Morphological characterization of abnormal human spermatozoa using transmission electron microscopy. Arch Androl 1980; 5:305-322.
15. Fredricsson B, Waxegard G, Brege S, Lundberg I. On the morphology of live spermatozoa of human semen. Fertil Steril 1977; 28:168-174.
16. Fredricsson B, Sennerstam R. Morphology of live seminal and postcoital cervical spermatozoa and its bearing to human fertility. Acta Obst. Gynec. Scand. (in press).
17. Makler A. Distribution of normal and abnormal forms among motile, non-motile, live and dead human spermatozoa. Int J Androl 1980; 3:620-628.
18. Anton-Lamprecht I, Kotzur B, Schopf E. Round-headed spermatozoa. Fertil Steril 1976; 27:685-693.
19. Eliasson R. Personal communication, 1981.
20. Afzelius BA, Eliasson R, Johnsen O, Lindholmer C. Lack of dynein arms in immotile human spermatozoa. J Cell Biol 1975; 66:225-232.
21. Afzelius BA. The immotile cilia syndrome and other ciliary diseases. Int Rev Exp Pathol 1979; 19:1-43.
22. Taylor CW, Shotton DM. Apparent aspermia due to retrograde ejaculation; successful insemination with semen recovered from the bladder. Stud. Fertil. 1955; 7:3-7.
23. Schirren C, Rehacek M, deCooman S, Widman HU. Die retrograde Ejakulation. Andrologia 1973; 5:7-14.

24. Wu, FCW, Edmond P, Raab G, Hunter WM. Endocrine assessment of the subfertile male. Clin Endocrinol 1981; 14:493-507.
25. Fredricsson B, Carlstrom K. Human testicular disorders: serum and urinary hormone patterns and in vitro conversion of (21-^{14}C,7-^{3}H)progesterone. Int J Androl 1979; 2:432-448.
26. Fredricsson B, Bjork G. Morphology of postcoital spermatozoa in the cervical secretion and its clinical significance. Fertil Steril 1977; 28:841-845
27. Ulstein M, Fjallbrant B. In vitro tests of sperm penetration in cervical mucus. In *Human Semen and Fertility Regulation in Men,* Hafez ESE (ed). Mosby, St Louis, 1976, pp 383-388.
28. Gaddum-Rosse P, Blandau RJ, Lee WI. Sperm penetration into cervical mucus in vitro. II. Human spermatozoa in bovine mucus. Fertil Steril 1980; 33:644-648.
29. Mangione CM, Medley NE, Menge AC. Studies on the use of estrous bovine cervical mucus in the human sperm-cervical mucus penetration technique. Int J Fertil 1981; 26:20-24.
30. Lorton SP, Kummerfeld HL, Foote RH. Polyacrylamide as a substitute for cervical mucus in sperm migration tests. Fertil Steril 1981; 35:222-225.
31. Barros C, Gonzales J, Herrera L, Bustos-Obregon E. Human sperm penetration into zona-free hamster oocytes as a test to evaluate the sperm fertilizing ability. Andrologia 1979; 11:197-210.
32. Binor Z, Sokoloski JE, Wolf DP. Penetration of the zona-free hamster egg by human sperm. Fertil Steril 1980; 33:321-327.
33. Overstreet JW, Yanagamachi R, Katz DF, Hayashi K, Hanson FW. Penetration of human spermatozoa into the human zona pellucida and the zona-free hamster egg: a study of fertile donors and infertile patients. Fertil Steril 1980; 33:534-542.
34. Hall JL. Relationship between semen quality and human sperm penetration of zona-free hamster ova. Fertil Steril 1980; 35:457-463.
35. Karp LE, Williamson RA, Moore DE, Shy KK, Plymate SE, Smith WD. Sperm penetration assay: useful test in evaluation of male fertility. Obstet Gynecol 1981; 57:620-623.

14

Vaginal Cytology and Endometrial Histology

Gabor Thomas Kovacs
Prince Henry's Hospital, Melbourne, Australia

I. VAGINAL CYTOLOGY

The first detailed report of the study of vaginal fluid smears during the sexual cycle in the guinea pig was by Stockard and Papanicolaou in 1917 (1). This was followed by several studies in rats, cows, and later monkeys.

During the 1920s, several articles appeared on the study of vaginal smears during the menstrual cycle in women, but it was not until 1933 that Papanicolaou (2) described the methodology for assessment of hormonal changes in "The Sexual Cycle in the Human Female as Revealed by Vaginal Smears," which is the basis for present-day cytological hormonal assessment.

A. Methodology

Stratified squamous epithelium is markedly influenced by hormones, and varies considerably during different phases of the menstrual cycle and during different stages of life. Therefore, the examination of the vaginal or buccal scrapings (cytogram) or exfoliated cells from the urinary tract (urocytogram) can be used as a bioassay to assess hormonal state. As this method measures the combined effect of several hormones on a target organ, and the sensitivity of this target organ is very variable, the results are not as reliable as those of direct hormone assays. Nevertheless, the cytohormonal assessment of vaginal smears has been widely used for the assessment of hormonal status, the diagnosis of ovulation, and to assess the response to ovulation induction (3).

On the microscopic examination of cytological specimens stained by Papanicolaou's stain, the stratified squamous epithelium can be divided into four characteristic cell types: (1) the primitive reserve cells, (2) basal and parabasal cells, (3) intermediate cells, and (4) superficial cells.

Estrogens promote the growth and maturation of stratified squamous epithelium up to and including the superficial layer. In the presence of high estrogen secretion (if unopposed by progesterone) superficial cells predominate.

The effect of progesterone on this epithelium, which has been matured by estrogen, is the rapid degeneration of the topmost layer and intermediate cells exfoliate as compact groups or clusters of cells, with few superficial cells being present in the smear. Progesterone alone promotes the storage of glycogen in squamous epithelial cells, producing a characteristic navicular appearance. For gynecological hormonal assessment vaginal wall smears are used most commonly. The cytohormonal patterns diagnosed on these smears can be quantitated in several ways.

1. Karyopyknotic Index

The karyopyknotic index (KI) is the number of pyknotic nuclei per 100 intermediate and superficial epithelial cells examined (4). The KI is zero if the epithelium is atrophic or during pregnancy. In patients who are on estrogen therapy or have estrogen-producing tumors, the KI is close to 100. During a normal menstrual phase the KI during the early follicular phase is between 0 and 32, at the preovulatory estrogen peak between 12 and 90, and in the luteal phase between 0 and 47. However, there are large individual variations from patient to patient.

2. Maturation Index

To determine the maturation index (MI), 100 squamous epithelial cells are classified as parabasal, intermediate, or superficial. The result is expressed as the ratio of parabasal:intermediate:superficial cells. A shift to the left means that parabasal cells predominate, whereas a shift to the right indicates a predominance of superficial cells.

3. Eosinophilic Index

To determine the eosinophilic index (EI), the number of squamous epithelial cells with an eosinophilic cytoplasm per 100 squamous epithelial cells examined is recorded. However, changes of pH and air drying prior to fixation influence the cytoplasmic coloring markedly. Therefore, the vaginal cytogram is less reliable when expressed this way. However, the EI is very suitable for assessment of urocytograms.

The changes in estrogen concentrations are best described by the KI. At ovulation there is a peak in both EI and KI followed by decrease in both after ovulation.

B. Clinical Applications

To obtain the most reliable information, the preparation, fixation, and staining of the smears should be carefully performed. The smear should be taken from the upper third of the lateral wall of the vagina, and care has to be taken not to contaminate it with cells from the cervix. The smear should be carefully spread so that it is even and thin onto a clean microscope slide. This should be immersed in fixative or covered with a spray fixative without delay. Fixation preserves the cells, prepares them for staining, kills bacteria and mould, and inactivates enzymes. If the cells are allowed to dry because of delay in fixation, the staining properties of the cytoplasm change. Staining is usually performed by Papanicolaou stain.

1. Cytohormonal Patterns at Different Stages of Life

From birth to the first 7 days of life, as sex hormones cross the placenta, the epithelium will provide a mature picture. From the second week of life to puberty, as no sex hormones are circulating, the picture is one of atrophy, with many parabasal cells being present. At puberty, the vaginal epithelium slowly reaches maturity. At first, many intermediate cells and superficial cells are evident as anovulatory cycles begin. The true progestogenic affect is not seen until sexual maturity.

Characteristic changes take place during the menstrual cycle. Days 1-5 during the menstrual phase, red blood cells, leukocytes, and endometrial cells predominate with some superficial and intermediate epithelial cells being present. During the proliferative phase, days 6-10 of the cycle, a large number of histiocytes appear, whose role is to clear up the debris. Intermediate cells are also apparent and toward the end of this phase the number of superficial cells increases. At ovulation, days 11-13, numerous superficial cells are seen and very few leukocytes or bacteria are present. During the secretory phase, days 14-28 of the cycle, intermediate squamous epithelial cells predominate. Within several days of ovulation the progesterone pattern appears with folding and clustering of the intermediate cells, the presence of navicular cells, leukocytes, and bacteria. Toward the end of the cycle cytolysis takes place, with many polymorphs being present. The KI increases and endometrial cells appear. In some women the progestogenic pattern is absent and only KI and EI point to the timing of ovulation. During pregnancy progestogenic pattern predominates, with the KI being less than 5. During the second month of pregnancy as the corpus luteum hands over hormonal production to the placenta sometimes a rise in the KI can be detected. This rise in KI seems to indicate that there is a threat to the pregnancy with inadequate progesterone production.

Prior to the onset of labor some women exhibit a rise in KI to 30 or so. This is said to herald the onset of labor, with a fall in progesterone production by the placenta. After the menopause, initially many intermediate cells predominate, but these are not folded nor do they form clusters. As aging continues, parabasal cells predominate, showing an atrophic pattern.

2. Use of Cytohormonal Assessment as a Reproductive Bioassay

Prior to the availability of urinary and plasma assays of estrogen and progesterone concentration, cytological assessment was the best method of assessing hormonal status (3). Today, with the development of radioimmunoassay methods, cytohormonal assessment has been mainly superseded. However, it may still be applicable in some situations. Vaginal smears can be taken by the patient herself daily if required, and stored until analysis can be performed. Thus it is suitable for patients in isolated areas. Its disadvantage is that the examination of the slides is very labor intensive and requires a highly skilled observer, and sets of slides are bulky and fragile.

It has been suggested by some workers that cytological assessment of vaginal smears is useful in assessing hormone replacement therapy during the menopause. However, as treatment of menopausal symptoms is symptomatic, and hormonal findings correlate poorly with symptomatology (5), cytology does not have much to offer in this situation.

II. ENDOMETRIAL HISTOLOGY

The menstrual cycle is the overt expression of the changing hormonal cycle of the female. Therefore, it is quite logical to utilize the endometrium as a gauge of hormonal function. The endometrium is also readily available and can be sampled with ease at curettage, and subsequently examined microscopically.

A. Methodology

Observations of histological changes of the endometrium appeared in the literature during the early twentieth century (6, 7). By 1920, Meyer (8) had established the preovulatory (proliferative) and postovulatory (secretory) patterns.

In 1935, Novak (9) described his suction-curet apparatus for endometrial biopsy without anesthesia. He called this the ovulation test, whereby a small amount of premenstrual endometrium is examined for secretory changes that only progesterone can evoke, thus confirming that ovulation has taken place and a corpus luteum has formed.

Vacuum curettage as an outpatient procedure without anesthesia was further refined (10) by using the Vabra apparatus.

By 1950, Noyes et al. developed a methodology to date histologically the endometrium within the menstrual cycle (11). They defined eight parameters which when examined in combination allowed accurate dating of endometrial specimens. These parameters are a combination of epithelial, glandular, and stromal detail:

Gland mitoses. These are indicative of proliferation and appear after menstruation and increase throughout the proliferative phase.

Pseudostratification of nuclei. This is characteristic of proliferation, but persists until active secretion begins.

Basal vacuolation. This is the earliest evidence that ovulation has taken place, and appears within 36-48 hr of ovulation.

Secretion. Secretions within the gland lumen become visible toward the midluteal phase, and decrease by the endluteal phase, as secretions become inspissated.

Stromal edema. Sometimes this appears during the proliferative phase also, but but is more constant during the middle and late secretory phase.

Pseudodecidual reaction. This appears around arterioles during the late secretory phase and progresses until just before menstruation, when the superficial compact layer forms.

Stromal mitoses. These are most abundant during the proliferative phase, absent during the midsecretory phase, but reappear during the pseudodecidual stage.

Leukocytic infiltration. During the cycle there are always a few lymphocytes present, but polymorphonuclear infiltration begins about 2 days before menstruation.

Using the foregoing criteria it is possible to date histologically endometrial biopsies into early, middle, or late proliferative and virtually to the day during the secretory phase. Noyes and Haman (12) reviewed the accuracy of endometrial dating using these criteria on over 1000 biopsies. Not only was there excellent correlation between endometrial dating when compared with menstrual date and basal temperature (60% within 1 day, 80% within 2 days), but also between the report by two different observers. They concluded that numerical endometrial dating was a sound and useful entity.

B. Clinical Application

The clinical application of endometrial histology in endocrinology is twofold. First its value in diagnosing that ovulation has taken place has been recognized since 1920 (8). However, this role has become less important by the development of assays of pregnanediol in urine (13) and progesterone in serum (14). Nevertheless, curettage is often combined with laparoscopy, and if this is performed in the luteal phase, endometrial histology can be used to confirm ovulation.

Second, Jones (15) described a syndrome of "luteal phase defect" (LPD), which she defined as inadequate progesterone secretion due to a defective corpus luteum. She suggested that this can be manifest as unexplained infertility or as recurrent first-trimester abortions. This syndrome has recently been reviewed (16) and the author maintains that the most efficient diagnosis of this syndrome is still by endometrial biopsy. She points out that although a basal temperature chart may alert suspicion about LPD, this is not reliable, and that many false positives will be diagnosed due to poor thermogenic response by some patients in the presence of normal progesterone levels. The only other alternative, collecting daily total urinary pregnanediol or serum progesterone levels, spanning the entire luteal phase, to detect statistical differences between normal and deficient cycles, is clinically impractical.

To make the diagnosis, a biopsy on day 26 of a 28-day cycle needs to be taken. This biopsy needs to be a full-thickness single swipe and should be obtained from the fundus of the uterus. The biopsy should then be dated and compared to the estimated day of ovulation and also to the onset of following menstruation. If the biopsy is more than 2 days out of phase, a repeated biopsy in the subsequent cycle should be taken, to confirm that it is a persistent phenomenon.

Although suggested treatment for LPD has included clomiphene citrate, human chorionic gonadotropin, and progestational agents as well as pure progesterone, Jones suggests that pure progesterone either by intramuscular injection or by pessary is the treatment of choice. For a recent review of the physiological and clinical aspects of LPD, the reader is directed to a review by Wentz (17).

REFERENCES

1. Stockard DR, Papanicoulaou GN. The existence of a typical oestrous cycle in the guinea pig with a study of its histological and physiological changes. Am J Anat 1917; 22:225-284.
2. Papanicolaou GN. The sexual cycle in the human female as revealed by vaginal smears. Am J Anat 1933; 52:519-637.
3. Murray M, Osmond-Clarke F. Pregnancy results following treatment with clomiphene citrate. J Obstet Gynaecol Br Commonw 1971; 78:1108-1114.

4. Pundel JD. *Acquisitions recentes en cytologie vaginale hormonale.* Masson, Paris, 1957, p 143.
5. James C, Breeson AJ, Kovacs GT, Grant C, Fry DE, Hill JG. The female climacteric—how much of a problem? (Submitted for publication.)
6. Hitchman F, Adler L. Monatsch Geburtsh Gynaekol 1908; 27:1-82.
7. Schroeder R. Arch Gynaekol 1915; 104:27-102.
8. Meyer R. Berl. Ges Geburtsch Gynaekol 1920; 27:2.
9. Novak E. A suction-curet apparatus for endometrial biopsy. JAMA 1935; 104:1497-1498.
10. Jensen JA, Jensen J. Abrasio mucosae uteri e aspiratione. Ugeskr Laeg 1968; 130:2124-2127.
11. Noyes RW, Hertig AT, Rock J. Dating the endometrial biopsy. Fertil Steril 1950; 1:3-25.
12. Noyes RW, Haman JO. Accuracy of endometrial dating. Fertil Steril 1953; 4:504-517.
13. Brown JB. A new method for the determination of oestrogens in urine and its application to a study of the oestrogen excretion in the menstrual cycle. Mem Soc Endocrinol 1955; 3:1-10.
14. Yoshimi T, Lipsett MB. The measurement of plasma progesterone. Steroids 1968; 11:527-540.
15. Jones GES. Some new aspects of the management of infertility. JAMA 1949; 141:1123-1129.
16. Jones GES. The luteal phase defect. Fertil Steril 1976; 27:351-356.
17. Wentz AC. Physiologic and clinical considerations. Clin Obstet Gynaecol 1979; 22:169-185.

BODY IMAGING METHODS

15
Photography

Stafford E. Brooks
North Canterbury Hospital Board, Christchurch, New Zealand

For the doctor fully to understand a patient, a mental picture is essential. Medical photography provides a record which is far more accurate than a subjective image based on frequently incomprehensible case notes and a fallible memory. The study of patients' photographs has several advantages. Repeated physical examinations by all those involved in the case may be avoided and previously unobserved signs may be apparent.

One or a series of clear, concise, accurately taken photographs can assist greatly in the diagnosis and treatment of patients, especially those with endocrine disorders (Figs. 1-3). Subsequent photographs provide a clinical comparison and an immediate assessment of any body or color changes (e.g. acromegaly, Cushing's syndrome, hypothyroidism). Serial photographs, (including those belonging to the patient) are particularly useful in assessing:

1. The development and progression of a patient's condition.
2. The age of onset of the disorder.
3. The severity of a patient's condition with reference to the normal appearance.
4. The family background. A photograph of relatives can often contribute to the doctor's knowledge of familial traits (e.g., short stature or facial features when abnormal growth hormone secretion is suspected).

I. TECHNIQUES

It is of the utmost importance that patients be fully informed by the doctor, and consent obtained, before full-length photographs are taken. The establish-

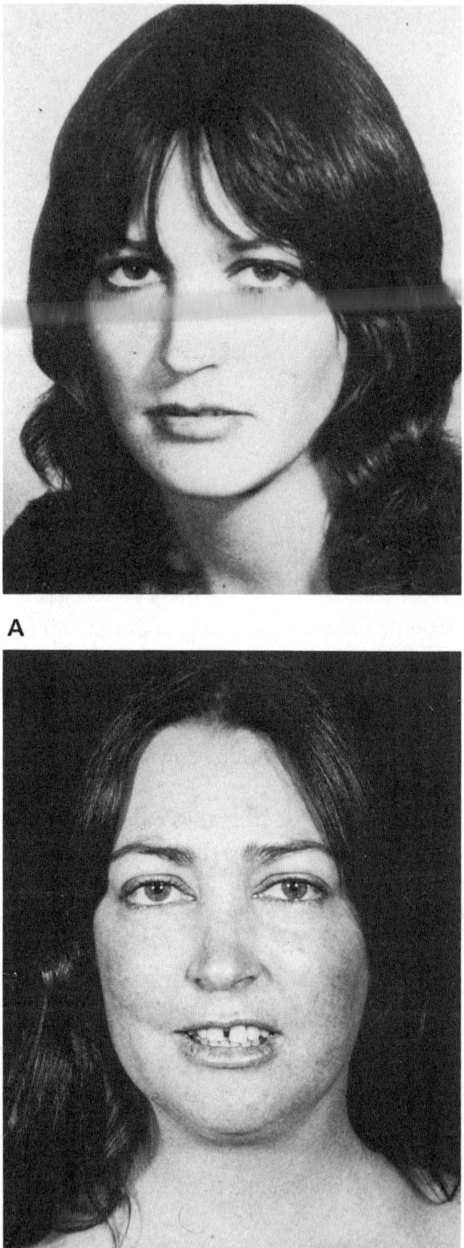

Figure 1 Cushing's syndrome. (A) Before onset of the disorder; (B) After onset and before treatment.

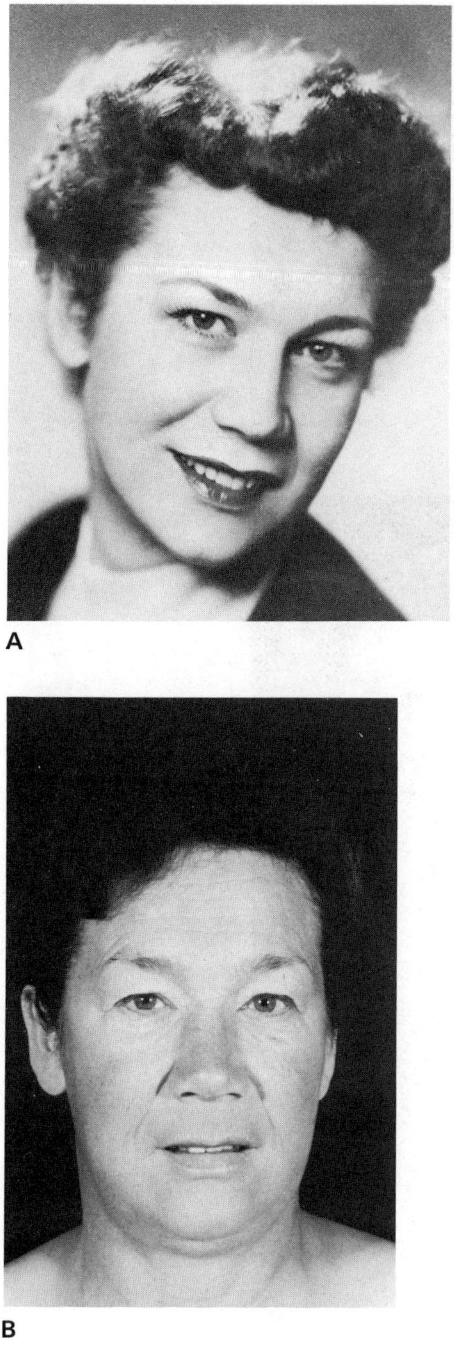

Figure 2 Hyperthyroidism. (A) Before onset of the disorder; (B) After onset and before treatment.

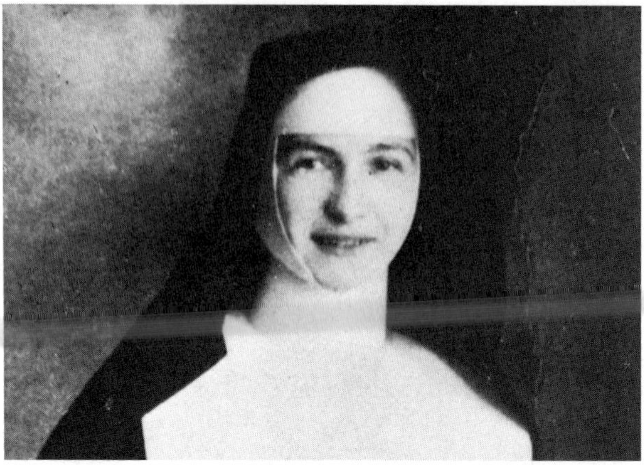

A

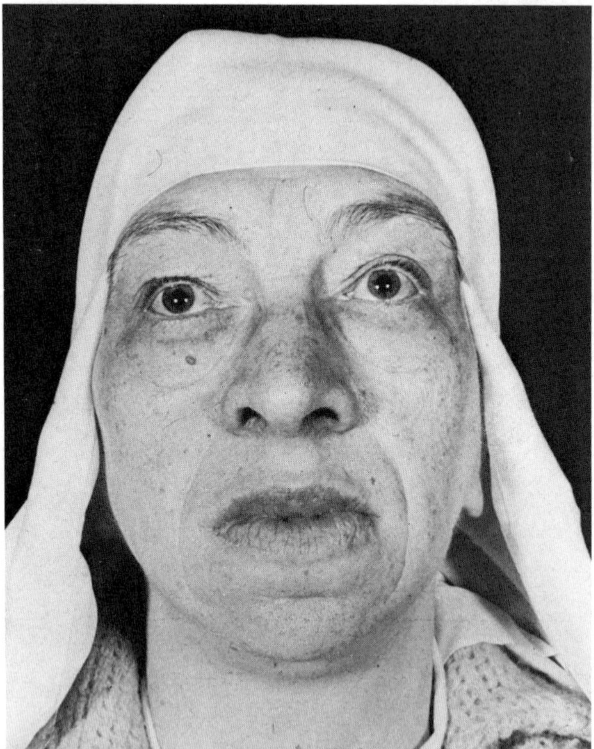

B

Figure 3 Acromegaly. (A) Before onset of the disorder; (B) After onset and before treatment.

ment of standardized methodology is essential. To ensure strict comparability, clinical photographs should be related in scale, size, and viewpoint from one patient to another and if possible from one hospital to another. Every patient who undergoes photography must be regarded as a potential candidate for subsequent serial records. For identification purposes it is suggested that a name and number be placed on the area of the negative which can be excluded in the print.

The following recommendations allow for easy measurement of any part of the body.

1. *Superimposing an accurately constructed standardized grid over the patient.* During printing, the grid positive is placed over the patient negative, ensuring that both negatives are lined up horizontally and vertically. By using black backgrounds the white grid gives clear-cut lines allowing easy measurement of any part of the body image, also eliminating shadows.
2. *Standardization of photographic techniques.* The camera tripod position should be permanently marked on the floor so that the exact position can be assured at any time. It is also essential to mark the position of the height scale and the position of the patient. The focal length of the lens and distance from lens to subject should be standardized.

The lighting position must also have permanent floor markings to ensure correct reproduction of exposure and color [essential when assessing pigment changes (e.g., Addison's disease)]. This relates especially to the main frontal lighting. Overhead and or back lighting is usually permanently fixed from the ceiling and does not appreciably affect the exposure or color balance.

Once the initial photographs are taken, an accurate record of the camera settings, distances, and so on, must be clearly set out on the patient's photographic requisition form. If there has been a variation from the accepted standard, exact photographs can be taken from the information on the form.

The retention of color balance from one negative process to another is extremely critical and difficult. Some suggestions may help to ensure this:

1. Control color processing within the photographic department and ensure strict adherance to every step of the process.
2. Ensure that the lighting and exposures are the same for all subsequent photographs.
3. Select one particular brand of color film and study its pecularities particularly from one batch to the other.
4. Use a color chart of three colors–white, red, and yellow–(or more if preferred) and place beside the patient when photographing changes in pigment.

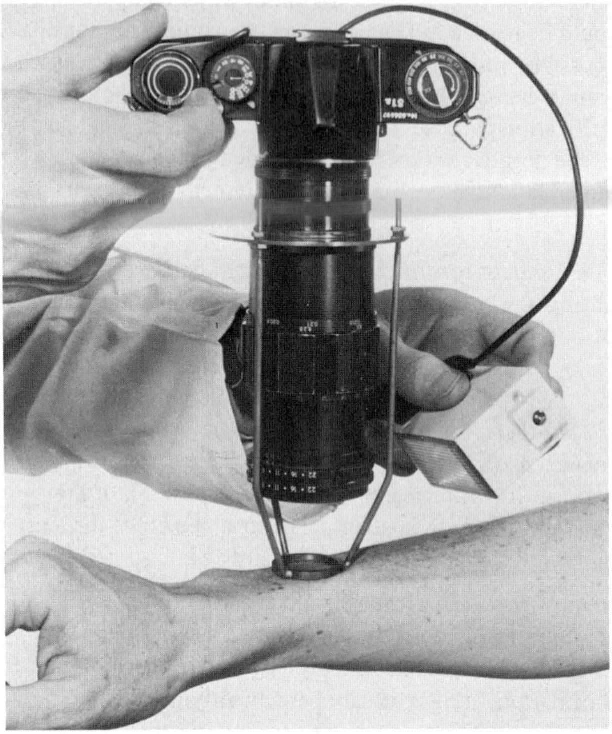

Figure 4A Hirsutism. The camera with extension rings and adjustable metal frame.

Satisfactory filing particularly of color transparencies is an important function of the photographic department. Provision for easy access and viewing is a major factor. This can be achieved by using a clear plastic holder especially manufactured to contain 20 transparencies and to fit the standard filing cabinet with a steel rod through the sleeve at the top of the holder. A complete file containing color transparencies of pathological specimens, old photographs, x-rays, and photographs of the patients can be observed in one glance by laying the holder over a viewing box. Finally, accurate coding of transparencies under the international code system facilitates the review of patients with a similar diagnosis.

II. SPECIAL TECHNIQUES

A. Hirsutism

A method of measuring hair growth rate has been developed based on repeated photographs with a special device. A tripod with built-in scale attached to the front of the camera largely eliminates errors of magnification and allows for accurate assessment of increase in length, diameter, bulk, and type of hair with no discomfort to the patient. It has been found that abnormal facial hirsutism in women is readily detected and assessed by this method.

Figure 4A shows the camera with extension rings and how the adjustable metal frame with the graduated ocular eye piece is fixed between extension tube 3 and the Macro-Takumar 1:4/50 mm fully extended lens. Figure 4B shows an example of photographs taken from the facial site in a hirsute woman, indicating hair growth over a 4-day period.

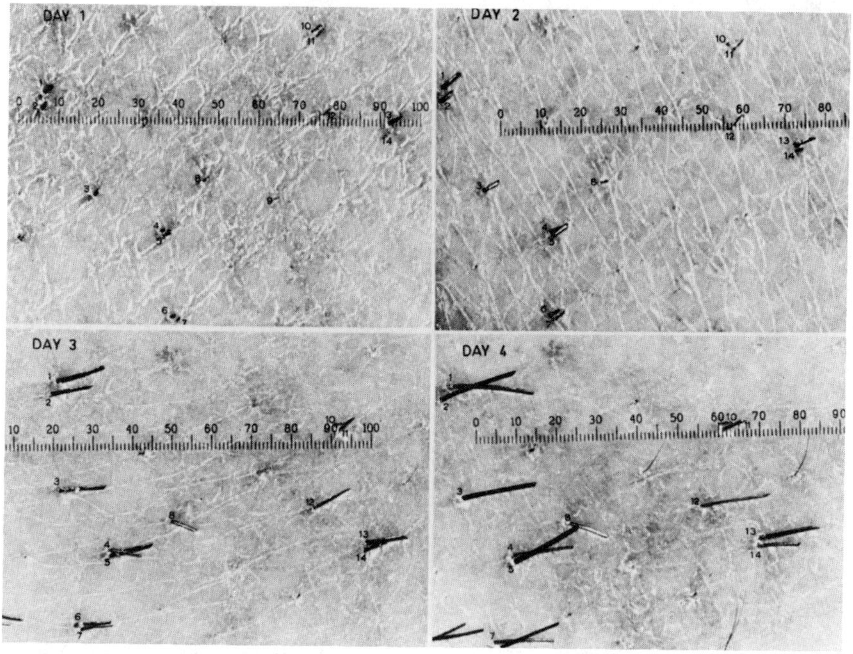

Figure 4B Photographs from a facial site in a hirsute woman, indicating hair growth over a 4-day period.

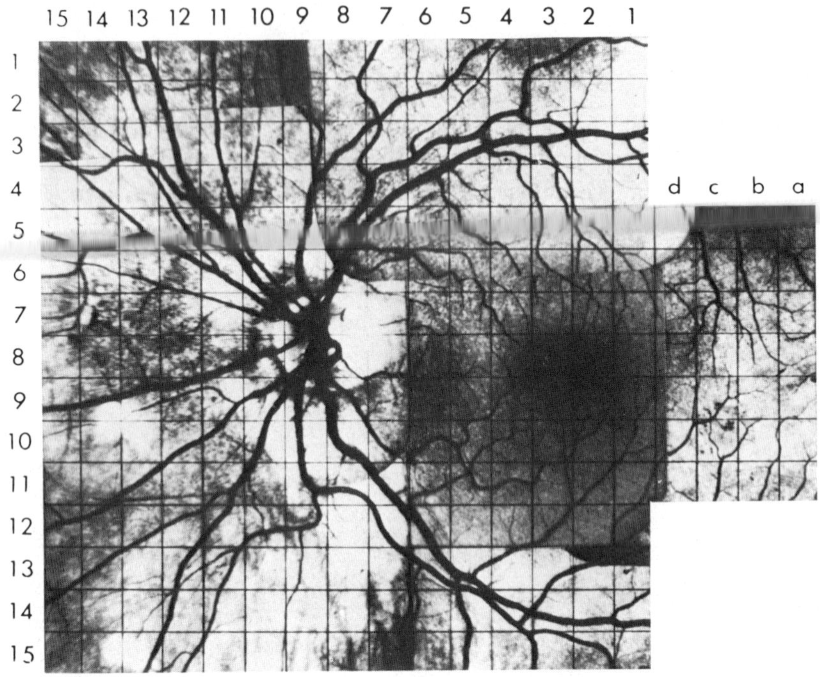

Figure 5 Photomontage of retinal photographs with superimposition of a grid to permit accurate quantitation of fundal abnormalities.

B. Infrared Photography

Black and white infrared photography has the ability to reveal vascular and other lesions more clearly than ordinary photography or visual observations. Color infrared photography extends the usefulness of the technique by introducing modified colors. There are many applications in research and diagnosis for this branch of medical photography (1).

C. Retinal Photography

Retinal photography, with or without the use of fluorescein, provides an objective record, particularly of the diabetic and hypertensive changes which are of interest to the endocrinologist. Photographs covering a 30° area of the retinal fundus are taken through the dilated pupil. A photomontage can be constructed from individual photographs, and superimposition of a grid allows accurate quantitation of fundal abnormalities (2) as shown in Figure 5. To provide a more detailed picture of the retinal vasculature, 10 ml of 10% fluorescein dye may be injected into an antecubital vein. Repetitive photographs are then taken with a fundus camera using a light source of the appropriate wavelength to excite fluorescence of the dye. Capillary dilatation, microaneurysms, capillary closure and leakage, and new vessel formation are seen in Figure 6.

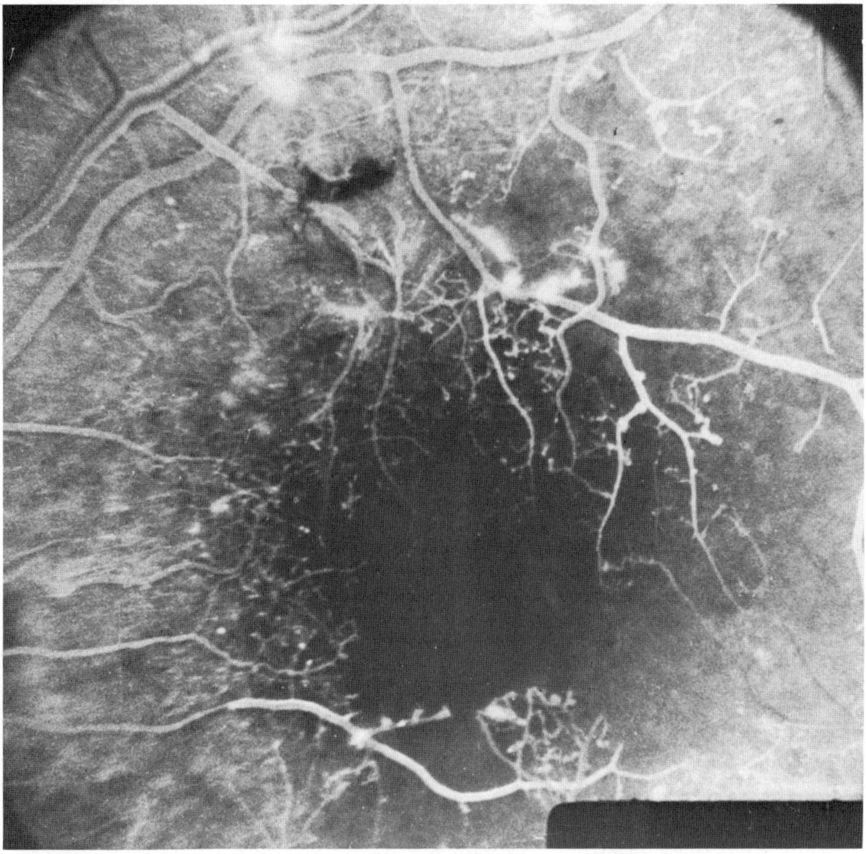

Figure 6 Fluorescein retinal photograph showing capillary dilatation, microaneurysms, capillary closure and leakage, and new vessel formation.

REFERENCES

1. Kodak. *Medical Infrared Photography.* Kodak Medical Publ No 1, Rochester, NY, 1967.
2. Parr JC, Spears GFS. Grading of diabetic retinopathy by point-counting on a standardised photographic sample of the retina. Am J Ophthalmol 1972; 74:459-465.

General Sources

Jacobson RE, Ray SF, Attridge GG, Axford NR. *The Manual of Photography* (formally *The Ilford Manual of Photography*). Focal Press, New York, 1978.

Langford MJ. *Basic Photography.* Focal Press, New York, 1971.

Langford MJ. *Advanced Photography.* Focal Press, New York, 1971.

Ollerenshaw R. *Longmore's Medical Photography.* Focal Press, New York, 1962.

16
Radiology and Ultrasound

A. Brian Ayers
St. Thomas' Hospital, London, England

In recent years the advent of computerized tomographic (CT) scanning and ultrasound has led to a reappraisal of the increasing role of radiology in the investigation of patients with endocrine disorders. However, these new techniques are not always universally available and traditional simple investigations can still give considerable information.

In general, radiology can assist the clinical endocrinologist in two major ways: First, it may demonstrate generalized changes which are subsequent to hormonal disturbance, and second, it can be used to identify local changes produced by enlargement of a particular endocrine gland. The recent advances in resolution of CT scanning and ultrasound have paid particular dividends in identifying local changes in an easier and less hazardous manner than the previous methods used.

I. PLAIN RADIOGRAPHS

A. Local Effects

1. Pituitary (1)

Initial investigation of patients with suspected pituitary or parapituitary tumors must include high-quality radiographs of the skull in true lateral projection supported by coned lateral, antero posterior (AP), and Towne's views of the pituitary fossa. In a true lateral film the anterior clinoid processes are exactly superimposed. The AP film is taken with a 7-8° tilt to project the petrous ridges into the lower third of the orbits. This view shows the floor. On the Towne's

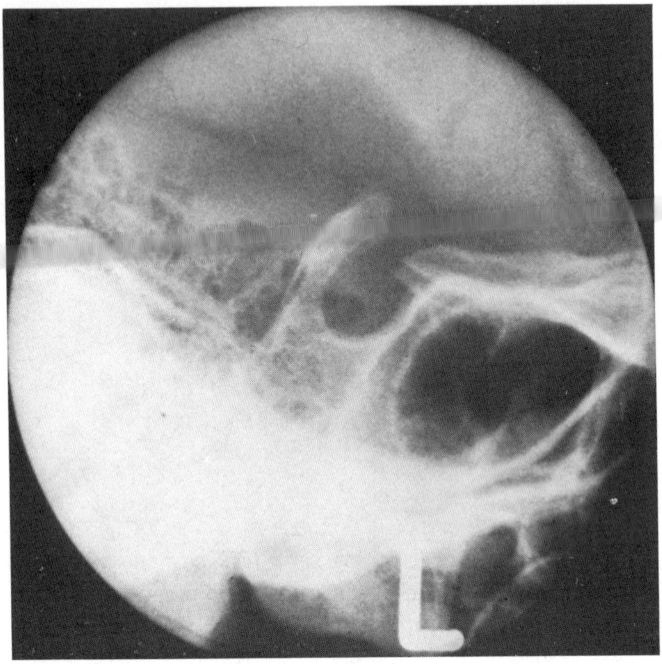

(a)

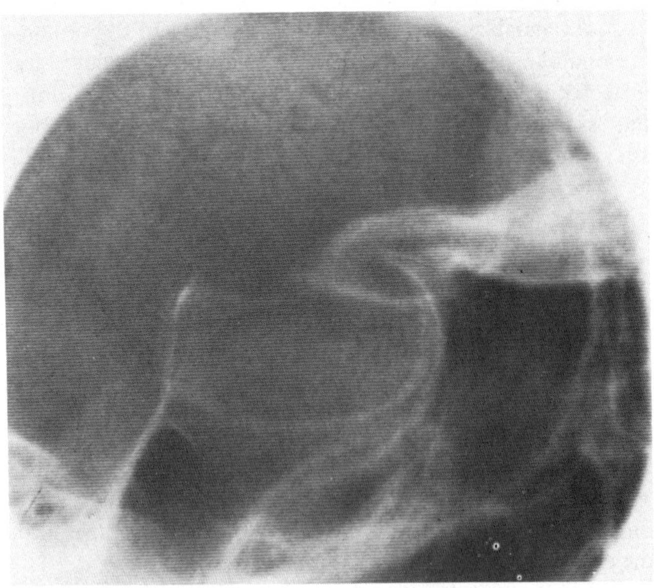

(b)

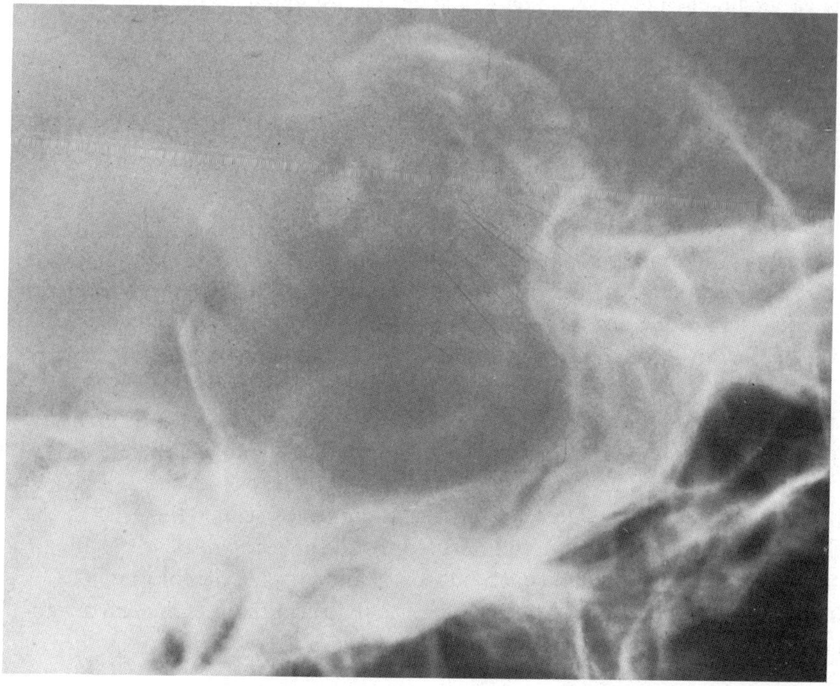

(c)

Figure 1 (a) Normal pituitary. Plain lateral. (b) Enlarged fossa–acromegaly. Lateral radiograph showing double floor anteriorly with erosion of margin inferiorly. (c) Craniopharyngioma. Lateral radiograph showing grossly enlarged fossa and extensive suprasellar calcification.

projection the dorsum sellae and posterior clinoid processes are projected into the foramen magnum or over the occipital bone. The radiographic signs to be identified are calcification, expansion of the fossa, erosion of the clinoid processes, and alterations in contour of the sella (Fig. 1).

Calcification is best visualized in the lateral view, but its midline position may be difficult to see on the other views. Tomography will be helpful in these cases, as it is important not to confuse calcification in other adjacent structures such as the carotid arteries with true pituitary or parapituitary tumor calcification. Calcification is most commonly seen in craniopharyngiomas.

The dimensions of the pituitary fossa can be measured from the three coned views by measuring the height, width, and AP diameters. Comparison of films from different centers may be difficult due to magnification factors produced by varying radiographic techniques, and in practice, these measurements are found to be of limited value, as by the time they become abnormal other fossa changes are obvious.

Erosion of the clinoid processes should be sought both in the lateral and frontal projections. The anterior clinoids can be best visualized on the AP film and the posterior clinoids on the Towne's view. Erosion commonly occurs with craniopharyngiomas. However, large suprasellar extensions of pituitary tumors may occur without erosion of the clinoid processes–"dumbbell" tumors. Erosion of a single process is a good localizing sign.

Pituitary tumors often initially cause asymmetry of the margins of the fossa by expansion producing the "double-floor" sign on the lateral film, with one part of the floor extending farther into the sphenoid bone or air sinus than the other. This should be confirmed by examining the floor of the fossa on the AP film using the anterior clinoid processes as anatomical landmarks. Asymmetry of the floor can, however, be seen in normal patients due to anatomical variations in shape (1). Categorization of the shape of a fossa as advocated by Doyle (1) is a most useful practice, with the final significance being influenced by the clinical findings. A further useful indicator of the presence of tumor is thinning or interruption of the lamina dura, but this is more readily demonstrated by tomography (see above). The value of the radiological findings in microadenomas has recently been reviewed (2).

2. Thyroid

Local radiographic examination of the thyroid requires three films: one AP and two lateral films of the neck. One lateral film is taken to show the soft tissues, while the second is a penetrated film.

Calcification is best identified on the soft tissue lateral film with the AP film used for localization. Calcification is most commonly seen in adenomas of the thyroid but is a well-recognized, although uncommon feature of malignant tumors. Attempts have been made to correlate the nature of the calcification with the histological type, but this is not entirely reliable (3). The lateral soft tissue film is useful also for the examination of soft tissue enlargement, particularly involving the isthmus. On the AP film soft tissue enlargement is often seen to be asymmetrical. The penetrated lateral film is taken to identify the lower limit of any retrosternal thyroid enlargement. The AP and lateral films are used in conjunction to detect local effects on the trachea which may be displaced, usually laterally, and/or stenosed by the enlarged thyroid.

3. Parathyroid

It is uncommon for parathyroid tumors to enlarge sufficiently to cause a local soft tissue mass, but when they do the effects are similar to those caused by localized thyroid enlargement and the same films are required. Calcification is not a feature.

4. Adrenals

Plain films of the upper abdomen may reveal a small area of calcification above the renal outline in one or both adrenal glands as an asymptomatic finding. Calcification may also be seen in relation to adrenal carcinoma or pheochromocytoma in a minority of cases. Rarely, a local mass effect will be seen with large tumors when the upper pole of either kidney is displaced laterally and downward.

5. Pancreas

Local effects in diseases of the endocrine pancreas are unusual. Calcification and pseudocysts secondary to pancreatitis are not specifically linked to endocrine disturbances and adenomas rarely reach a size to have plain film effects.

6. Miscellaneous

Chest radiographs are an important part of the endocrinological assessment, particularly in relation to the heart and thyroid (Fig. 2), but one must always remember that pulmonary and mediastinal tumors are one of the most common causes of ectopic hormone production. Calcification of carcinoid tumors, although uncommon, may be seen on abdominal radiographs.

B. General Effects

1. Skeletal

The skeleton is frequently affected by endocrine disturbances, particularly in the young, as normal growth requires many hormonal factors. Growth may be retarded in hypopituitarism or hypothyroidism or become excessive in juvenile acromegaly. Maturation of the long bones may be delayed in hypogonadism. The most useful method to assess bone age is to take a hand radiograph including the wrist and to compare the development of the bones on it with a set of standard films (4). Other more sophisticated methods exist, but this method is quick and easy and sufficiently accurate for most requirements. Films of the knees are useful additions when it is important to assess the remaining growth potential of the metaphyses before or during therapy. Early fusion and maturation occurs in hyperthyroidism and the adrenogenital syndrome.

Other skeletal abnormalities may be seen in cretinism on radiographs of the spine (Fig. 3a), hips, and knees (5). The vertebrae may be "tongue-shaped," simulating the changes seen with the mucopolysaccharidoses. Epiphyseal ossification is delayed and irregular, particularly involving the capital femoral and distal femoral epiphyses. Coxa vara may also be present.

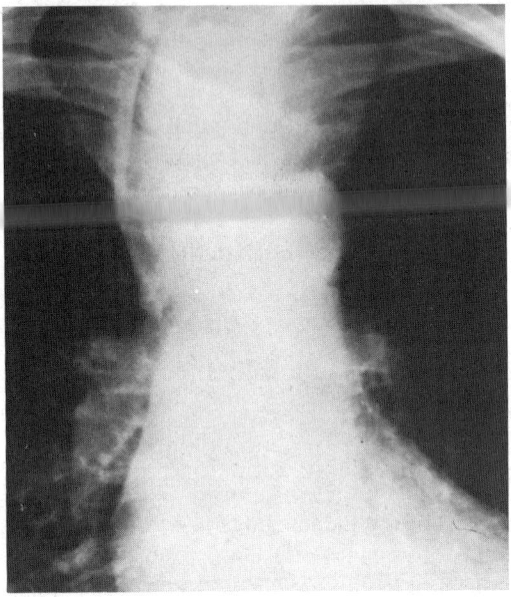

Figure 2 PA chest radiograph. The trachea is bowed to the right by a soft tissue mass representing an enlarged thyroid.

Lateral radiographs of the lumbar spine are used in patients suspected of osteoporosis (Fig. 3b), whether this is related to Cushing's disease or thyrotoxicosis. The radiological diagnosis of osteoporosis is difficult unless gross. The early signs of demineralization and cortical thinning are subjective and can be greatly influenced by technical factors. Specific methods for measuring bone density or cortical thickness are insensitive. The changes are also age related, particularly in females who undergo an early menopause. Vertebral collapse and rib fractures are more common in osteoporosis than in other forms of metabolic bone disease.

Demineralization of the skeleton and pathological fractures may also be present in hyperparathyroidism, but this is associated with trabecular changes and subperiosteal bone resorption, which is commonly found in the phalanges of the hands (Fig. 3c), the lateral ends of the clavicles, the symphysis pubis, and the ischial tuberosities. It is always true that a radiological opinion is limited by the quality of the radiographs, but this is never more true than when taking hand radiographs for metabolic bone disease. The finest-quality PA film is always essential using a very fine focal spot tube and film or film screen combinations designed for high definition (6). The earliest changes may require a magnifying glass and will be seen on the ulnar margins of the proximal and middle phalanges of the second and third fingers. Larger areas of trabecular bone resorption occur in flat and long bones, giving the "cystic" appearances of osteitis fibrosa cystica and are more common in primary than secondary hyperparathyroidism (Fig. 4). Sclerosis of these areas may occur after removal of the primary adenoma. Sclerosis is also a feature of renal osteodystrophy when the effects of bone resorption and sclerosis produce the pathognomonic "rugger-jersey" spine best identified on lateral films of the lumbar and thoracic spine (Fig. 3c). Cortical striation in the phalanges and metacarpals may also be evident, particularly in secondary hyperparathyroidism associated with osteomalacia (7).

One oddity is seen in the hand radiographs of patients who have been treated, usually by thyroidectomy, for thyrotoxicosis and consists of a florid periosteal reaction laying down layers of bone tangential to the metacarpal shafts. It is termed thyroid acropachy (Fig. 5d) (8).

Hand radiographs may also reveal changes in acromegaly (Fig. 5b), in which an increase in soft tissue thickness, an increase in the joint spaces, exaggeration of the musculotendinous insertions, and prominent terminal tufts are seen. The vertebrae may also be seen to have an increased AP diameter in florid acromegaly, but this is not a particularly sensitive sign.

AP radiographs of the feet will also show the changes described in the hands in hyperparathyroidism, acromegaly, and osteoporosis. In addition, oblique views are useful in demonstrating osteoarthritic changes at the tarsometatarsal joints, which may be severe in Cushing's syndrome or when associated with the peripheral neuropathy of diabetes mellitus. Charcot-type joints are also seen in the spine, hips, and knees. In addition, both these diseases are associated with an increased incidence of bone infection, which often involves the feet and may lead to bony ankylosis. Local areas of bone lysis are seen often associated with a periosteal reaction, although this may be absent in Cushing's disease.

Malignant tumors, particularly of the thyroid and adrenal glands, metastasise to bone and radiographs of the long bones, vertebrae, and ribs form the normal basis of a skeletal survey when metastases are suspected. The deposits are usually lytic with no significant bone reaction. Thyroid metastases are often large and are known to cause expansion of bone.

3. Soft Tissues

The soft tissue images on radiographs are often neglected with regret. Calcification in the soft tissues may be seen in a number of circumstances.

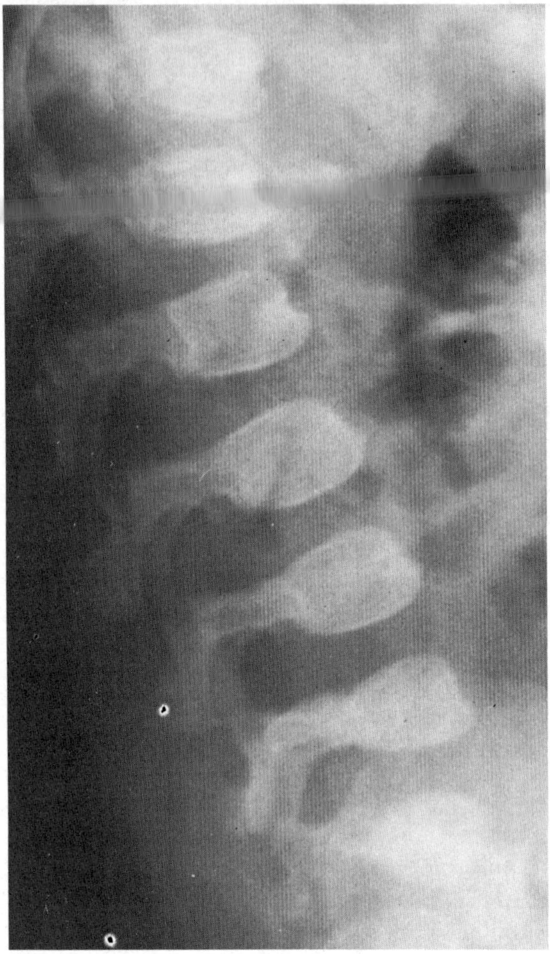

(a)

Figure 3 (a) Cretin. Lateral radiograph of lumbar spine showing deformity of the vertebral bodies. (b) Osteoporosis. Demineralization, "pencilled" cortices and partial vertebral collapse are shown. (c) Renal osteodystrophy. Rugger-jersey spine.

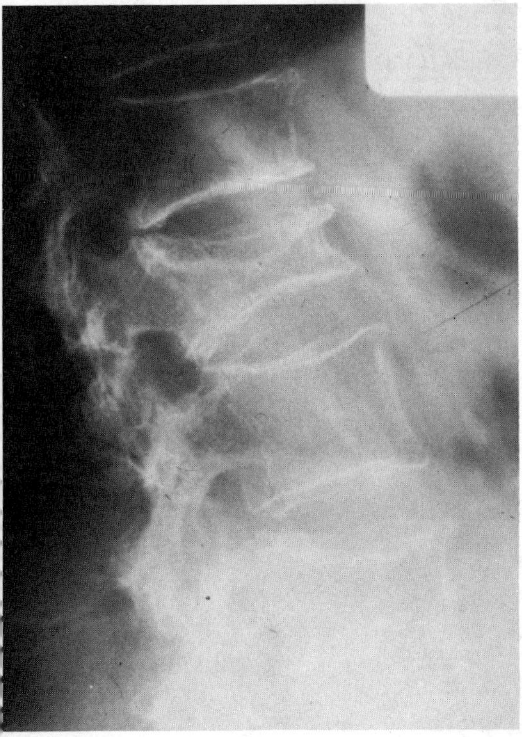

(b)

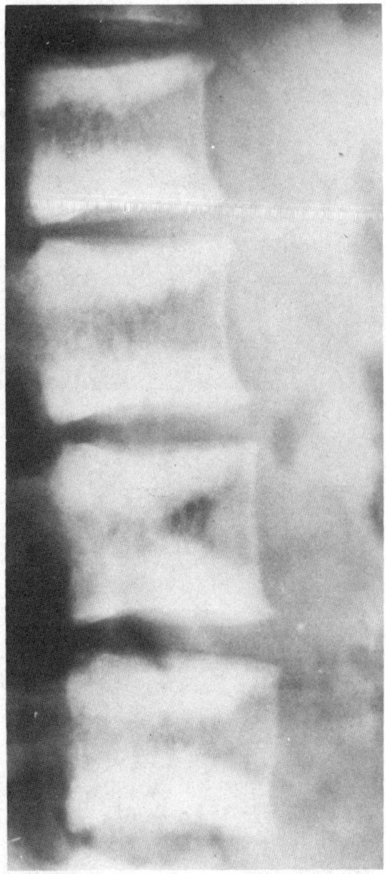

(c)

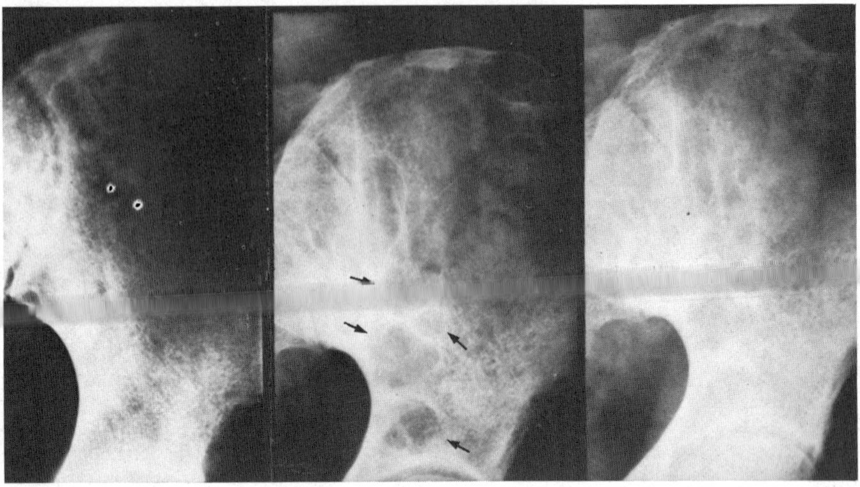

(a)

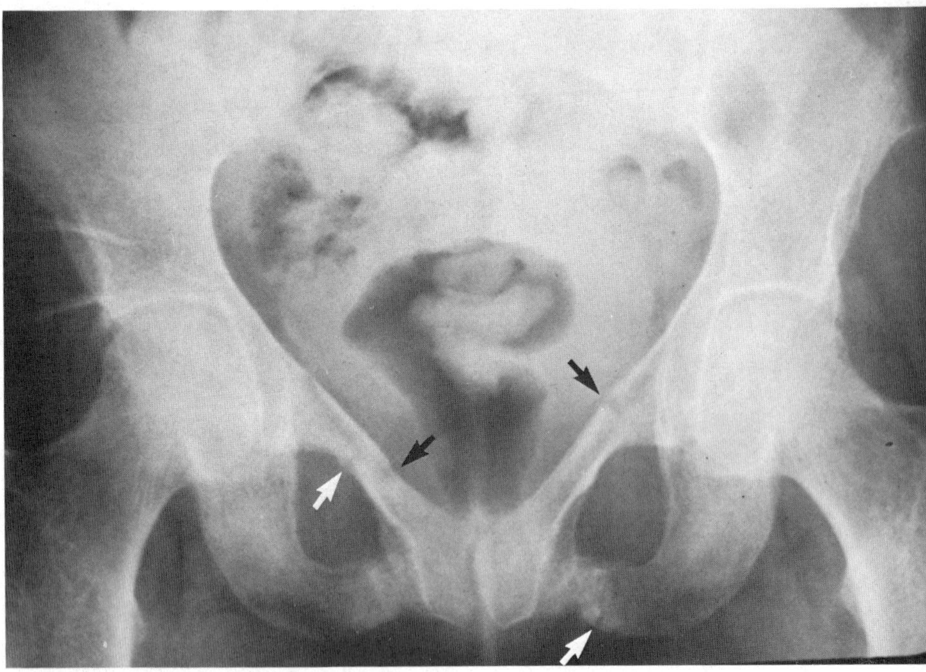

(b)

Figure 4 (a) Primary hyperparathyroidism. Coned views of left ilium, 1970, 1974, 1976, showing formation of the brown tumor followed by sclerosis of the margins following removal of a parathyroid adenoma in 1973. (b) Osteomalacia. Deformed pelvis with Looser's zone in both superior and inferior pubic rami.

Calcification of the large arteries from atheroma is a common feature in non-endocrine patients but is seen more floridly in diabetes mellitus. Calcification of the medium-sized and small arteries is seen extensively in diabetes mellitus, indicating Monckeberg's sclerosis. This is classically identified in the dorsalis pedis artery on radiographs of the feet. Similar arterial calcification is seen in the lower legs and forearms in patients with hyperparathyroidism. Periarticular soft tissue calcification is also a feature of renal hyperparathyroidism and may come and go quite quickly on dialysis. It is often painful.

Joint radiographs of the knees, wrists, or shoulders may reveal fine linear calcification in the cartilage called chondrocalcinosis and is seen following hypercalcemia, or Cushing's disease. Extensive fine linear calcification may be seen bilaterally in the pelvis in the vas deferens and is virtually seen only in tuberculosis and diabetes mellitus.

Two other soft tissue changes are very important. First, radiographs are often taken of an area related to a superficial ulcer in diabetes mellitus to look for evidence of osteomyelitis. These are usually radiographs of the feet and lower limbs. A specific effort must also be made to examine the soft tissues for evidence of bubbles of gas, which indicate the serious complication of anerobic infection. Of course, some air is seen in the soft tissue when an ulcer is present, but it should not track along the fascial or intramuscular planes. As the radiographs are usually taken to look at the adjacent bone, the soft tissues are overexposed and a bright light may well be required.

It has already been pointed out that the soft tissues become thickened in patients with acromegaly. This increase in thickness is best documented as the heel pad thickness, for which a lateral film of the heel is required using a focal-film distance of more than 3 ft to prevent magnification and care being taken not to disturb the soft tissues, in particular not to compress them (9). Measurement is made between the skin surface and the lowest part of the calcaneum. Excluding patients who habitually walk barefoot, the upper limit of normal is 23 mm. Acromegalics often demonstrate a heel pad thickness greater than this usually in the 30s but occasionally greater than 40. It often decreases with effective therapy.

4. Chest Radiography

A PA chest radiograph is a standard film in initial assessment of patients with endocrine disturbance. Cardiomegaly may be seen in Cushing's disease, acromegaly, thyrotoxicosis, myxedema, and diabetes mellitus. Calcification may be present in the aorta and coronary arteries due to atheroma. The chest is a common site for tumors producing ectopic hormones, and these may be either in the lungs or in the mediastinum.

In recent years the technique of chest radiography has altered in many departments to using a high kilovoltage (120-150 kV) in order to improve the over-

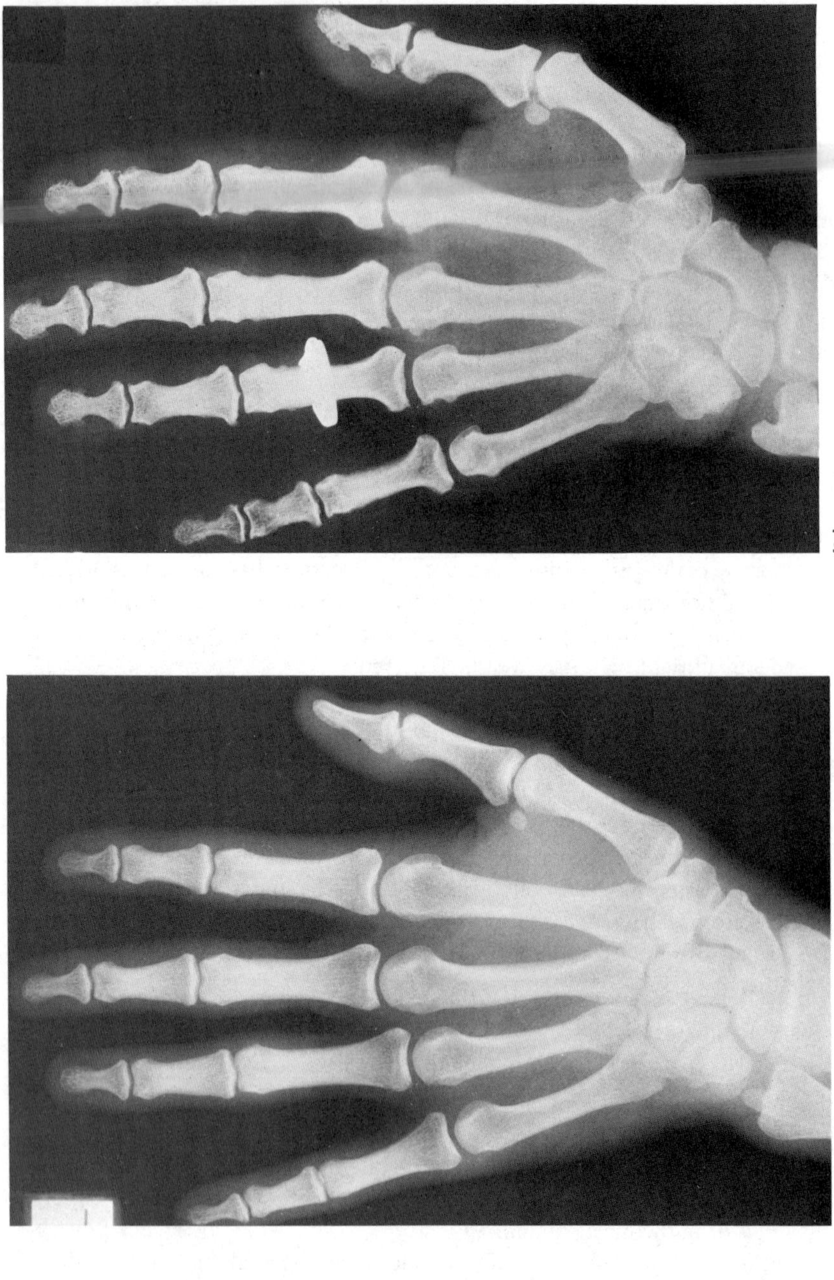

(b)

(a)

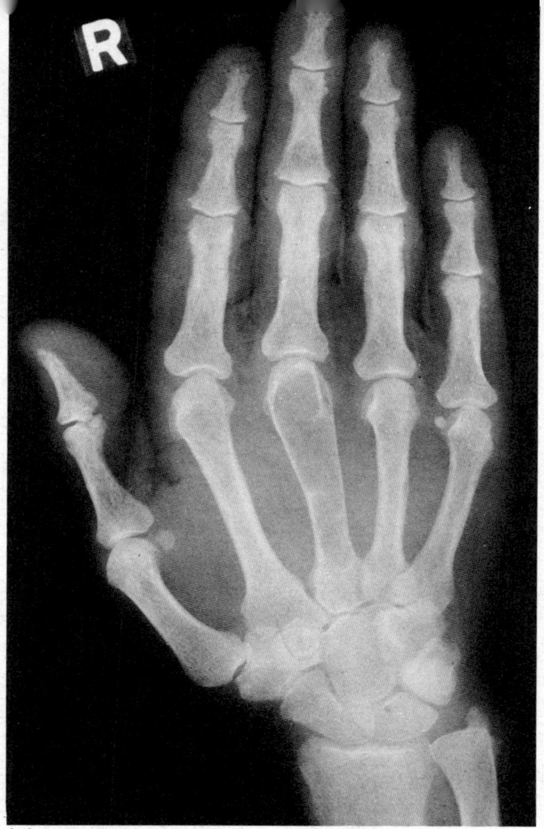

(c)

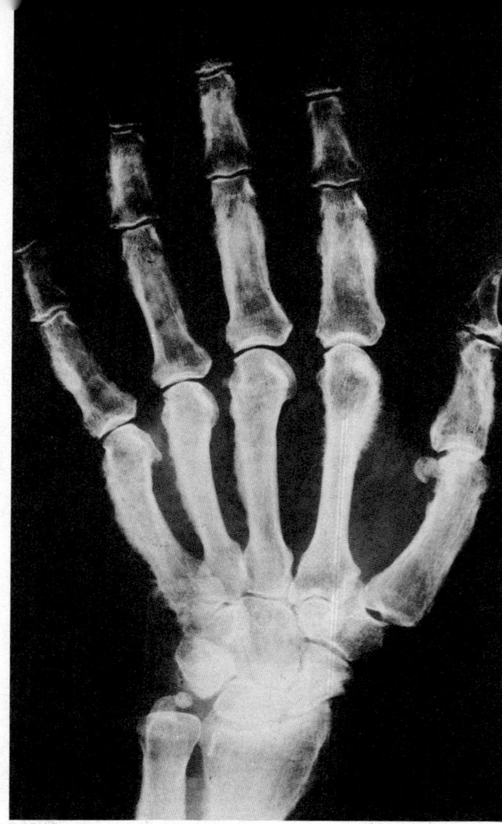

(d)

Figure 5 (a) Normal hand. (b) Acromegaly. Increased soft tissue thickness and widened joint spaces are evident. (c) Hyperparathyroidism. Extensive subperiosteal bone resorption is seen in the middle phalanges and terminal tufts. Note the large bone cyst in the third metacarpal. (d) Thyroid acropachy. (Courtesy of Dr. T. S. Weston, The Princess Margaret Hospital, Christchurch, New Zealand.)

all visualization of the mediastinum and lungs. This is a disadvantage when examining the bones of the thorax in endocrine patients, and a return to a chest radiograph using a low kilovoltage (70 kV) may be required to assess the ribs and scapulae when this is important.

5. The Skull

Apart from local changes of pituitary and parapituitary tumors previously discussed, lateral and AP skull films may show other changes. Calcification of the pineal may demonstrate an enlargement due to pinealoma (3) and calcification of the basal ganglia is seen in hypoparathyroidism and pseudo- and pseudopseudohypoparathyroidism (10). Acromegalic changes include enlargement of the paranasal air sinuses, prognathism with reversal of the bite, generalized hyperostosis of the vault, a prominent external occipital protuberance, and occasionally a frontal osteoma is seen. The skull vault may be demineralized in hyperparathyroidism, giving the so-called "pepper-pot" skull, but is present only when the other bony changes are severe.

II. TOMOGRAPHY

On plain radiographs there is superimposition of structures which often leads to interpretative difficulties. Tomography is a method of obtaining radiographs of planes or slices of the body by moving the x-ray focus (tube) and the film during exposure through a predetermined fulcrum. Varying the angle of movement alters the thickness of tissue in focus on the radiograph and raising or lowering the fulcrum changes the plane. The simplest form is horizontal linear tomography, which is often very satisfactory but linear artifacts are produced from adjacent bone or gas. Circular and hypocycloidal movements are available with better definition and fewer artifacts. However, these movements require more expensive equipment and increase the radiation dose to the patients.

1. Pituitary Fossa

Lateral tomography of the sella turcica is an important addition to the plain films. Hypocycloidal movement is preferred but linear tomography can produce good results. The fossa is tomographed from one anterior clinoid process to the other with the patient in a true lateral position. Ten to twelve sequential cuts 3 mm apart are taken and must be clearly labeled so that the midline cut and right and left sides can be identified. Coronal tomography is advocated by some (11) and will occasionally produce additional information but is not necessary as a routine. If performed, adequate protection for the eyes must be provided. Tomography of the sella will confirm many plain film findings about which one is not totally sure and give additional information regarding the thickness of the lamina dura, asymmetry of the fossa, and extensions into the sphenoid, which help in the difficult differentiation between anatomical variations and local effects of a small tumor (1).

2. Kidneys

Plain linear tomography of the kidneys in patients with Cushing's disease or hyperparathyroidism is used to confirm the presence of nephrocalcinosis, particularly in patients who have marked bowel shadows overlying the kidneys, and also can be used to assess renal size where renal failure is a complication of endocrine disease. AP tomograms through the kidneys are taken at 0.5-1.0 cm intervals with the patient supine.

3. Chest

Tomography, both of the lungs and mediastinum, is sometimes required when searching for sites of ectopic hormone production. AP linear tomography is used (12) for the lungs and central mediastinum, whereas lateral tomography is better for the anterior mediastinum, although sometimes both are required. It is not possible to generalize about technique, as this needs to be adapted to the particular clinical problem.

III. CONTRAST RADIOLOGY

Outlines of structures in the body are seen on plain radiographs because the difference in absorption between air, fat, soft tissue, and bone produces contrast. This natural contrast can be enhanced by air (negative) or barium and iodine (positive) contrast agents.

A. Air Contrast

Air contrast has been used in three main investigations for endocrinology, but all have been superseded almost completely by ultrasound and CT scanning.

1. Air Encephalography

This is performed by the injection of air into the subarachnoid space via lumbar puncture, and by positioning the patient, the air is encouraged to pass into the anterior end of the third ventricle and into the subarachnoid cisterns above the pituitary and surrounding the optic chiasma. In addition to plain films, lateral tomography of the fossa is performed in erect and supine positions in order to identify a suprasellar position or extension of tumor, particularly if visual field defects are present. AP tomograms (Fig. 6) can also be performed and are often useful in identifying the lateral margins of an upward extension and the position of the optic chiasma. Special maneuvers are required to encourage air into the fossa if the possibility of an "empty sella" is suspected (1).

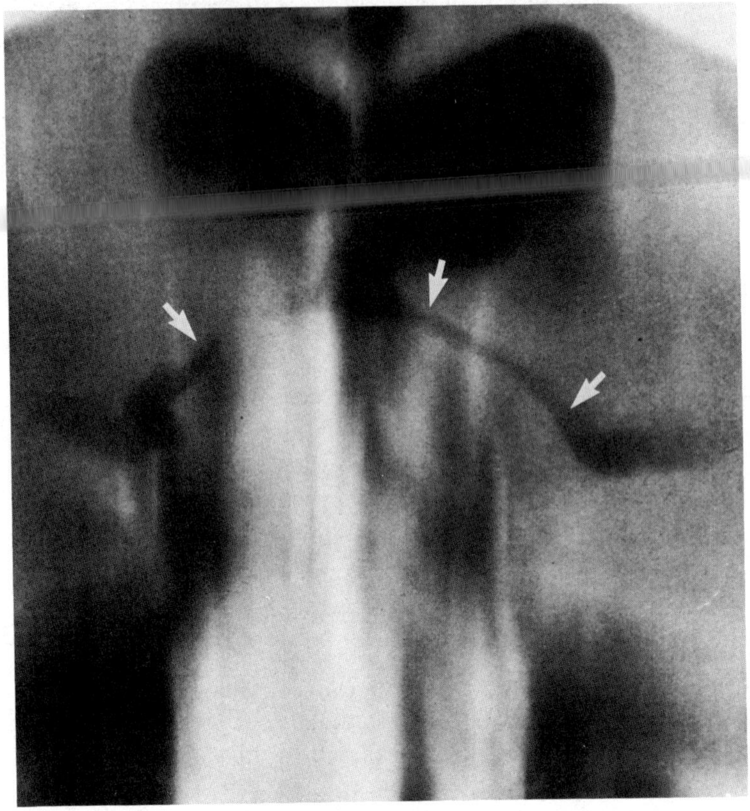

(a)

The examination often requires a general anesthetic, is dangerous in the presence of raised intracranial pressure, and many patients suffer an unpleasant few days of headaches and vomiting following the procedure. In the absence of good-quality CT scanning, it is still an essential investigation.

2. Retroperitoneal Air Insufflation

This technique was used to outline the adrenal glands by injecting air or carbon monoxide into the fascial plane between the coccyx and rectum and forcing it up the retroperitoneal space of the abdomen to surround the adrenal glands. Tomography of the suprarenal areas was then performed. This procedure was unpleasant, unreliable, and is not recommended.

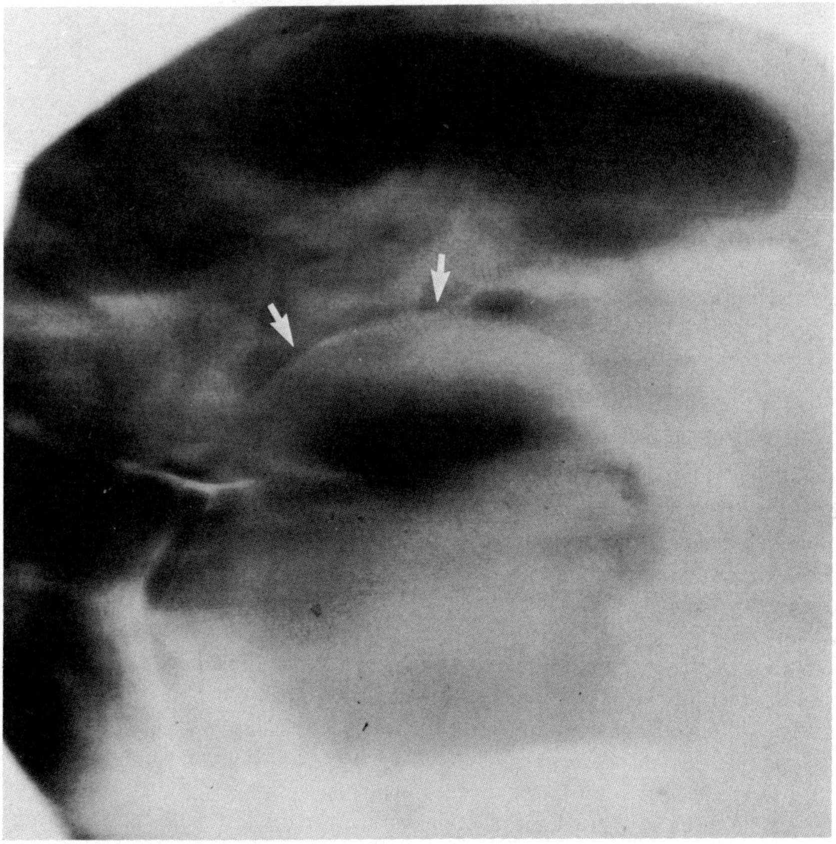

(b)

Figure 6 Air encephalogram. (a), AP and (b) lateral tomograms showing a large upward extension distorting the anterior half of the third ventricle.

3. Pelvic Gynecography

Air is introduced in the peritoneal space via the anterior abdominal wall, and by tilting the table air is introduced into the pelvis to outline the ovaries and uterus, which are recorded on plain films and tomography. Ultrasound and CT scanning have replaced this technique.

B. Positive Contrast

1. Barium

Preparations of barium sulfate are used widely in investigations of the gastrointestinal tract. The most important for the endocrinologist is the barium swallow, which is traditionally performed by a radiologist who takes spot films during fluoroscopy. Increasing use of videotape recording of fluoroscopy gives the opportunity for everyone concerned to see the swallow dynamically. The technique, which should include visualization of the esophagus in erect and supine positions, is used to assess the effects of thyroid enlargement and to localize parathyroid tumors.

Changes have also been described in the barium examination of the small bowel in relation to ileal carcinoid tumors, but this is uncommon (3).

2. Water-Soluble Contrast

The development of iodine-containing water-soluble agents tolerated systemically has led to their widespread use in intravenous urography, arteriography, venography, and other techniques in endocrinology. On the whole they are tolerated well, with minor common side effects of flushing and nausea, but occasionally severe adverse allergic reactions occur which may be fatal (13). Particular care must be taken to ascertain any previous history of contrast reaction and its severity. Emergency drugs and agents should be immediately available and extreme caution must be taken with any contrast injection in patients suspected of pheochromocytoma, as in the unblocked patient a hypertensive crisis can be initiated. Fast-acting blocking agents must be immediately at hand.

Tomography of the suprarenal areas immediately following an intravenous injection has been advocated in detecting adrenal tumors, particularly in Cushing's disease and pheochromocytoma, and will often help in localization if the tumors are large (>2 cm).

Arteriography has been performed widely and with great success in the investigation of endocrine tumors because they produce either displacement of vessels or a tumor "blush" (14). Techniques vary considerably and are too numerous for discussion here, but the aim is to introduce contrast into the arterial supply of a tumor, which usually requires a selective catheter procedure. Carotid angiography has long been a prerequisite to surgical intervention of pituitary tumors, whether by a cranial or a nasal approach. This is performed not only to demonstrate any tumor circulation but to exclude aneurysmal or ectatic carotid arteries and their displacement.

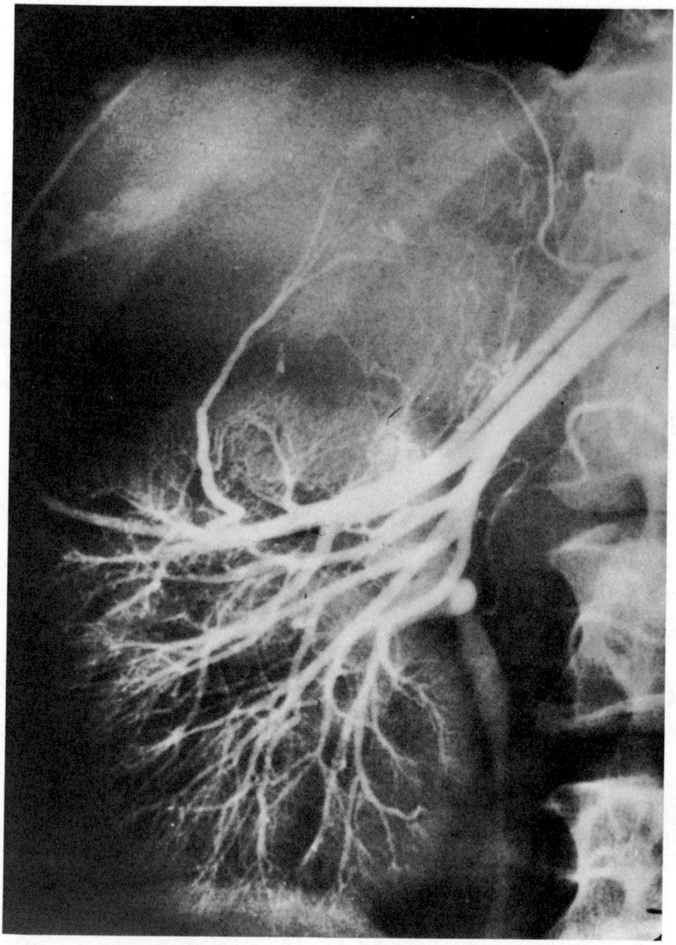

(a)

Figure 7 Adrenal tumor. Cushing's syndrome. (a) and (b) Arterial and capillary phases showing blood supply to the lower half of a right adrenal adenoma. (c) Pancreatic tumor. Vipoma in the head of pancreas.

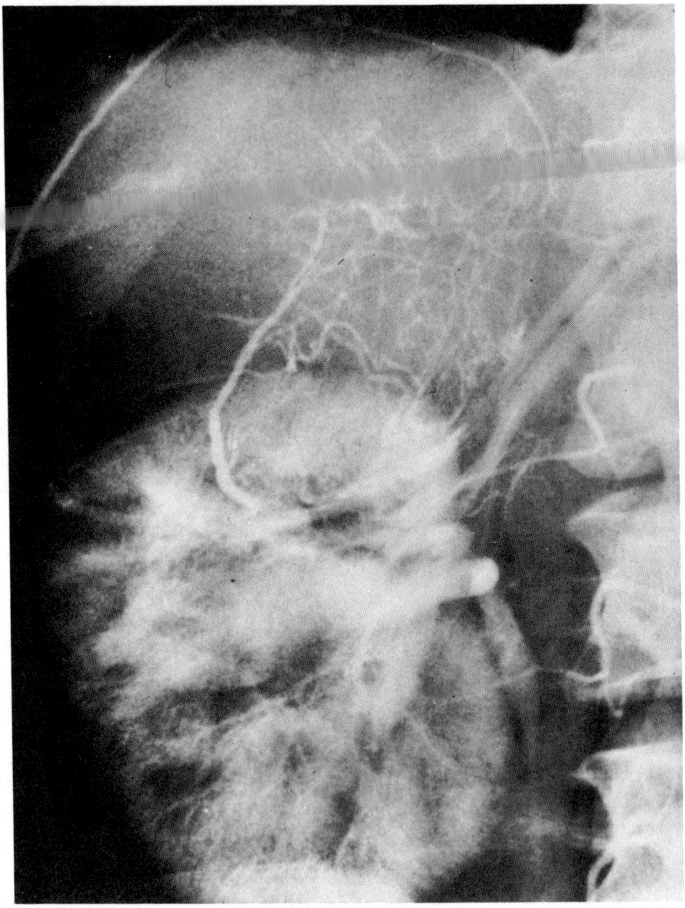

(b)

Figure 7 (Continued)

Selective catheter contrast studies are widely used to detect adrenal, pancreatic, and parathyroid tumors and occasionally for abdominal carcinoid tumors (Fig. 7) (14). They are often long, expensive, technically difficult, and involve a considerable radiation hazard. Complications are infrequent but include embolization and infarction, which may involve the whole adrenal gland. Selective arteriography of the adrenals is particularly unsuitable for the enthusiastic amateur. The radiographic signs are simply those of vessel displacement, tumor blush, and occasionally pathological circulation.

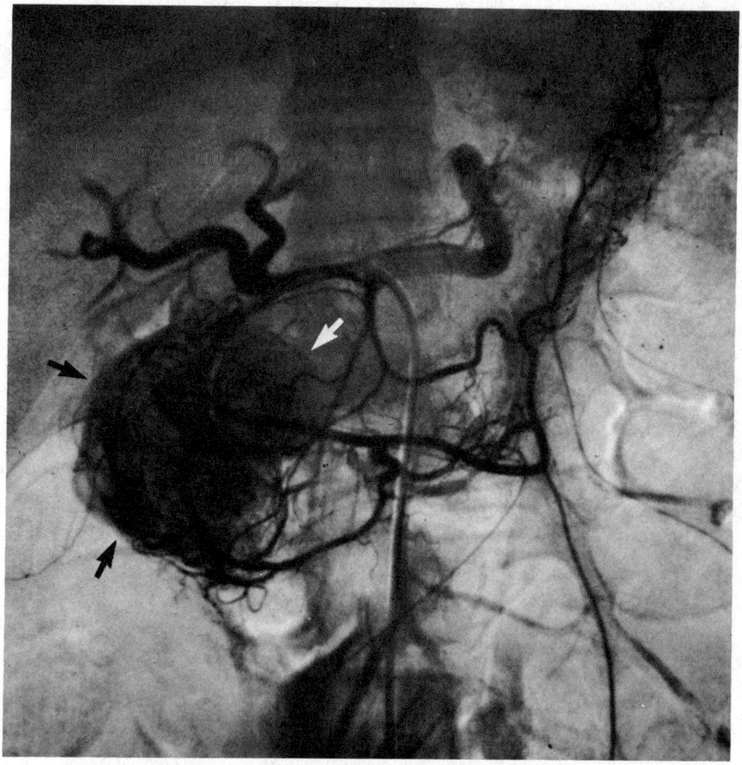

(c)

Venography is also used in the assessment of the size of pituitary tumors (1) and the diagnosis of adrenal tumors (15). Cavernous sinus venography is not widely used but has been shown to be able to demonstrate lateral extensions of pituitary tumors in patients with normal carotid arteriograms.

Adrenal venography requires selective catheterization of the adrenal veins with radiographs taken during retrograde injection. It is technically difficult and infarction of the adrenal glands may result (15). However, it is diagnostically useful and can be combined with venous sampling (see above). Therapeutic infarction by arterial and venous catheters is beginning to prove to be an additional management role for radiology (16,17).

Iodine-based contrast radiography is also useful in the investigation of infertility in the form of vasography in the male and hysterosalpingography in the female. Vasography is performed through a fine needle inserted into the vas deferens at the groin. The vas is normally very small and of little volume. All that is required to fill a normal vas is 1-2 cc of contrast (Conray 280). Spot films are taken as required.

IV. VENOUS SAMPLING

Improved techniques for the laboratory assessment of circulating hormones have led to the selective collection of venous samples of blood by catheter to identify the sites of highest hormone release from a secreting adenoma. The procedure should be performed under local anesthetic and the samples taken as quickly as possible from the selected areas. Small contrast injections are needed for localization. Peripheral and central venous samples should also be taken simultaneously. The end result will depend not only on the sampling technique, which must be meticulous, but also on the laboratory analysis. The laboratory should specify how the samples are to be handled from the time they are drawn into the syringe.

Localization of a single parathyroid can be achieved by this method but is often hindered by previous neck surgery, which obviously alters the venous anatomy and flow pattern in the neck. Samples are taken from both sides of the neck at a number of levels and from the mediastinum (14).

The technique has also been used for adrenal and pancreatic tumors, renal hypertension, and the investigation of ovarian dysfunction.

V. COMPUTERIZED TOMOGRAPHIC SCANNING

The first computerized tomographic (CT) scanner, produced by Godfrey Hounsfield, was designed to display slices of brain tissue in a transverse plane using the same principles of plain radiographic contrast but using a different method of recording the emerging x-ray beam. These principles have recently been reviewed by Pullan in simple mathematical language (18). The thickness of slice and resolution of the original scanners has been vastly improved over the last 5 years The new generation of general-purpose scanner also allows examination of the whole body and coronal slices of the head (Fig. 8), which can be achieved either by coronal positioning of the head or coronal reconstruction by computer from transverse cuts. Development of better resolution is in part limited by considerations of radiation dose to the patients, but in fact except where overlapping slices are used the radiation dose to the body is not great. Because of fine collimation the total body dose of a CT scan of the head is probably no greater than a normal series of plain skull radiographs. Tissue contrast enhancement by intravenous organic iodine agents is of great benefit in CT scanning and is necessary for nearly all endocrine applications.

A. Head Scanning

Pinealomas and craniopharyngiomas are easily identifiable by virtue of the displacement they produce and their frequent calcification. The CT scanner is about twice as efficient as a plain lateral skull radiograph at identifying calcification in tumors.

At first, only large upward extensions of pituitary tumors were confidently diagnosed (intrasellar masses were difficult because of artifacts produced by the partial volume effect from adjacent bone), but with better scanners and more experience it is possible to diagnose much smaller lesions, including microadenoma and the empty sella. Fine slices of <1 cm are taken sequentially from the base of the skull through the fossa and suprasellar region, but overlapping thick cuts are required on older scanners. Pituitary tumors are usually slightly denser than the normal brain tissue and frequently enhance with contrast. Expansion of the fossa is easily seen and any extension beyond the normal confines delineated. Enhancement may diminish following bromocryptine therapy. An empty sella can be confidently predicted, although the exact positions of the optic chiasma and internal carotid arteries are not visualized (19,20).

For most practical purposes of diagnosis and management of pituitary tumors, CT scanning has replaced pituitary fossa tomography, carotid arteriography, and air encephalography except as a preoperative assessment, where the latter investigations are still required by our surgical colleagues. However, three-dimensional reconstruction from CT scanning may yet become practical.

B. Body Scanning

The general purpose CT scanner has made us reassess the value of complicated invasive procedures such as arteriography and venography. In the neck, difficulties were experienced initially with resolution and artifacts because of contour, size, and position in the scan field, but some success has been reported in the detection of parathyroid adenomas (21,22). Thyroid enlargement and in particular the extent of any retrosternal extension is easily visualized. Calcification is more readily identified than on plain films. Hemorrhage into cysts can be difficult to assess.

Visualization of large (>2 cm) adrenal tumors such as pheochromocytomas and carcinomas has been possible from the old generation of scanner, but adrenal adenomas in primary aldosteronism of less than 10 mm have been demonstrated on the newer machines. CT scanning is much less hazardous than adrenal selective arteriography or venography. The main difficulties lie in patients with little retroperitoneal fat and movement blur (23-25).

Lack of retroperitoneal fat is also a limiting factor in visualization of small pancreatic adenomas. Although these tumors usually enhance well, the contrast

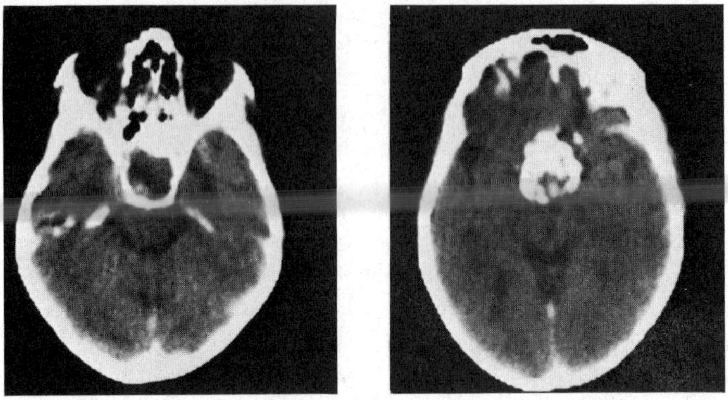

(a)

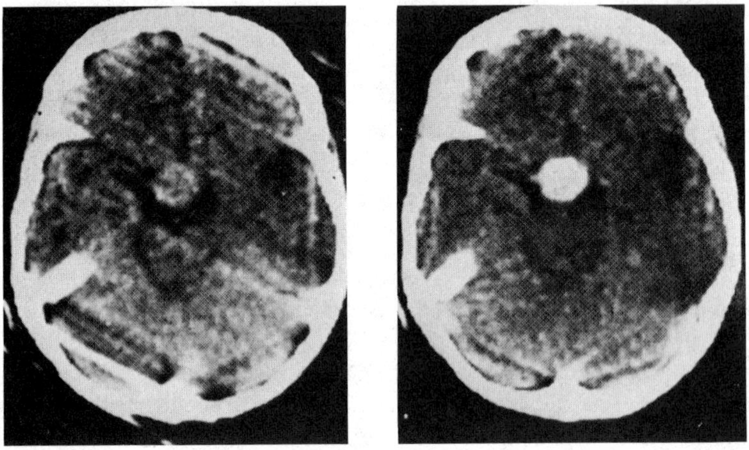

(b)

Figure 8 CT scanning. (a) Craniopharyngioma. An enlarged fossa with dense suprasellar calcification is shown. (b) Pituitary tumor before and after contrast enhancement. (c) Pancreatic vipoma of Fig. 7c. (d) Left adrenal tumor with diameter indicated.

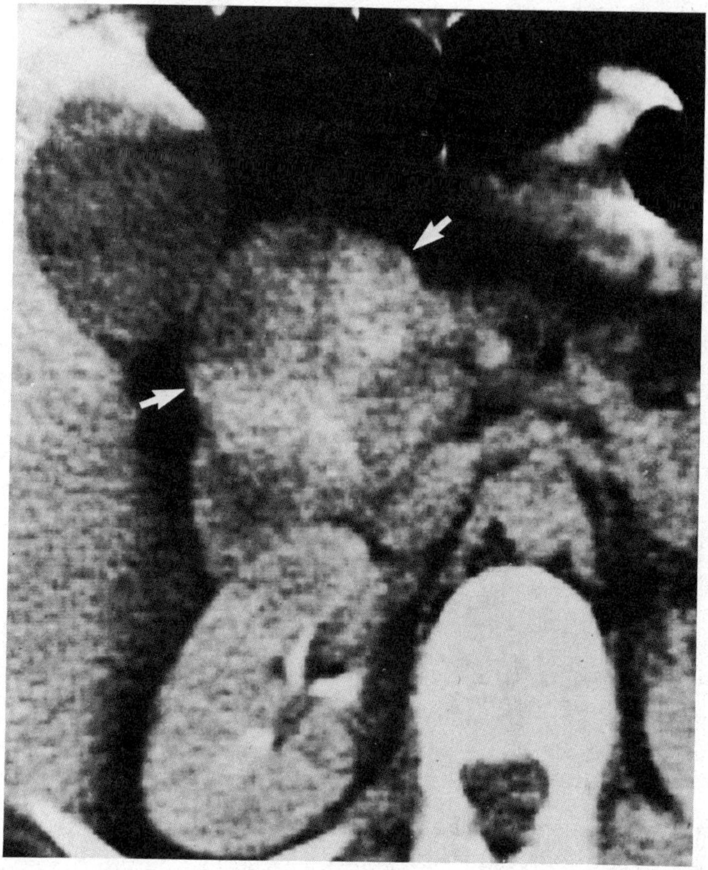

(c)

has to be given by infusion rather than by injection. Selective arteriography is still an important procedure in this area.

In the presence of ectopic hormone production, CT scanning of the chest and abdomen may be performed in a tumor search and is particularly useful in the chest. As stated previously, such extensive scanning by CT delivers a much smaller total body dose to the patient than many people expect. Pheochromocytomas may be multiple, not in the adrenal glands, and anywhere along the sympathetic chain. In these circumstances extensive CT scanning of the chest and abdomen may be necessary if the clinical situation is life threatening.

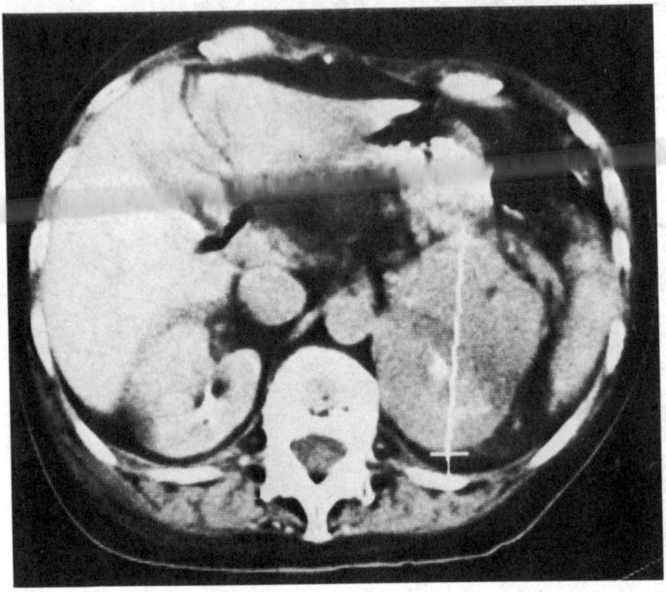

(d)

Figure 8 (Continued)

VI. ULTRASOUND

Ultrasound is a new imaging technique and one that uses completely different principles to radiography (26). The images produced represent a totally different physical phenomenon to radiographs including CT scan pictures, and clinicians have often been confused by the modality, which is not as widely accepted as CT scanning. It has advantages and disadvantages. The advantages are that it is quick and relatively cheap. It is becoming less operator dependent with better equipment and has generally better definition. It has no proven detrimental effect in diagnostic use and therefore has to be very seriously considered in the investigation of children. The plane of scanning is infinitely variable. Its disadvantages are that it is difficult to interpret and open to operator-dependent technical error. Because of the physical principles of the technique, one cannot use it accurately through bone or gas. It is therefore limited to certain areas of the body. Modern high-resolution gray scale systems are essential. It has no application in pituitary tumors.

In the neck the thyroid can be recognized with ease and enlargement due to cyst or tumor differentiated. Because of the irregular contour of the neck it was

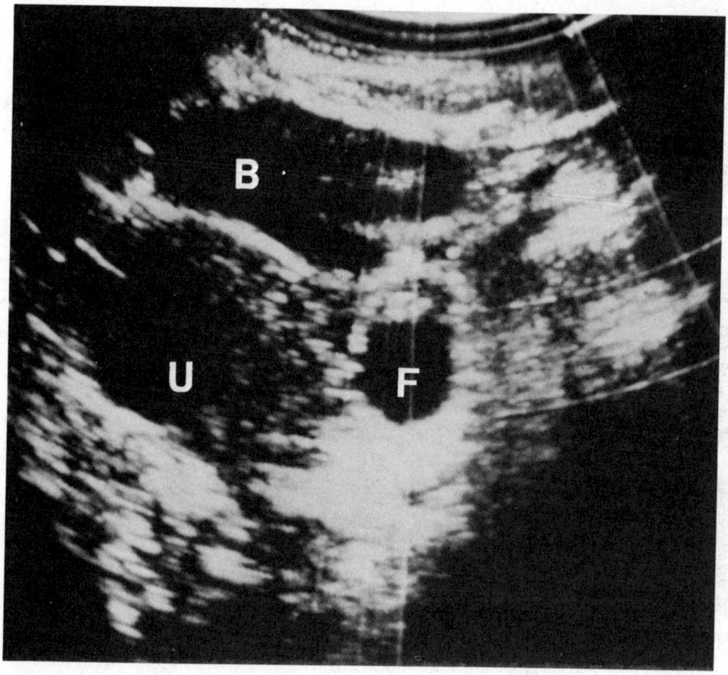

(a)

Figure 9 Ultrasound. (a) Day of LH peak. Ovarian follicle, 25.4 mm in diameter. (b) One day later. Follicle now collapsed. B, bladder; U, uterus; F, follicle; CF, collapsed follicle. (Courtesy of Dr. G. Duff, Christchurch Women's Hospital, Christchurch, New Zealand.)

necessary, with the older static B scanners, to make a water bath to scan the neck in longitudinal and lateral planes (27). However, with the development of small-headed sector scanners, real-time direct contact scanning can produce excellent results. A 5-MHz probe is used for high definition. The full extent of a retrosternal thyroid may be impossible to identify because of the manubrium. It is not yet possible to distinguish between different types of solid neoplastic enlargement of the thyroid (28). Parathyroid tumors have been localized by ultrasound examination of the neck using a technique similar to that used for the thyroid, with a high accuracy rate (29).

Ultrasound detection of adrenal tumors may be achieved if the mass is greater than 2 cm in diameter (30,31). The right adrenal gland can be visualized from the front, scanning through the liver, with the patient's right side raised,

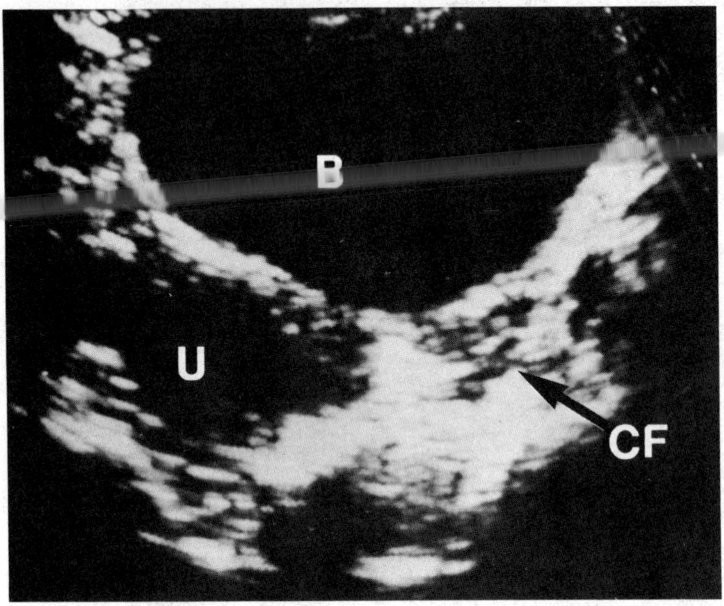

(b)

Figure 9 (Continued)

but often a posterior or posterolateral approach is required for both adrenals. Scans are taken in longitudinal, oblique, and transverse planes in varying stages of arrested respiration using 2.5- or 3.5-MHz probes with appropriate focusing. Difficulties are produced by the posterior aspects of the lower ribs and high diaphragms. On the whole, ultrasound in the abdomen is easier on thin patients. Send those with a lot of retroperitoneal fat for CT scanning!

The pancreas is not an easy organ to visualize by any technique, and although ultrasonography can be very successful it can fail in a significant number of cases due to upper abdominal bowel gas lying anterior to the pancreas. The position and shape of the normal pancreas vary a good deal and tumors have to be large enough to distort the outline of the gland, although adenomas have a lower echogenicity than the normal gland (32). The gland is visualized by oblique transverse scans using the hilum of the right kidney and the superior mesenteric vessels as initial anatomical landmarks. If a tumor is found in the pancreas the liver can be examined at the same time by taking longitudinal, transverse, and subcostal oblique scans to identify any metastases or local invasion into the porta hepatis.

The Female Pelvis. Ultrasound was initially developed as a diagnostic tool for gynecology and extensive experience of ovarian visualization has been obtained, including normal follicular development (33). It is extremely important that when scanning the ovaries the bladder is distended with urine to produce an ultrasound "window" into the pelvis. Normally, a 3.5-MHz probe will give good results, but a 2.5-MHz probe may be needed in large patients. Radial scanning systems using 3.5-MHz probes with short focus have been designed for rectal insertion but have not become popular, although they can give good detail (34).

Normal uterus and ovaries can be visualized in a high proportion of young women. The shape and size of a normal adult uterus is easily recognized. In cases of infertility, congenital anomalies can be recognized as can fibroids. An infantile uterus may be seen in Turner's syndrome. Normal ovarian size (1 x 2 x 3 cm) and shape can be determined regularly and more easily than with pelvic pneumography, with which measurements compare favorably. Physiological changes of the follicle and corpus luteum can be monitored to predict ovulation (Fig. 9) (35). Small ovaries may be found in Turner's syndrome and enlarged polycystic ovaries in the Stein-Leventhal syndrome (36).

REFERENCES

1. Doyle FH. Radiology of the pituitary. In *Recent Advances in Radiology and Medical Imaging,* Lodge, Sir Thomas, Steiner, RE (eds). Churchill Livingstone, Edinburgh, 1979.
2. Teasdale E, MacPherson P, Teasdale G. The reliability of radiology in detecting prolactin-secreting microadenomas. Br J Radiol 1981; 54:566-571.
3. Teplik JG, Haskin ME. *Diseases of the Endocrine System in Roentgenologic Diagnosis.* Saunders, Philadelphia, 1976, vol II.
4. Greulich WW, Pyle SI. *Radiographic Atlas of Skeletal Development of the Hand and Wrist,* 2nd ed. Stanford University Press, Stanford, Calif, 1959.
5. Murray RO, Jacobson HG. *The Radiology of Skeletal Disorders.* Churchill Livingstone, Edinburgh, 1977, vol. 1.
6. Carr D, Davidson JK, McMillan M, Davidson M. Renal osteodystrophy an underdiagnosed condition. Clin Radiol 1980; 31:55-59.
7. Meema HE, Meema S. Improved roentgenologic diagnosis of osteomalacia by microradioscopy of hand bones. Am J Roentgenol 1975; 125:925-935.
8. Moule B, Grant MC, Boyle IT, May H. Thyroid acropachy. Clin Radiol 1970; 21:329-333.
9. Kho KM, Wright AD, Doyle FH. Heel pad thickness in acromegaly. Br J Radiol 1970; 43:119-125.

10. Steinbach HL, Young DA. The Roentgen appearance of pseudohypoparathyroidism (PH) and pseudo-pseudohypoparathyroidism (PPH). Am J Roentgenol 1966; 97:49-66.
11. Vezina JL, Sutton TJ. Prolactin-secreting pituitary microadenomas. Am J Roentgenol 1974; 120:46-54.
12. Sonksen PH, Ayers, AB, Braimbridge M, Corrin B, Davies DR, Jeremiah GM, Oaten SW, Lowy C, West TET. Acromegaly caused by pulmonary carcinoid tumours. Clin Endocrinol 1976; 5:503-513.
13. Ansell G. *Complications in Diagnostic Radiology.* Blackwell, Oxford, 1976.
14. In Angiography. *Radiologic Clinics of North America,* Lang EK (ed). Saunders, Philadelphia, 1976, vol XIV.
15. Davidson JK, Morley P, Hurley GD, Holford NGH. Adrenal venography and ultrasound in the investigation of the adrenal gland: an analysis of 58 cases. Br J Radiol 1975; 48:435-450.
16. Timmis JB, Brown MJ, Allison DJ. Therapeutic embolization of phaeochromocytoma. Br J Radiol 1981; 54:420-422.
17. Rosenstock J, Allison DJ, Joplin GF, Lewis PD, Mashiter K, Welbourn RB, White MC. Therapeutic adrenal infarction in ACTH-dependent Cushing's syndrome. Br J Radiol 1981; 54.
18. Pullan BR. The scientific basis of computerized tomography. In *Recent Advances in Radiology and Medical Imaging.* Lodge Sir Thomas, Steiner RE (eds). Churchill Livingstone, Edinburgh, 1979, vol. 6.
19. Banna M, Baker HL, Houser OW. Pituitary and parapituitary tumors on computed tomography. Br J Radiol 1980; 53:1123-1143.
20. Kuuliala I. Computed axial tomography of pituitary adenomas. Clin Radiol 1981; 32:259-264.
21. Doppman JL, Brennan NF, Koehler JO, Marx SJ. Computed tomography for parathyroid localisation. J Comput Assist Tomogr 1977; 1:30-36.
22. Adams JE, Adams PH, Mamtora H, Isherwood I. Computed tomography and the localisation of parathyroid tumours. Clin Radiol 1981; 32:251-254.
23. Dunnick NR, Schaner EG, Doppman JL, Strott CA, Gill JR, Javadpour N. Computed tomography in adrenal tumours. Am J Roentgenol 1979; 132:43-46.
24. Korobkin M, White EA, Kressel HY, Moss AA, Montagne JP. Computed tomography in the diagnosis of adrenal disease. Am J Roentgenol 1979; 132:231-238.
25. Meek D, Duncan JG, McAreavey D. Computed tomography in the localisation of aldosterone-secreting adrenal adenomas. Br J Radiol 19XX; 54.
26. Wells PNT (ed). *Ultrasonics in Clinical Diagnosis,* 2nd ed. Churchill Livingstone, Edinburgh, 1977.
27. Berger LA, Lister A, Lilley AC. A water bath for thyroid scanning with ultrasound. Br J Radiol 1981; 54:630-631.

28. Propper RA, Skolnick ML, Weinstein BJ, Dekker A. The nonspecificity of the thyroid halo sign. J Clin Ultrasound 1980; 8:129-132.
29. Scheible W, Deutsch AL, Leopold GR. Parathyroid adenoma: accuracy of preoperative localization of high-resolution real-time sonography. J Clin Ultrasound 1981; 9:325,330.
30. Sample WF. Adrenal ultrasonography. Radiology 1978; 127:461-466.31
31. Yeh H-C, Mitty HA, Rose J, Wolf BS, Gabrilove JL. Ultrasonography of adrenal masses: usual features. Radiology 1978; 127:467-474.
32. Raghavendra BN, Glickstein ML. Sonography of islet cell tumour of the pancreas: report of two cases. J Clin Ultrasound 1981; 9:331-333.
33. Hall DA, Hann LE, Ferrucci JT, Black EB, Braitman BS, Crowley WF, Nikrui N, Kelley J. Sonographic morphology of the normal menstrual cycle. Radiology 1979; 133:185-188.
34. Morley P. Pelvic echography. In *Recent Advances in Radiology and Medical Imaging,* Lodge Sir Thomas, Steiner RE (eds). Churchill Livingstone, Edinburgh, 1979, vol 6.
35. Fleischer AC, Daniell JF, Rodier J, Lindsay AM, Jones AE. Sonographic monitoring of ovarian follicular development. J Clin Ultrasound 1981; 9:275-280.
36. Swanson M, Sauerbrei EE, Cooperberg PL. Medical implications of ultrasonically detected polycystic ovaries. J Clin Ultrasound 1981; 9:212-222.

17
Radionuclide Imaging

Keith E. Britton
St. Bartholomew's Hospital and Medical College, London, England

Radionuclide images are to function what x-ray films are to structure. Both pictures are obtained using electromagnetic radiation. This radiation is called x-radiation when it comes from the electron rings of certain atoms and gamma radiation when it comes from the nucleus—hence nuclear medicine. The atoms that give off gamma rays are part of a class of atoms called radionuclides. When such radionuclides are administered and taken up by organs in the body the gamma rays penetrate the body wall and are detectable externally by a gamma camera—hence radionuclide imaging. The resulting picture is a two-dimensional representation of the distribution of a particular function of an organ and is called a *scan* or static image.

Radionuclide imaging does not demonstrate structure, does not demonstrate pathology, and does not diagnose disease. Radionuclide imaging does demonstrate the distribution of a particular function of an organ and how that distribution of function is altered in disease. It is important to the understanding of radionuclide imaging to be aware that the function of an organ chosen in order to image the organ with radionuclides is not necessarily the function of the organ that is most relevant to the particular clinical problem at hand. Whereas the amount taken up and the distribution of radioactive iodine may well be the most clinically important function to image in thyroid disease, the uptake of radioactively labeled cholesterol may not equate with the output rate of aldosterone in an adrenal adenoma, nor the uptake of radioselenium-labeled methionine with the output rate of parathyroid hormone. This limitation is also aggravated by the fact that no radioactively labeled compound (radiopharmaceutical) is totally taken up by or totally specific to a particular organ. Thus iodine is taken up not only by the thyroid, but by the stomach mucosa, salivary, and sweat glands and choroid plexus of the ventricles, as well as remaining in the blood and extracellular fluid and being excreted by the kidneys and in the feces. A further problem is that gamma rays used in nuclear medicine are not very penetrating and are attenuated and partly scattered as they pass through tissues. The depth of the organ is thus important and the sensitivity with which gamma rays are detected falls off inversely with the square of the distance between the detector and the organ. These factors make the measurement of the absolute amount of radionuclide in an organ difficult and, in static imaging, either these measurements are not made and an indirect semiquantitative "analog" image is produced, or the measurements have to be made with reference to some standard source, or relative to some feature on the static image. As examples, the amount of activity detected in an adrenal gland is related to the amount of activity of the tracer injected at the start of the test, whereas when the pituitary is imaged in transverse section through the head, its activity is compared with that in a tissue background area around it and measured as a pituitary-to-background ratio.

I. THE PITUITARY

This organ has been difficult to image noninvasively, particularly for the confirmation of microadenoma. X-ray computerized tomography (CT) is limited by artifacts due to the boney cage around the pituitary and by the fact that the attenuation properties of an adenoma are similar to those of the normal pituitary. Conventional radionuclide brain scanning is unreliable unless there is suprasellar extension. In this case there may be apparent prolongation and thickening inferiorly of the anterior sagittal sinus activity. However, the development of transverse section single photon emission tomography (SPET), the radionuclide equivalent of x-ray CT, has changed this. A microadenoma is physically small but functionally very active if it is causing an endocrine syndrome and thus very vascular. Uptake of [^{99m}Tc] pertechnetate is high (Fig. 1).

After oral administration of 400 mg of potassium perchlorate to suppress choroid plexus and salivary uptake, about 15 mCi(550 MBq) [^{99m}Tc] pertechnetate is given intravenously. Conventional brain imaging is undertaken 20 min later with a gamma camera and then SPET is commenced at 40 min. For small suspect tumors a region of interest is set over it and the activity compared with that in the pituitary environment (1). A pituitary-to-background ratio of over 1.28 is abnormal, and using this technique in 19 patients with pituitary adenomata and in two patients without tumors, all confirmed by air encephalography, conventional brain imaging was correct in 35%, x-ray CT in 50%, and SPET in 71%, a significant improvement. Six tumors missed by SPET were also not evident on x-ray CT. The change in function (e.g., of prolactinoma treated by bromocrip-

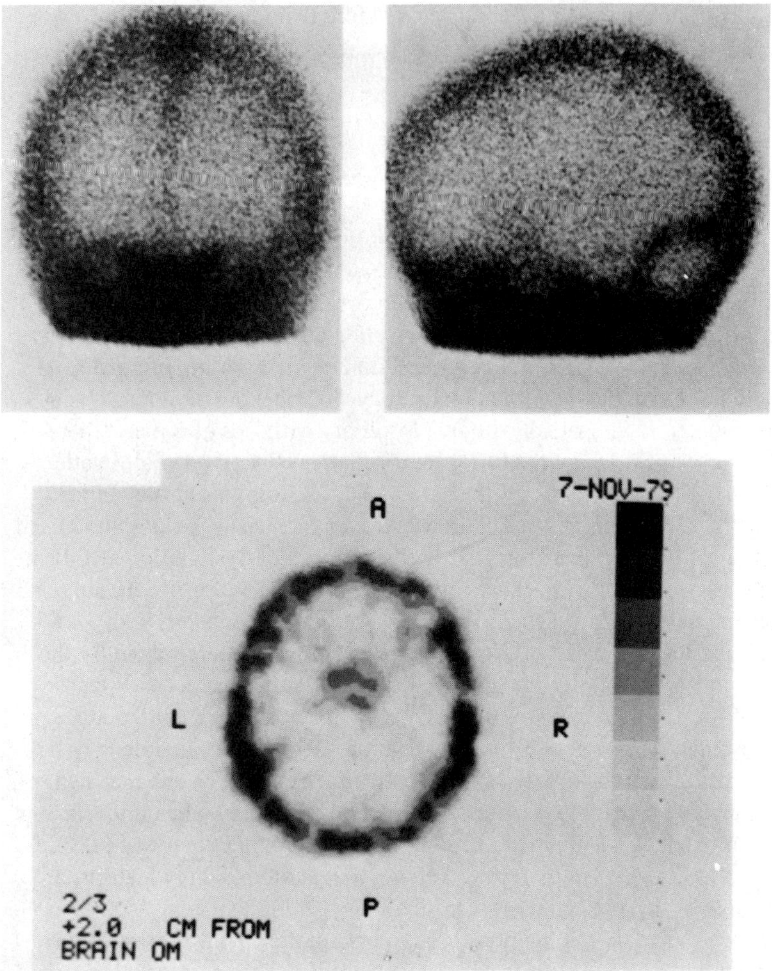

Figure 1 Pituitary adenoma, [^{99m}Tc] pertechnetate study. Top: anterior and right lateral views of the conventional brain scan are normal. Bottom: transverse section emission tomography shows increased uptake in the pituitary adenoma.

tine) may be followed by SPET and occurs before radiological change. Now pituitary imaging agents based on pituitary receptor binding are under study.

II. THE THYROID

It is essential to remember that a thyroid image, obtained using radioiodine, ^{131}I- or ^{123}I-, or ^{99m}Tc-labeled pertechnetate, does not demonstrate the structure of the thyroid and cannot be used to confirm that a cancer of the thyroid is present. In the case of radioiodine the demonstrated function is that of the iodine trap and organification and storage processes, whereas for pertechnetate it is only of the iodine trap which takes up pertechnetate, since the size of these two molecules is similar. An area of loss of function (e.g., at the site of a palpable thyroid nodule) may be due to hemorrhage, cyst (simple or compound), adenoma, or cancer. If the palpable nodule is solitary with loss of uptake, there is a 1 in 25 chance of it being due to cancer in a patient from a general practice population and a 1 in 5 chance if the patient is from hospitals in the United Kingdom. The diagnosis of thyroid cancer is a clinical one by palpation (2) and the thyroid scan merely confirms that there is an area of dysfunction at this site. Any lump suspected of being cancer clinically requires histology to be obtained whatever the thyroid scan shows.

The smallest size of a focal defect in the thyroid scan is determined by the physical characteristics of the imaging system and, in the past, a lesion causing a defect of less than 7.5 mm was unlikely to be detected. As a consequence of the improvement in imaging techniques an apparently solitary nodule may be associated with small focal defects previously undetected. The enhancement of a thyroid image using computer-assisted analysis is necessary when undertaking a search for a defect possibly representing cancer in a patient exposed in childhood to external radiation therapy, where there is a strong family history, or when medullary thyroid cancer is suspected.

As well as giving off gamma rays, ^{131}I is a beta-particle emitter, and these particles are destructive. It gives one of the highest radiation doses of any nuclear medicine test, thus its use for thyroid imaging is being phased out. It should now be reserved for the staging and therapy of thyroid cancer and the treatment of thyrotoxicosis, its use being replaced by pertechnetate imaging and by ^{123}I imaging where pertechnetate imaging gives problems. For similar reasons ^{131}I uptake as an estimate of thyroid function at 4, 24, and 48 hr after ingestion is being replaced by the use of thyroid hormone radioassay on blood samples and by measurement of pertechnetate or ^{123}I uptake during imaging at 20 min or 2-4 hr, respectively, after their intravenous injection. It should be remembered that iodine-containing preparations inhibit the uptake of radiolabeled iodine by the thyroid, including many medications and many radiological contrast media.

A. The Thyroid Image

There is no normal pattern of distribution of thyroid uptake due to the considerable variation in lobe size, lobularity, and indentation, and the presence or absence of an isthmus or pyramidal lobe. A familiar shape is of a right lobe of slightly greater functioning mass than the left with a small linking functioning mass due to the isthmus. When a pertechnetate scan is to be undertaken 20 min after the intravenous injection of [^{99m}Tc] pertechnetate 2.7 mCi(100 MBq), it is helpful to give the patient a glass of water to drink to clear the esophagus of salivary excretion of pertechnetate. The patient lies supine with the neck extended and a gamma camera, on which a pinhole collimator is mounted is set at a fixed distance (by means of a former) from the thyroid. When ^{123}I is used, imaging is taken 2-4 hr after injection of 0.5-1.1 mCi(20-40 MBq). The total counts and imaging time should be recorded.

The thyroid scan, being a test of function, can never give a certain pathological diagnosis. Thus its best use is in terms of questions such as: "Does this mass in the neck contain normally functioning thyroid tissue?" or "Is this solitary nodule hyperactive?" Some indications for thyroid imaging are given in Table 1 and some situations are presented where thyroid imaging is not cost effective.

B. Pertechnetate, ^{123}I, or ^{131}I

^{99m}Technetium generators are generally available and the most cost effective agent for thyroid imaging is [^{99m}Tc] pertechnetate, with its 6-hr half-life and 0.14-MeV energy gamma ray, which is suitable for imaging with the gamma camera or rectilinear scanner. In countries where such generators are unavailable or excessively expensive, ^{131}I has to be used for thyroid imaging, 24 hr after its oral administration. Such centers are not likely to have a gamma camera, for which the relatively high energy of ^{131}I of 0.364 MeV is unsuitable, and traditional rerectilinear imaging of the thyroid would be undertaken. Its use as an uptake test for thyroid function should be replaced by blood estimations of triiodothyronine (T_3), thyroid stimulating hormone (TSH), and thyroxine (T_4). Except in patients with known thyroid cancer its use as an imaging agent should be discontinued. A safer isotope is ^{123}I (free of ^{124}I). This radionuclide has no beta-ray emission, a short half-life of 13 hr, and a high abundance pure gamma-ray emission of 0.159 MeV, rather similar to that of ^{99m}Tc. The radiation dose to the thyroid from 500 μCi (20 MBq)^{123}I is 10 times less than that from 50 μC2(2 MBq) of ^{131}I. After intraveous administration of ^{123}I imaging may be undertaken between 2 and 4 hr later. The lower energy of ^{123}I compared with ^{131}I makes background correction less important when looking for increased iodine uptake. It is a better Thyroid imaging agent than [^{99m}Tc] pertechnetate,

Table 1 Main Indications and Lack of Indications for Imaging the Thyroid

1. Extrathyroidal mass thought to contain functioning thyroid tissue	At thoracic inlet, retrosternal, thyroglossal cyst, lingual mass
2. Hypothyroid	
Simple goiter	When thyroiditis is expected
Multinodular goiter	Iodine deficient
	Before cosmetic surgery
3. Euthyroid	
Smooth goiter	No indication
Solitary nodule	No indication if surgery is already decided
	To indicate lack of function compatible with malignancy if surgery is undecided
	For autonomous nodule
	For adenoma
Multinodular goiter	Before surgery, to indicate nonfunctioning areas
4. Hyperthyroid	
Smooth goiter	No indication
Solitary nodule	For toxic adenoma or associated cold nodule
Multinodular goiter	For sites of toxic nodules
5. Painful thyroid	To distinguish thyroiditis from focal change such as hemorrhage
6. Evaluation of known thyroid cancer	

because it is organified as well as trapped, both in terms of interobserver agreement when reporting thyroid scans and in terms of correlation with the final clinical diagnosis (3). Cost-effective practice is to undertake pertechnetate imaging for all thyroid requests and repeat the test in about 1 in 6 to 1 in 10 with ^{123}I. The main reasons for choosing ^{99m}TC or ^{123}I are set out in Table 2, given the indications set out in Table 1.

C. Warm and Hot Nodules

The thyrotoxic patient with biochemical confirmation of this diagnosis has a smooth goiter in Graves' disease. If a nodule is palpated, this is an indication for imaging. A single focal area of activity, with lack of uptake elsewhere in the gland due to suppression of TSH secretion by excess circulating T_3 and thyroxine, is typical of a toxic nodule (Fig. 2). In the equivocally thyrotoxic or as an incidental finding, a nodule may be palpated which on imaging is more active than its environment whose uptake is not suppressed. If radioiodine has been used, it may be worth testing whether such a "warm" nodule is autonomous or not by administering 40 μg of T_3 three times a day for a week and on the morning of the scan. If the nodule is autonomous its uptake is not suppressed, whereas the uptake by the rest of the gland is totally suppressed. However, if [^{99m}Tc] pertechnetate has been used, it is essential to repeat the study with radioiodine, for three reasons: (1) the pertechnetate uptake may only represent vascularity, and certain thyroid cancers may be very vascular but unable to take up iodine; (2) the radioiodine scan may be quite normal, indicating lobulation or a benign adenoma; and (3) the T_3 suppression test is unreliable with pertechnetate imaging.

The multinodular goiter in a thyrotoxic patient contains one or more toxic nodules unsuppressible with T_3. The environment of the toxic nodules may not show uptake because of suppression of TSH secretion or because of associated

Table 2 Choice of ^{99m}Tc or ^{123}I

Condition	[^{99m}Tc] pertechnetate	[^{123}I] iodine (^{131}I)
Extrathyroidal mass	Mass in neck between hyoid and thyroid	Lateral neck, lingual, retrosternal regions Doubt about Tc result
Hypothyroid	Yes	No, except if Tc uptake is too poor for detail
Goiter, simple or nodular	Yes	Yes, only if solitary warm nodule on Tc, or palpable nodule with normal Tc result
Hypothyroid on T_3/T_4, hyperthyroid on carbimazole	Yes	No, organification of iodine is suppressed
Factitious thyrotoxicosis	No	Yes, to show lack of uptake
Suppression and stimlation tests	No	Yes
Known thyroid cancer	No	Yes, ^{131}I

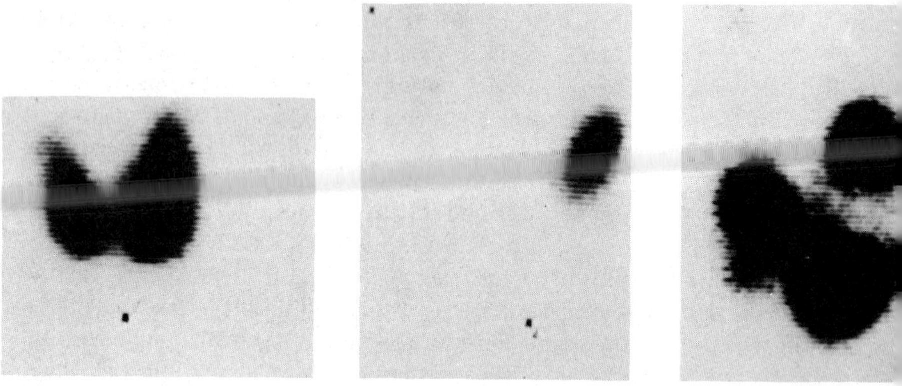

Figure 2 Thyroid imaging in thyrotoxicosis, [^{99m}Tc] pertechnetate studies. Left: Graves' disease. Middle: toxic nodule with suppression of other uptake. Right: toxic multinodular goiter.

nonfunctioning nodules. TSH stimulation will show which areas are suppressed and need to be left behind at surgery and which are not.

D. Thyroiditis and Goiter in Children

The appearance of the thyroid scan during subacute viral thyroiditis is of generally reduced uptake distributed patchily through an apparently enlarged gland. In autoimmune thyroiditis, the gland is usually increased in size with a more irregular patchy distribution of uptake. Occasionally, there may be discrete areas of deficient uptake simulating a multinodular goiter and the thyroid scan may not allow this distinction to be made. Acute viral thyroiditis and de Quervain's thyroiditis may result in such a low thyroid uptake that it is hardly visualized.

Simple goiter in children is usually physiological and requires no imaging. Occasionally, it may be due to enzyme deficiencies preventing organification. The [^{99m}Tc] pertechnetate distribution may be normal, but radioiodine uptake is reduced. The lack of organification, which is also often seen with thyroiditis and with carbimazole treatment, may be tested using perchlorate discharge. Perchlorate, like pertechnetate, is a molecular competitor with iodine for the trap; 500 μCi (20 MBq) of ^{123}I is given intravenously and uptake measurements are made at 10-min intervals for the first hour. Potassium perchlorate 400 mg is then given orally and uptake measurements are continued for a further hour. A fall in radioiodine content of the gland by 50% below the 1-hr uptake level is evidence of a major defect in organification. A fall of less than 10% of the 1-hr uptake level is normal.

E. Suspected Thyroid Cancer

The solitary nodule in a euthyroid patient does not need imaging if surgery is already decided upon. However, the demonstration of a classical "cold nodule", that is, a single palpable mass shown to be unable to take up pertechnetate or radioiodine, may with consideration of the patient's age group, history, and examination findings, encourage the obtaining of a histological diagnosis (Fig. 3). The nonspecific scan appearance has lead to further thyroid imaging with a number of different radiopharmaceuticals: $[^{75}Se]$ selenomethionine (4), $[^{64}Ga]$ gallium (5), and $[^{201}Tl]$ thallium (6). Although all series show some advantages for

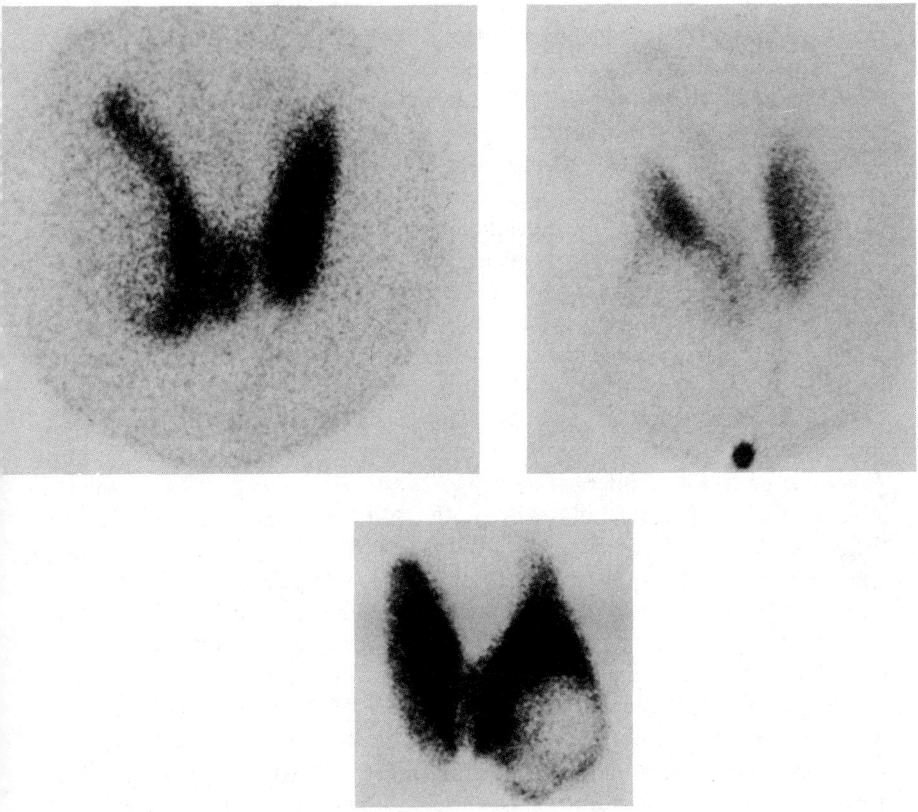

Figure 3 Nonfunctioning solitary thyroid nodule, $[^{99m}Tc]$ pertechnetate studies. Top left: simple cyst. Top right: thyroid carcinoma. Bottom: nodular colloid goiter.

these techniques, none are sufficiently reliable to alter clinical management. An alternative approach is to use fluorescent thyroid imaging. In this technique *stable* iodine in the thyroid is forced to fluoresce under bombardment with gamma rays from one or more [^{241}Am] americium sources. The fluorescent rays are recorded and the amount and distribution of stable iodine estimated. Thyroid cancer is usually iodine deficient, and such a finding would indicate the need for histology. Ultrasound may exclude the 9% of simple cysts (see Chap. 16), but no imaging modality so far has been shown to be an adequate substitute for clinical suspicion of cancer as an indication for needle biopsy and/or surgery.

F. Known Thyroid Cancer

The confirmation of a clinical diagnosis of thyroid cancer is a histological one, whether a previous thyroid scan has shown a cold nodule or not. Except in the case of inoperable or anaplastic carcinoma where external irradiation of the neck may be the only answer, the first principle is to carry out total thyroidectomy to prevent competitive uptake of ^{131}I by normal tissue, which inhibits the demonstration of any potential functioning metastasis. The residual thyroid tissue after recovery from such surgery may be imaged using about 0.3 mCi (10 MBq) of ^{131}I 2 or 3 days after oral administration. If found, an ablation dose of about 80 mCi is given using a closed system. The patient must be in a single-bed suite with shower and toilet, and all the necessary statutory requirements regarding high-dose ^{131}I therapy must be observed. Three to four days after this, a whole body survey is undertaken, preferably using a whole-body counter-profiling system, followed by local imaging of any peaks of activity that are seen. These studies are undertaken to demonstrate the possible presence of functioning metastases. A whole-body bone scan with [^{99m}Tc] methyldiphosphonate is undertaken either before or a little after this to demonstrate possible sites of nonfunctioning metastases in addition. In the absence of metastases, the patient is made euthyroid with T_3 and followed up. This also suppresses any TSH dependency of the cancer. At 3 months after stopping T_3 for 2 weeks, the bone scan and then the iodine survey are repeated using 1–5 mCi (40–200 MBq).

Some authorities recommend giving two intramuscular injections of TSH 10 units, one 12 hr and one just before the iodine survey to stimulate any possible iodine uptake. A positive result is more than 0.5% of the administered iodine in a metastasis, and this is the indication for [^{131}I] iodine therapy. The patient is readmitted to the designated suite and given 150–200 mCi (6–7.5 MBq). Replacement T_3 is then reinstituted. The imaging procedures are repeated at 3-, 6-, and 12-month intervals according to length of absence of recurrence and ^{131}I therapy repeated as above if a functioning metastasis is seen.

III. THE PARATHYROID

In hyperparathyroidism, biochemical confirmation is essential before parathyroid adenoma imaging is undertaken. It is one of the most difficult of radionuclide imaging techniques but is worthwhile, particularly in patients in whom neck exploration has been unsuccessful, because of the morbidity of thyroid-parathyroid venous sampling. There is no specific radiopharmaceutical and so [^{75}Se] selenomethionine (SM) is used. This is a radiolabeled analog of the amino acid methionine, which is a constituent of most proteins. The uptake of SM is not only by the parathyroid adenoma but also by the thyroid, cervical vertebrae, sternum, clavicles, and hyoid. After injection of SM, blood activity is high, falling to rise again as SM-labeled proteins enter the circulation. The minimum is at about 30 min and this is the optimum time for imaging after injection.

The patient is given about 100 μCi(4 MBq) of ^{125}I orally a day before the test. The low energy of ^{125}I allows a thyroid scan to be undertaken without scatter into the energy windows of ^{75}Se. No special preparation has been found convincing, although EDTA infusion may be advised (8). The next day, about 150 μCi(9 MBq) of ^{75}Se is injected intravenously. Two images are recorded at 20-30 and 30-40 min and stored so that they can be superimposed on the thyroid image. A modern double isotope channel gamma camera allows these images to be obtained simultaneously with those of the thyroid.

The most active spots on the parathyroid image are obtained by progressive background subtraction. Those in the line of the cervical spine, sternum, and clavicles are excluded. The most active spots on the thyroid image are obtained and those that coincide with active parathyroid spots are excluded. Ideally, this leaves one hot parathyroid spot at a site of relatively low thyroid uptake, and this is the most probable site of the adenoma (Fig. 4). Retrosternal adenomas cannot be diagnosed, but [^{201}Tc] Thallium imaging is promising.

In conclusion, parathyroid imaging with radionuclides is being reintroduced partly because of improvements in the technique, partly because a positive result saves time and trouble, and partly because the morbidity of thyroid-parathyroid venous sampling, and the delay in obtaining the results is being increasingly recognized.

IV. THE ADRENALS

From the point of view of radionuclide imaging each adrenal gland may be considered as being made up to two organs: the adrenal cortex, which is imaged using radiolabeled cholesterol derivatives, in particular [^{75}Se] selenomethylcholesterol (SMC); and the adrenal medulla, which is imaged using radioiodinated meta-iodobenzylguanidine, (MIBG). The difficulties in localizing and lateralizing

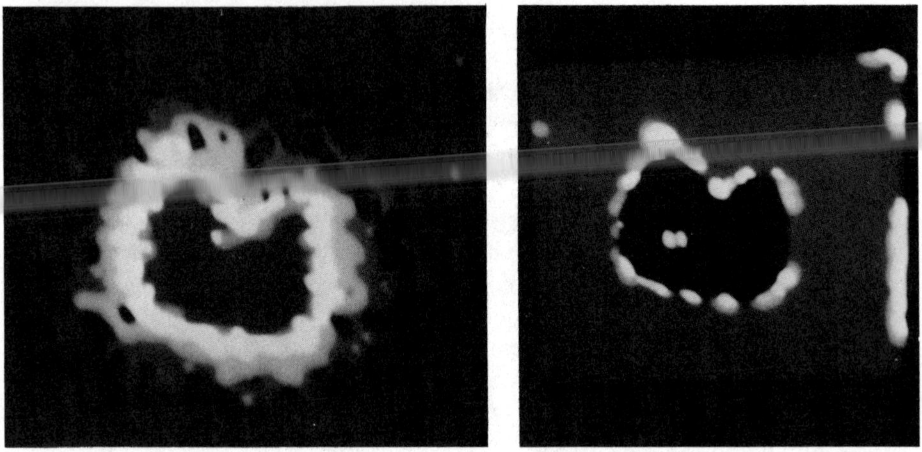

Figure 4 Parathyroid adenoma, [^{75}Se]selenomethionine study. Left: ^{125}I thyroid scan. Right: [^{75}Se]selenomethionine scan from which the thyroid scan has been subtracted, leaving a focal spot of high uptake in the parathyroid adenoma, confirmed surgically.

the site of adrenal pathology are the principal reasons for radionuclide adrenal imaging once biochemical results have confirmed the clinical diagnosis. The advantage of adrenal imaging over x-ray CT is that it can detect the physically small hyperfunctioning adenoma, particularly the adenoma causing Conn's syndrome, whereas x-ray CT is the method of choice for suspected adrenal cancer.

[^{75}Se] SMC has a better uptake and longer half-life than the ^{131}I-labeled cholesterols. It can be stored at room temperature and autoclaved. Its use does not require thyroid suppression, so it is preferred at present.

First the patient undergoes kidney imaging using a computer-linked gamma camera a minute after injection of about 2 mCi (75 MBq) [^{99m}Tc] diethylenetriamine pentacetic acid (DTPA). A posterior view is taken. Then two true lateral views of the kidney are obtained with a radioactive linear marker on the skin so that the skin-upper renal pole distance may be measured. This is an indicator of adrenal depth, which varies in adults from between 5 and 13 cm and compares well with depth obtained by transverse single photon emission tomography (SPET) (9). After the kidney studies are complete, the SMC is administered intravenously in a dose of about 250 μCi(9 MBq). The patient is sent home and returns for imaging at 7 and 14 days. These late imaging times ensure the virtual absence of nonadrenal activity, particularly in the liver and gut, but imaging first at 3 days may be effective. The imaging data are stored in the computer and corrected for background. Using the measured adrenal depth and standard curve relating depth to activity (10), the percentage of the administered SMC in each adrenal is determined. The normal range is 0.07-0.30% of the injected dose.

A. Cushing's Syndrome

The findings in bilateral hyperplasia are the same whether it is pituitary dependent, due to ectopic adrenocorticotropic hormone (ACTH), or congenital. Both glands are hyperactive, each with an average uptake of about 0.6% of the dose injected. Asymmetrical uptake is common, with one gland having an uptake in the upper normal range. Adrenal adenoma gives a specific picture of complete suppression of uptake by the contralateral normal gland (due to suppression of ACTH secretion by the high cortisol levels) and gross hyperactivity in the affected gland, averaging 0.9% of the injected dose (Fig. 5). Hyperplasia of a post-adrenalectomy recurrence also gives unilateral uptake after bilateral adrenalectomy. Infarction of one hyperplastic adrenal after venography, metastasis to one adrenal, or a large pheochromocytoma may prevent unilateral uptake.

Adrenal carcinoma gives a complex range of pictures, ranging from an adenoma-like picture for a well-differentiated cortisol-producing cancer, to absence of uptake. Occasionally, metastases may take up SMC, but this is not specific since granulomas may also show activity. Radiological CT scanning is preferred for adrenal cancer and is successful in Cushing's syndrome. The combination of these two noninvasive techniques has reduced the need for venous catheterization and/or angiography in the majority of cases.

B. Conn's Syndrome

The findings in bilateral hyperplasia (and in Bartter's syndrome) are of two hyperfunctioning glands with an average uptake of 0.35% of the injected dose by each. Overlap with the normal range is seen in 20%. A unilateral adenoma is reliably diagnosed (unless it is ectopic in the pelvis) with an average uptake of 0.47% and the contralateral gland is always visible, with uptake in the normal range using this technique (Fig. 6). X-ray CT scanning is less reliable in the diagnosis of Conn's adenoma. Positive lateralization and the distinction of adenoma from hyperplasia was correct in 18 or 21 patients, the three errors being due to not distinguishing bilateral hyperplasia from normal (11).

Dexamethasone suppression has its advocates but is not recommended because a normal result is "no uptake," so that technical failure cannot be excluded; and because dexamethasone "escape" occurs if adrenal imaging is delayed more than 5 days, so that a normal adrenal may be seen and interpreted as an adenoma.

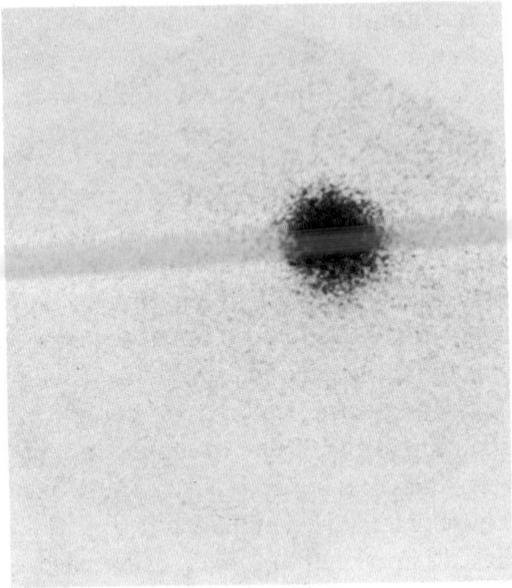

Figure 5 Right adrenal adenoma, posterior view, [^{75}Se]selenomethylcholesterol study. There is complete suppression of uptake by the left adrenal.

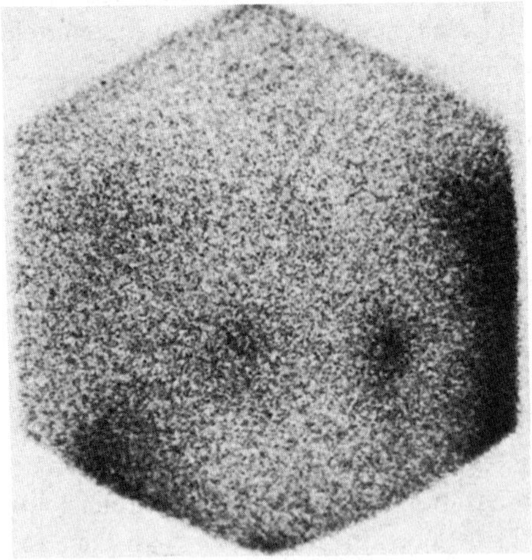

Figure 6 Bilateral adrenal hyperplasia causing Conn's syndrome, [^{75}Se]selenomethylcholesterol study. High uptake in both adrenals is seen (0.4% of the dose injected in each) and also in the colon.

C. Pheochromocytoma

The recent demonstration by Sisson et al. (12) of imaging the pheochromocytoma with [^{131}I] MIBG, not only in the adrenal but elsewhere in the abdomen, both benign and malignant and both adrenaline and noradrenaline secreting, will revolutionize the approach to localizing this tumor. These authors show it to be more reliable than x-ray CT. It is also thought that paraganglionomas along the thoracic and abdominal sympathetic chain take up MIBG. It is not reliable to use radiolabeled cholesterol to demonstrate adrenal pheochromocytoma as an absence of uptake by an adrenal.

D. Conclusion

Adrenal imaging with radiopharmaceuticals is a routine procedure in Cushing's and Conn's syndromes. A quantitative approach is more reliable than analog imaging, because of the great variation in depth of adrenals, so that a normal gland that is closer to the skin surface appears larger. Combinations of noninvasive radionuclide and x-ray CT imaging may avoid the need for invasive radiology in most cases.

V. OTHER ENDOCRINE DISORDERS

There is no radiopharmaceutical yet available to image insulinomas, glucagonomas, or endocrine adenomas of the intestinal tract. Ovarian imaging is not undertaken because of the potential radiation hazard to germ cells. Testicular imaging is undertaken not for endocrine reasons but to distinguish torsion from epididymitis (13).

REFERENCES

1. Britton KE, Shapiro B. Single photon emission tomography of the pituitary. J R Soc Med 1981; 74:667-669.
2. Staunton MD, Greening WP. Clinical diagnosis of thyroid cancer. Br Med J 1973; 4:532-535.
3. Shapiro B, Britton KE, Fountos A, et al. A multiobserver comparison of $^{99m}TcO_4$ and ^{123}I thyroid imaging. Eur J Nucl Med 1981; 6:135-137.
4. Spencer R, Holroyd AM. The value of ^{75}Se selenomethionine scanning in solitary nodules of the thyroid gland. Br J Radiol 1974; 47:457-463.
5. Kaplan WD, Holman BL, Selenkow HA, et al. ^{67}Ga-citrate and the nonfunctioning thyroid nodule. J Nucl Ned 1974; 15:424-425.
6. Harada T, Ito Y, Shimaoka K, Taniguchi T, Matsudo A, Senoo T. Clinical evaluation of ^{201}thallium chloride scan for thyroid nodule. Eur J Nucl Med 1980; 5:125-130.

7. Britton KE, Pearce PC. A method of dispensing ^{131}I therapy doses. Br J Radiol 1975; 48:687.
8. Elte JWF, Goslings BM, Pauwels EKJ. Parathyroid scanning with ^{75}Se selenomethionine after EDTA infusion. Nucl Med Commun 1980; 1:282-290.
9. Britton KE, Shapiro B, Hawkins LA. Emission tomography for adrenal imaging. Nucl Med Commun 1980; 1:37-40.
10. Hawkins LA, Britton KE, Shapiro B. Selenium 75 selenomethylcholesterol: a new agent for quantitative functional scintigraphy of the adrenals: physical aspects. Br J Radiol 1980; 53:883-889.
11. Shapiro B, Britton KE, Hawkins LA, Edwards CRW. Clinical experience with ^{75}Se selenomethyl cholesterol adrenal imaging. Clin Endocrinol 1981; 15:19-27.
12. Sisson JC, Frager MS, Valk TW, et al. Scintigraphic localisation of pheochromocytoma. N Engl J Med 1981; 305:12-17.
13. Lopez-Majano V, Salvatore M. Testicular imaging. Nucl Med Commun 1981; 2:221-226.

Further Reading

Maisey MN, Britton KE, Gilday D (eds). *Clinical Nuclear Medicine*. Chapman & Hall, London, 1983.

18
Laparoscopy

Roger J. Pepperell
University of Melbourne, Melbourne, Australia

Laparoscopy is a technique that enables direct visualization of intra-abdominal organs and allows biopsies to be taken from such organs if considered appropriate. The technique is widely used in the assessment of women with infertility, as it enables the external appearance and patency of the fallopian tubes to be assessed, the presence of endometriosis to be excluded, and the macroscopic and microscopic normality of the ovaries to be determined.

Evaluation of infertility is certainly not complete until a laparoscopy has been performed as, even when a hysterogram shows no apparent tubal abnormality, it is not uncommon to find extratubal adhesions or clubbing of the fimbriae, which may be interfering with fertility. It is also well known that even severe pelvic endometriosis may only be able to be diagnosed at the time of laparoscopy, as it is frequently asymptomatic and not evident on pelvic examination. The vast majority of women being subject to diagnostic laparoscopy for infertility do not have an endocrine problem, however.

The use of laparoscopy as an aid to endocrine diagnosis is virtually confined to the conditions listed in Table 1. Not all patients in each of the subgroups listed require laparoscopy; in fact, it is usual to be able to make a diagnosis by clinical assessment and hormone assays, and laparoscopy is then reserved for the more difficult diagnostic dilemmas.

I. PRIMARY AMENORRHEA

Three distinct subgroups of patients with primary amenorrhea require laparoscopy: those with probable mullerian duct abnormalities, those with a normal 46XX chromosome analysis but elevated serum follicle stimulating hormone

Table 1 Use of Laparoscopy for Endocrine Diagnosis

Condition	Reason for laparoscopy
Primary amenorrhea	To assess mullerian duct development To assess ovarian development (± biopsy)
Secondary amenorrhea	Ovarian visualization Biopsy (if serum FSH level elevated)
Hirsutism	Ovarian visualization ± biopsy
Menstrual disorders	To diagnose hormone-producing ovarian tumors
Intersex	To determine sex of rearing
Precocious puberty	To diagnose hormone-producing ovarian tumors

(FSH) levels, and those whose chromosome analysis shows a Y chromosome to be present.

Mullerian duct absence or extreme hypoplasia can usually be diagnosed prior to laparoscopy by the presence of normal secondary sexual characteristics, evidence of ovulation, and the absence of a palpable uterus on vaginal or rectal examination. Laparoscopy is required, however, if a full assessment of the extent of the abnormality is necessary in order that an accurate prognostic statement can be made.

The presence of elevated FSH levels usually indicates an abnormality of ovarian development or function. Such subjects may have complete ovarian absence, streak gonads, or have "ovarian resistance." The former conditions can be clearly defined by laparoscopy, and biopsy of a streak gonad is not required to confirm the absence of Graafian follicles. In fact, laparoscopic ovarian biopsy of such gonads is associated with a considerable risk of hemorrhage due to the close proximity of the vascular supply, and can rarely be justified. Where the ovary appears to be of normal or near normal in size, however, a biopsy should be taken. If this biopsy shows the presence of a normal number of Graafian follicles, the diagnosis of ovarian resistance can be made. Such information is of limited use to the clinician as, while the FSH levels remain elevated, ovulation induction is doomed to failure. It does allow the patient to be informed accurately about the exact diagnosis, however.

Patients with known X-chromosome abnormalities (e.g., XO, XO/XX mosaic) rarely require laparoscopy, as if the serum FSH level is elevated, streak gonads will be shown to be present. If the serum FSH level is normal (e.g., in some patients with XO/XX mosaicism), Graafian follicles are presented in the ovaries and ovarian biopsy is not required to confirm this. Such subjects usually have smaller ovaries than normal, often subsequently develop a premature menopause, and removal of any ovarian tissue for biopsy can rarely be justified.

Except in patients with the testicular feminization syndrome and whose gonads are clearly palpable in the pubic region, laparoscopy or laparotomy is required for all phenotypically female subjects shown to have a Y chromosome. Such subjects are at increased risk for the development of gonadal tumors (1) (usually gonadoblastoma or dysgerminoma) and it is usual to recommend gonadectomy at or before the age of puberty. Where gonadectomy is refused, or its timing delayed, laparoscopy is advisable to ensure that a tumor is not already present.

II. SECONDARY AMENORRHEA

The usual reasons for laparoscopy in patients with secondary amenorrhea are to diagnose polycystic ovarian disease (PCO) and to perform an ovarian biopsy in patients with elevated serum FSH levels. Many patients with PCO have mild hirsutism, moderately enlarged ovaries, slightly elevated serum luteinizing hormone (LH) levels, and a clinical diagnosis can readily be made. Where laparoscopy is performed, the appearance of the ovaries is virtually diagnostic for the condition as the ovaries are enlarged, smooth, pearly white in color, and often small cysts are able to be identified beneath the surface (2). Ovarian biopsy, although not usually necessary to confirm the diagnosis, is sometimes therapeutic with reestablishment of ovulatory cycles following the procedure (3).

Where the FSH levels are elevated, the diagnosis could be that of ovarian failure or ovarian resistance. It is important to differentiate between the two conditions if the patient is concerned about her fertility potential, as spontaneous resolution occurs in about 25% of patients with apparent ovarian resistance (4). This would not be recognized if the patient was assumed to have ovarian failure and given hormone replacement therapy. In the presence of ovarian failure the ovaries usually appear to be small, shriveled up, and pale in color (2), whereas in ovarian resistance the ovaries are often of normal size but show no evidence of follicular growth. Ovarian biopsy will usually clarify the diagnosis; however, the biopsy should be obtained with Palmer forceps and should measure at least 0.8 x 0.6 x 0.4 cm (2). If the biopsy is not large enough it may not be representative of the whole ovary and incorrect advice may then be given to the patient. This applies particularly where a small biopsy shows no Graafian follicles and the patient is labeled as having premature ovarian failure, only to commence menstruating again and sometimes conceiving at a later date (4-6).

III. HIRSUTISM

Where the hormone assays indicate a probable ovarian cause for the hirsutism, it has been common for gynecologists to perform a laparoscopy and ovarian biopsy to make a diagnosis of PCO and exclude an androgen-producing tumor of the ovary (e.g., arrhenoblastoma). Androgen-producing tumors are extremely rare and are often too small to be identified separately from surrounding normal ovarian tissue. Blind biopsy of an apparently normal ovary is not justified to exclude such a tumor and biopsy is usually not required to make a diagnosis of PCO because of the classical macroscopic features of the ovary in patients with this condition. As indicated earlier, this diagnosis can usually be made clinically, supported by the presence of elevated serum LH levels, and laparoscopy is usually not required at all.

IV. MENSTRUAL DISORDERS

The vast majority of patients with menstrual irregularity have an endocrine cause for their problem and have some disturbance of their hypothalamic-pituitary-ovarian axis. This can be clarified with hormone assays and laparoscopy is rarely required in the diagnostic evaluation of such patients. The only subjects in whom laparoscopy is indicated are those shown to have persistent marked elevation of their estrogen levels, in whom an estrogen-producing tumor of the ovary is suspected. Such patients are uncommon and, as the tumor may be small and not easily identified from surrounding normal ovarian tissue, ovarian biopsy may not enable the diagnosis to be made anyway.

V. INTERSEX

Laparoscopy has been used in the diagnostic evaluation of patients with intersex to determine the presence or absence of mullerian duct structures, the macroscopic features of the gonads, and to enable biopsies to be taken from the gonads (7). All of these features may aid the clinician in determining the sex of rearing. It is often more appropriate for these assessments to be made at the time of laparotomy however, as gonads or other structures which are inappropriate for the chosen sex of rearing can then be removed.

VI. PRECOCIOUS PUBERTY

Laparoscopic assessment of girls with precocious puberty would allow recognition of an estrogen-producing ovarian tumor if one was present and of sufficient size to be differentiated from surrounding ovarian tissue (7). The procedure can only be justified if the elevated estrogen levels are associated with prepubertal levels of FSH and LH and there is no evidence of an adrenal tumor.

Although laparoscopy is a relatively simple technique, severe complications can occur during and after its performance. Death or severe morbidity has been reported due to anesthetic accidents, gas embolism, peritonitis due to perforation of gastrointestinal organs, and hemorrhage following ovarian biopsy (2,8). Laparoscopy should not be performed unless the diagnosis is uncertain and cannot be clarified using less invasive procedures.

REFERENCES

1. Fathalla MF, Rashad MN, Kerr MG. The relationship between ovarian tumors and intersex states with special reference to the disgerminoma and arrhenoblastoma. J Obstet Gynaecol Br Commonw 1966; 73:812–820.
2. Fayez JA, Jonas HS. Assessment of the role of laparoscopic ovarian biopsy. Obstet Gynecol 1976; 48:397-402.
3. Yuzpe AA, Rioux JE. The value of laparoscopic ovarian biopsy. J Reprod Med 1975; 15:57-59.
4. O'Herlihy C, Pepperell RJ, Evans JH. The significance of FSH elevation in young women with disorders of ovulation. Br Med J 1980; 281:1447-1450.
5. Sutton C. The limitations of laparoscopic ovarian biopsy. J Obstet Gynaecol Br Commonw 1974; 81:317-320.
6. Shangold MM, Turksoy RN, Bashford RA, Hammond CB. Pregnancy following the "insensitive ovary syndrome." Fertil Steril 1977; 28:1179-1181.
7. Cognat M, Papathanassiou Z, Gomel V. Laparoscopy in infants and adolescents. J Reprod Med 1974; 13:11-12.
8. Loffer FD, Pent D. Indications, contraindications and complications of laparoscopy. Obstet Gynecol Surv 1975; 30:407-427.

PITUITARY DISORDERS

19

Corticotropin, Lipotropins, and Endorphins

Don H. Nelson and A. Wayne Meikle
University of Utah School of Medicine, Salt Lake City, Utah

The anterior pituitary gland secretes (ACTH), adrenocorticotropic hormone, which has as its primary function the control of corticosteroid secretion by the adrenal cortex. In addition to ACTH, however, recent evidence has demonstrated the production and secretion of a number of other peptides, including β-lipotropin (β-LPH) and β-endorphin. These peptides and others have as a common precursor a 239-amino acid peptide which has been named proopiocortin (see Fig. 1). This large precursor corresponds to the 31K glycosylated precursor of Mains and Eipper (2). ACTH and β-lipotropin are cleaved from this large molecule by trypsin-like activity. Although there are some species variations, ACTH and β-LPH may be secreted or broken down further to give β-endorphins, α-melanocyte stimulating hormone (MSH), β-MSH, or α-endorphin. β-MSH has not been positively identified in humans and earlier studies suggesting its presence in either the gland or in plasma were probably confused by reaction of antisera with other peptides. In the monkey, pig, and sheep, however, large concentrations of β-MSH are found which are restricted mainly to the pars intermedia (which is rudimentary in the adult human). α-MSH and corticotropin-like intermediary lobe peptide (CLIP) have been found in all species studied, although the levels in adult, nonpregnant humans are difficult to detect.

Large molecules with ACTH immunoreactivity have been described in patients with Cushing's disease, Nelson's syndrome, and in "ectopic" ACTH-producing tumors obtained from lung or other nonpituitary tissues (3-5). The "big ACTH" extracted from a number of tumors lacked biological activity, but activity was present after treatment with trypsin, suggesting identity with proopiocortin.

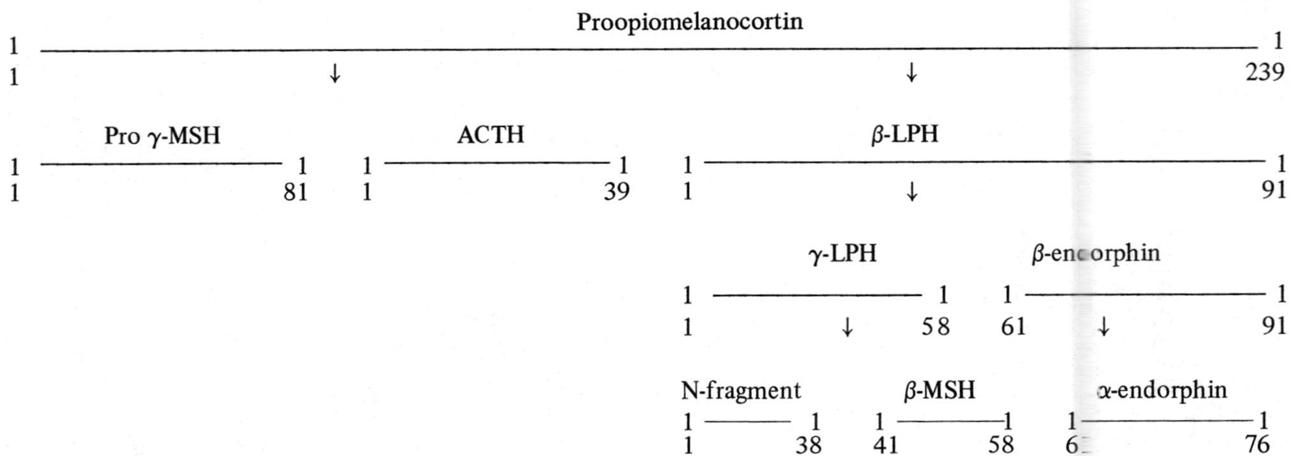

Figure 1 Breakdown of the common precursor for ACTH and LPH. (Adapted from Ref. 1.)

Many studies have now demonstrated a significant correlation between plasma levels of ACTH, LPH, and β-endorphin (5-7). Both in vitro and in vivo studies demonstrate release of ACTH, β- and γ-LPH, and β-endorphin following stimulation by corticotropin releasing factor (CRF) (8). β-LPH conversion to β-endorphin is increased in ACTH-secreting adenomas, with suppression of ACTH and β-endorphin in surrounding nonadenomatous tissues (9). Isolation of an end-terminal peptide similar to the pro-γ-MSH proposed by Nakao from a Cushing's-producing pituitary adenoma has also been reported (11, 12).

Secretion of corticotropin and related peptides by the anterior pituitary gland appears to be largely under the control of CRF produced by the anterior hypothalamus. Although vasopressin and other peptides have the ability to stimulate ACTH and β-lipotropin secretion under a variety of circumstances, the probable true CRH is a recently isolated, identified, and synthesized 41 residue peptide, as shown in Figure 2. Of interest are the many similarities in structure between this peptide and angiotensinogen and sauvagine. The latter is a 40-residue peptide isolated from the skin of the South American frog *Phylomedusa sauvagei*, which causes release of ACTH and β-endorphin in vivo and in vitro and inhibits thyrotropin, somatotropin, and prolactin secretion. CRF and sauvagine cause lowering of blood pressure when used in quantities 100 times greater than that necessary to stimulate ACTH and β-endorphin secretion.

I. CUSHING'S DISEASE

The primary clinical syndrome resulting from the oversecretion of corticotropin and related peptides is Cushing's disease or pituitary-dependent Cushing's syndrome (14).

Cushing's syndrome is due to cortisol overproduction by the adrenal glands, or administration of excessive quantities of glucocorticoids. Spontaneous or endogenous oversecretion of cortisol is produced by excessive secretion of ACTH from the pituitary gland or by autonomous adrenal tumors or non-pituitary tumors. Hypothalamic secretion of corticotropin releasing hormone (CRF) may be responsible in some cases, but definite proof of this etiology has been difficult to establish.

Drug-induced causes (exogenous) of Cushing's syndrome are more common than endogenous causes of the disorder. Corticosteroid administration is the most common cause of the syndrome. Etiologic determination usually presents no difficulty due to the history of drug administration. However, surreptitious use of glucocorticoids may require careful evaluation. A particular problem arises when patients are receiving "small" doses of glucocorticoids, such as 5 mg of prednisone twice daily, and present with the syndrome. It is our experience that "small" divided doses are more likely to produce the syndrome than a

H-Ser-Gln-Glu-Pro-Pro-Ile-Ser-Leu-Asp-Leu-Thr-Phe-His-Leu-Leu-Arg-
Glu-Val-Leu-Glu-Met-Thr-Lys-Ala-Asp-Glu-Leu-Ala-Gln-Gln-Ala-His-
Ser-Asn-Arg-Lys-Leu-Leu-Asp-Ile-Ala-NH_2

Figure 2 Structure of CRF. (From Ref. 13.)

comparable single daily dose (15). The problem presented by these cases is whether there is an endogenous or exogenous cause for the disorder. Although the incidence is unknown, pseudo-Cushing's syndrome produced by chronic alcohol abuse is recognized with increased frequency (16). In milder forms of depression (particularly of the familial type), the differentiation of endogenous Cushing's syndrome and depression may be a challenge. In both conditions the dexamethasone suppression test is abnormal (17, 18).

The clinical features of Cushing's syndrome range from a few of the signs and symptoms to a florid picture. Weight gain, acne, back pain, hirsutism, amenorrhea, and proximal muscle weakness are common symptoms and signs. Excess fat is typically distributed over the trunk, head, and neck, with prominent supraclavicular fat pads and a "buffalo hump." The face is plethoric and moon-shaped. Proximal muscle wasting results in thin arms and legs. The skin may be thin and bruise easily and purple striae may be observed on the lower abdomen and upper thighs. Mild hirsutism is common and is produced by excess adrenal androgen secretion. If a marked degree of virilism is present (clitoral enlargement, increased muscle mass, and voice change), an adrenal cortical adenoma or carcinoma producing androgens is more likely. Pigmentation of the buccal mucosa, palmar creases, sun-exposed areas, knuckles, and recent scars may be found in patients with ACTH-dependent Cushing's syndrome. Hypertension is common and it is unclear whether it is caused by cortisol excess alone or by other adrenal steroids. Overt diabetes is uncommon but glucose intolerance may be present. Osteoporosis may produce loss of height through collapse of vertebrae, and other pathologic fractures may occur in the syndrome of longer duration.

Glucocorticoid excess has profound effects on the metabolism of carbohydrates, lipids, and proteins and also stimulates the appetite. Its metabolic effects promote the increased synthesis of fat. Catabolism of protein results in muscle wasting and weakness; loss of collagen in the skin produces striae, bruising, and poor wound healing; and loss of protein of the bone matrix contributes to osteoporosis. The anti-insulin effect of cortisol produces glucose intolerance or contributes to the occurrence of overt diabetes. Those patients with the syndrome caused by ectopic ACTH production may present with weight loss, hyperpigmentation, muscle weakness, edema, and hypertension with hypokalemia. In these cases excess mineralocorticoid production apparently is more profound than in those with pituitary-dependent Cushing's syndrome. The majority of the signs and symptoms of pituitary-dependent Cushing's syndrome result from the increased secretion of corticosteroids secondary to excessive secretion of ACTH. In most cases this can be demonstrated to be secondary to a small adenoma of the anterior pituitary gland. Although these adenomas are occasionally large enough to be seen by conventional x-ray examination, computerized axial tomography (CAT) scans of the pituitary gland with enhancement have greatly increased our ability to demonstrate the presence of these adenomas. Of interest are occasional reports of patients with corticotroph cell hyperplasia of the pituitary and no demonstrable adenoma. It is patients of this type in whom the etiology may be hypothalamic oversecretion of CRF. Such patients are unlikely to respond to surgery of the pituitary gland unless total hypophysectomy is performed (19). In a number of cases multiple ACTH-secreting microadenomas have been described or the reappearance of Cushing's syndrome following the removal of a single adenoma has occurred (20). The occasional report of patients with intermittent Cushing's disease also is suggestive of stimulation of the pituitary gland by exogenous factors such as CRF (21). In large pituitary tumors, such as those associated with Nelson's syndrome, pituitary apoplexy may occur acutely (22) or silently (23), followed by considerable fall in plasma ACTH levels. Spontaneous remission of Cushing's disease may occur secondary to infarction of a pituitary tumor or due to as yet unidentified factors (24-26).

Selective venous sampling for ACTH may be useful in demonstrating the pituitary source of the ACTH (27). Studies of this type are difficult to perform, however, and should be carried out only with the aid of a radiologist experienced with venous catheterization. Even with expert help the results have often been difficult to interpret in our experience with the technique.

Increased secretion of ACTH is usually associated with large quantities of β-lipotropin. Both molecules have melanocyte stimulating activity, which produces varying amounts of pigmentation. As the amount of β-lipotropin and ACTH produced is roughly correlated with the size of the tumor, the degree of pigmentation also increases as tumor size increases. This is particularly true in Nelson's syndrome (see below), in which large tumors are associated with a marked degree of pigmentation.

β-Endorphin, which is also increased in the plasma of patients with pituitary-dependent Cushing's disease, has been demonstrated to have profound effects on mental function (28, 29). This, and similar peptides, produce behavioral changes when injected intracerebrally or intraventricularly in animal models and may produce alterations in schizophrenic states (30, 31). Although a direct relation between increased amounts of β-endorphins and the mental disturbances of Cushing's syndrome has not been demonstrated, many instances of improved mental function occurring following correction of Cushing's disease have been reported. These have been attributed to reduced levels of corticosteroids, which can influence mental function when present in pharmacological amounts, but change in mental status following the removal of ACTH-secreting tumors occurring in patients who have previously undergone bilateral adrenalectomy strongly suggests these peptides as etiologic factors in the mental disturbance of some patients with Cushing's disease. An active field of investigation at present is the influence of ACTH, β-lipotropin, and β-endorphin-like peptides not only on mental disturbance but also on attention and memory (32, 33).

Laboratory diagnosis of pituitary-dependent Cushing's syndrome is dependent on demonstrating increased secretion of cortisol by hyperplastic adrenal glands, and ACTH levels which are higher than normal for the level of cortisol secretion. The increased ACTH is due in most cases to a small adenoma of the pituitary gland, which is less sensitive to suppression by cortisol than is normal ACTH-secreting pituitary tissue. The approach to demonstrating these abnormalities consists of (1) measurement of elevated levels of cortisol or increased secretion; and (2) demonstration of ACTH secretion which is not suppressed by moderately elevated corticosteroid levels. Increased cortisol secretion is usually demonstrated by the presence of high normal to slightly elevated plasma cortisol levels with loss of diurnal variation. Plasma cortisol levels are highly dependent on the amount of corticosteroid binding globulin (CBG) in the plasma, and thus all elevations in cortisol should be viewed with the possibility that they may have occurred secondary to an increase in the CBG. CBG levels are increased in patients receiving estrogens or during pregnancy. A rare familial condition occurs in which there is a peripheral tissue insensitivity to the corticosteroids produced (34). High plasma cortisol levels may be present in these subjects in the absence of elevated CBG and yet not produce Cushing's syndrome.

Total free cortisol measured in the urine will demonstrate adrenal hyperactivity and is the most useful of the urinary corticosteroid determinations. If the urine is adequately collected, and this is sometimes difficult, an elevation in excretion is highly suggestive of the diagnosis. Other urinary determinations, such as 17-ketogenic steroids and 17-hydroxycorticosteroids, have the disadvantage that obese patients have higher than normal levels and a number of drugs may interfere with the determination. Aspirin in doses exceeding 4.8 g daily inhibits the β-glucuronidase employed in some urinary measurements and will thus result in low levels of hormone being measured. Propoxyphene and pentazocine will suppress urinary corticoids, as do chlorpromazine and hydroxyzine. Phenylbutazone produces increased 6β-hydroxylation, which may interfere with the extraction by organic solvents of cortisol and its metabolites, and phenobarbital and diphenylhydantoin also stimulate hepatic oxygenases involved in drug hydroxylation and in large doses may influence urinary findings. As there is day-to-day variation in the excretion of these hormones, all elevations should be confirmed and a likely diagnosis not ruled out on the basis of a single normal value.

Plasma ACTH and/or β-lipotropin levels are characteristically elevated to a moderate extent and fail to suppress when moderate amounts of corticosteroids are administered. ACTH, like the corticosteroids, undergoes both circadian and episodic variation in the blood. Patients with pituitary-dependent Cushing's disease will usually be found to have slightly elevated ACTH levels, although normal levels may be present. An elevated level may be found on a single measurement coincident with an episodic peak in a normal individual. A group of hospitalized patients have been shown to have higher levels than do normal control subjects, presumably secondary to the stress of their illness and hospitalization (35). Samples are particularly likely to be demonstrably elevated if obtained during the late evening (8-12 P.M.), as ACTH normally is very low during this time period. A greater than normal ACTH response to metyrapone administration is highly suggestive of pituitary hyperactivity in patients demonstrated to have Cushing's syndrome. As autonomous adrenal tumors have low to absent ACTH secretion, even normal plasma ACTH values greatly increase the possibility that the disease is pituitary dependent. ACTH is a highly labile molecule and thus great care must be taken in obtaining samples and transporting them for ACTH determination. The blood is normally drawn with heparin, kept in ice, and the plasma is separated in a refrigerated centrifuge and then frozen. To prevent ACTH binding to glass, syringes and tubes employed in the entire procedure are plastic. As β-lipotropin is a much more stable molecule than is ACTH, and is elevated with ACTH, it has been suggested that measurement of β-lipotropin replace routine ACTH measurements.

Suppression tests are some of the most useful of the tests employed in the diagnosis of Cushing's disease and in its differentiation from adrenal tumors. Although there are both false positive and false negative tests (as explained more completely in Chapter 38), resistance to suppression by dexamethasone or other potent corticosteroid in a patient who has an elevated plasma ACTH is highly suggestive of the diagnosis of Cushing's disease. Our commonly used screening test is the 1-mg dexamethasone suppression test, although 0.5 mg of dexamethasone every 6 hr for eight doses is also an adequate test. Failure to suppress following the 1-mg administration is presumptive evidence of Cushing's syndrome. Suppression of cortisol levels by this dose rules out the diagnosis in 95% of cases. The multiple-dose suppression test is usually carried out using urinary 17-hydroxycorticosteroids or 17-ketogenic steroids, but plasma levels of cortisol also have been employed. Significant suppression largely rules out the disease, while failure to suppress is highly suggestive of Cushing's syndrome. Most patients who fail to suppress endogenous secretion with a 1-mg overnight suppression test, or the low-dose multiple dexamethasone suppression test will suppress when a higher dose of dexamethasone is administered. For the overnight test this consists of 4 mg or even 8 mg given in a single dose. For the multiple dose the standard test is 2 mg every 6 hr for 48 hr (high-dose suppression test) (36). Failure to suppress with high doses of dexamethasone is most consistent with the presence of an autonomous tumor, but some tumors of the adrenal and ectopic ACTH-producing tumors will suppress with very high doses of dexamethasone (37, 38).

Of interest in the employment of the dexamethasone test in Cushing's syndrome are the group of patients who have an acute increase in cortisol secretion following administration of dexamethasone. Continued administration of dexamethasone to most of these patients will produce suppression. An occasional patient will be found dexamethasone nonsuppressible and yet will show suppression when large amounts of cortisol are administered. It is postulated that in these cases the "receptors" in the pituitary gland which are sensitive to corticosteroid levels in the plasma fail to respond normally to dexamethasone, but may still respond to cortisol. Factors that influence the metabolism of dexamethasone may have considerable effect on these suppression tests (these are covered more fully in Chapter 38).

The use of metyrapone as a pharmacologic stimulator of adrenal pituitary secretion has proven to be a highly useful test in the differential diagnosis of the etiology of Cushing's syndrome (39, 40). Whether the single- or multiple-dose test is performed, an active to a hyperactive increase in secretion of 11-desoxycortisol and ACTH following administration of metyrapone is highly suggestive of the presence of pituitary-dependent Cushing's syndrome (41). Failure to respond is characteristic of patients who have autonomously secreting adrenal tumors or ectopic ACTH-secreting tumors (14). The sequential evaluation of patients with suspected Cushing's syndrome is outlined in Diagnostic Summary I.

II. ACTH-SECRETING PITUITARY TUMORS ASSOCIATED WITH INTENSE PIGMENTATION (NELSON'S SYNDROME)

The initial patient found to have this syndrome was a patient with apparent pituitary-dependent Cushing's syndrome who underwent bilateral adrenalectomy for her disease in the mid-1950s (22). Three years following total adrenalectomy, she was found to have extremely marked generalized pigmentation of the skin and a pituitary tumor. Plasma levels of ACTH as determined by bioassay were found to be 400 mU/dl (normal is less than 1 mU/dl). Following removal of the pituitary gland there was a marked decrease in skin pigmentation and also in plasma ACTH values.

Diagnostic Summary 1 Cushing's syndrome.

Test and results	Probable diagnosis
1. Dexamethasone suppression (1 mg overnight)	
8 A.M. cortisol	
<5 μg/dl	Normal
>5 μg/dl	Inadequate test, Cushing's syndrome, endogenous depression, or acute alcoholism
2. Urinary free cortisol, >normal	Stressed patient or Cushing's syndrome
3. 8 A.M. plasma ACTH (or β-lipotropin)	
Elevated ACTH	Stressed patient, pituitary dependent Cushing's disease; acute alcoholism, endogenous depression, or ectopic tumor
Very high ACTH, >500 pg/ml	Ectopic ACTH tumor
Low ACTH	Adrenal tumor producing Cushing's syndrome, or poor sample preparation
4. Metyrapone (single-dose test)	
Lack of response 11-Desoxycortisol, <7 μg/dl Plasma ACTH, <100 pg/ml	Adrenal tumor, ectopic tumor, drug interference with test
Active response 11-desoxycortisol, >7 μg/dl ACTH, >150 pg/dl	Normal or pituitary-dependent Cushing's disease
5. High-dose dexamethasone suppression (4 mg or more)	
Lack of suppression of 8 A.M. cortisol	Adrenal tumor, ectopic tumor, rare pituitary-dependent Cushing's disease
6. a. CAT scan of pituitary if pituitary dependent Cushing's disease likely b. CAT scan of adrenal if adrenal tumor is suspected	
7. Selective venous catheterization; for determination of ACTH or cortisol if tests above are not definitive	

Note: For further details regarding the interpretation of the investigations above, see Ref. 14.

Approximately 10% of patients who underwent bilateral adrenalectomy during the period of time that this form of therapy was widely used have been seen to develop pituitary tumors of this type. It is generally believed that these tumors result from continued growth of microadenomas present and responsible for the development of the initial Cushing's disease. The recent description of similar tumors, in rare instances, in patients with Addison's disease lends support to the concept that hypothalamic stimulation or lack of corticosteroid feedback suppression on the pituitary gland contributes to the production of the pituitary tumors (42). The high levels of ACTH occasionally are associated with the development of testicular or paraovarian tumors. These tumors are thought to arise from adrenal cells, although the exact origin is controversial (43).

Although it has been suggested that pituitary irradiation may decrease the incidence of these pituitary tumors, this has not been a consistent finding and at present there is no preventive measure known. These tumors may be rapidly growing and they may undergo spontaneous infarction or extend outside the sella. It is advisable, therefore, to undertake surgical removal if growth is found to be present.

III. NODULAR ADRENAL CORTICAL HYPERPLASIA

Multiple hyperplastic nodules and adenomas have been seen in a number of patients with Cushing's syndrome (44). In the most common variety there is hyperplastic tissue associated with the adenomas, suggesting that ACTH has not been suppressed (45). In some cases elevated ACTH has been demonstrated (46). In a few cases the adenomas have failed to respond to metyrapone and ACTH levels were found to be suppressed (47). It is not clear at present whether this represents the same disease as the pituitary-dependent variety.

IV. SPECIFIC ACTH DEFICIENCY

An extremely rare pituitary associated adrenal disorder is specific ACTH deficiency. These patients have normal production of other pituitary hormones, but are found to be deficient in ACTH secretion. As a result of this deficiency, the adrenals undergo atrophy and the patient has adrenal insufficiency of the type seen in panhypopituitarism. The condition is difficult to diagnose, as the patient does not develop the pigmentation or electrolyte disturbances of primary adrenal insufficiency or the decreased thyroidal or gonadal function typical of panhypopituitarism. Diagnosis is made by finding that a patient who becomes hypotensive or extremely ill when stressed has low plasma cortisol, a failure to respond to metyrapone, and a low plasma ACTH. It is not unusual for such patients to become hyponatremic when stressed. The hyponatremia is dilutional in type and appears to result from increased secretion of antidiuretic hormone with water retention in an attempt to compensate for the vascular collapse characteristic of acute adrenal insufficiency.

REFERENCES

1. Lowry PJ, Cillio G, Hope J, Jackson S. Structure and biosynthesis of peptides related to corticotrophin and lipotrophin. Horm Res 1980; 13:201-210.
2. Mains RE, Eipper BA. Biosynthesis of adrenocorticotropic hormone in mouse pituitary tumor cells. J Biol Chem 1976; 251:4115-4120.
3. Yalow RS, Berson SA. Size heterogeneity of immunoreactive human ACTH in plasma and in extracts of pituitary glands and ACTH producing thymoma. Biochem Biophys Res Commun 1971; 44:439-445.
4. Wolfsen AR, Odell WD. ProACTH: use for early detection of lung cancer. Am J Med 1979; 66:765-772.
5. Krieger DT, Liotta AS, Suda T, Goodgold A, Condon E. Human plasma immunoreactive lipoprotein and adrenocorticotropin in normal subjects and in patients with pituitary-adrenal disease. J Clin Endocrinol Metab 1979; 4:566-571.
6. Gewirtz G, Schneider B, Krieger DT, et al. Big ACTH: conversion to biologically active ACTH by trypsin. J Clin Endocrinol Metab 1974; 38:227-230.
7. Bertagna X, Luton J-P, Binoux M, Bricaire H, Girard F. Characterization of lipotropin-, corticotropin-, and β-endorphin-immunoreactive materials secreted in vitro by a human pituitary adenoma responsible for a case of Nelson's syndrome. J Clin Endocrinol Metab 1979; 49:527-532.
8. Gillies G, Ratter S, Grossman A, Gaillard R, Lowry PJ, Besser GM, Rees LH. ACTH, LPH and β-endorphin secretion from perfused isolated human pituitary tumour cells in vitro. Horm Res 1980; 13:280-290.
9. Suda T, Abe Y, Demura H, Demura R, Shizume K, Tamahashi N, Sasano N. ACTH, β-LPH, and β-endorphin in pituitary adenomas of the patients with Cushing's disease: activation of β-LPH conversion to β-endorphin. J Clin Endocrinol Metab 1979; 49:475-477.
10. Chan JSD, Seidah NG, Gianoulakis C, Belanger A, Chretien M. Chemical characterization of adrenocorticotropin and a novel peptide biosynthesized from a pituitary adenoma of a patient with Cushing's disease. J Clin Endocrinol Metab 1980; 51:364-367.
11. Nakao K, Oki S, Tanaka I, Nakai Y, Imura H. Concomitant secretion of γ-MSH with ACTH and β-endorphin in humans. J Clin Endocrinol Metab 1980; 51:1205-1207.
12. Shibasaki T, Masui H, Sato G, Ling N, Guillemin R. Secretion pattern of proopiomelanocrotin-derived peptides by a pituitary adenoma from a patient with Cushing's disease. J Clin Endocrinol Metab 1981; 52:350-353.

13. Vale W, Spiess J, Rivier C, Rivier J. Characterization of a 42-residue ovine hypothalamic peptide that stimulates secretion of corticotropin and β-endorphin. Science 1981; 213:1394-1397.
14. Nelson DH. Cushing's syndrome. In *The Adrenal Cortex: Physiological Function and Disease.* Saunders, Philadelphia, 1980, pp 134-176.
15. Meikle AW, Nelson DH. Unpublished observations, 19XX.
16. Smals AG, Kloppenborg PW, Njo KT, Knoben JM, Ruland CM. Alcohol induced cushingoid syndrome. Br Med J 1976; 2:1298.
17. Starkman MN, Schteingart DE, Schork MA. Depressed mood and other psychiatric manifestations of Cushing's syndrome: relationship to hormone levels. Psychosom Med 1981; 43:3-18.
18. Carroll BJ, Schroeder K, Mukhopadhyay S, Greden JF, Feinberg M, Ritchie J, Tarika J. Plasma dexamethasone concentrations and cortisol suppression response in patients with endogenous depression. J Clin Endocrinol Metab 1980; 51:433-437.
19. Schnall AM, Kovacs K, Brodkey JS, Pearson OH. Pituitary Cushing's disease without adenoma. Acta Endocrinol 1980; 94:297-303.
20. Lamberts SWJ, Stefanko SZ, deLange SA, Germin H, van der Vijer J-CM, deJong FH. Failure of clinical remission after transsphenoidal removal of a microadenoma in a patient with Cushing's disease: multiple hyperplastic and adenomatous cell nests in surrounding pituitary tissue. J Clin Endocrinol Metab 1980; 50:793-795.
21. Bochner F, Burke CJ, Lloyd HM, Nurnberg BI. Intermittent Cushing's disease. Am J Med 1979; 67:507-510.
22. Nelson DH, Meakin JW, Dealy JB, Jr, et al. A corticotropin producing tumor of the pituitary gland. N Engl J Med 1958; 259:161-164.
23. Findling JW, Tyrrell JB, Aron DC, Fitzgerald PA, Wilson CB, Forsham PH. Silent pituitary apoplexy: subclinical infarction of an adrenocorticotropin-producing pituitary adenoma. J Clin Endocrinol Metab 1981; 52: 95-97.
24. Jordan RM, Cook DM, Kendall JW, Kerber CW. Nelson's syndrome and spontaneous pituitary tumor infarction. Arch Intern Med 1979; 139:340-342.
25. Kammer H, Barter M. Spontaneous remission of Cushing's disease. A case report and review of the literature. Am J Med 1979; 67:519-523.
26. Scott RS, Espiner EA, Donald RA. Intermittent Cushing's disease with spontaneous remission. Clin Endocrinol 1979; 11:561-566.
27. Findling JW, Aron DC, Tyrrell JB, Shinsaki JH, Fitzgerald PA, Normal D, Wilson CB, Forsham PH. Selective venous sampling for ACTH in Cushing's syndrome. Ann Intern Med 1981; 94:647-652.
28. Bloom F, Segal D, Ling N, et al. Endorphins: profound behavioral effects in rats suggest new etiological factors in mental illness. Science 1976; 194: 632-635.

29. Jacquet YF, Marks N. The C-fragment of β-lipotropin: an endogenous neuroleptic or antipsychotogen? Science 1976; 194:632-635.
30. Beckwith BE, Sandman CA, Kastin AJ. Influence of three short-chain peptides (α-MSH, MSH/ACTH 4-10, MIF-I on) dimensional attention. Pharmacol Biochem Behav 1976; 5:11-16.
31. Verhoeven WMA, van Praag HM, van Ree JM, de Wied D. Improvement of schizophrenic patients treated with [des-tyr[1]]-γ-endorphin (DTγE). Arch Gen Psychiatry 1979; 36:294-298.
32. Rigter H, Shuster S, Thody AJ. ACTH, α-MSH and β-LPH: Pituitary hormones with similar activity in an amnesia test in rats. J Pharm Pharmacol 1977; 29:110-111.
33. Miller LH, Harris LC, Van Riezen H, et al. Neuroheptapeptide influence on attention and memory in man. Pharmacol Biochem Behav 1976; 5:17-21.
34. Schweizer-Cagianut M, Froesch ER, Hedinger C. Familiar Cushing's syndrome with primary adrenocortical microadenomatosis (primary adrenocortical nodular dysplasia). Acta Endocrinol (Copenh) 1980; 94:529-535.
35. Berson SA, Yalow RS. Radioimmunoassay of ACTH in plasma, J Clin Invest 1968; 47:2725-2751.
36. Liddle GW. Test of pituitary-adrenal suppressibility in the diagnosis of Cushing's syndrome. J Clin Endocrinol Metab 1960; 20:1539-1560.
37. Kendall JW, Sloop PR, Jr. Dexamethasone-suppressible adrenocortical tumor. N Engl J Med 1968; 279:532-535.
38. Matthews JI, Fariss BL, Chertow BS, et al. Adrenal adenoma with variable response to dexamethasone suppression and metyrapone stimulation. J Clin Endocrinol Metab 1972; 34:902-905.
39. Jenkins JS, Meakin JW, Nelson DH, Thorn GW. Inhibition of adrenal steroid 11-oxygenation in the dog. Science 1958; 128:478-480.
40. Liddle GW, Island D, Lance EM, Harris AP. Alterations of adrenal steroid patterns in man resulting from treatment with a chemical inhibitor of 11β-hydroxylation. J Clin Endocrinol Metab 1958; 19:906-912.
41. Jubiz W, Meikle AW, West CD, et al.: Single-dose metyrapone test. Arch Intern Med 1970; 125:472-474.
42. Himsworth RL, Lewis JG, Ress LH. A possible ACTH secreting tumour of the pituitary developing in a conventionally treated case of Addison's disease. Clin Endocrinol 1978; 9:131-139.
43. Baranetsky NG, Zipser RD, Goebelsmann U, Kurman RJ, March CM, Morimoto S, Stanczyk FZ. Adrenocorticotropin-dependent virilizing paraovarian tumors in Nelson's syndrome. J Clin Endocrinol Metab 1979; 49:381-386.
44. Kirschner MA, Powell RD Jr, Lipsett MB. Cushing's syndrome: nodular cortical hyperplasia of adrenal glands with clinical and pathological features suggesting adrenocortical tumor. J Clin Endocrinol Metab 1964; 24:947-955.

45. Fraser R, James VHT, Landon J, et al. Clinical and biochemical studies of a patient with a corticosterone-secreting adrenocortical tumour. Lancet 1968; 2:1116-1120.
46. Aron DC, Findling JW, Fitzgerald PA, Brooks RM, Fisher FE, Forsham PH, Tyrrell JB. Pituitary ACTH dependency of nodular adrenal hyperplasia in Cushing's syndrome. Am J Med 1981; 71:302-306.
47. Hidai H, Fujii H, Otsuka K, et al. Cushing's syndrome due to huge adrenocortical multinodular hyperplasia. Endocrinol Jpn 1975; 22:555-560.

20
Disorders of Pituitary-Gonadal Function

David M. Hurley and Henry G. Burger
Prince Henry's Hospital, Melbourne, Australia

I. NORMAL DEVELOPMENT AND FUNCTION

It is necessary to have a clear understanding of the events of sexual differentiation, the normal functions of the testis and ovary, and the means by which these functions are regulated if disorders of gonadal function are to be properly assessed.

A. Sexual Differentiation

Sexual differentiation occurs in three stages which normally follow each other in an orderly sequence. Chromosomal sex, established at the time of fertilization, determines gonadal sex, which subsequently determines phenotypic sex.

1. Chromosomal Sex

At fertilization, the hitherto haploid egg with its X chromosome receives an X or Y chromosome from the fertilizing sperm, which therefore determines the chromosomal sex. In humans, the heterogametic sex (XY) is male and the homogametic sex (XX) female. Sexual development is apparently identical in males and females for the first 40 days of gestation, during which the wolffian and mullerian duct systems and the common external genital structures are formed.

2. Gonadal Sex

At about 40 days of gestation, the gonadal sex is established. Testicular development appears to be determined by the H-Y antigen, the product of a gene on the Y chromosome. If the H-Y antigen is present, the gonad will differentiate into a testis. If not, it will become an ovary.

3. Phenotypic Sex

The definitive gonad determines internal and external genital development.

Internal Genitalia. The internal genital organs are derived from the wolffian and mullerian ductal systems. In the male, the wolffian ducts form the epididymis, vas deferens, and seminal vesicles, while the mullerian ducts disappear. In the female, the mullerian ducts become the fallopian tubes, uterus, and upper vagina, while the wolffian ducts regress.

External Genitalia. The external genital organs and urethra arise from the urogenital sinus and the genital tubercle, folds, and swelling. The urogenital sinus forms the prostate gland and prostatic urethra in the male, forming the urethra and part of the vagina in the female. The genital tubercle becomes the glans penis in the male and the clitoris in the female, while the urogenital folds develop into the shaft of the penis and the labia minora, respectively. The urogenital swellings form the scrotum and labia majora.

In the absence of a testis, a female phenotype develops. The male pattern of development is determined by hormones of the fetal testis; the gonad does not appear to be needed for female development, however. In the male, secretion of mullerian inhibiting factor (MIF) by the fetal testis leads to regression of the mullerian ductal system. The fetal testis also secretes testosterone, which is responsible for differentiation of the wolffian system into the epididymis, vas, and seminal vesicles, but development of external genitalia occurs only after local 5α reduction of testosterone to dihydrotestosterone.

Phenotypic sex is established by the middle of the second trimester. In the second half of pregnancy, testicular descent and differential growth of male external genitalia occur.

Sexual differentiation is completed at puberty, when activation of hypothalamic gonadotropin releasing hormone (Gn RH) secretion leads to increased gonadotropin secretion and hence increased gonadal steroid production, resulting in the development of secondary sexual characteristics and fertility.

B. Normal Gonadal Function

The testis and the ovary have two major functions, hormone secretion and gamete production. In the testis, there is an anatomical separation of hormone-secreting Leydig cells, in an interstitial compartment, from a sperm-producing tubular compartment composed of seminiferous tubules and other ductal structures (Fig. 1a). The functions of these compartments are regulated in a partly independent manner by the pituitary gonadotropic hormones, luteinizing hormone (LH) acting mainly on the interstitial compartment and follicle stimulating hormone (FSH) acting predominantly on the tubular compartment (Fig. 1a).

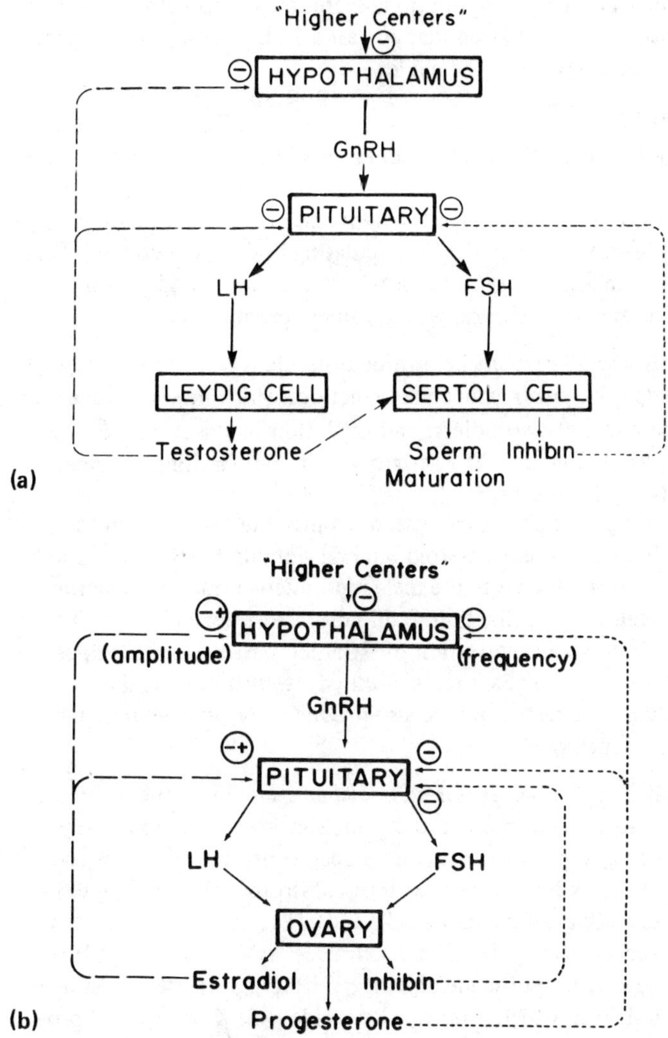

Figure 1 (a) Regulation of testicular function. (b) Regulation of ovarian function.

This specificity is increased by the action of separate feedback signals from each compartment which permit differential control of LH and FSH secretory rates (Fig. 1a). However, testosterone secreted by the Leydig cells under LH control is an essential regulator of spermatogenesis.

In the case of the ovary (Fig. 1b), hormone secretion and gamete production are much more closely interrelated, so that corresponding anatomical and regulatory distinctions cannot as readily be made.

1. Hormone Secretion

Synthesis and secretion of sex steroid hormones, principally testosterone in the male and estradiol and progesterone in the female, are the means by which the gonad brings about normal pubertal development and maintains secondary sexual characteristics and fertility. In addition to circulating in the bloodstream, these hormones are present in high concentrations within the gonad, and have important local actions, particularly with respect to gamete production.

Testis. In the testis, the 27-carbon cholesterol molecule is converted to 19-carbon carbon testosterone in five enzyme-mediated reactions which involve cleavage of the cholesterol side chain at two points, and oxidation of the A ring to the Δ^4-3-keto configuration (Fig. 2). The activity of the rate-limiting enzyme, 20,22-desmolase, is regulated by LH.

Approximately 6 mg of testosterone is secreted into the bloodstream each day, where 98% is bound to the sex steroid binding globulin (SSBG) and albumin. In a number of target tissues in the male reproductive tract, testosterone acts only after intracellular 5α reduction to dihydrotestosterone (Fig. 3). Testosterone may also undergo aromatization to estradiol, particularly in adipose tissue (Fig. 3). In addition, small amounts of dihydrotestosterone and estrogen are secreted directly by the testis, and are also produced by peripheral metabolism of adrenal androstenedione.

Ovary. 17β-Estradiol, the principal steroid hormone secreted by the ovary during the follicular phase, is synthesized in the granulosa cells of the follicle by aromatization of androgen precursors that have been formed in the theca cells (Fig. 4). These events are stimulated by both gonadotropins, FSH acting to increase the aromatase activity of granulosa cells and LH to enhance production of androgens by thecal cells (Fig. 4). FSH also induces synthesis of the LH receptor. Rising estrogen levels subsequently trigger pituitary release of a midcycle surge of LH and FSH, which leads to a "steroidogenic shift" so that progesterone is secreted in increasing amounts; aromatase activity remains maximal, however, so that, after a transient decrease at midcycle, estrogen secretion continues in the luteal phase (Fig. 6). The daily production of estradiol is approximately 40 μg (100 nmol) in the early follicular phase, 400 μg (1000 nmol) in the preovulatory period, and 280 μg (770 nmol) in the midluteal phase. The corresponding figures for progesterone are approximately 2 mg per day in the follicular phase and 25 mg per day in the midluteal phase.

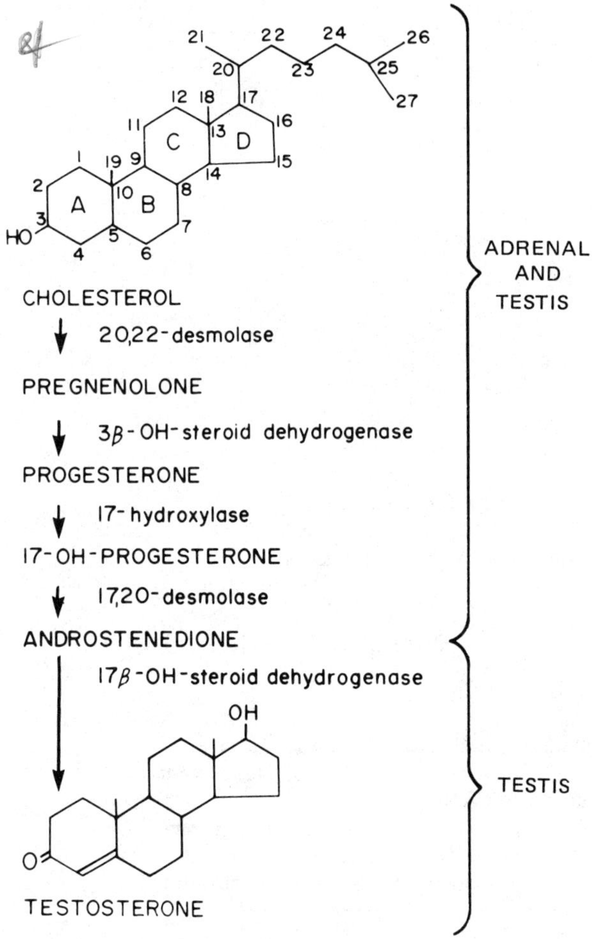

Figure 2 Synthesis of testosterone.

Mechanism of Steroid Hormone Action. The male sex hormones, testosterone and dihydrotestosterone, and the female sex hormones, estradiol and progesterone, act on their target tissues to bring about the phenotypic, reproductive, and psychological changes that constitute puberty, and continue to act thereafter to maintain these secondary sexual characteristics and hence fertility. Each class of sex steroid acts by binding to specific cytoplasmic hormone receptors; the hormone-receptor complex then migrates to the nucleus, binding to

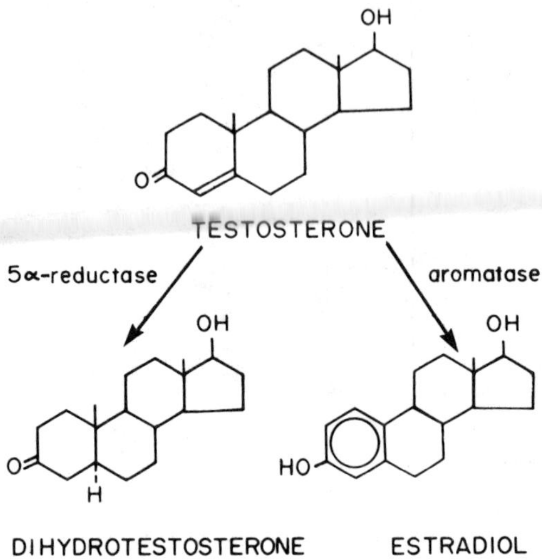

Figure 3 Metabolism of testosterone in peripheral tissues.

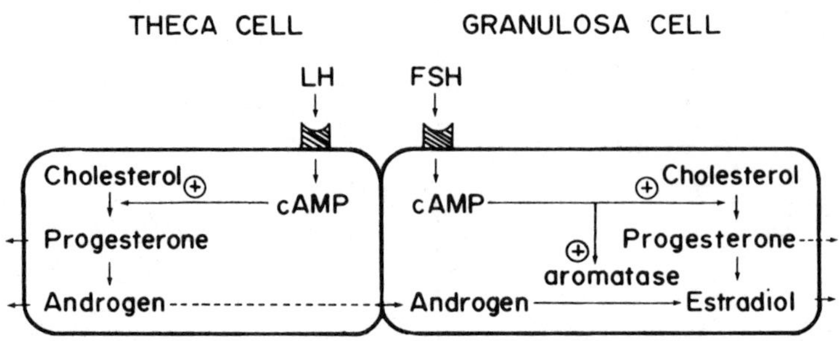

Figure 4 Steroid synthesis in the ovarian follicle.

specific chromatin acceptor sites, acting there to regulate the expression of specific sets of genes.

2. Gamete Production

Testis. In the postpubertal male, spermatozoa are produced continuously from germ cells lining the seminiferous tubules.Spermatogonia, arising from germ cells, divide mitotically to form spermatocytes, which undergo meiotic division to form haploid spermatids. These small round cells are transformed into spermatozoa, a process apparently dependent on the Sertoli cell. Once released from the Sertoli cell, these spermatozoa travel along the tubule, through the rete testis, and into the epididymis, where further maturation occurs and where sperm are stored, ready for ejaculation. The process of spermatogenesis takes about 72 days, and the spermatozoa reach the tail of the epididymis 7-10 days after they detach from the epithelium. FSH and intratesticular testosterone are essential for these processes. A major part of the action of FSH is due to effects on the Sertoli cell, which is known to play an essential local role in the support of spermatogenesis and is the probable source of the protein feedback signal, inhibin, a specific inhibitor of pituitary FSH secretion (Fig. 1).

Ovary. Gamete production in the female involves cyclical maturation of an ovarian follicle under the influence of LH and FSH. Following a midcycle surge of LH and FSH, the ripened follicle ruptures, releases the enclosed ovum, and is transformed into a corpus luteum. Estrogen and progesterone secreted by the corpus luteum prepare the endometrium for implantation, should conception occur. If conception does not take place, the corpus luteum involutes, leading to a fall in estrogen and progesterone, menstruation, and initiation of a new cycle. These events are dependent on appropriate patterns of pituitary gonadotropin secretion, which are in turn determined by negative and positive feedback effects of changing profiles of ovarian steroid and nonsteroidal hormones (Figs. 1b, 6) (see below).

C. Regulation of Gonadal Function

1. Gonadotropins

In both sexes, hormone secretion and gamete production by the gonads are dependent on appropriate circulating concentrations of the pituitary gonadotropic hormones, LH and FSH. It is believed that both are secreted from a single cell type, the gonadotrope. LH and FSH are members of the glycoprotein family of hormones, together with thyroid stimulating hormone (TSH) and human chorionic gonadotropin (hCG). The molecules of these hormones are composed of two polypeptide subunits, designated α and β. All members of the family share a common α subunit, but each has a specific β subunit. There is nonetheless considerable amino acid sequence homology between the various β subunits and also to a lesser extent between α and β subunits. These sequences are encoded in separate genes whose expression is regulated in a partly independent manner. Following translation, the α and β polypeptides are glycosylated, a necessary step for biological activity, and then combine to be stored in vesicles as intact LH or FSH, ready for release. Like other peptide hormones, LH and FSH act on their target cells by combining with specific cell surface receptors. Receptor binding is followed by activation of membrane-bound adenylate cyclase, a step requiring cyclic GMP; the resulting rise in intracellular cyclic AMP levels activates a cyclic AMP-dependent protein kinase, leading to phosphorylation of many proteins which subsequently promote steroid hormone secretion and gamete production by largely unknown mechanisms.

2. Gonadotropin Releasing Hormone

In the adult, stored gonadotropin is discharged episodically into the bloodstream in response to intermittent stimulation of the gonadotrope by the gonadotropin releasing hromone (GnRH), a decapeptide which is released from hypothalamic neuroendocrine cells at intervals of 60–120 minutes into the hypothalamohypophyseal portal venous system. GnRH also stimulates synthesis of LH and FSH, presumably by increasing transcription of the α and β subunit genes.

Recent evidence suggests that GnRH must be provided in a pulsatile fashion of an appropriate frequency for the gonadotrope to remain responsive; precise regulation of the size of GnRH pulses is apparently less important.

GnRH secretion is kept to a low level in childhood by inhibitory central nervous system (CNS) influences which are independent of other feedback signals and which are mediated at least in part by monoamines and probably also by opiate peptides. The onset of puberty follows a reduction in the level of CNS inhibition, allowing pulsatile GnRH secretion to emerge. At first the gonadotrope responds with predominant FSH secretion, but gradually switches to LH predominance as puberty progresses. The result is gonadal maturation, establishment of sex hormone secretion, development and maintenance of secondary sexual characteristics, gamete production, and fertility.

3. Feedback Regulation of Gonadotropin Secretion

The size and LH/FSH ratio of each pulse of gonadotropin depend not only on the size and frequency of the GnRH pulses arriving from the hypothalamus, but also on the level of specific humoral feedback signals secreted by the testis and ovary.

In the male, LH acts on and is regulated by the hormone-secreting compartment of the testis. The specific feedback signal is testosterone, acting predominantly at the level of the pituitary to reduce the LH secretory response to GnRH. The tubular compartment is dependent on FSH, and regulates the rate of FSH synthesis by means of a specific negative feedback signal, the protein hormone, inhibin, believed to be secreted by the Sertoli cell (Fig. 1a).

In the female, estradiol inhibits gonadotropin secretion, mainly by reducing gonadotrope sensitivity to GnRH but probably also by inhibiting hypothalamic GnRH secretion. However, once estradiol levels exceed a critical value, the feedback effect becomes a positive one, resulting in a striking increase in gonad-

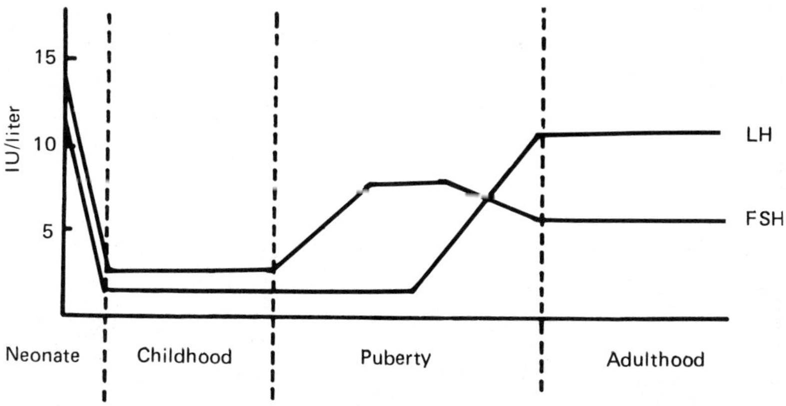

Figure 5 Changing gonadotropin patterns with age.

otrope sensitivity to GnRH, and to a lesser extent, in increased amplitude of GnRH pulse secretion. These changes lead to discharge of very large quantities of LH and FSH at midcycle, leading to rupture and luteinization of the follicle. Progesterone is subsequently secreted by the corpus luteum in addition to estradiol, and also acts as a feedback regulator of gonadotropin secretion, reducing the frequency of GnRH pulses in the second half of the menstrual cycle. It is likely that inhibin, secreted by the granulosa cells, is also involved in regulation of FSH secretion, as in the male (Fig. 1b).

D. Normal Patterns of Gonadotropin and Gonadal Hormone Secretion

It is apparent from the preceding discussion that changes in the various factors regulating GnRH, gonadotropin, and gonadal hormone secretion will result in characteristic hormone patterns at each stage of development (Fig. 5). In infancy, gonadotropin levels are comparable to those in adults, but soon decline as central nervous system inhibition increases, and remain low throughout childhood. FSH levels are higher than those of LH. With the onset of puberty, pulsatile gonadotropin secretion appears at night, and eventually occurs throughout the day. At first FSH secretion predominates, but the pattern is reversed as FSH levels decline and LH levels exceed those of FSH. In the male, testosterone rises steadily to adult levels. In the female, the cyclical events of follicle maturation, ovulation, corpus luteum formation, and menstruation begin, paralleled by rising estradiol levels in response to small increases in pulsatile LH secretion early in the cycle, a midcycle surge of LH and FSH as estrogen feedback becomes positive, and increasing progesterone levels which reduce the gonadotropin pulse

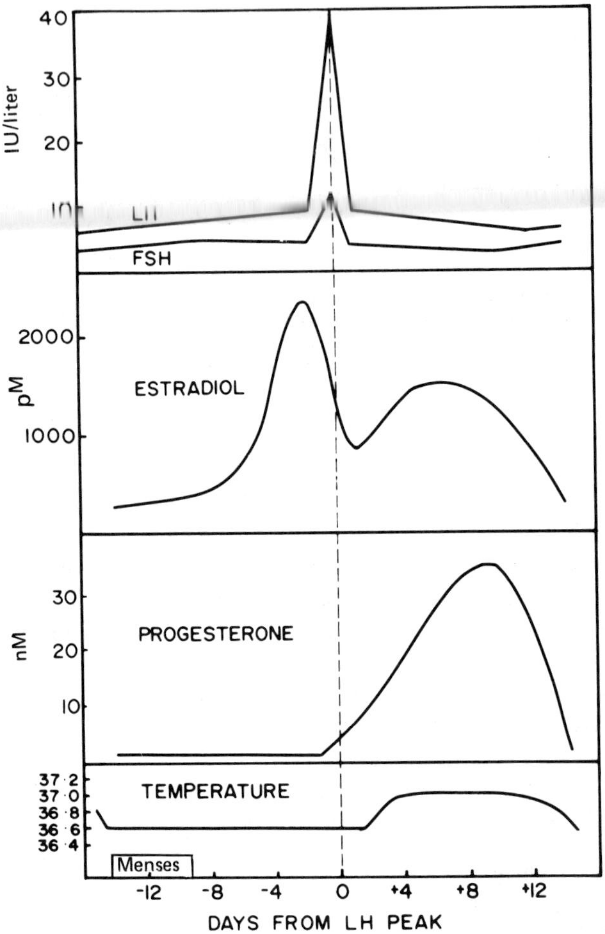

Figure 6 Schematic diagram of changes in blood hormone levels and body temperature during the menstrual cycle. It should be noted that although the pattern of changes is relatively uniform, the absolute hormone levels vary greatly between individuals.

frequency; as menstruation approaches, progesterone levels fall and FSH levels begin to rise (Fig. 6). Should pregnancy occur, progesterone levels rise still higher, and pituitary gonadotropins are suppressed as human chorionic gonadotropin assumes the role of corpus luteum maintenance.

In the fifth or sixth decade, ovarian function declines, resulting in anovulation, amenorrhea, and reduced steroid hormone and presumably inhibin levels. With the loss of feedback inhibition, large-amplitude gonadotropin pulses are seen, resulting in the high serum levels of LH, and especially FSH, characteristic of the postmenopause.

II. PATHOPHYSIOLOGY AND CLINICAL PRESENTATION

A variety of lesions at the level of the hypothalamus, pituitary, or gonad may lead to disordered gonadal function, resulting in one or more of a number of specific clinical syndromes, depending on the nature of the disorder and the patient's sex and stage of sexual development at the time of its onset. The pathophysiology and clinical features of these syndromes are considered in this section.

A. Sexual Ambiguity

Sexual ambiguity at birth reflects abnormalities of fetal sexual differentiation (see Sec. I.A). Most cases of sexual ambiguity represent disorders of phenotypic sex in patients whose chromosomal and gonadal sex are concordant and clearly male or female. The clinical syndromes resulting from such disorders are designated male and female pseudohermaphroditism, respectively. Disorders of gonadal and chromosomal sex are much rarer causes of sexual ambiguity and produce a somewhat different clinical picture.

1. Female Pseudohermaphroditism

Female pseudohermaphroditism results from virilization of an otherwise normal female fetus by excessive levels of androgen. Such infants have ovaries, fallopian tubes, uterus, and vagina, but the clitoris is hypertrophied, and the labia majora rugose and bulbous, with variable degrees of fusion, resulting in an appearance similar to that of males with hypospadias and bilateral cryptorchidism. The commonest cause is congenital adrenal hyperplasia, although treatment of threatened abortion with progestagens which have significant androgenic activity may also cause female pseudohermaphroditism in the infant.

Approximately 50% of infants with congenital adrenal hyperplasia due to 21-hydroxylase deficiency develop adrenal crisis in the first weeks of life due to lack of adrenal glucocorticoid and mineralocorticoid hormones (see Chap. 25). If milder forms are not recognized in the neonatal period, the child will develop hirsutism and virilization (see Sec. II.F). Growth will initially be very rapid, but premature fusion of epiphyses leads ultimately to short stature. Other clinical features of untreated congenital adrenal hyperplasia include pigmentation due to long-standing ACTH excess and hypertension in those with the relatively uncommon 11-hydroxylase deficiency. Occasional cases that were recognized for the first time in adolescent or early adult years have been regarded by some as late onset "acquired" adrenal hyperplasia, but are probably mild forms of classical congenital adrenal hyperplasia which have escaped earlier detection. Such patients undergo a relatively normal puberty, but are amenorrheic.

Although spontaneous mutation leads to new cases, a careful family history should reveal other affected members in this inherited autosomal recessive condition. A positive family history greatly facilitates correct diagnosis, particularly in the milder forms where other conditions enter the differential diagnosis. The family history may be extended to include measurement of 17-hydroxyprogesterone responses to ACTH to demonstrate heterozygosity in patients, siblings, and other relations (1).

2. Male Pseudohermaphroditism

Male pseudohermaphroditism represents failure of the testis to bring to completion the processes of differentiation of internal and external genital organs into the male form. The clinical consequences depend on the nature of the defect and the stage of development at which it arises.

Idiopathic bilateral cryptorchidism associated with hypospadias is the most common variety. Other important causes are anorchia and inborn errors of metabolism affecting enzymes of testosterone synthesis, 5α-reductase, or the testosterone receptor.

In the case of anorchia, testicular failure occurs in 46 XY males after MIF secretion has accomplished mullerian duct regression, but before testosterone secretion can complete virilization of external genitalia. In the pure form, the clinical result is a 46XY phenotypic female with no testes but male internal genital organs and no evidence of mullerian structures. If the testicular failure occurs later in development or is only partial, incomplete virilization will lead to difficulty in assigning a male or female sex. The mildest forms will result in a clearly male phenotype with absent testes and perhaps a microphallus.

46XY individuals who lack the enzyme 5α-reductase in the tissues which normally give rise to the external genitalia undergo normal male internal genital development, having well-developed testes, vasa deferentia, and seminal vesicles, but have severe perineoscrotal hypospadias and a blind vaginal pouch. Substantial masculinization usually occurs at puberty, however.

Total lack of a functional androgen receptor results in the syndrome of complete testicular feminization. Although mullerian ductal regression occurs, lack of testosterone action prevents wolffian ductal development, so that there is total absence of internal genital organs. Furthermore, lack of action of testosterone and dihydrotestosterone in the presence of appreciable levels of estrogen results in a normal female external phenotype, with a shallow, blind-ending vagina. Rudimentary undescended testes are present. Such individuals usually undergo a relatively normal female pubertal development except for primary amenorrhea, thereby coming to medical attention for the first time. Others may present at an earlier age with inguinal herniae, and are found to have undescended testes. Occasional girls with tall stature and primary amenorrhea are found to have testicular feminization.

A number of syndromes of partial androgen receptor deficiency have been described in which the phenotype may be female, male, or indeterminate, depending on the severity of the lesion. Like complete testicular feminization, these are inherited in an X-linked recessive manner.

Hypospadias and bilateral cryptorchidism without other abnormalities of sexual differentiation is the most common form of male pseudohermaphroditism. Although deficient androgen action is postulated, the cause is unknown. If testicular descent has not occurred by the age of 3 months, it is unlikely to do so. The major clinical consequences are infertility due to impaired spermatogenesis and an increased risk of testicular malignancy. Androgen secretion is usually normal.

3. Chromosomal and Gonadal Disorders of Sexual Differentiation

The most important condition in this category is mixed gonadal dysgenesis, a relatively common cause of ambiguous genitalia. Affected individuals usually have 45X/46XY mosaicism, with a testis on one side and a streak gonad on the other. Both mullerian regression and external genital masculinization are deficient, apparently the result of a defect in the magnitude or timing of testicular secretion of both MIF and testosterone. The clinical features consist of a male, female, or intermediate phenotype with one testis, incomplete virilization, and the presence of uterus, vagina, and at least one fallopian tube. Approximately 60% are raised as females.

B. Precocious Puberty

The normal process of puberty and its clinical staging are discussed in Chapter 2. In developed Western countries, the onset of puberty in boys, defined as the earliest detectable testicular enlargement, occurs between the ages of 10 and 13 years, while in girls puberty normally begins between the ages of 9 and 12 years, breast development usually being the earliest sign. The mean age at menarche is about 12.5 years, ranging from 9 to 16 years. Puberty may therefore be regarded as precocious if it begins before the age of 10 in boys and 9 in girls.

The syndrome of true precocious puberty is believed to result from premature activation of hypothalamic GnRH secretion due to a premature reduction in the inhibitory influence normally exerted by higher centers of the brain during childhood. In a number of cases this is related to an identifiable structural lesion of the central nervous system. In other cases, no such lesion can be found.

It is important to distinguish between true precocious puberty and pseudoprecocious puberty resulting from autonomous extragonadal or gonadal sex hormone secretion. Boys with true precocious puberty have testicular volumes exceeding 4 ml, associated with normal spermatogenesis and fertility. In pseudoprecocious puberty, however, testicular volumes are less than 4 ml, with no tubular development. A cerebral lesion will be evident in some cases of true precocious puberty, and an adrenal lesion will be apparent in many boys with pseudoprecocious puberty.

In girls, true precocious puberty leads to regular ovulatory menses and fertility; these will be absent in girls with pseudoprecocious puberty, who will often have a palpable ovarian tumor. True precocious puberty in girls should also be distinguished from the apparently benign conditions of premature adrenarche and premature thelarche, in which growth of secondary body hair and breast development, respectively, begin at an early age as isolated events, which are not followed by complete premature pubertal development.

Precocious puberty is twice as common in girls as in boys, with idiopathic premature activation of hypothalamic GnRH secretion accounting for 80% of cases in girls and 40% in boys. The idiopathic form is often familial. A further 15% of cases in girls are due to estrogen-secreting ovarian tumors, especially the granulosa cell tumor, the remaining 5% being due to hypothyroidism, Albright's fibrous dysplasia, and other conditions. The mechanisms by which these latter conditions cause precocious puberty are not well understood. Structural cerebral lesions are a rare cause of precocious puberty in girls. In boys, however, an underlying cerebral lesion is present in 20% of cases, while a further 25% are due to congenital adrenal hyperplasia. Functioning testicular tumors account for fewer than 10% of cases. Precocious puberty of both types is associated with an acceleration of growth which leads to tall stature at first, but premature epiphyseal fusion results ultimately in short stature.

C. Delayed Puberty

As is apparent from Section II.B, puberty may be regarded as delayed in boys if it has not started by the age of 14 years. It should be emphasized that testicular enlargement is the earliest sign, volumes greater than 4 ml being a reliable indication that puberty has begun. In girls, puberty may be regarded as delayed if it has not commenced by 13 years of age. Primary amenorrhea should not be diagnosed before the age of 16 years if other aspects of pubertal development are normal and if there is no uterine or vaginal obstruction. It is important to recognize that primary amenorrhea is not necessarily synonymous with delayed puberty.

A number of clinical features may be present in addition to the lack of pubertal development. Increased limb length due to delayed epiphyseal fusion results in a characteristic "eunuchoid habitus" when puberty is delayed, so that arm span is greater than height and the ratio of lower segment height to upper segment height is greater than unity (see Chap. 2). Short stature associated with delayed puberty usually reflects a "constitutional delay" of both growth and pubertal development, but may also reflect growth hormone deficiency, hypothyroidism, or Turner's syndrome.

Delayed puberty is the result of delay in or failure of the increased gonadal steroid secretion that normally brings about the changes of puberty. This may reflect a lesion at the level of the hypothalamus, pituitary, or gonad.

Delayed puberty in girls is often associated with stress, weight loss, chronic illness, or high levels of physical activity. Persisting inhibition of hypothalamic GnRH secretion by the central nervous system is thought to be the mechanism involved in such cases. Idiopathic, often familial, delayed puberty in boys and girls appears to have a similar basis and is the most common variety. Puberty will eventually occur in such cases. Much less frequently, delayed puberty is a manifestation of Kallman's syndrome, in which impaired hypothalamic GnRH secretion leads to isolated gonadotropin deficiency, often associated with anosmia and other midline developmental defects. Puberty will not begin spontaneously in this condition.

Structural lesions of the hypothalamus and pituitary which may impair gonadotropin secretion and lead to failure of pubertal development include tumors, especially the craniopharyngioma, granulomatous disorders, trauma, and irradiation. Hyperprolactinemia, whether due to a functioning pituitary tumor or other factors (see Chap. 22), may also produce this syndrome.

There are a number of rare but conceptually important eponymous syndromes which have in common a failure of normal development of the hypothalamus, leading to impaired GnRH secretion.

The main primary ovarian cause of failure to enter puberty is Turner's syndrome, in which lack of an X chromosome is associated with failure of normal ovarian development, so that only "streak" ovaries are present. Other abnormalities include short stature, facial changes, short webbed neck, shieldlike chest, and cubitus valgus. Cardiovascular abnormalities, especially aortic coarctation, and renal anomalies are common. Ovarian failure may also result from autoimmune mechanisms, sometimes in association with autoimmune failure of other endocrine glands. Primary testicular disease is not a major cause of delayed puberty, although occasional patients with Klinefelter's syndrome may present in this way.

D. Primary Amenorrhea

Amenorrhea is usefully characterized as primary, in which menstruation has never occurred in a girl aged 16 years or more, and secondary, where menarche has occurred but menses have subsequently ceased (see Sec. II.E). Primary amenorrhea is a part of the syndrome of delayed puberty (see Sec. II.C), but may also occur in the presence of otherwise normal pubertal development when the impairment of ovarian function is mild, particularly in functional hypothalamic disturbances and in hyperprolactinemia (see Sec. II.E). Structural abnormalities of the uterus and vagina which obstruct menstrual flow will also cause primary amenorrhea with otherwise normal pubertal development, so that genital anatomy should be properly assessed in such cases, recognizing that it may sometimes be difficult to distinguish clinically between hypoplasia of the genital tract resulting from estrogen deficiency and congenital structural abnormalities.

E. Secondary Amenorrhea

Impaired ovarian function arising in the adult female who has undergone normal puberty may cause no clinical features other than amenorrhea and infertility. In less severe disturbances, occasional, usually anovulatory cycles occur. Symptoms of estrogen deficiency, such as loss of libido, reduction in breast size, dyspareunia, and hot flashes, may also be present.

The major causes of this syndrome are functional disorders of hypothalamic GnRH secretion and hyperprolactinemia, although the possibilities of pregnancy, polycystic ovarian disease, structural lesions of the pituitary and hypothalamus, isolated gonadotropin deficiency, and primary ovarian failure should be considered.

1. Functional Hypothalamic Amenorrhea

The reduced secretion of gonadotropins which occurs in women suffering stress, anorexia nervosa, endogenous depression, weight loss, systemic illness, or idiopathic hypothalamic amenorrhea is attributable to impaired hypothalamic secretion of GnRH due to inhibition by higher centers. So-called ballet dancer's and jogger's amenorrhea also fall into this category. Although estrogens exert inhibitory actions at both pituitary and hypothalamic levels, the syndrome of post-pill amenorrhea reflects prolonged inhibition of GnRH secretion, tending to occur in women whose GnRH secretion is already marginal for other reasons, such as those already mentioned.

2. Hyperprolactinemia

Elevated prolactin levels, whether due to pituitary tumor, drugs, or other causes, may inhibit gonadal hormone secretion directly, but also inhibit gonadotropin secretion at a hypothalamic level, probably by actions affecting monoamine metabolism. Galactorrhea is a common accompaniment (see Chap. 22).

3. Obesity and Polycystic Ovary Syndrome

In amenorrhea associated with obesity and the polycystic ovary syndrome, the normal cyclical changes in ovarian hormone secretion which ensure appropriate gonadotropin secretion and hence ovulation do not occur because of relatively unchanging extraovarian production of large amounts of estrogen by aromatization of weak androgens. This situation is the result of excessive secretion of weak androgens by the ovary in the case of the polycystic ovary syndrome, while the defect in obesity appears to be increased aromatase activity in adipose tissue, perhaps combined with increased adrenal secretion of weak androgens. In both cases, the result is a qualitative rather than quantitative defect, in which feedback effects of the estrogen appear to sensitize the pituitary and hypothalamus, leading to large-amplitude GnRH pulses and increased LH secretion, but suppression of FSH release. LH further stimulates ovarian androgen secretion, establishing a vicious cycle.

4. Structural Hypothalamic Lesions

Craniopharyngiomas and granulomas of histiocytosis X or sarcoidosis arise primarily in the hypothalamus, and pituitary tumors may spread locally to involve this area. Other important causes of hypothalamic damage are cranial irradiation and surgery. In all these cases, other features of hypothalamic disturbance may be present (see Sec. III.C).

5. Hypopituitarism

Gonadotropin secretion may be impaired as the result of a number of disease processes affecting the pituitary gland. The most important of these are postpartum necrosis (Sheehan's syndrome), pituitary tumor, whether functional or nonfunctional, surgery, irradiation, and trauma. The gonadotropin deficiency is often part of a more general impairment of pituitary hormone secretion, but may be relatively specific. In the case of an expanding pituitary tumor, headache and bitemporal hemianopia may be present.

6. Primary Ovarian Failure

Acquired ovarian failure may be caused by autoimmune mechanisms, and is often associated with autoimmune failure of other endocrine glands, while other cases may simply reflect relatively early onset of an otherwise normal menopause. In the resistant ovary syndrome, follicles are present within the ovary but are unresponsive to gonadotropins.

F. Hirsutism and Virilization

Exogenous or endogenous androgen excess in the female fetus or young child results in female pseudohermaphroditism, whereas androgen excess in older girls or adult women results in hirsutism, amenorrhea, and virilization, which are superimposed on preceding normal female development.

If androgen excess is mild, hirsutism may develop without other features (see below). This is best assessed by the method of Ferriman and Gallwey (2), in which the severity of hair growth in each of nine sites on the face, chest, abdomen, back, and limbs is graded on a scale of 0 to 4 and scores summed.

When androgen levels are higher, clinical features of virilization appear. These include a male pattern of muscle development, skin oiliness and acne due to increased sebum production, frontal balding and temporal hair recession, deepening of the voice, and clitoral hypertrophy. Psychological changes, particularly increased aggression, may also develop.

Hirsutism is most often idiopathic or familial in origin, sometimes associated with increased secretion of weak androgens, mainly dehydroepiandrosterone, its sulfate, and androstenedione, produced by the adrenals and/or the ovaries. Specific adrenal conditions which cause hirsutism and virilization include Cushing's syndrome of all types, especially adrenal carcinoma, and congenital adrenal hyperplasia due to deficiency of the 21-hydroxylase or 11-hydroxylase enzymes (see Chaps. 19 and 25). Hirsuitism may also be the result of ovarian androgen secretion in polycystic ovarian disease and functioning ovarian tumors, especially the granulosa cell tumor. Finally, drugs such as diphenylhydantoin, diazoxide, minoxidil, metyrapone, and androgen-related progestins can cause hirsutism.

Hirsutism present since puberty is likely to be benign in origin, while sudden onset of hirsutes and virilization at a later stage suggests a functioning adrenal or ovarian tumor. Where an ovarian or adrenal tumor is the cause of the androgen excess, the tumor is often easily palpable.

G. Impotence, Male Infertility, and Androgen Deficiency

In the adult male, reduced androgen secretion by the Leydig cells of the interstitial compartment of the testis will lead to impotence and loss of secondary sexual characteristics, while impaired function of the tubular compartment will result in infertility.

1. Impotence

Normal sexual potency implies adequate libido, the achievement and maintenance of an erection satisfactory for vaginal intercourse, and the ability to ejaculate and experience orgasm. Libido is predominantly a psychological phenomenon which is dependent on adequate levels of androgen. Erection, also androgen dependent, is a vascular event which is initiated and terminated by the autonomic nervous system, particularly the parasympathetic component, under the direction of higher centers which are again strongly influenced by psychological factors.

It is therefore not surprising that most cases of impotence are psychological in origin. It is characteristic of psychogenic impotence that spontaneous nocturnal erections continue to occur, unlike the situation in organic impotence. Other clinical features suggesting a psychogenic basis include sudden onset at the time of identifiable psychological stress and a fluctuating or intermittent course according to varying levels of guilt and anxiety, often associated with different partners.

Neurological disturbances, drugs, and endocrine disease are the principal causes of organic impotence. Impotence occurs very commonly in male diabetics and is thought to reflect autonomic neuropathy; impotence resulting from damage to autonomic nerves is common after prostatic, aortoiliac, and large bowel surgery. A large number of drugs cause impotence by interfering with autonomic nervous function, particularly antihypertensives such as methyldopa, reserpine, guanethidine, and to a lesser extent, β-adrenergic antagonists. Alcohol, narcotics, benzodiazepines, major tranquilizers, tricyclic antidepressants, and monoamine oxidase inhibitors may also result in impotence. Finally, impotence may be caused by testosterone deficiency or prolactin excess, the latter apparently acting directly on the testis to inhibit hormone synthesis, in addition to interfering with GnRH secretion by the hypothalamus.

It is therefore apparent that the cause can be identified clinically in most cases, the first step being to distinguish between psychogenic and organic impotence. Specific features suggesting testosterone deficiency (see below) or prolactin excess (especially galactorrhea) should always be sought but will rarely be found.

2. Androgen Deficiency

Reduction in androgen secretion after pubertal development will result in loss of secondary sexual characteristics, normally maintained by testosterone. The clinical consequences include reduced potency and libido, reduced muscle mass and strength, loss of aggression, slowing of beard growth, variable loss of pubic and axillary hair, and penile atrophy.

Pituitary, hypothalamic, and primary testicular disorders should be considered. Important causes of pituitary lesions include functioning and nonfunctioning tumors, trauma, surgery, and irradiation. Impaired hypothalamic GnRH secretion occurs in Kallman's syndrome and may also be the result of compression by a pituitary tumor, granulomatous disease, irradiation, surgery, or trauma. The major primary testicular cause of androgen deficiency is Klinefelter's syndrome, in which a variable testosterone deficit is associated with complete tubular hyalinization and azoospermia (see below). It should be noted that androgen deficiency associated with hyperprolactinemia may not only reflect hypopituitarism caused by a prolactin-secreting pituitary tumor, but may also be the result of inhibition by prolactin itself of both GnRH secretion and testicular steroidogenesis.

3. Male Infertility

Male infertility, defined as the inability to father children and correlated with reduced sperm numbers and impaired sperm motility, most often reflects primary failure of seminiferous tubular function, with normal androgen secretion, and is usually otherwise asymptomatic.

Known causes of seminiferous tubular disease include testicular maldescent, testicular torsion or injury, mumps orchitis, prostatitis, hernia surgery, chronic renal failure, cytotoxic drugs, and other toxins, but the majority of cases are idiopathic. The testes are usually soft in consistency and often reduced in volume in such patients. Varicocele is also believed to be associated with impaired spermatogenesis, but this remains controversial. In Klinefelter's syndrome, tubular hyalinization and fibrosis results in small firm testes and azoospermia. Azoospermia may also reflect obstruction, usually within the epididymis, in which case testicular size is normal. A past or family history of chronic sinusitis or bronchiectasis, including fibrocystic disease, is often present in such patients, and may also be present in patients with the immotile cilia syndromes, in which a generalized cilial disorder affects both sperm and respiratory ciliated epithelium. Some will have the complete syndrome of Kartagener, consisting of chronic sinusitis, bronchiectasis, and situs inversus, inherited in an autosomal dominant manner. Much less frequently, male infertility is the result of gonadotropin deficiency or hyperprolactinemia.

III. DIAGNOSTIC TESTS

The evaluation of patients suspected of having disordered gonadal function should include an objective assessment of gonadal function, identification of the locus of the abnormality (whether at the level of gonad, pituitary, or hypothalamus), and elucidation of the nature of the defect at that site.

Much of this information may be apparent from the clinical assessment and knowledge of the likely differential diagnosis. Nevertheless, specific investigations are usually necessary. These investigations and their usefulness are discussed below, grouped according to their objective.

A. Determination of Sex

Where there is any possibility of sexual ambiguity, careful documentation of the sexual phenotype is essential, with particular attention to details of the external genital anatomy (see Sec. II.A). Assessment of internal genital organs by ultrasound, endoscopy, radiological procedures, or examination under anesthetic may be necessary. Genotype is best assessed by modern staining techniques using cultured lymphocytes, but examination of buccal scrapings for the presence or absence of Barr bodies, representing a second X chromosome, is useful where these facilities are not available. These investigations are discussed in detail in Part I.

B. Assessment of Gonadal Function

1. Hormone Secretion

Androgens. The adequacy of testosterone secretion in the adult male can usually be assessed quite accurately by means of a careful history and physical examination. Not infrequently, however, denial of sexual dysfunction and minimal changes in secondary sexual characteristics may conceal clearly subnormal hormone secretion. Measurement of the testosterone concentration in blood is therefore an essential part of the evaluation of testicular function. The standard radioimmunoassay (RIA) measures the total serum concentration of testosterone rather than the biologically active free concentration, which is usually about 2% of the total. Values are therefore influenced by variations in the level of the serum binding proteins, mainly sex steroid binding globulin (SSBG) and albumin, which do not, however, alter the steady-state free testosterone concentration. Total testosterone concentrations may be "corrected" for changes in serum binding by a number of methods, including charcoal or resin uptake tests and equilibrium dialysis. This does not appear to be necessary in routine clinical practice, but it should be appreciated that SSBG levels are increased by estrogen and reduced by androgen. Testosterone levels in saliva are a more accurate reflection of free levels and may become more widely used in the future.

Reference ranges for serum total testosterone vary and should be determined for each laboratory. In the authors' laboratory, the range in normal men is from 10 to 33 nmol/liter. In prepubertal boys, testosterone levels are less than 1 nmol/liter.

Serum testosterone RIA is most useful in the following situations:

1. Assessment of suspected hypogonadism in adult males.
2. Monitoring of testosterone replacement therapy.

3. Confirmation that puberty has not started in boys in whom delayed puberty is suspected.
4. Establishment of the presence of testes in apparent cryptorchidism.
5. Assessment of pre- or postpubertal females with clinical features of androgen excess. Measurement of other androgens may be helpful in this group, patticularly dihydrotestosterone, androstenedione, dehydroepiandrosterone and its sulfate in blood, and androsterone and etiocholanolone (the major 17-ketosteroids) in urine. A normal level of 17-hydroxyprogesterone in blood or pregnanetriol in urine excludes congenital adrenal hyperplasia due to 21- or 11-hydroxylase deficiency.

Estrogen. Ovarian estradiol secretion in adult women can usually be assessed with reasonable accuracy by means of a careful history and physical examination, together with a basal temperature chart, which provides evidence regarding ovulation (see Sec. III.B.2). Self-assessment of vaginal mucus is also helpful (see Chap. 5). More direct assessments of estrogen secretion are therefore often not required.

The progestagen test and endometrial biopsy (see Chap. 14) give an indication of endogenous estrogen secretion in terms of the degree of endometrial proliferation that is revealed, but the use of these indirect tests has declined in favor of direct assay of estrogens in blood or urine. Radioimmunoassay (RIA) is now the main method of estrogen assay, having largely replaced the earlier chemical methods. RIAs measuring estradiol in blood have been developed using antibodies which are highly specific in the case of plasma estradiol, but less so for the urinary metabolites (4). Of the various estrogen metabolites and conjugates which may be assayed in a 24-hr urine collection, the most useful appear to be total estrogen, estradiol, or estrone after hydrolysis or unhydrolyzed estrone-3-glucuronide (3, 4). Rapid urinary estrogen assays providing a same-day result have been an important advance in ovulation induction with human gonadotropins (5).

In the normal menstrual cycle, plasma estradiol levels vary from 150 to 500 pmol/liter in the early follicular phase, rising to 500 to 1000 pmol/liter in the late follicular phase, and reach a preovulatory peak of up to 2500 pmol/liter. In the luteal phase the levels are 300-1500 pmol/liter. Levels in postmenopausal women and men are less than 150 pmol/liter. The mean 24-hr urinary total estrogen in the early follicular phase is 25 nmol (range 14–50 nmol), rising to a mean preovulatory level of 180 nmol (range 110-280 nmol), mean luteal phase peak levels being 100 nmol (range 55-160 nmol). In postmenopausal women and adult men, 24-hr urinary total estrogen varies from 5 to 60 nmol. Levels of 24-hr urinary estrone-3-glucuronide are approximately 75%-90% of the total estrogen values.

The main clinical applications of these assays are:

1. Confirmation of estrogen deficiency and determination of its severity in women with suggestive clinical features (see Sec. III)
2. Monitoring of ovulation induction
3. Investigation of suspected estrogen excess in males (e.g., gynecomastia)

Progesterone. Direct chemical and, more recently, RIA methods of assay of progesterone and its metabolites and conjugates in blood and urine are available. The most useful of these are assay of total progesterone levels in blood and assay of total pregnanediol after hydrolysis or unhydrolyzed pregnanediol-3-glucuronide in urine by specific RIA (4). The main applications of these assays are in confirming whether or not ovulation has occurred and in assessing the adequacy of corpus luteum function (Sec. III.B.2, Ovulation).

2. Gamete Production

Spermatogenesis. As indicated in the Section I, spermatogenesis should be considered separately from hormone secretion, and should be assessed in its own right when fertility is in question. Testicular size and consistency generally reflect the state of spermatogenesis, as the tubular compartment makes up most of the volume of the testis, and must be carefully measured and recorded in all assessments of gonadal function (see Chap. 3).

Semen analysis is the most important test of seminiferous tubular function. The parameters that should be evaluated include details of collection, volume, sperm concentration, total sperm number, sperm motility and morphology, and the presence of inflammatory cells. These are discussed in Chapter 13. It is essential that this analysis be carried out in a laboratory experienced in these techniques, using standardized criteria and appropriate quality controls.

Further information on spermatogenesis can be obtained by testicular biopsy, but as the histological picture can often be accurately predicted from serum FSH concentrations (see below), this is generally unnecessary (6). This approach may need to be modified, however, in view of recent evidence that primary testicular disease is associated with an increased risk of testicular tumors which may be readily detected at an early "carcinoma in situ" stage by testicular biopsy.

Ovulation. The occurrence of ovulation can be detected retrospectively by a number of clinical and laboratory means of varying reliability. A normal menstrual cycle is good presumptive evidence of regular ovulation. Midcycle pain, so called Mittelschmerz, may be a symptom of ovulation, but is only noticed by a small proportion of women. Other symptoms implying prior ovulation are breast swelling and primary dysmenorrhea, both related to rising progesterone levels. Changes in cervical mucus reflect elevated estrogen levels late in the follicular phase (see Chap. 5), and can be used in predicting ovulation in women who ovulate regularly, but are not in themselves signs that ovulation will definately occur. Plasma and urinary estrogen assays have similar predictive value (4). The most useful clinical sign of ovulation is the rise in basal body temperature which follows in 80-90% of ovulations, averaging 0.4°C (7). This is attributable to increased progesterone secretion. In many cases, the rise is preceded by a brief temperature fall which usually occurs at about the time of ovulation. The absence of a temperature rise in the second half of the cycle is good evidence that ovulation has not occurred, although no rise is seen in 10-20% of women shown to have ovulated by other criteria (7).

The most widely used laboratory test of ovulation is assay of progesterone or its metabolites in blood or urine, a rise indicating corpus luteum formation and therefore implying prior ovulation. The height of the progesterone peak which follows ovulation varies considerably, both within and between individuals, but a plasma value greater than 16 nmol/liter (5 ng/ml) or a 24-hr urinary pregnanediol above 6 nmol (2 ng) is a reliable index of prior ovulation (8). Rapid assay of LH in blood or urine can also be used in predicting ovulation, the median interval between the earliest clear-cut rise in plasma LH and ovulation being 32 hr (95% confidence limits 24-38 hr) (9).

Perhaps the most direct assessment of ovulation, short of visualization at laparoscopy, is visualization by ultrasound. Recent technical advances have made this a reliable procedure. Follicles greater than 12 mm in diameter can be seen easily, and followed daily until rupture, when they can no longer be demonstrated. An average rate of increase in diameter is 2.5 mm per day, with ovulation likely once the diameter exceeds 20 mm (10).

C. Assessment of Hypothalamus and Pituitary

That disturbed gonadal function is secondary to a lesion in the pituitary or hypothalamus can often be established by clinical criteria and knowledge of the likely differential diagnosis. Clinical features of hypopituitarism indicate a lesion in the pituitary, hypothalamus, or both. The presence of diabetes insipidus is a clear indication of a hypothalamic lesion, however. Pituitary tumors may be recognized clinically by evidence of hypersecretion of pituitary hormones, particularly growth hormone and prolactin, or by the consequences of local expansion, notably headache, bitemporal visual field loss, and palsies of the third, fourth, and fifth cranial nerves, which pass through the cavernous sinus. Major hypothalamic damage results in a characteristic syndrome in which gross obesity and somnolence are the predominant features.

In many cases, however, distinction between primary and secondary hypogonadism requires further investigation. Additional tests are needed to determine the nature of lesions in the pituitary and hypothalamus.

1. Pituitary Hormone Secretion

Gonadotropins. The interpretation of the results of FSH and LH assays must take into account the pulsatile nature of gonadotropin secretion and the variations in the normal pattern that are determined by sex, age, stage of sexual development, and stage of the menstrual cycle (see Sec. I). The particular reference preparation of LH or FSH being used must be clearly stated, as preparations vary considerably in their biological and immunological potency. In general, the sensitivity of these assays enables high levels to be clearly distinguished from normal values, but low levels may not be separated as readily from the normal range.

Primary hypogonadism is readily identified by the marked increase in gonadotropin levels in blood and urine which results from loss of gonadal feedback inhibition and is accompanied by low sex steroid levels. In men, damage to both interstitial and tubular compartments of the testis results in elevated levels of LH and FSH; where tubular function is selectively impaired, only FSH levels rise, presumably reflecting loss of inhibin but not testosterone feedback (see Sec. I), (11). It should also be noted that clear-cut rises in gonadotropin levels may not be seen in primary gonadal failure in children between the ages of 2 and 9 because of dominance of central nervous system inhibition of gonadotropin secretion, which is independent of gonadal feedback mechanisms (12).

Impaired gonadal function that is accompanied by low gonadotropin levels may be attributed to a lesion in the pituitary or hypothalamus–hence the terms hypogonadotropic hypogonadism and secondary hypogonadism. The further characterization of such lesions is discussed in the following paragraphs.

In addition to the absolute levels of LH and FSH, attention should be given to the LH-FSH ratio. In the polycystic ovary syndrome, for example, LH levels are much higher than FSH level, although both are usually within the normal range (13). In anorexia nervosa and other causes of reduced GnRH secretion, a return to the prepubertal pattern of low gonadotropin levels and FSH preponderance occurs (14).

Other Pituitary Hormones. The assay of other pituitary hormones may yield important information in patients in whom secondary hypogonadism is suspected.

An elevated serum prolactin level may reflect the presence of a small or large prolactin-secreting pituitary tumor or a hypothalamic lesion resulting in the loss of the normal inhibition of pituitary prolactin secretion. Assay of prolactin in blood is therefore an important investigation in this context, bearing in mind that hyperprolactinemia may also be due to drugs or hypothyroidism and that the influence of stress, nipple stimulation, and pulsatility of secretion need to be taken into account in drawing blood for prolactin assays and in interpreting the results.

The remaining pituitary hormones should be assessed if a more general impairment of pituitary function is likely, or if a hyperfunctioning pituitary tumor is suspected (see Chaps. 36–42).

2. Hypothalamic Releasing Hormones

Direct assay of endogenous GnRH secretion would be expected to be a very useful test in assessing disturbances of gonadal function, but is exceedingly difficult because of the very small amounts that reach the peripheral circulation. Some authors have reported successful GnRH assays of blood (15), and have found the expected pattern of GnRH levels in various conditions, namely elevated levels in primary hypogonadism and pituitary disease, and undetectable levels in hypothalamic disease. Direct assay of GnRH in human pituitary portal blood has been attempted (16); interpretation of the results is made difficult by the very low levels and the admixture of arterial and venous blood with that from the portal system.

To the extent that pituitary responsiveness depends in part on the level of prior exposure to GnRH, endogenous secretion rates can be inferred from the pattern of LH and FSH responses to a standard dose of GnRH. As indicated in Chapters 36 and 37, however, this approach has many shortcomings and is of limited usefulness.

3. Assessment of Hypothalamic and Pituitary Anatomy

In parallel with the tests of hypothalamic and pituitary function described above, an assessment of the anatomy of the region should be made, looking particularly for evidence of a tumor (see Chap. 16). A wholly intrasellar lesion cannot be displayed reliably by currently available techniques, although modern contrast-enhanced CAT scans are approaching this degree of resolution. Intrasellar lesions which indent the normal smooth contour of the pituitary fossa are detectable by coned lateral and anteroposterior skull x-rays, with or without tomography, but several studies have shown that many apparently normal individuals have similar radiological appearances, casting considerable doubt on the specificity of this observation in patients suspected of harboring pituitary tumors (17). Larger lesions which cause greater expansion of the pituitary fossa are readily detected by plain skull x-rays and can usually be visualized by CAT scan.

A lesion occupying a suprasellar position, whether originating from within or outside the pituitary fossa, may be clinically apparent as loss of the temporal visual fields; formal charting, including the use of small and colored targets, should be routinely performed if a pituitary or hypothalamic lesion is suspected. Clinical involvement of the cranial nerves in the cavernous sinus indicates a parasellar lesion. In general, however, modern CT scanning is the best method of assessing lesions in these situations. Coronal views are particularly useful in this respect. The resolving power of this technique is improved by the intravenous administration of iodine-containing contrast medium; introduction of metrizamide or air into the subarachnoid space has also been helpful. CAT scanning has now all but replaced the much more invasive procedure of pneumonoencephalography. The radiation exposure to the lens, maximal in coronal views, and the risks of iodine sensitivity are the main hazards of CAT scanning.

IV. APPROACHES TO CLINICAL PROBLEMS

In the investigation of disordered gonadal function, a strategy should be adopted which is appropriate to the particular clinical problem, based on knowledge of the likely differential diagnosis. Sometimes a careful clinical assessment is all that is needed. Suitable approaches to the various clinical syndromes that may be encountered are outlined in this section.

A. Sexual Ambiguity

In addition to a careful clinical assessment (see Sec. III), a small number of relevant investigations will provide correct diagnosis of sexual ambiguity in most cases. Determination of karyotype will indicate the chromosomal sex. If 46XX is found, the plasma level of 17-hydroxyprogesterone or 24-hr urinary excretion of pregnanetriol should be determined, elevated values indicating congenital adrenal hyperplasia. Further tests will be needed to distinguish between 21- and 11-hydroxylase deficiency (see Chap. 25).

If the karyotype is 46XY, assessment of external and internal genital anatomy will usually lead to the correct diagnosis. In testicular feminization, high levels of testosterone and gonadotropins will be associated with inability of cultured genital skin fibroblasts to bind testosterone, whereas failure of in vitro conversion of testosterone to dihydrotestosterone confirms 5α-reductase deficiency.

Although sexual ambiguity is usually recognized in the neonatal period, it should be kept in mind that congenital adrenal hyperplasia in the female may not be identified until later in childhood or adolescence as hirsutes and virilization. While partial deficiency of the androgen receptor may cause male pseudohermaphroditism, complete testicular feminization most often presents as primary amenorrhea, infertility, or tall stature in a phenotypically normal female.

B.. Precocious Puberty

The diagnosis of precocious puberty is a clinical one (see Sec. II), supported by characteristic growth charts and radiological evidence of advanced bone age (see Chap. 2). In true precocious puberty in girls, as indicated by cyclical menses, evidence of ovulation, and adult gonadotropin levels, an idiopathic basis is likely and a structural cerebral lesion very unlikely. In cases of pseudoprecocious puberty, an ovarian tumor can be reliably excluded by careful palpation and pelvic ultrasound. Albright's fibrous dysplasia may be recognized clinically by the characteristic skin pigmentation and bone lesions, and hypothyroidism should be excluded by thyroid function testing (see Chap. 8).

In view of the relatively high incidence of organic disease in boys, however, a careful search should be made for a cerebral lesion if uniform testicular enlargement indicates true precocious puberty (see Chap. 3), while adrenal hyperplasia or tumor should be excluded if the testes are less than 4 ml in volume (see Chap. 25). Functioning testicular tumors may secrete sufficient quantities of α-fetoprotein, hCG, or its β-subunit for these to be measured in blood. It should be noted that measurement of the gonadotropin responses to GnRH has little advantage over measurement of basal levels in the assessment of precocious puberty.

C. Delayed Puberty

Only those subjects who meet the strict criteria for the diagnosis of delayed puberty (see Sec. II.C.) should be investigated. In particular, boys with testicular volumes of greater than 4 ml can be confidently assumed to have entered puberty, even if no other signs of puberty are present. The degree of developmental retardation can be assessed from growth charts and by comparison of chronological age with bone age (see Chap. 2).

Although hypothalamic, pituitary, and primary gonadal disorders need to be considered, a functional delay or failure of hypothalamic GnRH secretion is the usual cause of delayed puberty in boys. The principal problem is to differentiate between normal variant delayed puberty, often familial, and isolated gonadotropin deficiency (Kallman's syndrome), often associated with loss of olfaction and other midline developmental abnormalities. Assays of LH, FSH, and testosterone and GnRH tests cannot reliably distinguish between these possibilities (see Chaps. 36 and 37), so that only the passage of time will resolve the dilemma.

Structural hypothalamic and pituitary lesions should be considered, particularly if there are clinical features suggesting loss of other pituitary functions. In their absence, a lateral skull x-ray and serum prolactin level are a reasonable minimum.

The main primary testicular cause of delayed puberty is Klinefelter's syndrome, in which the karyotype is 47XXY; rarely, syndromes of testicular dysgenesis or absence and gonadotropin resistance need to be considered. In these cases, clinical features and high gonadotropin levels will indicate the primary testicular basis.

In girls with delayed puberty, the karyotype should always be determined in order to exclude Turner's syndrome. Otherwise, the differential diagnosis lies between a functional disturbance of hypothalamic GnRH secretion, isolated gonadotropin deficiency (Kallman's syndrome), hypopituitarism, and hyperprolactinemia. Often a clinical diagnosis of functional hypothalamic disturbance can be made, in which case puberty will eventually commence; if not, Kallman's syndrome remains a possibility. In the absence of specific clinical pointers, a lateral skull x-ray and serum prolactin level will exclude structural pituitary lesions and hyperprolactinemia. As in boys, basal and GnRH stimulated gonadotropin levels are usually not helpful in differentiating between functional delay and isolated gonadotropin deficiency. Finally, it should be noted that isolated growth hormone deficiency (see Chap. 29) and hypothyroidism (see Chap. 21) may result in delayed puberty.

D. Primary Amenorrhea

Primary amenorrhea, as defined in Section II.D, is one of the consequences of delayed puberty (see above), but may occur in the presence of otherwise apparently normal pubertal development. In addition to the investigations outlined in the preceding section, a careful clinical assessment of genital anatomy is important, often best conducted under anesthesia. Pelvic ultrasound, hysterosalpingography, and laparoscopy may also be used to define the internal genital organs.

E. Secondary Amenorrhea

A careful clinical assessment may indicate the cause of impaired ovarian function arising in the adult female, always remembering that pregnancy is by far the most common cause of secondary amenorrhea. Conditions associated with a functional disturbance of hypothalamic GnRH secretion should be noted (see Sec. II.E), and the breasts examined for galactorrhea. Clinical signs of hypopituitarism, perhaps associated with headache and visual field disturbance, should not be overlooked. Hirsutes, obesity, and cystic ovarian enlargement suggest polycystic ovarian disease.

If menses are occurring, it is important to demonstrate failure of ovulation in order to exclude other causes of female infertility, particularly disease of the fallopian tubes. Lack of a rise in basal body temperature or in progesterone levels in plasma or urine confirm anovulation. Assay of plasma or urinary estrogen levels may also be helpful in assessing impaired ovarian function.

Basal LH and FSH levels should be determined and will usually be normal or low, excluding primary ovarian failure. A high LH/FSH ratio is characteristic of polycystic ovarian disease, whereas low levels with FSH predominance suggest deficiency of hypothalamic GnRH secretion, usually functional in origin.

Appropriate blood samples for prolactin assay should be taken in all cases. If factors such as stress, nipple stimulation, drugs, and hypothyroidism can be excluded, hyperprolactinemia appears to reflect a pituitary microadenoma in most cases, although a large tumor should be excluded by means of a lateral skull x-ray. Where features of hypopituitarism or pituitary tumor are present, formal visual field assessment, lateral skull x-ray, CAT scan, and thorough testing of pituitary function are necessary.

F. Hirsutism and Virilization

Mild hirsutism of gradual onset, which is not associated with menstrual disturbance or virilization and which is often familial, can be safely assumed to be benign and probably does not warrant laboratory investigation, as this is unlikely to influence the patient's management. Plasma 17-hydroxyprogesterone or 24-hr urinary pregnanetriol should be determined if mild forms of congenital adrenal hyperplasia are suspected (18). A high LH/FSH ratio and enlarged cystic ovaries, demonstrated by palpation and pelvic ultrasound, are characteristic of the polycystic ovary syndrome. Cushing's syndrome should be excluded in patients with suggestive clinical features (see Chap. 19).

In virilized patients in whom congenital adrenal hyperplasia has been excluded, elevated plasma or urinary androgens suggest an adrenal or ovarian tumor which can best be localized by palpation, abdominal CAT scan, and ultrasound of abdomen and pelvis. It should be kept in mind that certain drugs, such as diphenylhydantoin, diazoxide, minoxidil, metyrapone, and androgen-related progestins, can cause hirsutism and that hirsute patients may present with infertility or menstrual disturbance.

G. Impotence and Male Infertility

In all men in whom impaired testicular function is suspected, a careful history (see Sec. II) and a thorough physical examination are essential. In addition to checking height and weight, the span and lower segment height should be determined in men who appear to have a eunuchoid habitus. An assessment of androgen status should be made, paying attention to potency, muscle development, beard and other hair growth, voice, and penile size. Clinical features of adrenal and thyroid insufficiency should be sought and visual acuity, fields, and fundi checked. Olfaction should be tested if Kallman's syndrome is suspected. The breasts should be carefully examined, looking for gynecomastia or galactorrhea, and the chest examined for evidence of chronic upper or lower respiratory tract disease, known to be associated with the immotile cilia syndromes and obstructive azoospermia. Finally, the scrotum should be carefully examined. Testicular size should be determined by means of the Prader orchiometer, a set of ellipsoids of known volume, and testicular consistency noted. As seminiferous tubules make up most of the volume of the testis, primary or secondary tubular damage usually results in loss of volume and a soft testicular consistency. In Klinefelter's syndrome, the testes are typically less than 6 ml in volume and of firm consistency, associated with tall stature, a eunuchoid habitus, and variable androgen deficiency. In obstructive azoospermia, testicular size is normal. In most cases, the epididymis is the site of the obstruction, but congenital absence of the vas should be excluded by palpation of the cord. The epididymis should also be palpated for evidence of distention or inflammation. If prostatitis is suspected, a rectal examination should be performed.

Examination of the spermatic cord with the patient standing may reveal a varicocele, identified as a visible or palpable swelling of the veins surrounding the cord or as an impulse palpable on coughing or during the Valsalva maneuver.

If the clinical assessment suggests impaired testicular function, both compartments should be checked by means of plasma testosterone assay, semen analysis, and measurement of plasma LH and FSH levels. A primary testicular lesion can be readily distinguished from hypofunction secondary to a hypothalamic or pituitary lesion on the basis of gonadotropin levels, which will be high in the former case and low in the latter.

If the clinical and biochemical evidence indicates a pituitary or hypothalamic lesion, tests of pituitary and hypothalamic function and anatomy should be carried out as already described, looking particularly for a large prolactin-secreting pituitary tumor, other pituitary lesions, and isolated gonadotropin deficiency (Kallman's syndrome).

Primary testicular lesions are much commoner, and may be subdivided into those which only affect tubular function, with impaired sperm production and elevated FSH levels but normal testosterone and LH levels, and those which affect both compartments of the testis. Karyotype should be checked in all cases in which azoospermia or severe oligospermia is associated with testicular volumes of loss than 6 ml and elevated levels of FSH, in order to exclude Klinefelter's syndrome (47XXY). In this condition, there may also be variable degrees of impairment of hormone secretion.

Although many causes of impaired sperm production are known (see Sec. II.G), these can usually be identified clinically; as no specific etiology can be found in the remaining majority of cases, further investigations beyond those already mentioned are of little clinical assistance. If surgical treatment of varicocele is contemplated, radiological confirmation of reflux from the renal vein into the internal spermatic vein should be obtained. Whether such surgery is beneficial is not yet firmly established, however.

Diagnostic Summary 1 Sexual Ambiguity

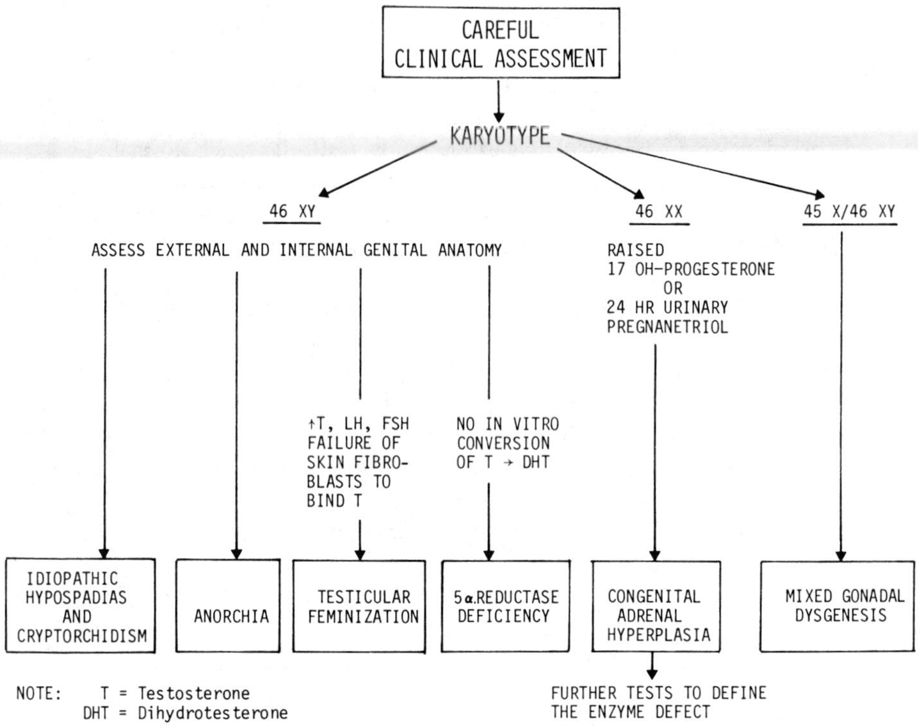

NOTE: T = Testosterone
DHT = Dihydrotesterone

Diagnostic Summary 2 (a) Precocious Puberty—Boys; (b) Precocious Puberty—Girls

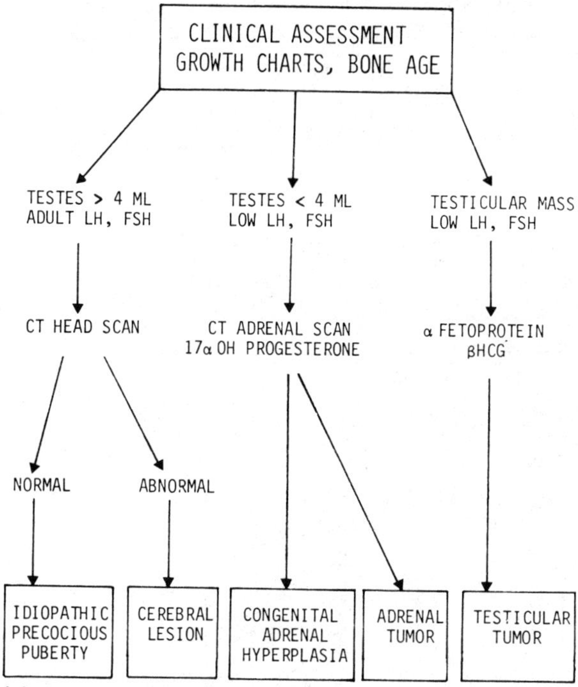

(a)

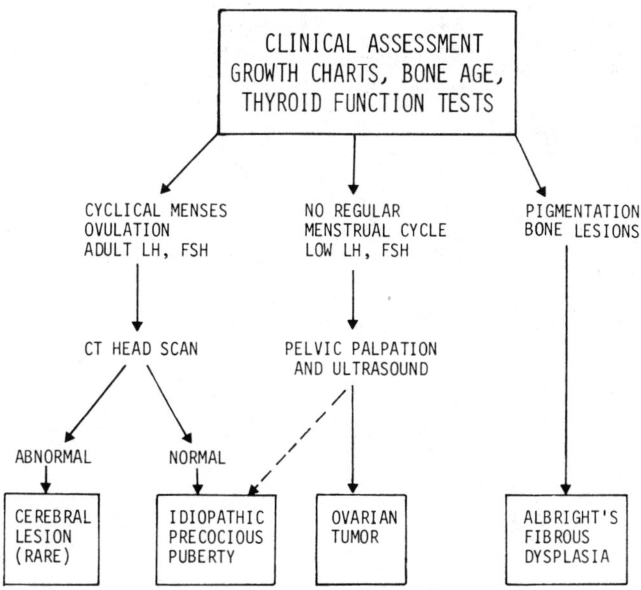

(b)

Diagnostic Summary 3 Delayed Puberty

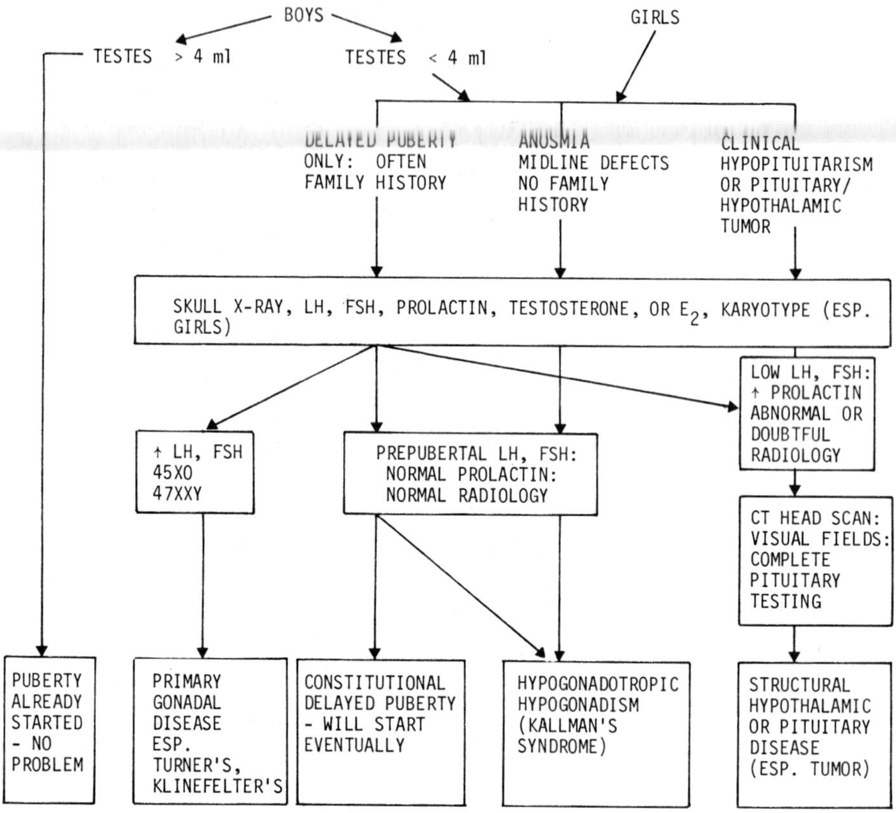

Diagnostic Summary 4a Primary Amenorrhea

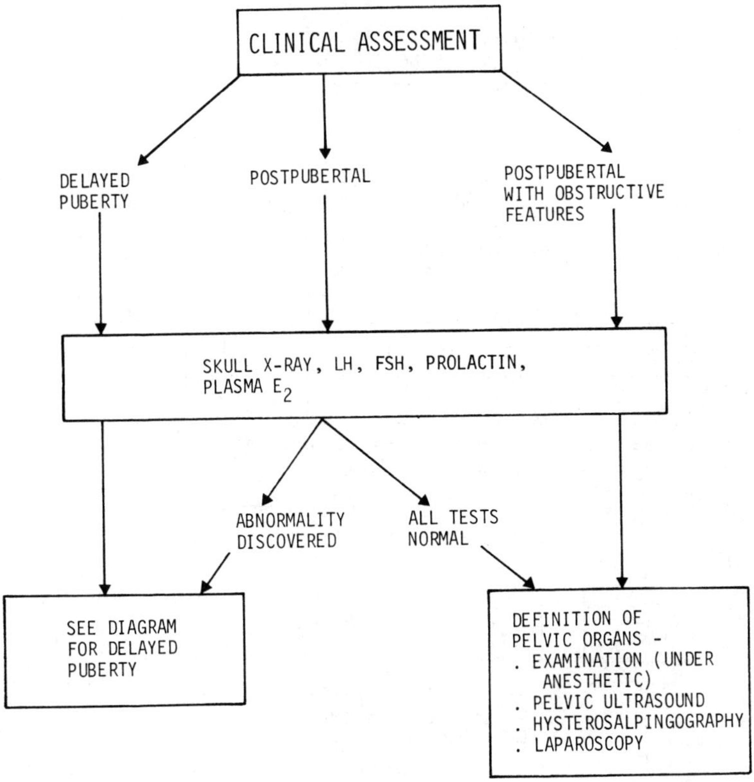

Diagnostic Summary 4b Secondary Amenorrhea

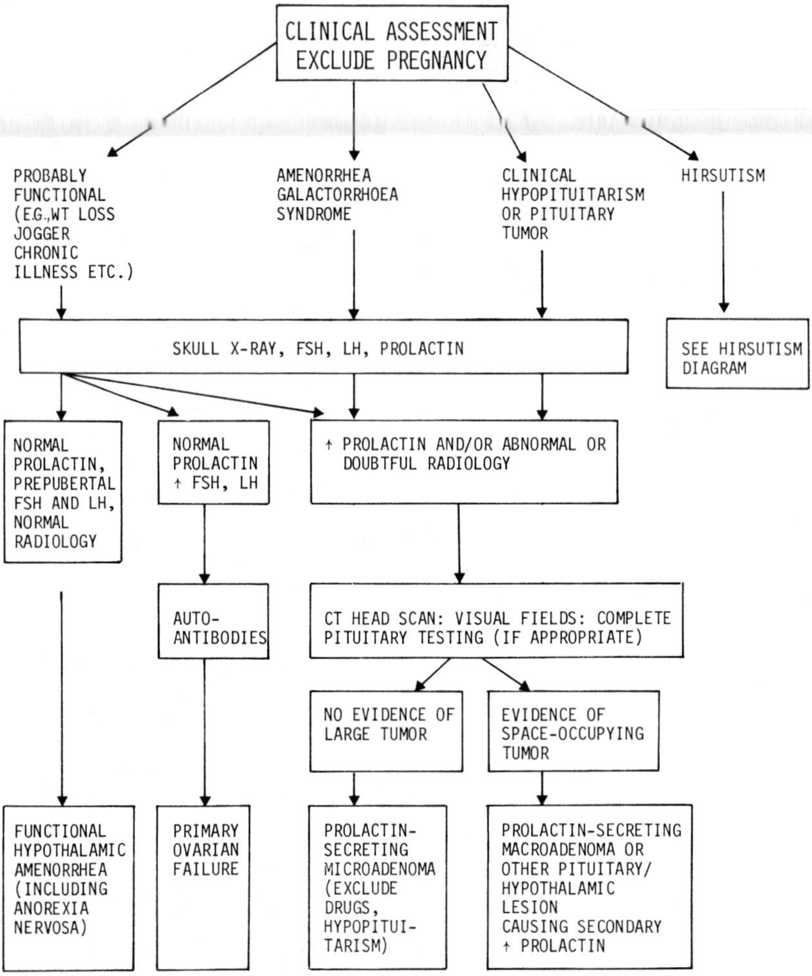

Diagnostic Summary 5 Hirsutism and Virilization

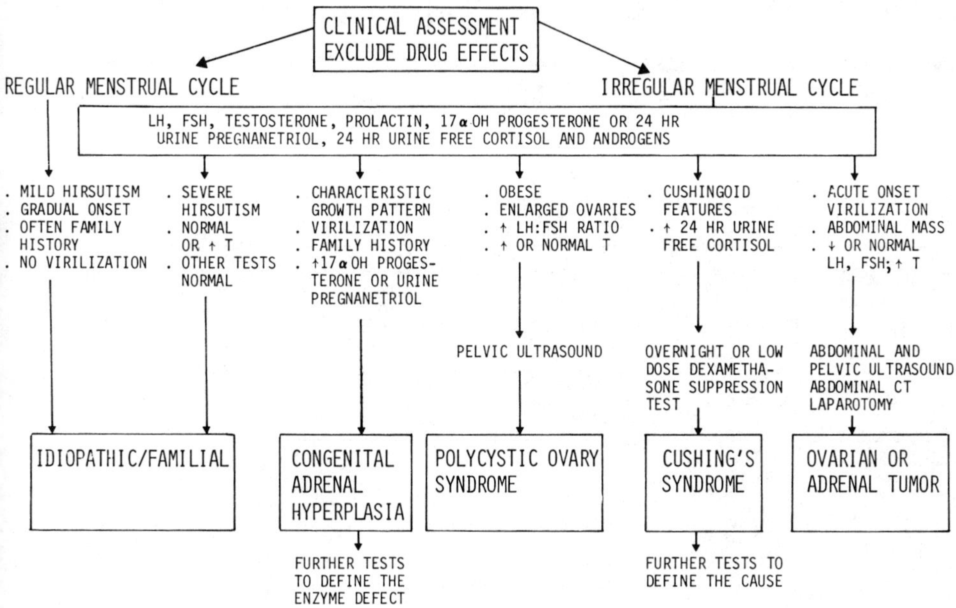

Diagnostic Summary 6 (a) Infertility—Assessment of the Male; (b) Infertility—Assessment of the Female

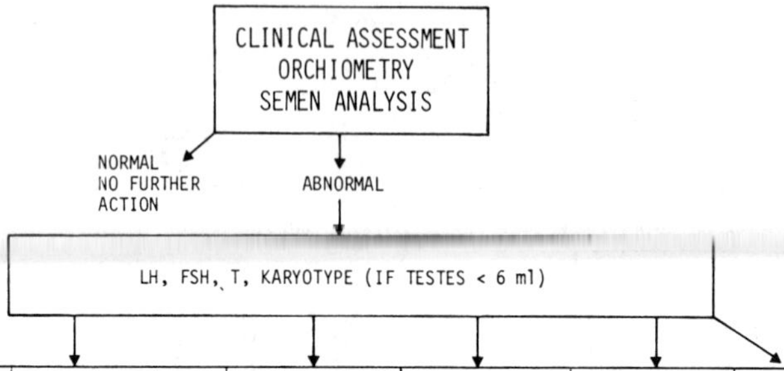

SEMEN ANALYSIS:	OLIGOSPERMIA AND/OR ↓ MOTILITY	AZOOSPERMIA	OLIGO- OR AZOOSPERMIA	AZOOSPERMIA	OLIGO- OR AZOOSPERMIA
TESTICULAR VOL:	↓ OR NORMAL	NORMAL	↓ OR NORMAL	< 6 ml	↓ OR NORMAL
FSH:	NORMAL	NORMAL	↑	↑	↓
LH:	NORMAL	NORMAL	NORMAL OR ↑	↑	↓
T:	NORMAL	NORMAL	NORMAL OR ↓	↓ OR NORMAL	↓
↓	IDIOPATHIC OLIGOSPERMIA OR MOTILITY DISORDER, VARICOCELE, PROSTATITIS	OBSTRUCTION, USUALLY EPIDIDYMAL, OR IDIOPATHIC DISORDERS OF SPERMATOGENESIS	PRIMARY SEMINIFEROUS TUBULAR FAILURE	KLINEFELTER'S SYNDROME OR OTHER PRIMARY TESTICULAR DISEASE	KALLMAN'S SYNDROME OR HYPOPITUITARISM ↓ PROLACTIN, CT HEAD SCAN, VISUAL FIELDS, COMPLETE PITUITARY TESTING

(a)

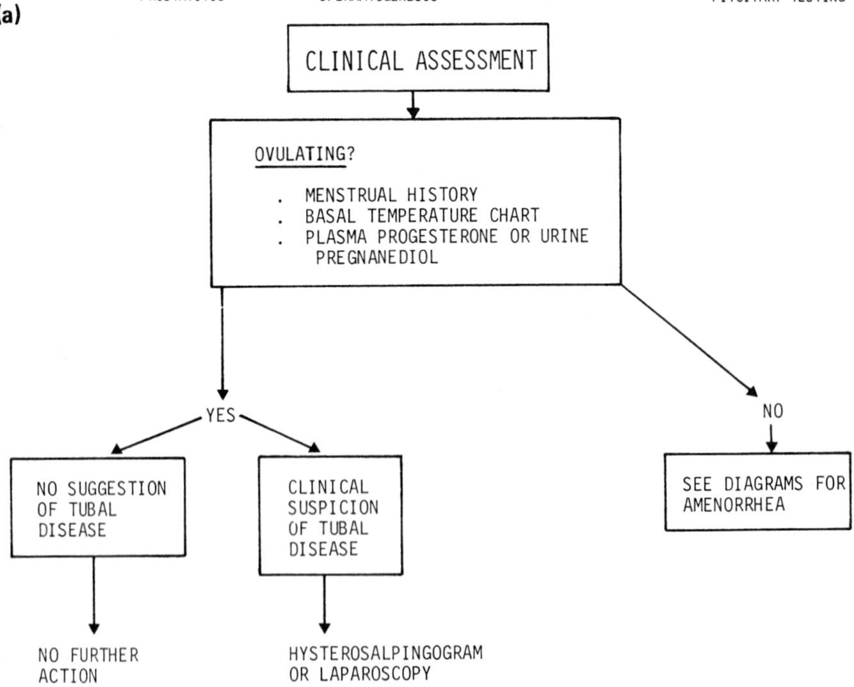

(b)

REFERENCES

1. Gutai JP, Kowarski AA, Migeon CJ. The detection of the heterozygous carrier for congenital virilizing adrenal hyperplasia. J Pediatr 1977; 90: 924-929.
2. Ferriman D, Gallwey JD. Clinical assessment of body hair growth in women. J Clin Endocrinol Metab 1961; 21:1440-1447.
3. Collins WP, Collins PO, Kilpatrick MJ, Manning PA, Pike JM, Tyler JPP. The concentrations of urinary oestrone-3-glucuronide, LH and pregnanediol-3-glucuronide as indices of ovarian function. Acta Endocrinol 1979; 90: 336-348.
4. Adlercreutz H, Lehtinen T, Kairento A. Prediction of ovulation by urinary estrogen assays. J Steroid Biochem 1980; 12:395-401.
5. Brown JB, Beischer NA. Current status of estrogen assays in gynecology and obstetrics. Obstet Gynaecol Surv 1972; 27:205-235.
6. de Kretser DM, Burger HG, Fortune D, Hudson B, Long AR, Paulsen CA, Taft HP. Hormonal, histological and chromosomal studies in adult males with testicular disorders. J Clin Endocrinol Metab 1972; 35:392-401.
7. Moghissi KS. Accuracy of basal body temperature for ovulation detection. Fertil Steril 1976; 27:1415-1421.
8. Abraham GE, Maroulis GB, Marshall JR. Evaluation of ovulation and corpus luteum function using measurements of plasma progesterone. Obstet Gynecol 1974; 44:522-525.
9. World Health Organization, Task Force on methods for the determination of the fertile period. Temporal relationships between ovulation and defined changes in the concentration of plasma estradiol-17β, luteinizing hormone, follicle stimulating hormone and progesterone. I. Probit analysis. Am J Obstet Gynecol 1980; 38:383-390.
10. Kerin JF, Edmonds DK, Warnes GM, Cox LW, Seamark RF, Matthews CD, Young GB, Baird DT. Morphological and functional relations of graafian follicle growth to ovulation in women using ultrasonic, laparoscopic and biochemical measurements. Br J Obstet Gynaecol 1981; 88:81-90.
11. Scott RS, Burger HG. Inhibin is absent from azoospermic semen of infertile men. Nature 1980; 285:246-247.
12. Conte FA, Grumbach MM, Kaplan SL, Reiter EO. Correlation of luteinizing hormone-releasing factor-induced luteinizing hormone and follicle-stimulating hormone release from infancy to 19 years with the changing pattern of gonadotropin secretion in agonadal patients: relation to the restraint of puberty. J Clin Endocrinol Metab 1980; 50:163-168.
13. Rebar RW, Judd HL, Yen SSC, Rakoff J, Vandenberg G, Naftolin F. Characterization of the inappropriate gonadotropin secretion in polycystic ovary syndrome. J Clin Invest 1976; 57:1320-1329.
14. Warren MP, Jewelewicz R, Dyrenfurth I, Ans R, Khalaf S, Vande Wiele RL. The significance of weight loss in the evaluation of pituitary response to LH-RH in women with secondary amenorrhea. J Clin Endocrinol Metab 1975; 40:601-611.

15. Kawamura Y, Miyake A, Aono T, Kurachi K. Plasma luteinizing hormone-releasing hormone levels in normal women and patients with amenorrhea. Fertil Steril 1980; 34:444-447.
16. Carmel PW, Antunes JL, Ferin M. Collection of blood from the pituitary stalk and portal veins in monkeys, and from the pituitary sinusoidal system of monkey and man. J Neurosurg 1979; 50:75-80.
17. Burrow GN, Wortzman G, Rewcastle NB, Holgate RC, Kovacs K. Microadenomas of the pituitary and abnormal sellar tomograms in an unselected autopsy series. N Engl J Med 1981; 304:156-158.
18. Rosenwaks Z, Lee PA, Jones CS, Migeon CJ, Wentz AC. An attenuated form of congenital virilizing adrenal hyperplasia. J Clin Endocrinol Metab 1979; 49:335-339.

21
Growth Hormone

Leslie Lazarus
St. Vincent's Hospital, Sydney, Australia

The growth-promoting ability of aqueous extract of bovine pituitaries was first demonstrated by Evans and Long in 1921 (1) but it was not until 1944 that bovine growth hormone (GH) was isolated (2). Failure of investigators to induce the anticipated change in primates with bovine GH raised doubts regarding the role of GH in humans until 1957, when Knobil et al. (3) demonstrated that this was due to species specificity and subsequently Raben prepared biologically active growth hormone from human pituitaries (4). The structure of human GH was finally elucidated by Li and Dixon in 1971 (5) and modified by Niall et al. in 1973 (6).

Human growth hormone (hGH) consists of a single peptide chain of 191-amino acid residues with two intrachain disulfide bridges and a molecular weight of 22,005 daltons. The structure of hGH resembles that of placental lactogen, with which it shares 161 out of 191 identical amino acid residues. hGH also shares structural homology with human prolactin (hPrl), which consists of 198 amino acid residues of which 49 are in identical positions. Biologically active hGH has been produced from *Escherichia coli* using recombinant DNA methodology (7). Relatively large amounts of hGH are stored in the pituitary and may make up as much as 10% of the dry weight of tissue and yielding 8-10 mg of hGH on extraction.

The hGH isolated from pituitary glands has been found not to be a single substance but a mixture of variants differing in amino acid sequence, posttranslational modified forms, and fragments (8). Lewis et al. (8) have identified several classes of hGH variants, including single-chain forms, an S-S dimer, and two-chain forms. The single-chain forms are recognized by their electrophoretic characteristics and have been referred to as fast, slow, slow-slow, and deamidated hGH. The S-S form is a dimer of hGH formed by intermolecular disulphide linkage and is biologically inactive. The two-chain variant of hGH is formed by selective removal of amino acid residues 135-149 by proteinases, resulting in two chains held together by a single disulfide bond between residues 53-165. If the disulfide bond is broken, two fragments are generated: F1, consisting of the residues 1-135, and F2, from residues 150-191. Each of these fragments is relatively inactive biologically. The hGH variants are of variable immunological potency in hGH radioimmunoassay (RIA), which cannot be used for their assays. The most interesting of the hGH variants is the 20,000-dalton (20K) form. It is found in all human pituitaries and may account for as much as 15% of the pituitary content of hGH. It differs from hGH by the deletion of 15 amino acid residues between 32 and 46. The 20K form possesses growth-promoting activity with a potency similar to that of normal hGH but lacks the insulin-like activity and FFA-mobilizing activity normally seen with hGH. The circulating form of hGH in serum has also been shown to be a heterogeneous mixture of the hGH monomer and polymeric forms (9).

Although the pituitary contains large stores of hGH the daily secretion rate is low and has been calculated by Alford et al. (10) to be about 400 μg per day in healthy young adults and about 700 μg per day in adolescents by Finkelstein et al. (11). The characteristic secretory pattern is one of low basal levels with discrete secretory episodes associated with sleep, exercise, stress, and high-protein meals. The secretory peaks are larger in women than men. In children some 50% of the daily secretion occurs during sleep and is associated with the onset of slow-wave sleep about 60-90 min after its onset (12). Using a continuous sampling technique, Plotnick et al. (13) estimated the mean serum hGH level during a 24-hr period to be 6.94 ± 3.34 (± SD) mU/liter in young adults and 14.7 ± 3.4 mU/liter in adolescents. The hGH response to stimuli during adolescence is significantly greater than that seen in prepubertal children (14). Several workers have recorded a decrease of GH secretion with age (11, 15, 16) and a loss of the sleep-related growth hormone peaks in old age (17). This reduced secretion of GH in old age is not associated with a change in the size of the pituitary (18) or GH content (19), suggesting that it is related to a change in neurosecretory mechanisms. Obesity is also associated with a reduction in GH release (20).

Growth hormone secretion by the pituitary gland is influenced by the hypothalamus, although to date no GH releasing hormone has been isolated*. The

---

*Recently, Thorner, MO, Rivier, J., Spiess, J. et al. (Lancet 1983, i, 24–28) have characterized and sequenced a growth hormone releasing factor from the pancreatic tumor of a patient with acromegaly.

tetradecapeptide somatostatin is an inhibitor of GH release and while it was originally isolated from the hypothalamus, it has since been identified widely throughout the central nervous system and the gastrointestinal tract. Hypothalamic biogenic amines have a major role in the control of GH secretion and a number of drugs which have an effect on brain biogenic amine turnover or receptors have been noted to influence GH secretion in both normal and pathological states. Many of the standard provocative tests of GH secretion are based on these observations.

After secretion GH binds to receptors on target tissue, such as the liver. The GH receptor from rabbit liver has been solubilized and purified to a considerable extent by Waters and Friesen (21). It is a sialoglycoprotein of 300,000 daltons, composed of four nonidentical subunits of 70,000 daltons. The binding site of the hGH receptor is unique in that it recognizes only primate GH, and thus the expression of the species specificity resides at the level of the GH receptor.

I. MEASUREMENT OF GROWTH HORMONE

The GH content of human serum may be measured by bioassay, radioreceptor assay, or radioimmunoassay. Bioassays using as an end point the widening of the tibial epiphyseal cartilage in the hypophysectomized rat have demonstrated the presence of bioassayable GH in a concentration several hundredfold greater than that which can be accounted for by RIA (22). The bioassays, however, require the extraction of large volumes of plasma, thus restricting their use to research protocols. RIA was first applied to hGH in 1963 by Hunter et al. (23) and since then has had a major impact on physiological studies and clinical practice. Results may be reported in mU/liter of the WHO First International Reference Preparation of hGH for immunoassay (66/217) or in ng/ml. As most highly purified hGH preparations have an immunological potency of 2 mU/mg, the results reported in ng/ml may be multiplied by 2.0 to give an equivalent potency in mU/liter. There is, however, a considerable interlaboratory bias due to the use of different antisera, standards, and separating techniques. In a recent survey the Australian Human Pituitary Advisory Committee asked 22 laboratories to assay the hGH content of a serum sample and the results ranged from 22 to 53 mU/liter with a consensus figure of 34. For these reasons clinicians should be extremely cautious in the use of reference ranges from the literature rather than the laboratory performing the assay. A further source of error in the interpretation of RIA data results from the heterogeneity of circulating hGH, especially in patients with acromegaly and spuriously elevated results may be reported following serial dilution of a serum sample with high levels. Fortunately, hGH is relatively stable in serum and samples may be collected without additives and maintained stable for prolonged periods if frozen at −20°C.

Growth hormone has been identified also in lymph (24), cerebrospinal fluid (CSF) (25), and urine (26). Elevated levels have been noted in CSF of patients with suprasellar extension of pituitary tumors and hGH in CSF has been suggested for the diagnosis and management of GH-secreting pituitary adenomas (27). hGH has been identified in the urine and some workers have suggested its measurement as a measure of GH secretion rates. A comprehensive study by Bala et al. (26) revealed that less than 0.01% of injected hGH appeared in the urine and that the excretion of radioimmunoassayable hGH in urine was very low, ranging from 35 ng per day in the hypopituitary subject, 79 ng per day in the normal to 254 ng per day in the acromegalic.

Growth hormone binds to specific receptors on many tissues and assays utilizing the binding of ^{125}hGH to liver membrane receptors or a human lymphocyte line (IM-9) have been used to compare RIA and RRA. The RRA assays have provided data different from that of RIA and have been interpreted to demonstrate that not all of the circulating hGH is biologically active (28).

II. TESTS OF GH SECRETION

Because of low basal secretion of hGH in the normal subject it is not possible to differentiate normal from hypopituitarism by the measurement of basal samples. The measurement of hGH secretory rates has been achieved by the use of continuous sampling (13), but this is far too expensive and time consuming for routine diagnostic use. Measurement by RIA of the hGH responses to stimulation or suppression tests has now become established as an effective means to assess the GH secretory capacity of the pituitary or the presence of an abnormality of the GH control mechanism.

The tests used may be classified as physiologic stimuli, nutrient challenge, pharmacologic agents, or hormonal (Table 1).

A. Physiologic

1. Sleep

The sleep-associated peak of hGH occurs during the onset of slow-wave sleep electroencephalograph (EEG) stages 3 and 4, and it has been suggested that a single sample appropriately obtained might serve as a physiologic screening test of GH secretion in children with short stature. A number of groups (29-31) have reported that a single sample taken 60-90 min after the onset of sleep will reveal a hGH level of > 10 mU/liter in up to 75% of normal controls but no significant peak in GH-deficient children. While the test can be performed without frequent sampling or EEG monitoring, it does require hospitalization and is useful only as a screening procedure to demonstrate that the child is *not* GH deficient. A sup-

Table 1 Tests of Growth Hormone Secretion

1. Physiologic stimuli	
	Sleep
	Exercise
2. Nutrient challenge	
	Hypoglycemia
	Arginine infusion
	Hyperglycemia
3. Pharmacologic agents	
	L-dopa
	Clonidine
	Diazepam
	Metoclopramide
	Propranolol
4. Hormonal	
	TRH
	Sex steroids
	Glucagon
5. Miscellaneous	
	Vasopressin
	Tetracosactrin
	Prostaglandins
	Pyrogens
	Metyrapone

pression of the sleep-related hGH peak has been noted in obesity (32), old age (17), and acromegaly (17).

2. Exercise

Strenuous exercise has been recognized as a potent stimulus for GH release for many years, but it is important to note that the pattern of GH release is dependent on the work load and the duration of the exercise (see Fig. 1). Sutton et al. (33) showed that there was a similar hGH response in all subjects exercised to exhaustion but that exercise to only 80% of work capacity (W170) provoked *no* hGH response in fit subjects with a significant response in the unfit. It is therefore important to note that a negative hGH response to exercise may be due to an inadequate stimulus and this is particularly likely in small children, who are reluctant to exercise strenuously regardless of the mode of exercise. While the exercise test is now well established as a simple outpatient screening procedure (34, 35), it should be noted that a peak hGH level > 10 mU/liter may be noted in only 70-80% of normal subjects.

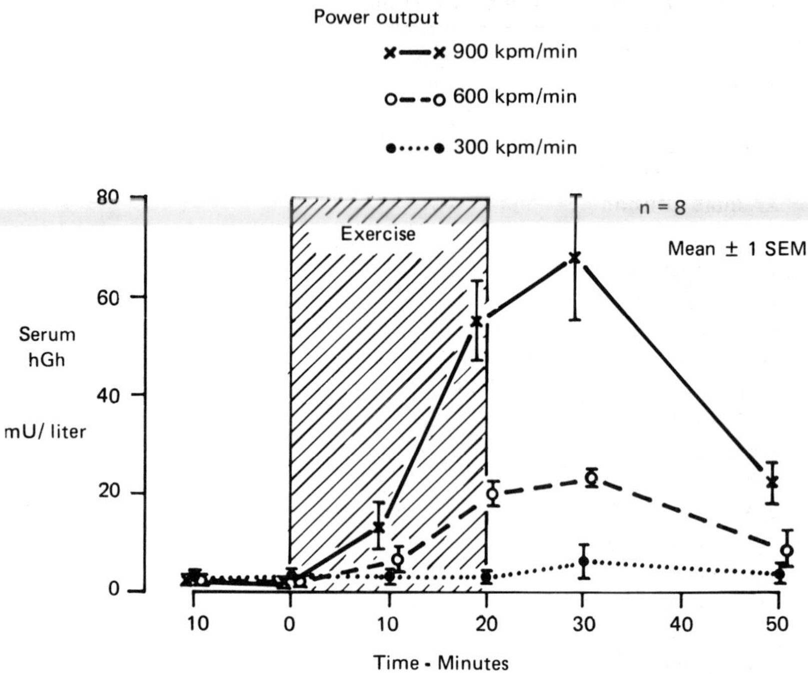

Figure 1 hGH response to various exercise work loads in normal subjects. (Adapted from Ref. 33.)

B. Nutrient Challenge

1. Hypoglycemia

Hypoglycemia is a potent stimulus to GH secretion and over the past 18 years insulin-induced hypoglycemia has become established as the standard GH stimulation test. Numerous studies (36) have reported hGH responses of > 15 mU/liter in from 75 to 90% of normal children following adequate hypoglycemia and all authors have reported a failure of response in children with hGH deficiency. The hypoglycemia is induced by the intravenous administration of an insulin dose of 0.05-0.1 U/kg body weight of purified neutral insulin and the measurement of hGH in serum samples for up to 90 min following the injection. The test has the advantage of permitting simultaneous measurement of cortisol to assess ACTH release and it may be given together with TRH or GnRH as a combined test of anterior pituitary function (37). The disadvantages are the potential dangers of profound hypoglycemia and the need for medical surveillance. It is important that a satisfactory degree of hypoglycemia be achieved and most workers accept a drop to at least 50% of the basal glucose level or to a level less than 2.2 mmol/liter (40 mg/dl). The hGH response to hypoglycemia is impaired in patients with depressive illnesses (38), obesity (20), hypothyroidism (39), or delayed puberty (14) and may be influenced by a number of pharmacologic agents (Table 2) (40-52).

2. Arginine Infusion

The GH releasing effect of amino acids was first noted by Knopf et al. (53). The amino acids may be given complexed in a protein meal, in a beef broth extract [Bovril (54)], or as an amino acid infusion. L-Arginine infusion has been the most widely used and will cause a peak GH level of ≥ 10 mU/liter in 80% of normal subjects (55) and a peak response of ≥ 15 mU/liter in 50% of normal subjects (56). All investigators have reported a failure of response in GH-deficient subjects. The arginine is given as an intravenous infusion of 0.5 g/kg body weight (to a maximum of 30 g) over 30 min and has the advantage of very few side effects. It is frequently used in a sequential test followed by insulin-induced hypoglycemia (57). Women respond more consistently and have a greater rise in GH than men (58). The response of men can be augmented by their pretreatment with estrogens (stilbestrol 2.5 mg twice daily for 2 days).

The mechanism of action of arginine differs from that of insulin as no fall in blood glucose is noted and the responses to hypoglycemia and arginine may be

Table 2 Effects of Pharmacologic Agents on Hypoglycemia-Induced GH Release

GH Response	Agent	Reference
1. Increase	Propranolol	40
	α-Methyldopa	41
2. Decrease	TRH	42
	Corticosteroids	43
	Reserpine	44
	Chlorpromazine	45
	Phentolamine	40
	L-Dopa	46
	Cyproheptadine	47
	Methysergide	48
	Ethanol	49
	Marijuana	50
	Acetylsalicyclic acid	51
	Theophylline	52

dissociated. The GH response to arginine is not influenced by a number of conditions which inhibit the response to hypoglycemia, including corticosteroid therapy and reserpine therapy (59).

3. Hyperglycemia

In the normal subject an elevation of blood glucose results in a suppression of hGH release. This suppression of hGH is followed by a compensatory rebound similar to that seen after the administration of somatostatin, suggesting that hyperglycemia acts via somatostatin. Measurement of the rebound peak of hGH during 5 hr of observation after an oral glucose load has been used to assess hGH secretion in short children but as only 70% of normal children respond and the test takes a prolonged time, it has not become well established (60).

The suppression of hGH levels during the course of a standard 2-hr oral glucose tolerance test has become established as a means of assessing the suppression of elevated basal levels of hGH. In acromegaly the elevated basal hGH either does not suppress or increases giving rise to a "paradoxical response." The latter response has become accepted as a diagnostic test for acromegaly, but it should be interpreted with caution, as a paradoxical response may be seen in normal adolescent children (61) and several pathological conditions (see Table 3).

By general consensus suppression of hGH levels to less than 10 mU/liter is considered "normal," but it should be noted that there is no statistical basis for this figure. To save assays some workers have suggested that only one hGH assay at 60 min postglucose ingestion will suffice, but this cannot be recommended due to the variability of the hGH response.

C. Pharmacologic Agents

1. L-Dopa

The finding of elevated levels of hGH in patients receiving L-dopa therapy for Parkinson's disease led to the use of this agent in the evaluation of GH secretion (72, 73). Peak hGH responses of $\geqslant$ 10 mU/liter have been reported in 90% of normal children and peak GH responses of $\geqslant$ 15 mU/liter have been reported in 70% (36, 74). The doses used range from 125 mg for 10 kg body weight to 500 mg for 30 kg, and the peak hGH responses occur 60-90 min after administration. While the test is well suited as an outpatient procedure, it induces vomiting and nausea in 10-15% of subjects.

2. Clonidine

Clonidine is an α-adrenergic drug used therapeutically as an hypotensive agent. In 1975, clonidine was observed to stimulate GH release in normal subjects (75), presumably via central biogenic amines. The drug was subsequently tested and proposed as a hGH stimulation test in children or adolescents (76). A single

Table 3 Conditions Associated with a Paradoxical hGH Response to a Glucose Load

Condition	Reference
1. Adolescence	61
2. Acromegaly	62
3. Cerebral gigantism	63
4. Hypothalamic tumors	62
5. Laron dwarfism	64
6. Diabetes mellitus	65
7. Chronic hepatitis	66
8. Renal failure	67
9. Thyrotoxicosis	68
10. Myocardial infarction	69
11. Endometrial carcinoma	70
12. Malnutrition	71

dose of 0.15 mg/m^2 is given orally and blood samples collected for 120 min. A peak of hGH occurs from 60 to 90 min following ingestion. In all subjects there is a fall in blood pressure of 20-25 mmHg and drowsiness which persists for 1-3 hr. Although it has been claimed by Gil-Ad (76) that clonidine is a more potent stimulus to hGH release than hypoglycemia, a comparative study (77) undertaken by the Health Services hGH Committee has not substantiated this claim and has also demonstrated a 25% failure rate, similar to that seen with other stimuli to hGH release. The Committee (77) concluded that clonidine may be safer than insulin-induced hypoglycemia but is no more effective. In one study a suppressed hGH response to clonidine was noted in subjects with endogenous depression (78).

3. Diazepam

Diazepam has been shown to stimulate hGH secretion (79) and has been advocated as a useful test of hGH secretory capacity by Kannan (80). Diazepam may be given either orally (0.2 mg/kg body weight) or intramuscularly (10 mg) and results in a peak of hGH at 40 min after oral or 20 minutes after intramuscular administration. The hGH responses have been considered to be similar to those observed with insulin-induced hypoglycemia. The mode of action of diazepam in influencing hGH release is not known but is postulated to be via potentiation of the γ-aminobutyric acid (GABA)-mediated neural function and changing turnover rates of dopamine, noradrenaline, and serotonin (81).

4. Metoclopramide

Metoclopramide, which is well established as a test of prolactin release, does not release GH in adult males but has been noted to stimulate the release of GH in hypogonadal males (82). On the basis of this latter observation Cohen et al. (83) have suggested its use as a test of hGH reserve in prepubertal or adolescent males. Given as an intravenous bolus of 10 mg it results in a significant release of hGH within 1 hr in 70% of normal subjects with no untoward side effects.

5. Propranolol

Propranolol, a β-adrenergic blocker, has been noted to augment the hGH responses to stimuli and thus to reduce the chance of false negative responses (74). Propranolol in a dose of 0.75 mg/kg body weight, but not exceeding 40 mg, is given 2 hr prior to L-dopa or glucagon. Propranolol may also be given as an intravenous infusion together with epinephrine (84) or together with epinephrine, while a sequential arginine infusion/insulin hypoglycemia test is undertaken (85). In a survey of 191 children studied with sleep, L-dopa or L-dopa/propranolol, Fass et al. (74) reported a 31.3% false hGH deficiency diagnosis rate with sleep, a 20.5% false rate with L-dopa alone, but only 5.2% for combined L-dopa/propranolol. Hypoglycemia may occur with propranolol-potentiated tests, and Pelsor et al. (86) have reported hypoglycemia as a frequent side effect occurring in 6 of 49 children. Pelsor et al. have noted that the hypoglycemia may occur in children with normal as well as abnormal hGH responses to either L-dopa/propranolol or glucagon/propranolol tests.

D. Hormonal

1. Thyrotropin-Releasing Hormone

Thyrotropin releasing hormone (TRH) was the first neurohormone to be isolated from hypothalamic tissue and shown to be effective in humans. Following the initial studies of thyroid stimulating hormone (TSH) release it was shown that TRH is a powerful releaser of prolactin and in some conditions hGH (87). With the availability of the synthetic tripeptide amide in pure form, TRH testing has become an important diagnostic procedure for the evaluation of patients with disorders of hGH secretion (88).

Although TRH does not stimulate the release of hGH in the normal subject, it does result in a significant hGH release in a number of conditions (Table 4), including acromegaly and several nonspecific disorders. The hGH response to TRH in acromegaly has been used for diagnostic purposes (87) and to indicate

Table 4 Paradoxical GH Responses to TRH

Condition	Reference
1. Acromegaly	87
2. Endogenous depression	95
3. Anorexia nervosa	96
4. Renal failure	97
5. Hepatic cirrhosis	98
6. Primary hypothyroidism	99
7. Cancer	100
8. Diabetic retinopathy	101

likely responses to bromocriptine (89) or the effectiveness of surgery (90, 91). While the mode of action of TRH in inducing this paradoxical release of hGH is obscure, it has been suggested that it is related to a disturbance of hypothalamic control as a similar paradoxical response to glucose may be seen in these conditions.

Further evidence of disturbed neuroendocrine control of hGH is provided by the observations that in the normal subject TRH inhibits the normal sleep-induced rise in hGH (92) and in normal rats it inhibits the pentobarbital-stimulated growth hormone release (93). Also, in experimental animals with disruption of the normal hypothalamic-pituitary pathways by severance of the stalk or transplantation of the pituitary to the renal capsule (94), TRH induces a rise in GH.

2. Androgens

The hGH secretion in adolescence is augmented (11) and the hGH response to stimuli in adolescent boys is greater than that in prepubertal boys or boys with delayed puberty (14). In a study of the hGH response to insulin-induced hypoglycemia, Eastman et al. (14) reported a mean peak hGH level of 2.64 mU/liter in eight prepubertal boys and a mean peak hGH level of 19.2 mU/liter in the same boys following either spontaneous puberty or hormone-induced puberty. Martin et al. (102) studied the hGH responses to insulin-induced hypoglycemia and arginine infusion in 22 young males (aged 8-17 years) with short stature and absent or delayed sexual development. In 21 of the 22 there was a subnormal hGH response to stimulation, but in each case this was corrected following androgen administration using either testosterone propionate intramuscularly or methyl testosterone orally for 4-5 days. Sustained improvement of the hGH response to stimulation was noted in 3 boys when repetitive studies were performed 8-12 months later following spontaneous sexual development (102).

3. Estrogens

Estrogen administration augments basal hGH levels in children (103) and adults (104). In women taking oral contraceptives (OC) the basal hGH and hGH production rate are elevated (105). Estrogens can also potentiate the hGH response to stimuli and the administration of diethylstilbestrol results in a positive response to arginine in men, who are usually unresponsive to this stimulus (54). In women on OC the responses to arginine (106) and to apomorphine (107) are enhanced.

Estrogens reduce somatomedin production (104) and there is in vitro evidence to support the concept that enhanced hGH secretion induced by estrogens is mediated by the negative feedback of lowered somatomedin levels on pituitary hGH release (108).

4. Glucagon

The use of glucagon to stimulate hGH release was first described by Mitchell et al. in 1970 (109) and refined by Vanderschueren-Lodeweyckx et al. in 1974 (110). Glucagon is given intramuscularly or subcutaneously as a single 1-mg dose and blood samples taken serially to 210 min. The hGH peak occurs at 120-180 min and is thought to be a response to the drop in blood glucose which follows the initial rise subsequent to the glucagon injection. The test has been reported to have only a 50% response in normal subjects, but the response may be substantially improved by pretreatment with propranolol (74).

E. Miscellaneous Stimuli

GH release has been reported in normal subjects following the administration of vasopressin (111), tetracosactrin (112), prostaglandin (113), pyrogens (114), and metyrapone (115). None of these procedures has become established as a diagnostic test.

III. SOMATOMEDINS

The somatomedins are a family of GH-dependent peptide growth factors of 7000-7500 daltons. At present, four such peptides have been purified from human plasma and named somatomedin-A (Sm-A), somatomedin-C (Sm-C), insulin-like growth factor-1 (IGF-1), and insulin-like growth factor-2 (IGF-2). The insulin-like growth factors resemble proinsulin and a close homology has been demonstrated between Sm-C and IGF-1. The somatomedins are transported bound to a carrier protein which itself is GH responsive. The carrier proteins

Table 5 Somatomedin Ranges

Assay	Growth hormone deficiency (U/ml)	Normal (U/ml)	Growth hormone excess (U/ml)
Bioassay	0.2-0.6	0.7-1.3	1.2-4.4
RRA	0.2-0.8	0.6-1.4	1.4-4.4
CPB assay	0.4-0.6	0.7-1.2	1.2-1.9
RIA	0-0.2	0.7-1.3	3.1-5.4

Source: Adapted from Refs. 117, 118.

appear to have two forms, of 120,000 and 70,000 daltons, respectively. The binding of Sm to carrier proteins may diminish the biological activity, and some workers consider that Sm should be dissociated from the carrier protein prior to assay, as assay of unextracted serum measures only 30-40% of Sm-C content. Clemmons et al. (116) refer to the unbound Sm-C as "available Sm" and consider that it adequately reflects the GH secretory status.

Somatomedins may be assayed by bioassay, radioreceptor assay, competitive protein binding assay, or radioimmunoassay. As there is no standard preparation available, the assays are compared with a normal young adult male pool which is allocated a potency of 1.0 U/ml. A summary of assay results in various conditions in the adult is shown in Table 5.

Sm-C levels are low in the newborn and rise during infancy to reach adult levels by age 9-11 years (119, 120). Peak levels of 1.5-2.5 U/ml are achieved during puberty, following which there is a tapering off in successive decades. During adulthood there is a log-normal distribution of Sm-C with 95% confidence limits of 0.4-2.0 U/ml (121). While the mean Sm-C for age 20-30 years is 1.2 U/ml, the level drops to 0.70 U/ml for subjects 50 and older. Rudman et al. (15) have reported a progressive decline of Sm-C after age 30 with some 50% of subjects 60 years and older having Sm-C levels of < 0.4 U/ml. At all age levels females have Sm-C some 10-20% greater than males (119). No acute fluctuations have been noted with feeding or exercise, and most observers have not detected a diurnal pattern in Sm-C.

During pregnancy there is an elevation of Sm-C (RIA) from about week 18 to a peak of 3-4 U/ml at term and a sudden drop postpartum similar to the pattern seen for hPL, which has been suggested as an Sm inducer in pregnancy (122). The Sm levels are lowered in starvation and poorly controlled diabetes mellitus due to both reduced production and the presence of an inhibitor (123). In renal failure there may be elevated Sm levels by RIA and reduced levels by bioassay due to the presence of circulating inhibitors which are removed by hemodialysis (124).

In GH-deficient states the Sm by both bioassay and RIA is low, but the range frequently overlaps that of the normal. Using SM (RIA), both Furlanetto et al. (120) and Copeland et al. (125) have claimed to be able to distinguish hypopituitary children from normals using a single basal sample. However, in a comparative study of 41 children undergoing clinical evaluation of short stature, Reiter and Lovinger (126) found discordant Sm-C and GH data in 27% of the children and expressed some doubts about the discriminant use of Sm-C RIA as a single screening test for GH deficiency. In order to overcome these constraints of low basal levels and discordant results, a number of workers have studied the Sm-C response to hGH administration. Rosenfeld et al. (127), however, found a lack of correlation between the Sm-C (RIA) response to hGH and growth rate in children with hypopituitary dwarfism. This poor correlation may be explained by a further study from the same group (128), which demonstrated a lack of correlation between Sm measured by RRA or RIA in response to hGH treatment. They suggested that the variability in the RRA/RIA ratio is due to the fact that the Sm-C (RIA) measures only one of a number of GH-dependent Sm peptides. Using the Sm response to hGH, Rudman et al. (129) have identified a group of children with short stature, a normal hGH response to stimuli, but a low Sm-C which responds well to GH administration. They have suggested that these children are a normal variant of the short-stature syndrome, which responds well to GH therapy but can only be detected by Sm-C assays.

Somatomedin assays may assist in the classification of a number of short-stature syndromes (Table 6), including growth hormone deficiency, normal variant short stature (129), Laron dwarfism (130), the Pigmy (131), and craniopharyngioma (132). In the Laron dwarf there is a familial inability to produce Sm, with resultant elevated levels of GH. In the African Pigmy there is failure to produce IGF-1. In some children following surgical correction of a craniopharyngioma there are very low levels of hGH but normal Sm and spontaneous growth without GH therapy.

Patients with acromegaly have been found by bioassays and some receptor assays to have an increase of Sm over normals. However, the results with protein binding assays and with an RIA for IGF-2 have not been elevated consistently. Using a RIA for Sm-C, Clemmons et al. (116) have reported a clear distinction between acromegaly (2.6 to 21.7 U/ml) and normals (0.3 to 1.4 U/ml) with a significant correlation between Sm-C levels and measures of clinical activity, such as heel pad thickness and glucose tolerance. Zapf et al. (133) and Bala and Bhaumick (134) have also reported that IGF-1 and basic somatomedin levels as measured by specific RIA are elevated in acromegaly. However, a cautious note has been sounded by Daughaday (135) regarding the diagnostic use of

Table 6 Sm-C Levels in Short Stature[a]

Group (reference)	GH basal	Stimulated	SM		Growth rate on GH treatment
			Basal	GH treatment	
GH deficient	↓	↓	↓	↑	↑
NVSS (129)	N	↑	↓	↑	↑
Laron (130)	↑		↓	↓	↓
Pigmy (131)	N	↑	↓	↓	
Craniopharyngioma (132)	↓	↓	N	N	b

[a]N: normal; ↑, increased; ↓, decreased.
[b]Spontaneous.

Table 7 Conditions That May Affect the hGH Responses to Stimulatory Tests

Condition	Reference
1. Decreased response	
Old age	15
Delayed puberty	102
Obesity	20
Hypothyroidism	39
Thyrotoxicosis	137
Endogenous depression	138
Cushing's syndrome	139
Stress	140
Maternal deprivation syndrome	141
2. Increased response	
Diabetes (poorly controlled)	142
Fasting	143
Malnutrition	144
Anorexia nervosa	145
Turner's syndrome	146
Endometrial cancer	147
Renal failure	148
Hepatic cirrhosis	149

Sm-C RIA in acromegaly. This caution has been supported by Stonesifer et al. (136), who found, in a study of 15 acromegalic patients, 3 months to 15 years after the onset of therapy, that the clinical responses were poorly correlated with Sm-C RIA and that the correlation between hGH and Sm-C was also poor. Stonesifer et al. concluded that Sm-C RIA offers no advantage over hGH assays in following patients treated for acromegaly. It would appear that further studies are required to define the role of Sm assays in the diagnosis and management of acromegaly.

IV. INTERPRETATION OF STIMULATION TESTS

The interpretation of hGH stimulation tests requires some knowledge of the adequacy of the test performed, the presence of conditions which may influence the hGH responses to stimuli, and the criteria to be applied in assessing the responses. As mentioned above, exercise should be undertaken to exhaustion, hypoglycemia of 2.2 mmol should be achieved and sleep should be monitored

Diagnostic Summary 1 Growth Hormone-Deficient Short Stature

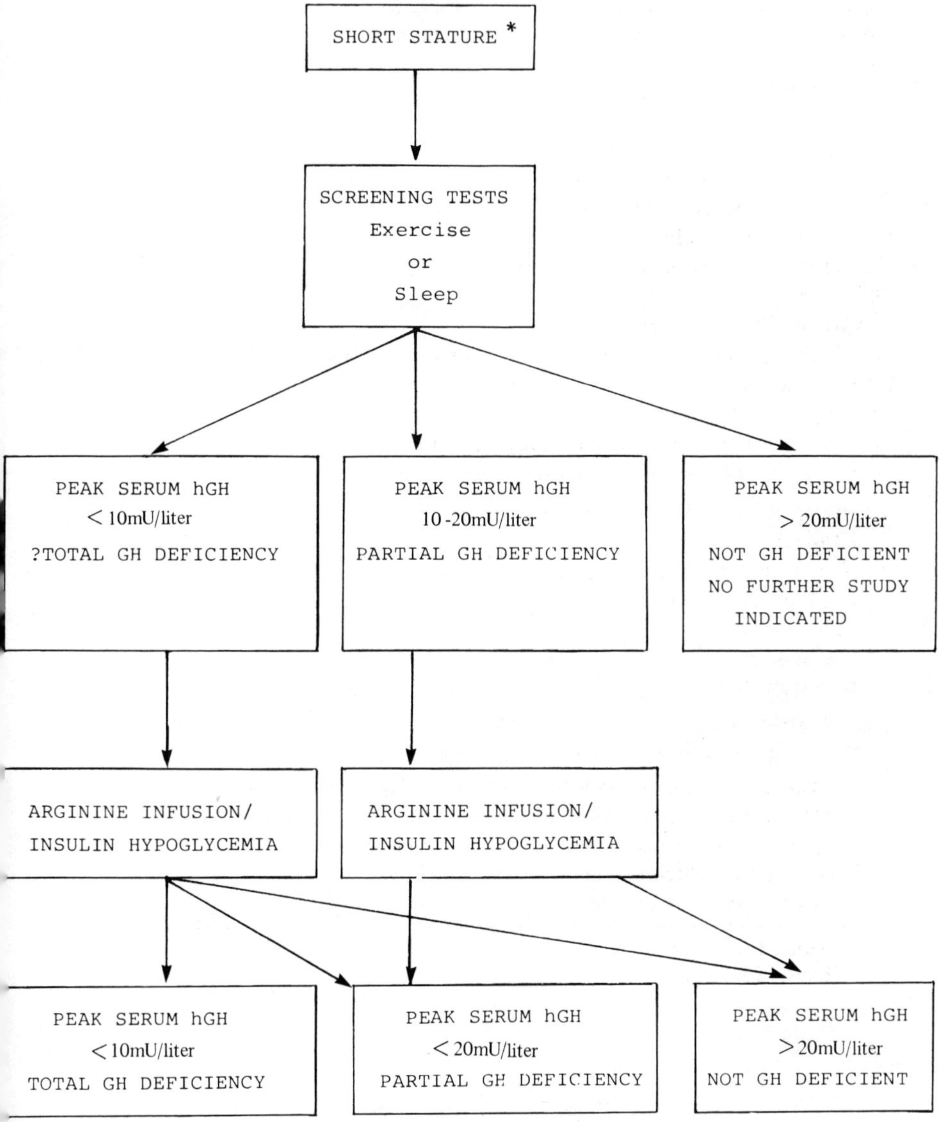

Diagnostic Summary 2a Acromegaly-Clinical Features

Overgrowth of soft tissues (face,[a] hands, heel pads)
Overgrowth of bone (prognathism, frontal sinuses)
Gigantism if bone development immature
Arthritis
Acroparesthesia and carpal tunnel syndrome
Enlarged glands (thyroid, lachrymal, salivary, and sweat), tongue, heart (cardiomyopathy), and viscera
Deep voice, barrel chest
Galactorrhea, amenorrhea, impotence
Skin tags, neck and axillae
Hirsutism, pigmentation
Impaired carbohydrate tolerance and diabetes mellitus
Hypertension
Hyperphosphatemia
Rare association with multiple endocrine adenoma (type 1) syndrome and other neoplasms

Complications of pituitary tumor growth
- Headaches
- Visual field impairment (often bitemporal)
- Pituitary apoplexy
- Epilepsy
- Papilledema
- Hypopituitarism

Radiological changes[b]
- Enlarged pituitary fossa, sinuses, and mandible
- Increased soft tissues and joint spaces (cartilage overgrowth)
- "Arrowheading" of terminal phalanges, muscle insertions prominent
- Thickening of cortical bone, porosis of cancellous bone
- Increased skin thickness and heel pad thickness
- CT scan important to assess tumor size

[a]See Chapter 15.
[b]See Chapter 16.

Diagnostic Summary 2b Growth Hormone Studies in Acromegaly

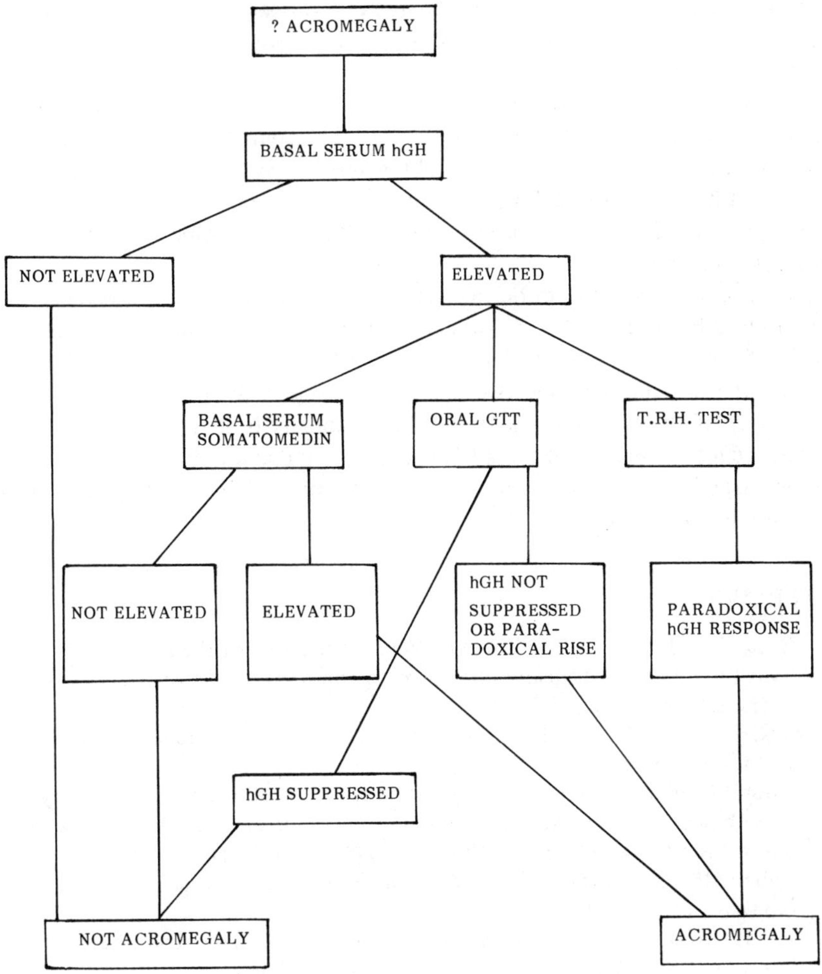

by EEG. It would appear that many of the negative responses are due to inadequately performed tests.

A number of conditions may affect the hGH responses to stimuli and these are listed in Table 7. It is important to note that the criteria applied to the assessment of hGH stimulation tests are largely empirical and based on accumulated evidence of subsequent responses to therapy. Most workers would accept the failure to achieve a peak level of 10 mU/liter as evidence of growth hormone deficiency. A further category of partial growth hormone deficiency has been accepted by consensus, although the cutoff for this group varies from 14 to 20 mU/liter in different centers. It should be noted that these are consensus figures that have no statistical basis and that the clinician must be cautious in their application due to the significant interlaboratory bias, which further complicates the interpretation.

The "normal" responses of normal subjects to hGH stimulation tests range from 50 to 90%, with most of the tests recording a positive response in approximately 75% of normal subjects if a peak of 15 mU/liter is to be achieved. This means that 1 in 4 normal subjects will have "partial growth hormone deficiency" on the basis of one test. For this reason it is customary to perform a series of tests to reduce the probability of a false interpretation and three tests (e.g., exercise, arginine/insulin infusion) will reduce the probability of a false diagnosis from 1 in 4 to 1 in 64.

REFERENCES

1. Evans HM, Long JA. The effect of the anterior lobe of the hypophysis administered intraperitoneally upon growth and maturity and oestrus cycles of the rat. Anat Rec 1921; 21:62-63.
2. Li CH, Evans HM. The isolation of pituitary growth hormone. Science 1944; 99:183-184.
3. Knobil E, Wolf RC, Greep RO, Wilhelmi AE. Effect of primate pituitary growth hormone preparation on nitrogen metabolism in the hypophysectomised rhesus monkey. Endocrinology 1975; 60:166-168.
4. Raben MS. Preparation of growth hormone from pituitaries of man and monkey. Science 1957; 125:883.
5. Li CH, Dixon JS. Human growth hormone. The primary structure of the hormone. Arch Biochem Biophys 1971; 46:233-236.
6. Niall HD, Hogan ML, Tregear GW, Segre GV, Hwang P, Friesen H. The chemistry of growth hormone and lactogenic hormones. Recent Prog Horm Res 1973; 29:387-416.
7. Olson KC, Fenno J, Lin N, Harkins RN, Snider C, Kohr WH, Ross MJ, Fodge D, Prender G, and Stebbing N. Purified human growth hormone from *E. coli* is biologically active. Nature 1981; 293:408–411.

8. Lewis, UJ, Singh RNP, Tutwiler GF, Sigel MB, Vanderlaan EF, Vanderlaan WP. Human growth hormone: a complex of proteins. Recent Prog Horm Res 1980; 36:477-504.
9. Yalow RS. Heterogeneity of human growth hormone. In *Advances in Human Growth Hormone Research,* Raiti S (ed). DHEW Publ (NIH) 74-612, 1974, p 483.
10. Alford FP, Baker HWG, Burger HG. The secretion rate of human growth hormone. 1. Daily secretion rates, effect of posture and sleep. J Clin Endocrinol Metab 1973; 37:515-520.
11. Finkelstein JW, Roffwarg WHP, Boyar RM, Kream J, Hellman J. Age-related change in the twenty-four-hour spontaneous secretion of growth hormone. J Clin Endocrinol Metab 1972; 35:665-670.
12. Takahashi Y, Kipnis D, Daughaday WH. Growth hormone secretion during sleep. J Clin Invest 1968; 47:2079-2090.
13. Plotnick LP, Lee PA, Migeon CJ, Kowarski, A. Comparison of physiological tests of growth hormone function in children with short stature. J Clin Endocrinol Metab 1979; 48:811.
14. Eastman CJ, Lazarus, L, Stuart MC, Casey, JH. The effect of puberty on growth hormone secretion in boys with short stature and delayed adolescence. Aust NZ J Med 1971; 2:154-159.
15. Rudman D, Kutnen MH, Rogers CM, Lubin MF, Fleming GA, Bain RP. Impaired growth hormone secretion in the adult population. J Clin Invest 1981; 67:1361-1369.
16. Bazzare TL, Johanson AJ, Huseman CA, Varma MM, Blizzard RM. Human growth hormone changes with age. In *Growth Hormone and Related Peptides,* Pecile A, Muller E (eds), Proc 3rd Int Symp, Milan, Int Congr Ser 381. Excerpta Medica, Amsterdam, 1976, pp 261-270.
17. Carlson HE, Gillin JC, Gorden P, Snyder F. Absence of sleep-related growth hormone peaks in aged normal subjects and in acromegaly. J Clin Endocrinol Metab 1972; 34:1102-1105.
18. Verzar F, Spichten H. The role of the pituitary in the ageing of collagen. Gerontologia (Basel) 1966; 12:48-56.
19. Gershberg H. Growth hormone content and metabolic actions of human pituitary glands. Endocrinology 1957; 61:160-165.
20. Glass AR, Burman KD, Dakins WT, Boehm TM. Endocrine function in human obesity. Metabolism 1981; 30:89.
21. Waters MJ, Friesen HG. Purification and partial characterisation of a non-primate growth hormone receptor. J Biol Chem 1979; 254:6815.
22. Ellis S, Vodian MA, Grindeland RE. Studies on the bioassayable growth hormone-like activity of plasma. Recent Prog Horm Res 1978; 34:213-234.
23. Greenwood FC, Hunter WM, Glover JG. The preparation of I^{131} labelled human growth hormone of high specific activity. Biochem J 1963; 89:114.

24. Santis MR, Lawrie EG, Hampers CL. Diffusion of growth hormone into thoracic duct lymph in man. J Clin Endocrinol Metab 1970; 31:632-639.
25. Linfoot JA, Garcia JF, Wei W. Human growth hormone levels in cerebrospinal fluid. J Clin Endocrinol Metab 1970; 31:230-232.
26. Bala RM, Ferguson KA, Beck JC. Growth hormone like activity in plasma and urine. In *Growth and Growth Hormone,* Pecile A, Muller E (eds), Int Congr Ser 244, Excerpta Medica, Amsterdam, 1972, pp 483–498.
27. Jordon RM, Kendall JW, Seaich JL, Allen JP, Paulson CA, Kerber CW, and Vanderlaan, WP. Cerebrospinal fluid hormone concentration in the evaluation of pituitary tumors. Ann Intern Med 1976; 85:49–55.
28. Herington AC, Jacobs LS, Daughaday WH. Radioreceptor and radioimmunoassay quantitation of human growth hormone in acromegalic serum: overestimation by immunoassay and systematic differences. J Clin Endocrinol Metab 1974; 39:257-262.
29. Underwood LE, Azumi K, Voina SJ, Van Wyk JJ. Growth hormone levels during sleep in normal and growth hormone deficient children. Pediatrics 1971; 48:946.
30. Mace JW, Gotlin RW, Beck P. Sleep related human growth hormone release: a test of physiologic growth hormone secretion in children. J Clin Endocrinol Metab 1972; 34:339.
31. Eastman CJ, Lazarus L. Growth hormone release during sleep in growth retarded children. ArchD is Child 1973; 48:502.
32. Othmer E, Levine WR, Malarky WB, Corvalan J, Haydem-Otto MP, Fishman PM, and Daughaday WH. Body build and sleep-related growth hormone secretion. Horm Res 1974; 5:156–166.
33. Sutton JR, Young JD, Lazarus L, Hickie JB, Maksvytis J. The hormonal response to physical exercise. Aust Ann Med 1969; 18:84-90.
34. Lacey KA, Hewison A, Parkin JM. Exercise as a screening test for growth hormone deficiency in children. Arch Dis Child 1973; 48:508.
35. Buckler JMH. Plasma growth hormone response to exercise as a diagnostic aid. Arch Dis Child 1973; 48:565.
36. Fraser SD. A review of growth hormone stimulation tests in children. Pediatrics 1974; 53:929-937.
37. Judd SJ, Lazarus L. A combined test of anterior pituitary response. Aust NZ J Med 1976; 6:30-36.
38. Gruen PH, Sachar EJ, Altman H, Sassin J. Growth hormone response to hypoglycaemia in depressed women. Arch Gen Psychiatry 1975; 32:31-33.
39. Iwatsuko H, Kiyokiko O, Yoshiaki O, Fukucki M, Miyai K, Hiroshi A, Kumakara Y. Human growth hormone secretion in primary hypothyroidism before and after treatment. J Clin Endocrinol Metab 1967; 27:1751-1754.
40. Blackard WG, Heidingsfelder SA. Adrenergic control mechanism for growth hormone secretion. J Clin Invest 1968; 47:1407-1411.
41. Steiner J, Cassar J, Mashiter K, Dawes I, Russel M, Fraser T, Breckenridge A. Effects of methyldopa on prolactin and growth hormone. Br Med J 1976; 1:1186-1188.

42. Maeda K, Kato Y, Chihara K, Ohgo S, Iwasaki Y, Abe H, Imura H. Suppression by thyrotropin-releasing hormone (TRH) of growth hormone release induced by arginine and insulin hypoglycaemia in man. J Clin Endocrinol Metab 1976; 43:453-456.
43. Frantz AG, Rabkin MT. Human growth hormone: clinical measurement, response to hypoglycaemia and suppression by corticosteroids. N Engl J Med 1964; 271:1375-1381.
44. Cavagnini F, Peracchi M. Effect of reserpine on growth hormone response to insulin hypoglycaemia and to arginine infusion in normal subjects and hypothyroid patients. J Clin Endocrinol Metab 1971; 51:651-655.
45. Sherman L, Kim J, Benjamin F, Kolodny HE. Effect of chlorpromazine on serum growth hormone concentration in man. N Engl J Med 1971; 284: 72-75.
46. Smythe GA, Compton PJ, Lazarus L. Serotoninergic control of human growth hormone secretion: the actions of L-dopa and 2-bromo-α-ergocryptine. In *Growth Hormone and Related Peptides,* Pecile A, Muller E (eds), Proc 3rd Int Symp, Milan, Int Congr Ser 381. Excerpta Medica, Amsterdam, 1976, pp 222-235.
47. Smythe GA, Lazarus L. Suppression of human growth hormone secretion by melatonin and cyproheptadine. J Clin Invest 1974; 54:116-121.
48. Bivens CH, Lebovitz HE, Feldman JM. Inhibition of hypoglycaemia induced growth hormone secretion by the serotonin antagonists cyproheptadine and methysergide. N Engl J Med 1973; 289:236-240.
49. Priem HA, Shanly BC, Malan C. Effect of alcohol administration on plasma growth hormone response to insulin-induced hypoglycaemia. Metabolism 1976; 397:403-407.
50. Berowitz NL, Jones RT, Lerner CB. Depression of growth hormone and cortisol responses to insulin induced hypoglycaemia after prolonged oral delta-9-tetrahydrocannabinol administration in man. J Clin Endocrinol Metab 1976; 42:938-941.
51. Cavagnini F, di Landro A, Invitti C, Raggi U, Alessandrini P, Pinto M, Girotti G, and Vigo P. Effects of acetylsalicylic acid and indomethacin on growth hormone secretion in man. Metabolism 1977; 26:193–200.
52. Peracchi M, Cavagnini F, Pontiroli AE, Raggiu, Malinuerni A, and Pinto M. Effect of aminophylline on growth hormone secretion in man. Acta Endocrinol (Copenh) 1974; 76:488–494.
53. Knopf RN, Conn JW, Fajans SS, Floyd JC, Guntsche EM, and Rull JA. Plasma GH response to intravenous administration of amino acids. J Clin Endocrinol Metab 1965; 25:1140–1144.
54. Jackson D, Grant DB, Clayton BE. A simple oral test of growth-hormone secretion in children. Lancet 1968; 2:373-375.
55. Raiti S, Davis WT, Blizzard RM. A comparison of the effects of insulin hypoglycaemia and arginine infusion on release of human growth hormone. Lancet 1967; 2:1182.

56. Frohman LA, Aceti T. Studies of growth hormone secretion in children: normal, hypopituitary and constitutionally delayed. J Clin Endocrinol Metab 1967; 27:1409.
57. Penny R, Blizzard RM, Davis WT. Sequential arginine and insulin tolerance tests on the same day. J Clin Endocrinol Metab 1969; 29:149.
58. Merimee TJ, Rabinowitz D, Fineberg SE. Arginine initiated release of human growth hormone. Factors modifying the response in normal men. N Engl J Med 1969; 280:1434-1438.
59. Cavagnini F, Peracchi M. Effect of reserpine on growth hormone response to insulin hypoglycaemia and to arginine infusion in normal subjects and hyperthyroid patients. J Endocrinol 1971; 51:651-656.
60. Okeda Y, Hikita T, Ishitobi K, Wada M, Santo Y, Harada Y. Human growth hormone secretion after exercise and oral glucose administration in patients with short stature. J Clin Endocrinol Metab 1972; 34:1055.
61. Pieters G, Smals A, Kloppenberg P. Defective suppression of growth hormone after oral glucose loading in adolescence. J Clin Endocrinol Metab 1980; 51:265.
62. Beck P, Parker ML, Daughaday WH. Paradoxical hypersecretion of growth hormone in response to glucose. J Clin Endocrinol Metab 1966; 26:463-469.
63. Hook EB, Reynolds JW. Cerebral gigantism: endocrinological and clinical observations of six patients, including a congenital giant, concordant monozygotic twins and a child who achieved gigantic size. J Pediatr 1967; 70: 900-914.
64. Najjar SS, Khachadurian AK, Ilbawi MN, Blizzard RM. Dwarfism with elevated levels of plasma growth hormone. N Engl J Med 1971; 284:809-812.
65. Yde H. Abnormal growth hormone response to ingestion of glucose in juvenile diabetics. Acta Endocrinol (Copenh) 1970; 64:339-345.
66. Becker MD, Cook GC, Wright AD. Paradoxical elevation of growth hormone in active chronic hepatitis. Lancet 1969; 2:1035-1039.
67. Kanis JA, Ledingham JG, Oliver DO, Walton RJ. Effect of bromocriptine on plasma growth hormone and glucose tolerance in chronic renal failure. Br Med J 1976; 1:879-883.
68. Cavagnini F, Peracchi M, Penerai AE, Pinto M. Alterazioni della secrezione di ormone somatotropo ed insulina. Quad Diagn Sclavo 1975; 11:372-381.
69. Lebovitz HE, Shultz KT, Matthews ME, Scheele R. Acute metabolic responses to myocardial infarction. Changes in glucose utilisation and secretion of insulin and growth hormone. Circulation 1969; 39:171-181.
70. Benjamin F, Casper D, Sherman L, Kolodny H. Growth hormone secretion in patients with endometrial carcinoma. N Engl J Med 1969; 281:1448-1452.
71. Pimstone B, Barbezat G, Hansen JD. Growth hormone and protein-calorie malnutrition: impaired suppression during induced hyperglycaemia. Lancet 1967; 2:1333-1334.

72. Boyd AE, Lebovitz HE, Pfeiffer JB. Stimulation of human growth hormone secretion by L-Dopa. N Engl J Med 1970; 283:1425.
73. Weldon VV, Gupta SK, Haymond MW, Pagliara AS, Jacobs LS, Daughaday WH. The use of L-dopa in the diagnosis of hyposomatotropism in children. J Clin Endocrinol Metab 1973; 36:42.
74. Fass B, Lippe BM, Kaplan SA. Relative usefulness of three growth hormone stimulation screening tests. Am J Dis Child 1979; 133:931-933.
75. Lal S, Tobis G, Martin JB, Brown GM, Guyda H. Effect of clonidine on growth hormone, prolactin, luteinising hormone, follicle stimulating hormone and thyroid stimulating hormone in the serum of normal men. J Clin Endocrinol Metab 1975; 41:827-832.
76. Gil-Ad I, Toffer E, Laron Z. Oral clonidine as a growth hormone stimulation test. Lancet 1979; 2:278-280.
77. Health Services Human Growth Hormone Committee. Comparison of intravenous insulin and oral clonidine. Arch Dis in Child 1981; 56:852-854.
78. Matussek M. Neuroendokrinalogische Untersuchungen bei depressiven Syndromen. Nervenarzt 1978; 49:569-575.
79. Taylor KM, Laverty R. The effect of chlordiazepoxide, diazepam and mitrazepam on catecholamine metabolism in regions of rat brain. Eur J Pharmacol 1969; 8:296-302.
80. Kannan V. Diazepam test of growth hormone secretion. Horm Metab Res 1981; 13:390-393.
81. Costa EA, Guidotti C, Mao C, Suria A. New concepts on the mechanism of action of benzodiazepines. Life Sci 1975; 17:167-170.
82. Cohen HN, Hay ID, Beastall GH, Thomson JH. Metoclopramide induced growth hormone release in hypogonadal males. Clin Endocrinol 1979; 11: 95-97.
83. Cohen HN, Hay ID, Thomson JA, Logue F, Ratcliffe WA, Beastall GH. Metoclopramide stimulation: a test of growth hormone reserve in adolescent males. Clin Endocrinol 1979; 11:89-93.
84. Massara F, Strunia E. Increase in plasma growth hormone concentration in man after infusions of adrenaline-propranolol. J Endocrinol 1970; 47: 95.
85. Lee PA, Thompson RG, Blizzard RM. Relationship of the adrenergic nervous system and growth hormone release in normal adults and children with various growth disorders. Metabolism 1974; 23:595–601.
86. Pelsor DA, Winter RJ, Green OC. Propranolol-induced hypoglycemia during growth hormone testing. J Pediatr 1981; 99(1):157-158.
87. Saito S, Abe K, Yoshida H, Kaneko T, Nakamura E, Shiruzu N, Yamainara N. Effects of synthetic thyrotrophin releasing hormone on plasma thyrotrophin growth hormone and insulin levels in man. Endocrinol Jpn 1971; 17:101-108.

88. Jackson IMD. Thyrotrophin-releasing hormone. N Engl J Med 1982; 306: 145-155.
89. Liuzzi A, Chiodini PG, Botalla L, Silvestrini F, Muller EE. Growth hormone-releasing activity of TRH and GH-lowering effect of dopaminergic drugs in acromegaly: homogeneity of the two responses. J Clin Endocrinol Metab 1974; 39:871-876.
90. Samaan SA, Leavens ME, Jesse RH. Serum GH and PRL response to TRH in patients with acromegaly before and after surgery. J Clin Endocrinol Metab 1974; 38:957-963.
91. Faglia G, Paracchi A, Ferrari C, Beck Pecoz P. Evaluation of the results of trans-sphenoidal surgery in acromegaly by assessment of the growth hormone response to thyrotrophin releasing hormone. Clin Endocrinol 1978; 8:373-380.
92. Chihara K, Kato Y, Maeda K, Abe H, Furomoto M, Imura H. Effects ot thyrotrophin-releasing hormone on sleep and sleep-related growth hormone release in normal subjects. J Clin Endocrinol Metab 1977; 44:1094-1100.
93. Brown M, Vale W. Growth hormone release in the rat: effects of somatostatin and thyrotrophin-releasing factor. Endocrinology 1975; 97:1151-1156.
94. Muller EE, Salern F, Coochi D, Locatelli V, Panerai AE. Interactions between the thyrotrophin-releasing hormone induced growth hormone rise and dopaminergic drugs: studies in pathologic conditions of the animal and man. Clin Endocrinol 1979; 11:645-656.
95. Maeda K, Kato Y, Ohgo S, Chihara K, Yoshimoto Y, Yamaguchi N, Kuromara S, Imura H. Growth hormone and prolactin release after injection of thyrotrophin-releasing hormone in patients with depression. J Clin Endocrinol Metab 1975; 40:501-505.
96. Maeda K, Kato Y, Yamaguchi N, Chihara K, Ohgo S, Iwasaki Y, Yoshimoto Y, Moridera K, Kuromaru S, and Imura H. Growth hormone release following thyrotrophin-releasing hormone injection into patients with anorexia nervosa. Acta Endocrinol (Copenh) 1976; 81:1–8.
97. Gonzales-Barcena D, Kastin AJ, Schalch DS, Torres-Zamora M, Perez-Pasten E, Kato A, Schally AV. Response to thyrotrophin releasing hormone in patients with renal failure and after infusion in normal men. J Clin Endocrinol Metab 1973; 36:117-120.
98. Panerai AE, Salerno F, Marneschi M, Cocchi D, Muller EE. Growth hormone and prolactin responses to thyrotrophin releasing hormone in patients with severe liver disease. J Clin Endocrinol Metab 1977; 45:134-140.
99. Hamada N, Uoi K, Nishizawa Y, Okamoto T, Hasegawa K, Morii H, Wada M. Increase of serum GH concentration following TRH injection in patients with primary hypothyroidism. Endocrinol Jpn 1976; 23:5-10.
100. Kaneijo K, Saito A, Yachi A, Wada T. Growth hormone responses to thyrotrophin-releasing hormone in cancer patients. Endocrinol Jpn 1980; 27:451-455.

101. Dasmahapatra A, Urdaniva E, Cohen MP. Growth hormone response to thyrotrophin-releasing hormone in diabetics. J Clin Endocrinol Metab 1981; 52:859.
102. Martin LG, Grossman MS, Commer TB, Levitsky LL, Clark JW, Camilla FD. Effect of androgen on growth hormone secretion and growth in boys with short stature. Acta Endocrinol (Copenh) 1979; 91:201-212.
103. Bacon GE, Lowrey GH, Knoller M. Comparison of diethylstilboestrol as a means of provoking growth hormone secretion. J Pediatr 1969; 75:385-392.
104. Wiedeman E, Schwartz E, Frantz AG. Acute and chronic estrogen effects upon serum somatomedin activity, growth hormone and prolactin in man. J. Clin Endocrinol Metab 1976; 42:942-952.
105. Thompson RG, Rodriguez A, Kowarski A, Blizzard RM. Growth hormone: metabolic clearance rates, integrated concentration and production rates in normal adults and the effect of prednisone. J Clin Invest 1972; 51:3193-3199.
106. Yen SSC, Vala P. Effects of contraceptive steroids on carbohydrate metabolism. J Clin Endocrinol Metab 1968; 28:1564-1570.
107. Ettigi P, Lal S, Martin JB, Friesen HG. Effect of sex, oral contraceptives and glucose loading on apomorphine-induced growth hormone secretion. J Clin Endocrinol Metab 1975; 40:1094-1098.
108. Berelowitz M, Szabo M, Frohman LA, Firestone S, Chu L. Somatomedin-C mediates growth hormone negative feedback by effects on both the hypothalamus and the pituitary. Science 1981; 212:1279-1281.
109. Mitchell ML, Byrne MJ, Sanchez Y, Sawin CT. Detection of growth hormone deficiency: the glucagon stimulation test. N Engl J Med 1970; 282: 539.
110. Vanderschueren-Lodeweyckx M, Walter R, Malvaux P, Eggermont E, Eeckels R. The glucagon stimulation test: effect on plasma growth hormone and on immunoreactive insulin, cortisol and glucose in children. J Pediatr 1974; 85:182-187.
111. Quabbe HJ. Plasma growth hormone response to vasopressin. Acta Endocrinol (Copenh) 1970; 63:359-377.
112. Bruno OD, Copinscki G, Leclercq R. Growth hormone response to rapid intravenous injection of various amounts of β^{1-24} ACTH. Horm Metab Res 1971; 3:318-320.
113. Ito H, Momose G, Katayama T. Effect of prostaglandin on the secretion of growth hormone. J Clin Endocrinol Metab 1971; 32:857-859.
114. Kohler PO, O'Malley BW, Rayford PL. Effect of pyrogen on blood levels of pituitary trophic hormones. J Clin Endocrinol Metab 1967; 27:219-226.
115. Takahara J, Ogawa N, Ofuji T. Extra-adrenal action of metyrapone upon human growth hormone secretion in man. Endocrinol Jpn 1972; 19:197-201.

116. Clemmons DR, Van Wyk JJ, Ridgway EC, Kliman B, Kjellberg RN. Evaluation of acromegaly by radioimmunoassay of somatomedin-C. N Engl J Med 1979; 301:1138-1142.
117. Phillips LS, Vassilopoulou-Sellin R. Somatomedins. N Engl J Med 1980; 302:371-380 (Part 1).
118. Phillips LS, Vassilopoulou-Sellin R. Somatomedins. N Engl J Med 1980; 302:438-446 (Part 2).
119. Bala RM, Lopatka J, Leung A, McCoy E, McArthur RG. Serum immunoreactive somatomedin levels in normal adults, pregnant women at term, children at various ages and children with constitutionally delayed growth. J Clin Endocrinol Metab 1981; 52:508-512.
120. Furlanetto RW, Underwood LE, Van Wyk JJ, E'Ercole AJ. Estimation of somatomedin-C levels in normals and patients with pituitary disease by radioimmunoassay. J Clin Invest 1977; 60:648-657.
121. Clemmons DR, Van Wyk, JJ. Somatomedin: physiological control and effects on cell proliferation. In *Handbook of Experimental Pharmacology,* vol 57: *Tissue Growth Factors,* Baserga R (ed). Springer Verlag, Berlin, 1981, pp 161-208.
122. Furlanetto RW, Underwood LE, Van Wyk JJ, Handwerger S. Serum immunoreactive somatomedin-C is elevated late in pregnancy. J Clin Endocrinol Metab 1978; 47:695-698.
123. Phillips LS. Nutritional regulation of somatomedin activity and growth. In *Somatomedins and Growth,* Proc. Serono Symposia, Giordano G, Van Wyk JJ, Minuto F (eds). Academic, New York, 1979, vol 23, p. 311.
124. Stuart M, Lazarus L. Somatomedins. Med J Aust 1975; 1:816.
125. Copeland KC, Underwood LE, Van Wyk JJ. Induction of immunoreactive somatomedin-C in human serum by growth hormone: dose response relationships and effect on chromatographic profiles. J Clin Endocrinol Metab 1980; 50:690-697.
126. Reiter EO, Lovinger RD. The use of a commercially available somatomedin-C radioimmunoassay in patients with disorders of growth. J Pediatr 1981; 99:720-724.
127. Rosenfeld RG, Kemp SF, Hintz RL. Constancy of somatomedin response to growth hormone treatment of hypopituitary dwarfism and lack of correlation with growth rate. J Clin Endocrinol Metab 1981; 53:611-617.
128. Kemp SF, Rosenfeld RG, Liu F, Gaspich S, Hintz RL. Acute somatomedin response to growth hormone: radioreceptor assay versus radioimmunoassay. J Clin Endocrinol Metab 1981; 52:616.
129. Rudman D, Kutner, MH, Goldsmith MA, Kenny J, Jennings H, Bain RP. Further observations on four subgroups of normal variant short stature. J Clin Endocrinol Metab 1980; 51:1378-1384.
130. Laron Z, Pertzelan A, Karp M, Kowaldo-Silbergard A, Daughaday WH. Administration of growth hormone to patients with familial dwarfism with high plasma immunoreactive growth hormone and measurement of

sulfation factor, metabolic and linear growth response. J Clin Endocrinol Metab 1971; 33:332.

131. Merimee TJ, Zapf J, Froesch ER. Dwarfism in the Pigmy. An isolated deficiency of insulin-like growth factor-1. N Engl J Med 1981; 305:965-968.
132. Kenny FM, Guyda H, Wright JC, Friesen HG. Prolactin and somatomedin in hypopituitary patients with "catch-up" growth following operations for craniopharyngioma. J Clin Endocrinol Metab 1973; 36:378.
133. Zapf J, Rinderkneckt E, Humbel RE, Froesch ER. Nonsuppressible insulin-like activity (NSILA) from human serum: recent accomplishments and their physiologic implications. Metabolism 1978; 27:1803-1828.
134. Bala RM, Bhaumick B. Radioimmunoassay of a basic somatomedin: comparison of various assay techniques and somatomedin levels in various sera. J Clin Endocrinol Metab 1979; 49:770-777.
135. Daughaday WH. New criteria for evaluation of acromegaly. N Engl J Med 1979; 301:1175-1176.
136. Stonesifer LD, Jordan RM, Kohler PO. Somatomedin-C in treated acromegaly: poor correlation with growth hormone and clinical response. J Clin Endocrinol Metab 1981; 53:931.
137. Giastina G, Reschini E, Valentina F. Growth hormone and cortisol responses to insulin-induced hypoglycaemia in thyrotoxicosis. J Clin Endocrinol Metab 1971; 32:571.
138. Sachar EJ, Muskrush G, Perlow M. Growth hormone responses to L-dopa in depressed patients. Science 1972; 178:1304-1305.
139. Hartog M, Gaafar MA, Fraser R. Effect of corticosteroids on serum growth hormone. Lancet 1964; 2:376.
140. Brown GM, Reichlin S. Psychologic and neural regulation of growth hormone secretion. Psychosom Med 1972; 34:45-61.
141. Powell GF, Brasel JA, Raiti S. Emotional deprivation and growth retardation simulating idiopathic hypopituitarism. II. Endocrinologic evaluation of the syndrome. N Engl J Med 1967; 276:1279-1283.
142. Hansen AP. Normalisation of growth hormone hyperresponse to exercise in juvenile diabetics after normalisation of blood sugar. J Clin Invest 1971; 50:1806-1811.
143. Galbo H, Christensen NJ, Mikines KJ, Sonne B, Hilsted J, Hagen C, Fahrenkrug J. The effect of fasting on the hormonal response to graded exercise. J Clin Endocrinol Metab 1981; 52:1106-1112.
144. Smith SR, Edgar PJ, Pozefsky T. Growth hormone in adults with protein calorie malnutrition. J Clin Endocrinol Metab 1974; 39:53.
145. Kanis JA, Brown P, Fitzpatrick K. Anorexia nervosa: a clinical, psychiatric and laboratory study. Q J Med 1974; 43:321.
146. Lindsten J, Cerasi E, Luft R, Hultquist G. The occurrence of abnormal insulin and growth hormone responses to sustained hyperglycaemia in a disease with sex chromosome aberrations (Turner's syndrome). Acta Endocrinol (Copenh) 1967; 56:107-131.

147. Benjamin F, Casper DJ, Sherman L. Growth hormone secretion in patients with endometrial carcinoma. N Engl J Med 1969; 281:1448-1452.
148. Feldman HA, Singer I. Endocrinology and metabolism in uraemia and dialysis: a clinical review. Medicine 1975; 54:345.
149. Conn HO, Daughaday WH. Cirrhosis and diabetes V. Serum growth hormone levels in Laennec's cirrhosis. J Lab Clin Med 1970; 76:678.

22
Prolactin

Stephen Franks
St. Mary's Hospital Medical School, University of London, London, England

Disorders of prolactin secretion are among the most common endocrine diseases seen in clinical practice; conditions associated with excessive prolactin secretion are the most prevalent of these disorders. Hyperprolactinemia is an important marker of a pituitary tumor and is associated with a characteristic disturbance of gonadal function which is reversible when prolactin concentrations are lowered. The importance of serum prolactin measurements in patients with pituitary disease and in those with amenorrhea or impotence is discussed and an approach to the further investigation of hyperprolactinemia is illustrated.

I. PATHOPHYSIOLOGY OF PROLACTIN SECRETION

A. Endogenous Factors Affecting Prolactin Secretion

The most important physiologic stimulus for prolactin release is suckling, but there are a number of other endogenous factors which influence prolactin secretion and which are important to consider in the interpretation of raised serum levels of prolactin. Both physical and psychological stress can cause moderate elevation of serum prolactin concentrations. Thus elevated prolactin levels may be found following surgery (1,2), gynecological examination, or even clinical interview (2). Breast examination does not seem to influence prolactin concentrations (2,3), and although venepuncture may cause a rise in prolactin in some cases (4), it usually has no effect (2). Prolactin secretion tends to be pulsatile both in normal subjects (5) and in those with hyperprolactinemia (6),

Table 1 Causes of Hyperprolactinemia

Drugs
Dopamine receptor antagonists
(e.g., phenothiazines, benzamides)
Dopamine depleting drugs
(e.g., α-methyldopa)
Estrogens
Primary hypothyroidism
Pituitary tumors
Destructive lesions of the hypothalamus
"Idiopathic"

although the pulses do not seem to occur at fixed intervals. There is a sleep-related rise in prolactin (5) which is usually lost in hyperprolactinemic patients. Endogenous estrogen stimulates prolactin secretion, explaining the somewhat higher levels in women compared with men (7) and the increasing plasma levels during pregnancy. There is some controversy as to whether there are significant changes in prolactin secretion during the menstrual cycle (8, 9), but there is a tendency for prolactin concentrations to be at their highest in the late follicular phase of the cycle.

B. Causes of Abnormal Prolactin Secretion

1. Hyperprolactinemia

The common causes of hyperprolactinemia are listed in Table 1. There are a number of drugs which elevate serum prolactin levels, the most important of these being the dopamine receptor blocking agents, such as phenothiazines, metoclopramide, and haloperidol. Prolactin secretion is under tonic inhibitory control, the predominant prolactin inhibiting factor (PIF) being dopamine (10). Thus,drugs which deplete the hypothalamic content of dopamine (e.g., α-methyldopa) or antagonize the action of dopamine at pituitary level (e.g., phenothiazines and benzamides) stimulate the secretion of prolactin. Dopamine receptor blocking agents have been used in dynamic tests of prolactin release (see Chap. 41). A careful drug history is clearly mandatory in the assessment of the hyperprolactinemic patient.

Tumors of the pituitary are an important cause of hyperprolactinemia. Elevated prolactin concentrations may result from primary hypersecretion by tumor cells (tumors producing either prolactin alone or prolactin and growth hormone) or may be secondary to upward extension of a nonprolactin-secreting tumor interfering with production or transport of PIF. Hypothalamic disease (e.g., tumors or granulomas) may cause hyperprolactinemia by this second mechanism (11, 12). Primary hypothyroidism may be associated with hyperprolactinemia and galactorrhea. In most of these cases prolactin levels fall to normal after treatment with thyroxine (6, 13).

In many patients there may be no obvious cause for the hyperprolactinemia. Up to two-thirds of women with hyperprolactinemic amenorrhea have normal pituitary x-rays (14). These patients may have small pituitary tumors but this cannot easily be proven and the cause of increased prolactin levels in this group remains uncertain.

2. Impaired Prolactin Secretion

The most common cause of impaired prolactin secretion is hypopituitarism. However, prolactin levels are rarely undetectable even in posthypophysectomy patients, and although the prolactin response to thyrotropin releasing hormone (TRH) may be blunted or absent, normal responses have been reported (15). Clinically, the only proven deleterious effect of impaired prolactin secretion is failure of lactation, as in Sheehan's syndrome (hypopituitarism associated with postpartum hemorrhage).

II. PREVALENCE AND CLINICAL PRESENTATION OF HYPERPROLACTINEMIA

A. Pituitary Tumors

The most frequent presenting symptom of patients with pituitary tumors and hyperprolactinemia is amenorrhea (with or without galactorrhea) or impotence. Patients with pituitary tumors may complain of local symptoms such as visual impairment or headache, but even in these patients symptoms associated with reproductive dysfunction are often present at the time of consultation. Analysis of a large series of patients with "functionless" tumors of the pituitary (11) at one London center showed that amenorrhea or impotence were the predominant symptoms in patients with hyperprolactinemia (over 70% presenting with reproductive problems), whereas local symptoms or the accidental finding of a large pituitary fossa (on a skull x-ray taken for other purposes) was the usual mode of presentation in those patients with normal prolactin levels (Fig. 1). Of 45 hyperprolactinemic patients with untreated pituitary tumors, only 10 complained of galactorrhea. It is important to note that elevated prolactin levels occurred in one-third of patients studied after pituitary surgery and that in many of these patients, persistent hyperprolactinemia, rather than gonadotropin deficiency, was the cause of continuing amenorrhea or impotence after surgical treatment. Prolactin-secreting pituitary tumors are diagnosed twice as often in women as in men. The mean age at diagnosis of a pituitary tumor is much

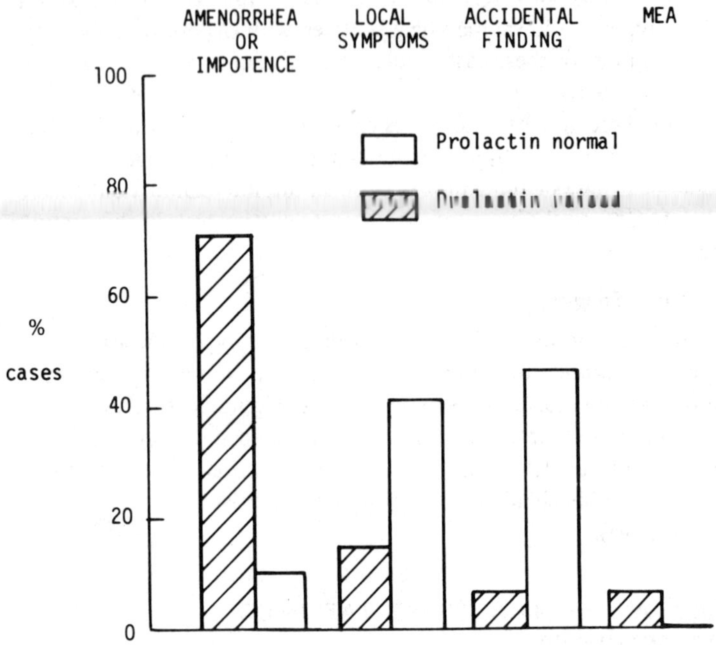

Figure 1 Presenting symptoms in 64 untreated patients with "functionless" tumors of the pituitary. The mode of presentation in the group of 45 hyperprolactinemic patients is compared with that in 19 with normal prolactin (MEA, multiple endocrine adenomata). The difference between the groups is significant ($\chi^2 = 23$; $p = < 0.001$). (From Ref. 11.)

higher in men than in women. It is noteworthy that, in the series above, although 8 of 21 men originally consulted their doctors because of impotence, in only one was the presence of a pituitary tumor recognized at an early stage.

Elevated prolactin levels are commonly found in patients with acromegaly. The prevalence of hyperprolactinemia in two large series of acromegalic patients was 26% and 30%, respectively (12, 16).

B. Hyperprolactinemic Amenorrhea

Hyperprolactinemia is a common cause of amenorrhea, occurring in 14-20% of patients (17-19). Pituitary tumors can be found in one-third to one-half of patients with hyperprolactinemic amenorrhea, but in most patients the cause of the elevated prolactin levels is not certain. Many patients also have galactorrhea, but hyperprolactinemia can occur in the absence of galactorrhea, which indeed may be found in only one-third of patients in some series (17). Patients with hyperprolactinemic amenorrhea are characteristically estrogen deficient (20) and may complain of vaginal dryness on intercourse or even of hot flushes. They rarely ovulate in response to clomiphene, but reproductive function can be restored by lowering prolactin levels by medical or surgical treatment.

C. Hyperprolactinemic Impotence

Hyperprolactinemia in men is associated with hypogonadism and impotence. In contrast to hyperprolactinemia in women, the syndrome of hyperprolactinemic impotence almost always occurs in men with obvious pituitary tumors (21-23). The prevalence of hyperprolactinemia in men presenting with impotence is, however, very low and it is probably only necessary to measure prolactin concentrations in those impotent men who have signs of hypogonadism. The finding of low testosterone levels is characteristic of hyperprolactinemia in men and, as well as impotence (or loss of libido), diminished facial and body hair and gynecomastia (but rarely galactorrhea) are common features of this syndrome.

III. DIAGNOSTIC TESTS

It can be seen from Section II that measurement of serum prolactin is important in patients with pituitary disease and in those with amenorrhea or hypogonadism. The history and examination may lead the clinician to suspect the diagnosis of hyperprolactinemia, but this can readily be confirmed by a simple blood test. The place of basal prolactin measurements and dynamic tests of prolactin secretion are discussed below and an approach to the further investigation of hyperprolactinemic syndromes is outlined.

A. Measurement of Serum Prolactin Concentrations

In recent years, the development of specific and sensitive radioimmunoassays for prolactin (24) has enabled physicians and gynecologists to have ready access to serum prolactin measurements. Despite the plethora of dynamic tests of prolactin secretion (Chap. 41) measurement of basal prolactin levels remains the most important test in the diagnosis of hyperprolactinemia.

1. Diagnosis of Hyperprolactinemia—How Many Blood Samples Are Needed?

A single prolactin measurement may sometimes be misleading; interpretation of a high prolactin level must take account of the possible endogenous and exogenous factors which may affect prolactin secretion (particularly pulsatility and stress) as well as possible methodological problems in the laboratory (25). The

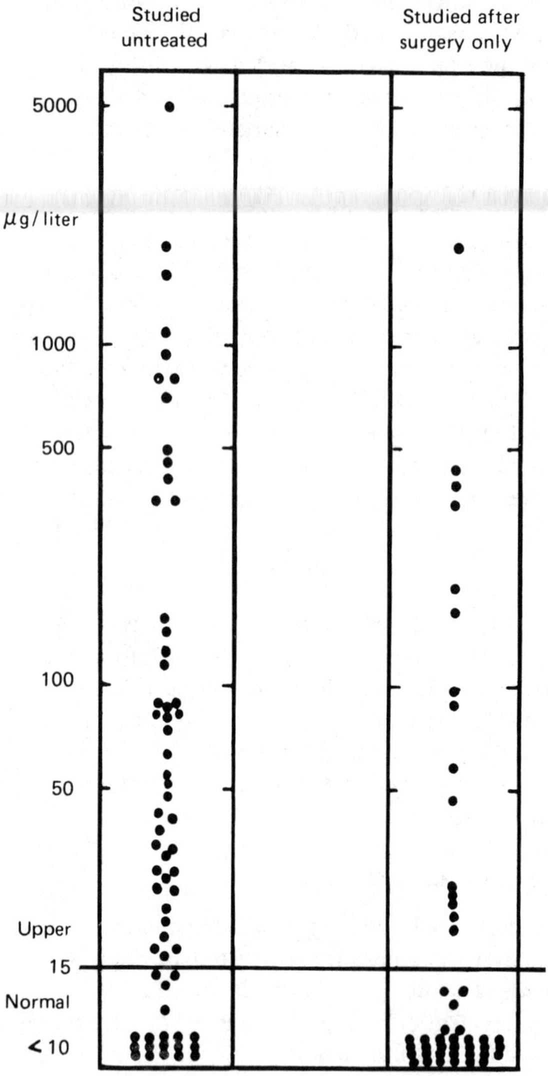

Figure 2 Prolactin concentrations in 111 patients with "functionless" pituitary tumors; horizontal line indicates upper limit of normal. (From Ref. 11.)

definition of hyperprolactinemia (i.e., the level at which prolactin levels are considered abnormally high) varies from laboratory to laboratory and it is important that each laboratory defines its own normal range. What, then, is the best method of confirming hyperprolactinemia? It has been suggested that multiple blood samples be taken through a venous cannula over the course of an hour (25), but a recent study has shown that sufficient information can be obtained from taking two or three random samples on different visits to the clinic [but preferably not on days when clinical examination is performed (26)], Prolactin measurements in women who present with amenorrhea or menstrual irregularities rarely present any problem in interpretation, but a significant number of patients with normal menses and unexplained infertility appear to have a high level of prolactin, which falls to normal during the course of sequential sampling. This is a particularly difficult group of patients in which to assess the etiological importance of raised prolactin levels and even in this group, multiple sampling does not provide any more useful clinical information than repeated random samples (26). Figure 2 shows the spectrum of serum prolactin levels in patients with pituitary tumors.

2. Dynamic Tests of Prolactin Secretion

Details of these tests and their application are given in Chapter 41. In general, these have not proved helpful in the diagnosis of abnormal prolactin secretion or in the definition of its cause. Twenty-four hour profiles of prolactin levels do not yield any clinically useful information.

B. Radiological Investigation of Hyperprolactinemic Patients

X-rays of the pituitary area are an important part of the investigation of hyperprolactinemia. In some cases the diagnosis of a pituitary tumor may have already been made on clinical, radiological, and sometimes histological criteria, and this may be the indication for measuring prolactin levels. In many patients, however, a raised prolactin level is found during the course of investigation of menstrual disturbance (with or without galactorrhea) and it is then important to go on to look for a pituitary or hypothalamic lesion. Galactorrhea in the absence of menstrual irregularities is rarely associated with hyperprolactinemia or pituitary tumor (27) and radiological examination should be reserved for those patients with elevated prolactin levels. A tumor may be apparent on simple lateral and posteroanterior views of the pituitary fossa; in some instances tomography of the sella turcica is helpful but, as discussed below, this is not advocated on a routine basis. If plain x-rays suggest the presence of a pituitary tumor further radiological examination, in the form of contrast studies or computerized tomography (CT), may be necessary to confirm the diagnosis and, particularly, to define any extrasellar extension of the tumor.

1. Plain X-rays and Tomography of the Pituitary Fossa

The characteristic feature of a prolactin-secreting tumor on plain lateral radiographs is a double floor due to asymmetric enlargement of the pituitary. A

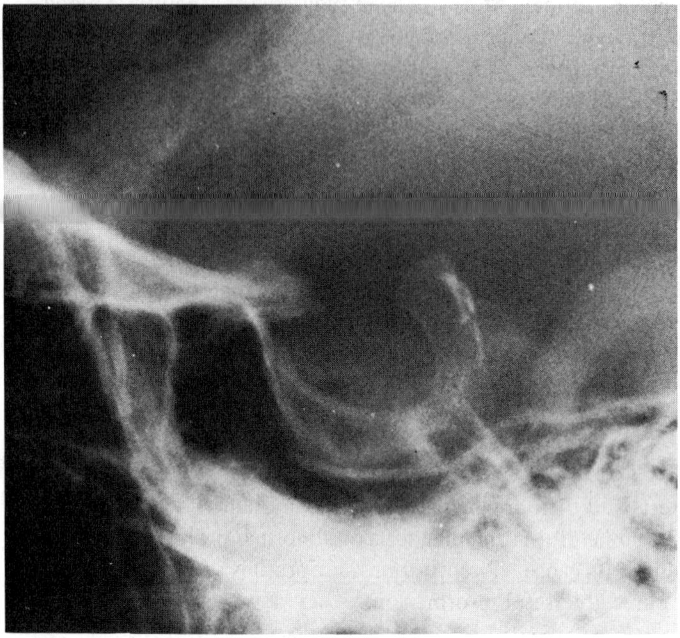

Figure 3 Plain lateral radiograph of the pituitary area of a 30-year-old woman with hyperprolactinemia and amenorrhea showing the "double floor" characteristic of a prolactinoma.

typical x-ray from a patient with a prolactin-secreting tumor is shown in Figure 3. It has been suggested that tomography of the sella is the only reliable means of defining an abnormal pituitary fossa in patients with galactorrhea and/or hyperprolactinemia (28). If, however, the plain radiograph is abnormal, there is little point in proceeding to tomography since this rarely gives further useful clinical information (29). It may be argued that exact definition of the contour of the fossa is important for the surgeon who is contemplating transsphenoidal surgery for a microadenoma (30), but in many centers the primary treatment of choice in patients with small tumors and hyperprolactinemia is bromocriptine (31). Tomography may be considered in patients with hyperprolactinemia who have normal plain radiography or in whom there is some doubt about the plain films (26, 29); Marrs and colleagues (29) found that 7 of 80 patients with hyperprolactinemia and normal plain x-rays had abnormal tomograms. However, detection of such slight abnormalities of the pituitary fossa is of questionable significance since recent studies have shown a poor correlation between minor radiological changes, serum prolactin levels, and the presence or absence of a pituitary adenoma (26, 32). Even in hyperprolactinemic patients such radiological findings are unlikely to influence management of the patient, since most endocrinologists would feel that medical treatment is both safe and effective. Formal classification of the size of the sella turcica has been advocated (30, 33). This may be useful in longitudinal study of a patient with a suspected pituitary tumor, but because of the disparity between minor radiological abnormalities and serum prolactin levels, it is not very helpful in patients with minor abnormalities of the pituitary fossa. In the case of larger prolactinomas with obvious sellar abnormalities there is quite a good correlation between the size of the fossa and the height of the prolactin level (34).

2. Air Encephalography, Metrizamide Cysternography, and CT Scan

In hyperprolactinemic patients with clear-cut abnormalities on plain radiograph suggestive of a pituitary tumor it is advisable to perform contrast studies to determine whether there is any extrasellar extension of the tumor. Lumbar air encephalography (AEG) has been successfully used for many years for this purpose (20) but is an uncomfortable procedure which is frequently followed by headache. Injection of the contrast medium, metrizamide, into the basal cistern is associated with less discomfort and gives excellent pictures of the outline of the tumor (35). However, this too is an invasive technique. In recent years the CT scan has been used to define pituitary tumors and although earlier studies gave disappointing pictures, improving resolution of the scan has led to its widespread use for this purpose. Definition of the tumor may be enhanced by the injection of contrast medium intravenously and precise assessment of upward extension of the lesion may be aided by coronal transformation of the tomographic cuts (see Fig. 4). Computerized tomography will also define primary hypothalamic lesions (such as craniopharyngioma) which may cause hyperprolactinemia. Such hypothalamic lesions may occur in the presence of a normal pituitary fossa, but routine CT scanning is not advocated in patients with hyperprolactinemia and normal pituitary x-rays unless there are other clues to suggest a hypothalamic lesion—such as hypopituitarism or diabetes insipidus and, particularly, a visual field defect. Infertile patients with hyperprolactinemia should have a CT scan before starting treatment.

C. Visual Fields

Formal evaluation of the visual fields should be made in patients with hyperprolactinemia and abnormal pituitary x-rays. Details of the methods are given in Chapter 4. This part of the investigation is particularly important in assessing

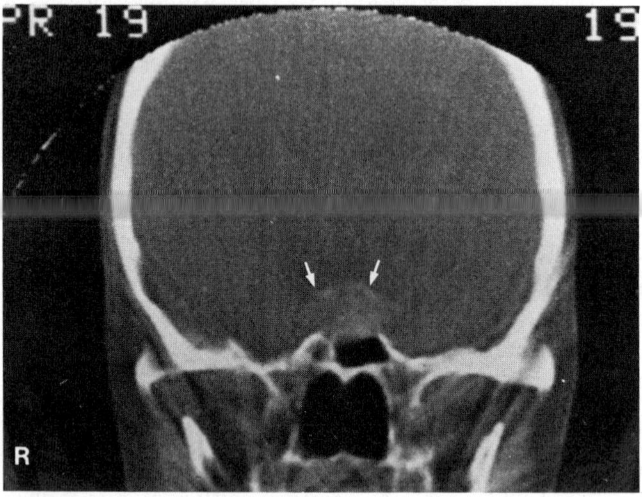

Figure 4 Coronal computerized tomography (CT) scan of the head in a 40-year-old woman with hyperprolactinemia. There is a large tumor arising from the pituitary fossa with significant suprasellar extension.

patients with prolactinomas during pregnancy. Special attention should be given to patients with large prolactinomas in whom ovulation has been induced by primary treatment with bromocriptine since the risk of expansion of the tumor, sufficient to cause visual impairment during late pregnancy, is probably greatest in this group (36).

D. Other Tests of Endocrine Function

Measurement of serum *thyroxine* should be made in all patients with hyperprolactinemia in order to exclude primary hypothyroidism as the cause of elevated prolactin levels. A serum *thyrotropin* (TSH) level may help to confirm the diagnosis and will differentiate between primary and pituitary-dependent hypothyroidism. Assessment of complete anterior pituitary function need not be undertaken on a routine basis. Significant hypopituitarism rarely occurs in the presence of small prolactinomas, but if there is radiological evidence of a large pituitary tumor and/or clinical evidence of hypopituitarism, a *combined anterior pituitary function test* should be performed (37). This is mandatory in patients who have had previous pituitary ablative treatment. The results of the test will determine the need for hormone replacement and, in the case of the response to luteinizing hormone releasing hormone (LHRH) will predict the chance of normal

Diagnostic Summary 1 Hyperprolactinemia

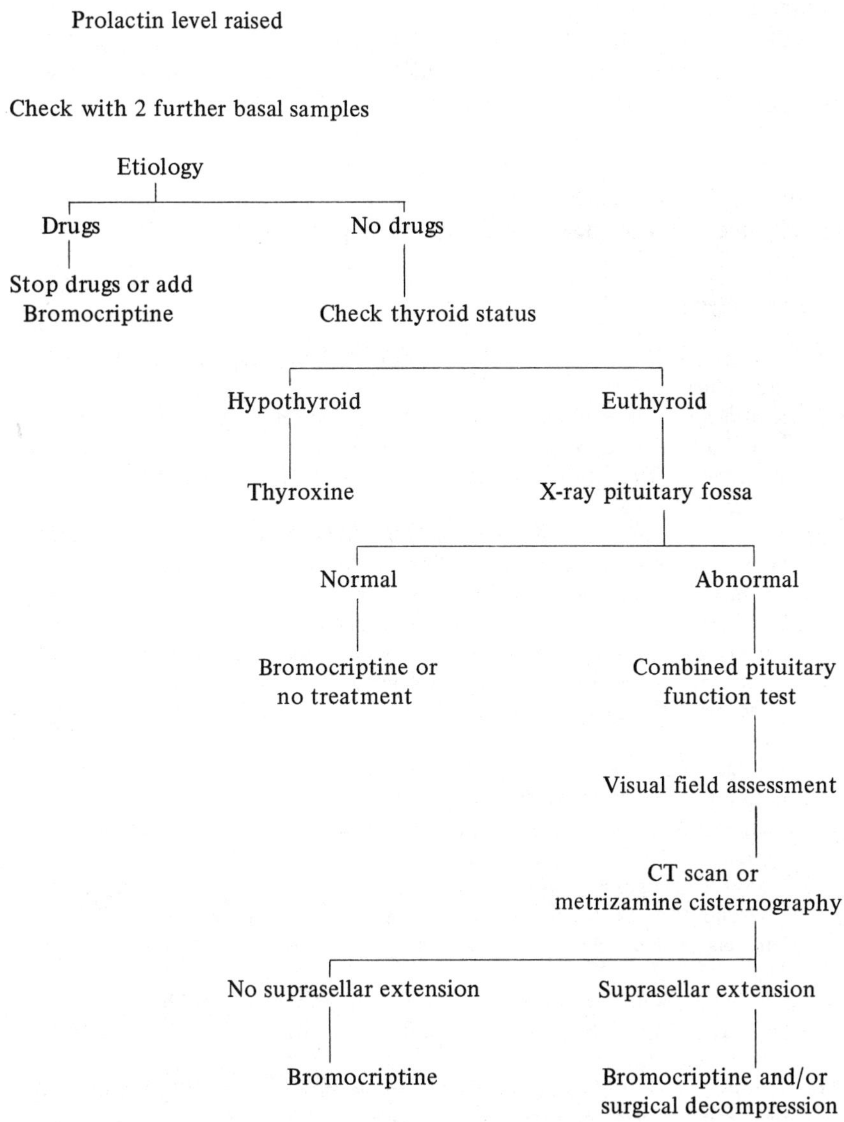

Suggested scheme for the diagnosis and management of hyperprolactinemia. The choice of treatment, particularly in patients with large pituitary tumors who desire pregnancy, is controversial. Details of the approach to the diagnosis of hyperprolactinemia may be found in Chapter 41.

reproductive function when the hyperprolactinemia has been treated by bromocriptine. Tests of posterior pituitary function are necessary only if there are symptoms of diabetes insipidus.

Measurement of gonadal steroids are useful in assessing the hyperprolactinemic patient who presents with reproductive problems. Women with hyperprolactinemia tend to have low *estradiol* levels and men low *testosterone.* During treatment, the most valuable biochemical index of response in women is a serum progesterone concentration in the putative luteal phase of the cycle to confirm ovulation. In men repeated measurement of *testosterone* is the most useful guide, supplemented, where necessary, by seminal analysis.

REFERENCES

1. Frantz AG, Kleinberg DL, Noel GL. Studies on prolactin in man. Rec Prog Horm Res 1972; 28:527-590.
2. Koninckx P. Stress hyperprolactinaemia. Lancet 1978; i:273.
3. Jarrell J, Franks S, McInnes R, Gemayel K, Guyda H, Arronet GH, Naftolin F. Breast examination does not elevate serum prolactin. Fertil Steril 1980; 33:49-51.
4. Adler RA, Noel GL, Wartofsky L, Frantz AG. Failure of oral water loading and intravenous hypotonic saline to depress plasma prolactin in man. J Clin Endocrinol Metab 1975; 41:383-389.
5. Sassin JF, Frantz AG, Weitzman ED, Kapen S. Human prolactin: 24-hour pattern with increased release during sleep. Science 1972; 177:1205-1207.
6. Franks S, Jacobs HS, Hull MGR, Steele SJ, Nabarro JDN. Management of hyperprolactinaemic amenorrhoea. Br J Obstet Gynaecol 1977; 84:241-251.
7. Friesen HG. Human prolactin in clinical endocrinology: the impact of radioimmunoassay. Metabolism 1973; 22:1039-1045.
8. McNeilly AS, Chard T. Circulating levels of prolactin in the menstrual cycle. Clin Endocrinol 1974; 3:105-112.
9. Robyn C, Delvoye P, Nokin J, Vekemens M, Badawi M, Perez-Lopez FR, L'Hermite M. Prolactin and human reproduction. In *Human Prolactin,* Pasteels JL, Robyn C (eds). Excerpta Medica, Amsterdam, 1973, pp. 167-188.
10. Gibbs DM, Neill JD. Dopamine levels in hypophysial stalk blood in the rat are sufficient to inhibit prolactin secretion in vivo. Endocrinology 1978; 102:1895-1900.
11. Franks S, Nabarro JDN, Jacobs HS. Prevalence and presentation of hyperprolactinaemia in patients with "functionless" pituitary tumours, Lancet 1977; 1:778-780.
12. Franks S, Jacobs HS, Nabarro JDN. Prolactin concentrations in patients with acromegaly: clinical significance and response to surgery. Clin Endocrinol 1976; 5:63-69.

13. Edwards CRW, Forsyth IA, Besser GM. Amenorrhoea, galactorrhoea and primary hypothyroidism with high circulating levels of prolactin. Br Med J 1971; 3:462-464.
14. Franks S, Disorders of human prolactin secretion. MD thesis. University of London, 1978.
15. Woolf PD, Jacobs LS, Donofrio R, Burday SZ, Schalk DS. Secondary hypopituitarism: evidence for continuing regulation of hormone release. J Clin Endocrinol Metab 1974; 38:71-76.
16. Moriondo P, Travaglini P, Rondena M, Beck-Peccoz P, Conti-Puglisi F, Ambrosi B, Faglia G. Prolactin secretion in acromegaly. In *Pituitary Microadenomas,* Faglia G, Giovanelli MA, MacLeod RM (eds). Academic, London, 1980, pp. 247-255.
17. Franks S, Murray MAF, Jequier AM, Steele SJ, Nabarro JDN, Jacobs HS. Incidence and significance of hypoprolactinaemia in women with amenorrhoea. Clin Endocrinol 1975; 4:597-607.
18. Glass MR, Shaw RW, Butt WR, Logan-Edwards E., London DR. An abnormality of oestrogen feedback in amenorrhoea galactorrhoea. Br Med J 1975; 3:274-275.
19. Van Look PFA, McNeilly AS, Hunter WM, Baird DT. The role of prolactin in secondary amenorrhoea. In *Prolactin and Human Reproduction,* Crosignani P, Robyn C (eds). Academic, London, 1977, pp 217-224.
20. Jacobs HS, Franks S, Murray, MAF, Hull MGR, Steele SJ, Nabarro JDN. Clinical and endocrine features of hyperprolactinaemic amenorrhoea. Clin Endocrinol 1976; 5:439-454.
21. Thorner MO, Besser GM. Hyperprolactinaemia and gonadal function: results of bromocriptine treatment. In *Prolactin and Human Reproduction,* Crosignani P, Robyn C (eds). Academic, London, 1977, pp 285-301.
22. Franks S, Jacobs HS, Martin N, Nabarro JDN. Hyperprolactinaemia and impotence. Clin Endocrinol 1978; 8:277-287.
23. Carter JN, Tyson JE, Tolis G, Van Vliet S, Faiman C, Friesen HG. Prolactin-secreting tumors and hypogonadism in 22 men. N Engl J Med 1978; 299:847-852.
24. Franks S, Prolactin. In *Hormones in Blood,* Gray CH, James VHT (eds). 3rd ed, Academic, London, 1979, vol I, pp 280-332.
25. Jeffcoate SL. Diagnosis of hyperprolactinaemia. Lancet 1978; 2:1245-1247.
26. Moult PJA, Dacie JE, Rees LH, Besser GM. Prolactin pulsatility in patients with gonadal dysfunction. Clin Endocrinol 1981; 14:387-394.
27. Kleinberg DL, Noel GL, Frantz AG. Galactorrhea: a study of 235 cases including 48 with pituitary tumors. N Engl J Med 1977; 296:589-600.
28. Vezina JL, Sutton TJ. Prolactin secreting pituitary microadenomas. Am J Roentgenol 1974; 120:46-54.
29. Marrs RP, Letzky OA, Teal J, Davajan V, March C, Mishell DR. Am J Obstet Gynecol 1979; 135:467-469.

30. Hardy J. Transsphenoidal surgery of hypersecreting pituitary tumors. In *Diagnosis and Treatment of Pituitary Tumors,* Kohler PO, Ross GT (eds), Int Congr Ser 303. Excerpta Medica, Amsterdam, 1973, pp 179-191.
31. McGregor AM, Grinsberg J. Dilemmas in the management of functioning pituitary tumors. Br J Hosp Med 1981; 25:344-352.
32. Burrow GN, Wortzman G, Rewcastle NB, Holgate RC, Kovacs K. Microadenomas of the pituitary and abnormal sellar tomograms in an unselected autopsy series. N Engl J Med 1981; 304:156-158.
33. Thorner MO, Edwards CRW, Charlesworth M, Dacie JE, Moult PJA, Rees LH, Jones AE, Besser GM. Pregnancy in patients presenting with hyperprolactinaemia. Br Med J 1979; 771-774.
34. Child DF, Nader S, Mashiter K, Kjeld M, Banks LF, Russell-Fraser T. Prolactin studies in "functionless" pituitary tumours. Br Med J 1975; i:604-606.
35. Thorner MO, Martin WH, Rogol AD, Morris JL, Perryman RL, Conway BP, Howards SS, Wolfman MG, MacLeod RM. Rapid regression of pituitary prolactinomas during bromocriptine treatment. J Clin Endocrinol Metab 1980; 51:438-445.
36. Bergh T, Nillus SJ, Wide L. Clinical course and outcome of pregnancies in amenorrhoeic women with hyperprolactinaemia and pituitary tumours. Br Med J 1978; i:875-880.
37. Harsoulis P, Marshall JC, Kuku SF, Burke CW, London DR, Fraser TR. A combined test for assessment of pituitary function. Br Med J 1973; iv: 1326-1329.

23
Thyrotropin

H. K. Ibbertson
University of Auckland School of Medicine, Auckland, New Zealand

Thyrotropin or thyroid stimulating hormone (TSH), a glycoprotein, is synthesized on the ribosomes of the anterior pituitary thyrotropes and stored there as the smallest of the pituitary granules. The molecule comprises two chains each of 14,000 daltons linked by disulfide bridges (1). The alpha chain is nearly identical to that of the other two-chain glycoprotein tropic hormones–follicle stimulating hormone (FSH), luteinizing hormone (LH), and human chorionic gonadotrophin (hCG)–and is biologically inactive. The β chain, which has minimal biological activity in isolation, is structurally distinct and confers specificity of action. Alpha and β subunits combine within the thyrotrope to form TSH before secretion (2), but release of isolated subunits also occurs with thyrotropin releasing hormone (TRH) stimulation (3).

I. CONTROLS

The synthesis of thyrotropin is directly stimulated by TRH, and the main control of both synthesis and secretion involves modulation of TRH action on the thyrotrope by the negative feedback inhibitory action of thyroid hormone.

A. Early Development

In the fetus during the first trimester there is a parallel but independent development of hypothalamic-pituitary-thyroid (HPT) components of the axis (4). By 10-12 weeks, hypothalamic nuclei and anterior pituitary cells are differentiated and TRH and TSH are detectable by radioimmunoassay in the respective tissues. Low levels of TSH and thyroxine (T_4) remain unchanged until 18-22 weeks, when a rise occurs. This marks the beginning of an active role for TSH in thyroid hormone biosynthesis and reflects the establishment of a permanent link between the hypothalamus and pituitary components of the pituitary portal venous system. Increasing TSH levels responsive to TRH reach a peak (15 μU/ml) early in the third trimester and then gradually fall to around 10 μU/ml at term. Full thyroid responsiveness is not immediate, and T_4 levels continue to rise despite the falling TSH during the third trimester. Maturation of thyroid responsiveness may be temporarily delayed into the neonatal period (below) or permanently in the rare syndrome of familiar thyroid unresponsiveness to TSH (5).

The second TSH surge occurs at the time of birth when exposure to low extrauterine temperatures invokes an acute TSH response with peak levels at 30 min, a rapid fall over 24 hr and a slower fall to normal during the first week (Fig. 1). There is a parallel TSH-dependent change in T_4 and a sixfold rise in triiodothyronine (T_3). In contrast to these mainly TSH-dependent changes,

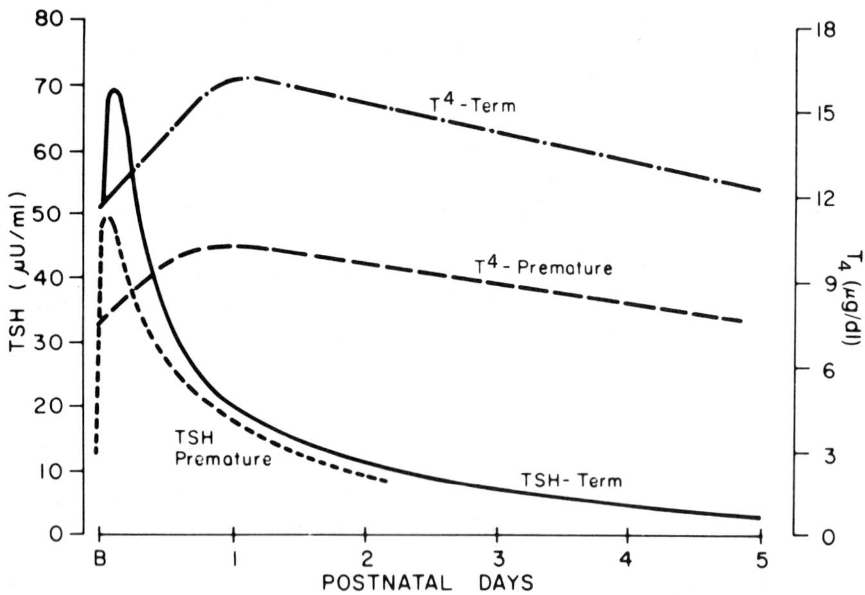

Figure 1 Changes in serum TSH and T_4 concentrations in full-term and premature infants during the first 5 days of life. The serum TSH reaches a maximum level at 30 min and the T_4 at 24–36 hr. These early changes are delayed and blunted in premature infants. (Reprinted from Ref. 4, by permission of The New England Journal of Medicine 1981; 304:706.)

reverse T_3 (rT_3) levels slowly decline during the last trimester and remain essentially unchanged during the neonatal period. All of these changes are delayed and blunted in the premature infant, but the general pattern is essentially the same.

B. Definitive Mechanisms

TRH is a tripeptide, pyroglutamyl histidyl prolinamide. Its synthesis by a non-ribosomal mechanism is widespread in the central nervous system and the hyophyseal portal venous blood provides access to receptor sites on specific pituicytes, the thyrotropes. Activation of adenyl cyclase and cyclic AMP generation leads to synthesis and secretion of TSH.

Available evidence suggests that the secretion of TRH is relatively constant, although cold exposure in the human neonate stimulates TSH release (6) and TSH levels are inversely related to core temperature in the human adult (7). A number of other suprahypothalamic neural inputs influence its production and the suppression of TSH secretion in fasting and in severe illness (8) are probable examples of this.

Thyroid hormone feedback on the thyrotrope blocks TRH action by a mechanism which involves protein synthesis. This process is in turn dependent on the binding of T_3 to nuclear receptors which have a 10-fold higher affinity for T_3 than T_4 (9). A high local concentration of T_3 is ensured by preferential 5-monodeiodination of T_4 to T_3 (10) and nuclear T_3 occupancy is approximately 80%, half of which is derived from T_4 (11). Thus thyroid function is finely modulated by this central mechanism, which depends on the local (thyrotrope) availability of the major thyroid hormone T_4 as a substrate for T_3. The theoretical and experimental basis for these conclusions have recently been reviewed by Larsen and co-workers (11). TSH secretion is subject to additional controls. There is a diurnal rhythm with a nadir during the afternoon and a peak around 3 A.M. which precedes that for ACTH and is probably independent (12). Somatostatin competes with TRH for thyrotrope receptors and lowers TSH in humans. Estrogen, glucocorticoids and β-adrenergic agonists all stimulate TSH secretion, while α-agonists have an inhibitory action. Their physiological signifiicance is uncertain. There is more evidence for a direct tonic inhibitory action of dopamine on the thyrotrope and blockade of dopamine by metaclopramide increases basal TSH levels (13). A positive T_3 feedback at hypothalamic level may enhance dopamine synthesis and thus exert a subsidiary control on TSH secretion. The *half-time of TSH turnover* is around 50 min and is prolonged in hypothyroidism and renal failure. With optimal radioimmunoassay conditions the normal euthyroid range is 0.1-3.2 μU/ml and levels may rise above 1500 μU/ml in severe primary hypothyroidism. TSH secretion is reduced approximately fivefold but is not totally inhibited in thyrotoxicosis. Using the ultrasensitive cytochemical bioassay the mean serum TSH in nine patients with untreated Graves' disease was 0.28 μU/ml (14).

The action of TSH on the thyroid involves binding to specific receptor sites stimulation of adenyl cyclase and augmentation of cyclic AMP concentration. This nucleotide acts to stimulate protein synthesis, iodide transport and binding, colloid resorption, and iodothyronine secretion—actions normally regarded as TSH effects. Lack of thyroidal response to TSH occurs in severe destructive disease, in the congenital syndrome of thyroidal TSH unresponsiveness (5), and in the presence of circulating thyroid receptor blocking antibodies (15). Disturbance at any level of the hypothalamic-pituitary-thyroid (HPT) axis can alter thyrotropin secretion. This can result from a disorder of TSH regulation or from a compensatory and appropriate adjustment to deviations in serum thyroid hormone levels.

II. DISORDERS OF TSH REGULATION

In the presence of an intact HPT axis there is a reciprocal relationship between serum TSH and free thyroid hormone levels. Serum TSH is thus low in thyrotoxicosis and high in primary hypothyroidism. Inappropriate TSH secretion is said to occur when this normal reciprocal relationship is disturbed or when serum levels are at variance with clinical expectation, as, for example, in hypothyroidism secondary to pituitary tumor when serum TSH may be elevated (Table 1). Such discordance usually results from functional or organic hypothalamopituitary disease but may occur in its absence. It is seen, for example, in "compensated hypothyroidism," when, despite normal T_4/T_3 levels, the serum TSH is elevated. Recent evidence indicates that this pattern is entirely appropriate, a reflection of the greater sensitivity of the thyrotrope compared with peripheral tissues to incipient hypothyroidism. Functional disorders of TSH secretion are particularly common during the neonatal period, and correct interpretation of data is essential to avoid inappropriate therapy.

A. Transient Neonatal Disorders

Neonatal screening programs indicate a prevalence of hypothyroidism of 1 in 4000 births (16). Defects in the early development of the HPT axis result in permanent abnormalities of TSH secretion (see below). More commonly (1-2%) the changes are temporary and result from immaturity of the secretory mechanisms. Such abnormalities are particularly common in premature infants and a number of syndromes have been identified (4).

Table 1 Disorders of TSH Regulation and Action

Reference	Disorder	fT_4
	Low or Normal TSH	
	Hypothalmopituitary dysfunction (active TSH)	
4	Neonatal transient hypothyroidism	↓
	Permanent secondary and tertiary hypothyroidism	↓
	Therapy-related	
36	Drug or destructive therapy of thyrotoxicosis	↓
37	Withdrawal of T_4 replacement	↓
38	Growth hormone therapy	↓
31,32	Nonthyroidal illness[a]	↑↓
	High TSH	
27	Hypothalamopituitary disease (inactive TSH)	↓
	Thyrotrope tumor	
41,42	Spontaneous (TSH-toxicosis)	↑
55,56	Complicating primary hypothyroidism	↓
	Tissue iodothyronine (T_4, T_3) resistance	
21	Infantile thyrotrope resistance	↑ (admin)
59,64	Local thyrotrope resistance (TSH-toxicosis)	↑
60,61,66	General tissue resistance (often familial)	N or ↑
	Thyroid gland thyrotropin resistance[b]	
4	Neonatal transient hypothyroidism	↓
4,5,Chap. 29, Ref. 131	Congenital dysgenesis or dyshormonogenesis	↓
	Acquired thyroid disease	↓
Chap. 29, Ref. 138	Compensated hypothyroidism[b]	N

[a] Also called "sick euthyroid" syndrome.
[b] In these disorders TSH regulation is normal.

1. Low T_4 and TSH levels have been observed in 25-50% of infants born before 37 weeks' gestation, the higher incidence occurring with increasing prematurity. Immaturity of TRH synthesis is held responsible. Serum T_4 levels return to normal within 4-20 weeks and subsequent growth and development is normal.
2. Transient TSH elevation with *normal* T_4 and T_3 have been reported particularly from Japan, where the prevalence approximates 1 in 9,000 births. Reduced thyroid responsiveness to TSH or immaturity of thyroid

hormone biosynthesis has been implicated in this disorder, which usually corrects itself within 9 months of birth. This condition could represent a less severe form of a third disorder.

3. Transient hypothyroidism with *low* serum T_4 and high TSH, which is reported with a prevalence of 1 in 60,000 to 460,000 newborn infants. The wide variation in reported prevalence may indicate that permanent hypothyroidism is often assumed and thyroxine replacement given without review from the time of diagnosis.

Immaturity or block of thyroid TSH receptors or hormone biosynthetic mechanisms seem the likely basis of this disorder. Transplacental passage of maternal TSH-binding inhibitor immunoglobulins was shown to cause temporary hypothyroidism in three infants delivered of mothers with Hashimoto's disease (17). Antithyroid drugs (18), iodine deficiency (19), and iodine excess have also been implicated. Neonatal hypothyroidism has been described following amniofetography (20), and careful inquiry should be made for these factors before the abnormality is attributed to intrinsic mechanisms.

In view of the temporary nature of these disorders a case can be made for the withdrawal of T_4 at 12 months or sooner, with formal retesting of all infants with congenital hypothyroidism receiving replacement therapy.

4. A fourth disorder of TSH regulation in the neonate may persist beyond the first year (21). Physiological doses of T_4 fail to suppress elevated serum TSH in some infants with congenital hypothyroidism and increasing dosage leads to symptoms and signs of thyrotoxicosis. This condition, which is probably permanent, represents a higher than normal set point of the servomechanism, presumably conditioned by intrauterine hypothyroidism.

B. Low TSH Syndromes

1. Organic

Genetic and Congenital Abnormalities. In addition to these transient disorders a number of neonatal syndromes are described of permanent or familial hypothyroidism attributable to anomalous hypothalamic or pituitary development. They include TRH deficiency, isolated TSH deficiency, familial panhypopituitarism, and congenital absence of the pituitary. The basis of these disorders is unknown but could include agenesis of hypothalamic neurones, defective TRH synthesis or delivery, thyrotrope agenesis, or receptor insensitivity to TRH. Their combined incidence is about 1 in 10,000 births, which contrasts with the total incidence of congenital primary hypothyroidism of 1 in 4000 births (4).

Acquired Abnormalities in the Adult. Acquired abnormalities of the hypothalamus and pituitary are more usual, although developmental lesions such as craniopharyngioma may present for the first time in adult life. Infiltrations such as sarcoidosis, tuberculosis, and histiocytosis may declare their presence by symptoms of hypopituitarism without other systemic manifestations. The mechanism of central hypothyroidism is not always evident, but an acquired isolated defect of TSH is likely to be secondary to a hypothalamic lesion, particularly if accompanied by appetite or sleep disturbance or polyuria. In hypothyroidism complicating Sheehan's syndrome, almost total anterior pituitary infarction is usual, although there may be evidence of associated hypothalamic TRH failure (22), and hypothalamic hypothyroidism has been reported (23).

TSH deficiency from an expanding tumor such as a chromophobe adenoma occurs relatively late (after growth hormone and gonadotropin), a consequence perhaps of the small numbers of thyrotropes (3-5% of the total cell population) and their "remote" localization in the anteromedial hypophysis (24). Thyrotrope destruction and absence of TSH response to TRH is in fact uncommon. More often, TSH response is normal or blunted and failure of TRH delivery from distortion of the portal venous system may be the basis of the hypothyroidism. A delay in TSH rise following TRH is said to be suggestive of a hypothalamic lesion (24) even when serum T_4 is normal. A similar pattern is, however, sometimes seen in pituitary disease (26) and in both is attributed to a sluggish T_4/T_3 release and hence feedback on the thyrotropes. To complicate the matter further, prolonged TRH stimulation may be necessary to elicit a TSH response in long-standing TRH deficiency (27). Failure of TSH response to the standard TRH test is thus compatible with primary thyrotropic failure, but a normal response has little localizing value (see Sec. II.C).

Serum TSH Elevation in Central Hypothyroidism. Serum TSH levels may be unexpectedly normal or even mildly elevated (in 25% of patients) in central hypothyroidism (27). This pattern has been described in children with hypothalamic hypopituitarism but also in many patients with pituitary tumors (29). In over half, the TSH response to TRH is normal or exaggerated, but the thyroidal response judged by a rise in T_3 is impaired or absent, particularly in those with elevated basal TSH. Such a discrepancy between TSH and T_3 response could indicate thyroid atrophy from chronic understimulation, but ^{131}I uptake and serum T_3 response to injected TSH are usually normal. Dilution curves of serum samples in the TSH radioimmunoassay (RIA) show parallelism with the TSH standard, but cytochemical bioassay has shown significantly lower levels in basal and stimulated samples (30). The immunoreactive material is thus biologically inactive, although it does respond to feedback stimuli and falls with administered T_3 or dexamethasone.

2. Functional

A variety of functional abnormalities of TSH secretion occur in association with systemic illness or in the course of therapy of thyroid or unrelated disease. Low or normal serum TSH occurs in association with low T_3 (31) and sometimes T_4 (32) in nonspecific acute or chronic nonthyroidal illnesses. The mechanism of this central inhibition of TSH secretion is unclear, but a similar pattern is seen in such diverse conditions as acute and chronic starvation (33, 10), hepatic cirrhosis (34), chronic renal failure (35), and critical illness of almost any cause (32). In most of these conditions the TRH-stimulated TSH response is blunted or normal. Similarly, inappropriately low TSH levels are seen in thyrotoxic patients who develop hypothyroidism from antithyroid drugs or destructive therapy (36). Prolonged TSH suppression leads to thyrotrope insensitivity which may persist for some months. A similar mechanism is involved following withdrawal of thyroxine replacement in patients with primary hypothyroidism (37). In both situations thyroid status is better assessed by the serum thyroxine level.

A different mechanism is concerned in the hypothyroidism which develops in growth hormone-deficient children receiving human growth hormone (hGH) therapy (38). hGH administration causes a reduction in serum T_4, FT_4, and rT_3 with variable change in serum T_3 (39). In addition, there is inhibition of the TSH response to TRH (40) and acceleration of peripheral conversion of T_4 to T_3 (41). These effects cause clinical hypothyroidism in about half the children treated with hGH, and routine T_4 administration has been advocated to avoid consequent impairment of growth response (38).

C. High Serum TSH Syndromes

1. TSH-Secreting Pituitary Adenoma (TSH-Toxicosis)

The association of thyrotoxicosis, pituitary tumor, and elevated or inappropriate levels of serum TSH has now been reported in more than 20 patients (42, 43). In earlier reports (44, 45) TSH elevation was inferred or measured by biological assay and on one occasion at least the association of tumor and hyperthyroidism was shown to be fortuitous (46). TSH has since been measured by specific radioimmunoassay and its pituitary origin has been documented by electron microscopy and/or immunocytochemistry (47, 48). Pure thyrotrope and mixed tumors containing prolactin and growth hormone-secreting cells are described. The tumor TSH concentration is usually low, but the total content is 10-15 times higher than in the normal pituitary gland. Pituitary fossa enlargement is usual and almost half the patients have presented with visual field defects. Thyrotrope microadenomata are common in primary hypothyroidism but have not yet been described in TSH-toxicosis. The clinical picture is variable but the thyrotoxicosis is often mild and the diagnosis made after years of recurrent hyperthyroidism. The age range of reported cases is 11-60 years and in contrast to Graves' disease, there is a slight male predominance. The thyroid gland is usually only slightly enlarged and exophthalmos and dermopathy are absent. Bilateral exophthalmos was present in one patient with associated acromegaly (49) and unilateral proptosis was a presenting sign in another patient (44). Hypopituitarism with gonadotrophin deficiency and/or growth hormone deficiency is uncommon, but acromegaly (49) and amenorrhea/galactorrhea syndrome (42) are well documented. Serum TSH is usually moderately elevated, but levels as high as 120 μU/ml have been reported (43). It is sometimes within the normal range (49, 50), although inappropriate for the level of serum thyroxine. When measured, serum LATS has been consistently negative (48, 51). In most patients serum TSH and radioiodine uptake fail to suppress with administered T_3 and the TRH-stimulated response is absent. In others there is partial T_3 suppression (50, 51) and a variable and usually blunted response to TRH (2), suggesting an abnormality in the thyroid hormone feedback. Despite this, normal suppression of TSH has been demonstrated with dexamethasone, (52) somatostatin, and bromoergocryptine. Elevation of serum glycoprotein α subunits is characteristic of most (2) but not all (51) patients with this syndrome. The levels are higher than those observed in primary hypothyroidism and the α subunit/TSH ratio is increased. TSH β is undetectable (2). Elevation of free α subunits is also seen in acromegaly and other non-TSH-secreting pituitary tumors; also in malignant ectopic tumors (53) as well as normal subjects infused with thyrotropin. In this instance there is a parallel increase in TSH β subunits (3). When the pituitary fossa is enlarged the demonstration of increased levels of isolated serum α subunits excludes an "empty fossa" and indicates the presence of a pituitary tumor.

TSH-toxicosis has been cured by hypophysectomy, but the incidence of postoperative hypopituitarism is high (42). Selective adenomectomy with pituitary irradiation (48, 52) has been more successful in restoring euthyroidism without hypopituitarism.

2. TSH-Secreting Tumor in Primary Hypothyroidism

In experimental hypothyroidism in rats and mice, protracted overstimulation of the thyrotropes from low thyroid hormone levels leads to the formation of pituitary tumors (54). A similar sequence is seen in human primary hypothyroidism and both thyrotrope hyperplasia (55) and adenoma formation (56) are described. The tumor thyrotropes contain active secretory granules and are distinct from the "thyroid deficiency" cells in the hypothyroid human pituitary gland (55). Sella enlargement from a pituitary adenoma is generally thought to be associated with long-standing hypothyroidism, but in some patients the duration of thyroid deficiency has been relatively short. Sella volume correlates directly with the severity of the hypothyroidism and most patients have visual field defects by the time the diagnosis is made. The serum TSH level is appropriate to the ambient serum T_4 and in contrast to TSH-toxicosis the servomechanism is intact and TSH dynamics are usually normal. Mixed tumors are seen, and as with TSH-toxicosis (41), amenorrhea-galactorrhea may be presenting symptoms. Treatment with thyroxine may cause regression of the tumor with correction of visual field defect (57) and remodeling of the expanded fossa, although surgery may also be necessary (58).

3. Iodothyronine Resistance Syndromes

Tissue insensitivity to thyroid hormones has been described in two main groups of patients. In one there is a local selective insensitivity of the pituitary thyrotropes to the negative feedback action of thyroid hormone with consequent TSH-dependent hyperthyroidism (59). In the other there is additional resistance to iodothyronines in selected peripheral tissues with variable occurrence of goiter and clinical hypothyroidism (60, 61). A third, though unsubstantiated syndrome is peripheral iodothyronine unresponsiveness with intact central mechanisms (62, 63).

Local (Thyrotrope) Iodothyronine Resistance. Local thyrotrope resistance with normal peripheral responsiveness to thyroid hormones is postulated as the basis of this rare syndrome of clinical and biochemical hyperthyroidism with elevated serum TSH (59, 64). TSH secretion is, with occasional exceptions (65), partially responsive to T_3 and TRH. The TRH-stimulated α subunit/TSH ratio is normal in contrast to the poor TSH response and increased α/TSH when hypersecretion of TSH is caused by a pituitary tumor. The resistance syndrome is further distinguished by the presence of a normal pituitary fossa. This condition might be diagnosed more often if serum TSH was measured in all young thyrotoxic patients who lack the classic features of Graves' disease.

General (Tissue) Iodothyronine Resistance. This rare syndrome has been described in a few families and in a similar number of sporadic patients. It is characterized by elevated serum thyroid hormones and TSH but clinical euthyroidism or hypothyroidism. The clinical spectrum is wide, with features ranging from a familial syndrome with deaf mutism, hypothyroidism, and eiphyseal dysgenesis (60, 61) to recurrent goiter (66) or short stature in an otherwise normal individual (67). In the original family (60), deaf mutism, epiphyseal dysgenesis, and small goiter was usual. In others, evidence of tissue hypothyroidism (66) or goiter (67) is absent. The differing clinical presentation reflects the extent of the end organ defect, and this may be quite variable. TSH is usually partially or completely suppressible by T_3 and the TRH response is normal or even exaggerated (68). Studies of nuclear binding of $[^{125}I]$ T_3 in cultured fibroblasts in these patients indicate normal affinity and capacity, suggesting an abnormality in nonnuclear T_3 receptors, or in postreceptor processes (69). Disorders of thyroid hormone biosynthesis in which serum TSH elevation is physiological and "appropriate" are discussed in Chapter 29.

REFERENCES

1. Cornell JS, Pierce JG. The subunits of human pituitary thyroid stimulating hormone (isolation, properties and composition). J Biol J Med 1973; 248: 4327-4333.
2. Kourides IA, Ridgeway EC, Weintraub BD, Bigos ST, Gershengern MC, Maloof F. Thyrotropin-induced hyperthyroidism: use of alpha and beta subunit levels to identify patients with pituitary tumours. J Clin Endocrinol Metab 1977; 45:534-543.
3. Chan V, Wang C, Yeung RT. Thyrotropin: alpha and beta subunits of thyrotropin, and prolactin responses to four-hour constant infusions of thyrotropin-releasing hormone in normal subjects and patients with pituitary-thyroid disorders. J Clin Endocrinol Metab 1979; 49:127-131.
4. Fisher DA, Klein AH. Thyroid development and disorders of thyroid function in the new born. N Engl J Med 1981; 304:702-712.
5. Cadaccioni JL, Carayon P, Michel-Bechet M, Foucault F, Lefort G, Piernon H. Congenital hypothyroidism associated with thyrotropin unresponsiveness and thyroid cell membrane alterations. J Clin Endocrinol Metab 1980; 50:932-937.
6. Fisher DA, Odell DW. Effect of cold on TSH secretion in man. J Clin Endocrinol Metab 1971; 33:859-862.
7. O'Malley BP, Davies TJ, Rosenthal FD. TSH responses to temperature in primary hypothyroidism. Clin Endocrinol 1980; 13:87-94.
8. Larsen PR, Dick TE, Markovitz BP, Kaplan MM, Gard TG. Inhibition of intrapituitary thyroxine to 3,5,3-triiodothyronine conversion prevents the acute suppression of thyrotropin release by thyroxine in hypothyroid rats. J Clin Invest 1979; 64:117-128.
9. Oppenheimer JH, Schwartz HC, Surks MI. Tissue differences in the concentration of triiodothyronine nuclear binding sites in the rat: liver, kidney, pituitary, heart, brain, spleen and testis. Endocrinology 1974; 95:897-903.
10. Croxson MS, Ibbertson HK. Low serum triiodothyronine (T_3) and hypothyroidism in anorexia nervosa. J Clin Endocrinol Metab 1977; 44:167-174.
11. Larsen PR, Enrique Silva J, Kaplan MM. Relationship between circulating and intracellular thyroid hormones: physiological and clinical implications. Endocr Rev 1981; 2:87-102.
12. Alford FP, Baker HWG, Burger HG, de Kretser DM, Hudson B, Johns MW, Masterson JP, Patel YC, Rennie GC. Temporal patterns of integrated plasma hormone levels during sleep and wakefulness. I. Thyroid stimulating

hormone, growth hormone and cortisol. J Clin Endocrinol Metab 1973; 36:841-847.

13. Feek M, Sawers JSA, Brown NS, Seth J, Irvine WJ, Toft D. Influence of thyroid status on dopaminergic inhibition of thyrotropin and prolactin secretion: evidence for an additional feedback mechanism in the control of thyroid hormone secretion. J Clin Endocrinol Metab 1980; 51:585-589.
14. Petersen V, Rees Smith B, Hall R. A study of thyroid stimulating activity in human serum with the highly sensitive cytochemical bioassay. J Clin Endocrinol Metab 1975; 41:199-204.
15. Konishi J. Kasagi K, Iida Y, Endo K, Matsumura N, Yamado Y, Nohara Y, Kojima H, Mori T, Tomizuka K. TSH-binding inhibitor immunoglobulins in Hashimoto's disease and neonatal transient hypothyroidism. In *Thyroid Research VIII*, Stockigt JR, Nagataki S (eds), Proceedings of the VIIIth International Thyroid Congress, Sydney. Australian Academy of Science, Canberra, 1980, pp 555-558.
16. Fisher DA, Dussault JH, Foley TPR, La Franch S, Mitchell ML, Walfish PG. Screening for congenital hypothyroidism: results of screening one million North American infants. J Pediatr 1979;94:700-705.
17. Matsuura N, Yamada Y, Nohara Y, Konishi J, Kasagi K, Endo K, Kohima H, Wataya K. Familial neonatal transient hypothyroidism due to maternal TSH-binding inhibitor immunoglobulins. N Engl J Med 1980; 303:738-741.
18. Chenon RG, Kaplan MM, Larsen PR, Selenkow HA, Crigler JF. Neonatal thyroid function after propylthiouracil therapy for maternal Graves' disease. N Engl J Med 1981; 304:525-528.
19. Silva H, Silva S. Interrelationships among serum thyroxine, triiodothyronine, reverse triiodothyronine and thyroid-stimulating hormone in iodine-deficient pregnant women and their offspring. J Clin Endocrinol Metab 1981; 51:671-677.
20. Rodesch F, Camus M, Ermans AM, Dodion J, Delange F. Adverse effect of amniofetography on fetal thyroid function. Am J Obstet Gynecol 1976; 126:723-727.
21. Redmond GP, Soyka LF. Abnormal TSH secretory dynamics in congenital hypothyroidism. J Paediatr 1981; 98:83-85.
22. Singer PA, Nestman JH, Manning PR, Nicoloff JT. Assessment of thyrotropin-releasing hormone and thyrotropin reserve in man. J Clin Invest 1973; 52:1099-1107.
23. Singer PA, Mestman JH, Manning PR, et al. Hypothalamic-hypothyroidism secondary to Sheehan's syndrome. West J Med 1974; 120:416-418.
24. Phifer RF, Spier S. Immunocytochemical and histologic demonstration of thyrotropic cells of the human adenohypophysis. J Clin Endocrinol Metab 1973; 36:1210-1221.
25. Pittman JA Jr, Haigher ED Jr, Hershman JM, Pittman CS. Hypothalamic hypothyroidism. N Engl J Med 1971; 285:844-845.

26. McLaren EH, Hendricks S, Pimstone BL. Thyrotropin response to intravenous thyrotropin-releasing hormone in patients with hypothalamic and pituitary disease. Clin Endocrinol 1974; 3:113-122.
27. Patel YC, Burger HG. Serum thyrotropin (TSH) in pituitary and/or hypothalamic hypothyroidism: normal or elevated basal levels and paradoxical responses to thyrotropin-releasing hormone. J Clin Endocrinal Metab 1973; 34:190-196.
28. Illig R, Krawczynska H, Torresani T, Prader A. Elevated plasma TSH and hypothyroidism in children with hypothalamic hypopituitarism. J Clin Endocrinol Metab 1975; 41:722-728.
29. Faglia G, Bitensky L, Pinchera A, Ferrari C, Paracchi A, Beck-Peccoz P, Ambrosi B, Spada A. Thyrotropin secretion in patients with central hypothyroidism: evidence for reduced biological activity of immunoreactive thyrotropin. J Clin Endocrinol Metab 1979; 48:989-998.
30. Petersen VB, McGregor AM, Belehetz PE, Elkeles RS, Hall R. The secretion of thyrotropin with impaired biological activity in patients with hypothalamic-pituitary disease. Clin Endocrinol 1978; 8:397-402.
31. Cavalieri RR, Rapopart B. Impaired peripheral conversion of thyroxine to triiodothyronine. Annu Rev Med 1977; 28:57-65.
32. Kapstein EM, Grieb DA, Spencer CA, Wheeler WS, Nicoloff JT. Thyroxine metabolism in the low thyroxine state of critical non-thyroidal illness. J Clin Endocrinol Metab 1981; 53:764-771.
33. Croxson MS, Hall TD, Kletzky OA, Jaramillo JE, Nicoloff JT. Decreased serum thyrotropin induced by fasting. J Clin Endocrinol Metab 1977; 45: 560-568.
34. Nomura A, Pittman CS, Chambers JB, Buck MW, Shimizn T. Reduced peripheral conversion of thyroxine to triiodothyronine in patients with hepatic cirrhosis. J Clin Invest 1975; 56:543-552.
35. Gomez-Pan A, Alvarez-ude F, Yeo PPB, Hall R, Evered DC, Kerr DNS. Function of the hypothalmo-hypophyseal-thyroid axis in chronic renal failure. Clin Endocrinol 1979; 11:567-574.
36. Toft AD, Seth J, Hunter WM, Irvine WJ. Plasma thyrotrophin and serum thyroxine in patients becoming hypothyroid in early months after iodine-I^{131}. Lancet 1974; 1:704-705.
37. Vagenakis AG, Braverman LE, Azizi F, Portnay GI, Ingbar SH. Recovery of pituitary thyrotrophic function after withdrawal of prolonged thyroid-suppression therapy. N Engl J Med 1975; 293:681-684.
38. Rosenbloom AL, Riley WJ, Silverstein JH, Garncia AD, Netzloff ML, Weber J. Low dose single weekly injections of growth hormone: response during first year of therapy of hypopituitarism. Pediatrics 1980; 66:272-276.
39. Gacs Banos CS. The effect of growth hormone on the plasma levels of T_4, free-T_4, T_3, reverse T_3 and TBG in hypopituitary patients. Acta Endocrinol (Copenh) 1981; 96:475-479.

40. Lippe BM, Van Herle J, LaFranchi H, Uller RP, Lavin N, Kaplan SA. Reversible hypothyroidism in growth hormone deficient children treated with human growth hormone. J Clin Endocrinol Metab 1975; 40:612-618.
41. Sato T, Suzuki Y, Taketroni T et al. Enhanced peripheral conversion of thyroxine to triiodothyronine during HGH therapy in GH deficient children. J Clin Endocrinol Metab 1977;45:326-329.
42. Bevoit R, Pearson-Murphy BE, Roberts F, Marcovitz S, Hardy J, Tsoukas G, Gardiner RJ. Hyperthyroidism due to a pituitary TSH secreting tumour with amenorrhoea-galactorrhoea. Clin Endocrinol 1980; 12:11-19.
43. Afrasiabi A, Valenta L, Givinup G. A TSH secreting pituitary tumour causing hyperthyroidism: presentation of a case and review of the literature. Acta Endocrinol (Copenh) 1979; 92:448-454.
44. Jailer JW, Halub DA. Remissional Graves' disease following radiotherapy of a pituitary neoplasm. Am J Med 1960; 28:47.
45. Lamberg BA, Ripatti J, Gordin A, Juustila H, Sivula A, Bjon Kensten G. Chromophobe pituitary adenoma with acromegaly and TSH induced hyperthyroidism associated with parathyroid adenoma. Acta Endocrinol (Copenh) 1969; 60:157.
46. Sandler R. Recurrent hyperthyroidism in an acromegalic patient previously treated with proton beam irradiation: Graves' disease as probable etiology based on followup observations. J Clin Endocrinol Metab 1976; 42:163-168.
47. Duello TM, Halmi NS. Pituitary adenoma producing thyrotropin and prolactin. An immunocytochemical and electron microscopic study. Virchows Arch A: Pathol Anat Histol 1977; 376:255-265.
48. Jolis G, Bind C, Bertrand G, McKenzie JM, Ezrin C. Pituitary hyperthyroidism: case report and review of the literature. Am J Med 1978; 64:177-181.
49. Hamilton CR Jr, Maloof F. Acromegaly and toxic goitre. Cure of the hyperthyroidism and acromegaly by proton-beam partial hypophysectomy. J Clin Endocrinol 1972; 35:659-664.
50. Faglia G, Ferrari C, Neri V, Beck-Peccoz P, Ambioso B, Valentin F. High plasma thyrotropin levels in two patients with pituitary tumour. Acta Endocrinol (Copenh) 1972; 69:649-658.
51. Baylis PH. Case of hyperthyroidism due to a chromophobe adenoma. Clin Endocrinol 1976; 5:145-150.
52. Hamilton CR Jr, Levi CA, Maloof F. Hyperthyroidism due to thyrotropin-producing pituitary chromophobe adenoma. N Engl J Med 1970; 283:1077-1080.
53. Dosogne-Guerin M, Stalarczyk A, Borkoski A. Prospective study of the alpha and beta subunits of human chorionic gonadotrophin in the blood of patients with previous benign and malignant conditions. Eur J Cancer 1978; 14:525-532.
54. Furth J, Clifton KH. Experimental pituitary tumours. In *The Pituitary Gland,* Harris GW, Donovan BT (eds). Butterworth, Kent, England, 1966; pp 460-497.

55. Bonnys M, Pasteels JL, Herlant M, Vanhaelst L, Bastenie PA. Comparison between thyrotropin concentration and cell morphology of anterior pituitary in a symptomatic atrophic thyroiditis. J Clin Endocrinol Metab 1972; 35:722-728.
56. Katz MS, Gregerman RI, Horvath E, Kovaks K, Ezrin C. Thyrotroph cell adenoma of the human pituitary gland associated with primary hypothyroidism: clinical and morphological features. Acta Endocrinol (Copenh) 1980; 95:41-48.
57. Leiba S, Landan B, Ber A. Target gland insufficiency and pituitary tumours. Acta Endocrinol (Copenh) 1969; 60:112-120.
58. Grosvalet A, Garel L, Ernest C, Sauvegrain J. Pituitary adenoma secondary to hypothyroidism; radiological changes during treatment. Ann Radiol (Paris) 1980; 23:159-162.
59. Gershengkorn MC, Weintraub BD. Thyrotropin-induced hyperthyroidism caused by selective pituitary resistance to thyroid hormone. A new syndrome of "inappropriate" secretion of TSH. J Clin Invest 1975; 56:633-642.
60. Refetoff S, De Wind LT, De Groot LJ. Familial syndrome combining deaf mutism, stippled epiphyses, goitre and abnormally high PBI: possible target-organ refractoriness to thyroid hormone. J Clin Endocrinol Metab 1967; 27:279-283.
61. Refetoff S, De Groot LJ, Barsano LP. Defective thyroid hormone feedback regulation in the syndrome of peripheral resistance to thyroid hormone. J Clin Endocrinol Metab 1980; 51:41-45.
62. Hutchison JA, Arneil GC, McGirn EM. Deficiency of an extrathyroidal enzyme in sporadic cretinism. Lancet 1957; 2:314-316.
63. Weiner JD, Lindeboom GA. Observations on an unusual case of myxoedema. Acta Endocrinol (Copenh) 1962; 39:439-442.
64. Norogroder M, Utiger R, Boyan R, Levine LS. Juvenile hyperthyroidism with elevated thyrotropin (TSH) and normal 24 hour FSH, LH, GH and prolactin secretory patterns. J Clin Endocrinol Metab 1977; 45:1053-1059.
65. Emerson CH, Utiger RD. Hyperthyroidism and excessive thyrotropin excretion. N Engl J Med 1972; 287:328-333.
66. Lamberg BA. Congenital euthyroid goitre and partial peripheral resistance to thyroid hormones. Lancet 1973; 1:854.
67. Schneider G, Keiser HR, Bardin CW. Peripheral resistance to thyroxine: a cause of short stature in a boy without goitre. Clin Endocrinol 1975; 4:111-115.
68. Elewaut A, Mussche M, Vermeulen A. Familial partial target organ resistance to thyroid hormones. J Clin Endocrinol Metab 1976; 43:575-581.
69. Eil C, Fein H, Smith T, Funlanetto R, Bourgeois M, Weintraub BD. Nuclear binding of ^{125}I-T_3 in intact skin fibroblasts from patients with peripheral thyroid hormone resistance (PTHR). Abstract, 57th Meeting American Thyroid Association, Inc. Abstract T-2. Minneapolis, Minnesota, Sept 1981.

24

Vasopressin and Oxytocin

Peter H. Baylis
Royal Victoria Infirmary, Newcastle-Upon-Tyne, England

I. PHYSIOLOGY OF NEUROHYPOPHYSIAL HORMONES

A. Biosynthesis

Arginine vasopressin (AVP) and oxytocin (OXT) are small nonapeptides, molecular weights 1086 and 1007, respectively, secreted by the posterior lobe of the pituitary gland. Their chemical structure is very similar, with substitutions taking place at positions 3 and 8 (Fig. 1). The hormones are synthesized in two distinct hypothalamic regions called the supraoptic (SON) and paraventricular nuclei (PVN), but each is derived from separate neurones. The nonapeptides are initially synthesized as part of large precursor molecules called propressophysin and prooxyphysin (1), which are degraded to give AVP and OXT with their own specific neurophysin (carrier protein). The latter complex migrates along the axons to the sites of release (Fig. 2). Following stimulation, the nonapeptide and its neurophysin are cleaved and then released into the circulation. No physiological function has been ascribed to neurophysin other than a carrier protein within axons.

B. Arginine Vasopressin

The factors that regulate the secretion of AVP are well established (Fig. 2). Plasma tonicity is the major determinant (2). Changes in plasma osmolality of less than 1% affect AVP release, and there appears to be a direct linear relation between plasma osmolality and plasma AVP concentration (3). Other factors affecting AVP release are probably important only under pathophysiological conditions. Pain, stress, and emotion do not appear to be important stimuli for

ARGININE VASOPRESSIN

Cys–Tyr–Phe–Glu(NH_2)–Asp(NH_2)–Cys–Pro–Arg–Gly(NH_2)

OXYTOCIN

Cys–Tyr–Ileu–Glu(NH_2)–Asp(NH_2)–Cys–Pro–Leu–Gly(NH_2)

Figure 1 Structure of vasopressin and oxytocin.

AVP secretion (4). The hormone is cleared extremely rapidly from the circulation by the liver and kidneys, so that changes in plasma AVP are reflections of altered neurohypophysial secretion rather than clearance (5). The major physiological function of AVP is the absorption of solute-free water by the collecting tubules in the renal medulla, thus concentrating the urine. Increasing body water loss leads to hypertonicity of extracellular fluid, so stimulating the release of the hormone, which, in turn, conserves renal water loss. Under conditions of severe dehydration when the urine is maximally concentrated, another factor is required to maintain water balance (i.e., thirst). This sensation only becomes apparent at plasma osmolalities that stimulate sufficient AVP to cause maximally concentrated urine (3). Under similar conditions, plasma AVP may rise to levels that maintain blood pressure (6). Other functions of AVP remain controversial (e.g., memory) or are probably not relevant to physiological hormone concentrations (e.g., lipolysis).

C. Oxytocin

The stimuli that release OXT have been reviewed by Roberts (7). Little is known about OXT secretion in healthy men, but in lactating women suckling is a major stimulus. Estrogen, progesterone, and prostaglandin all modulate OXT release (8). Like AVP, the half-life of plasma OXT is extremely short, due to rapid clearance by the kidneys and liver. Oxytocinase, an enzyme present in the serum of pregnant humans, contributes to degradation (9). The physiologically significant actions of OXT appear to be confined to the female at term and during lactation (Fig. 2). No role has been found for the hormone in males.

II. INVESTIGATION OF DISORDERS OF POSTERIOR PITUITARY FUNCTION

A. Polyuria

Polyuria may be arbitrarily defined by a urine output greater than 2 liters per day and is caused by only three types of functional defect: (1) a deficiency of

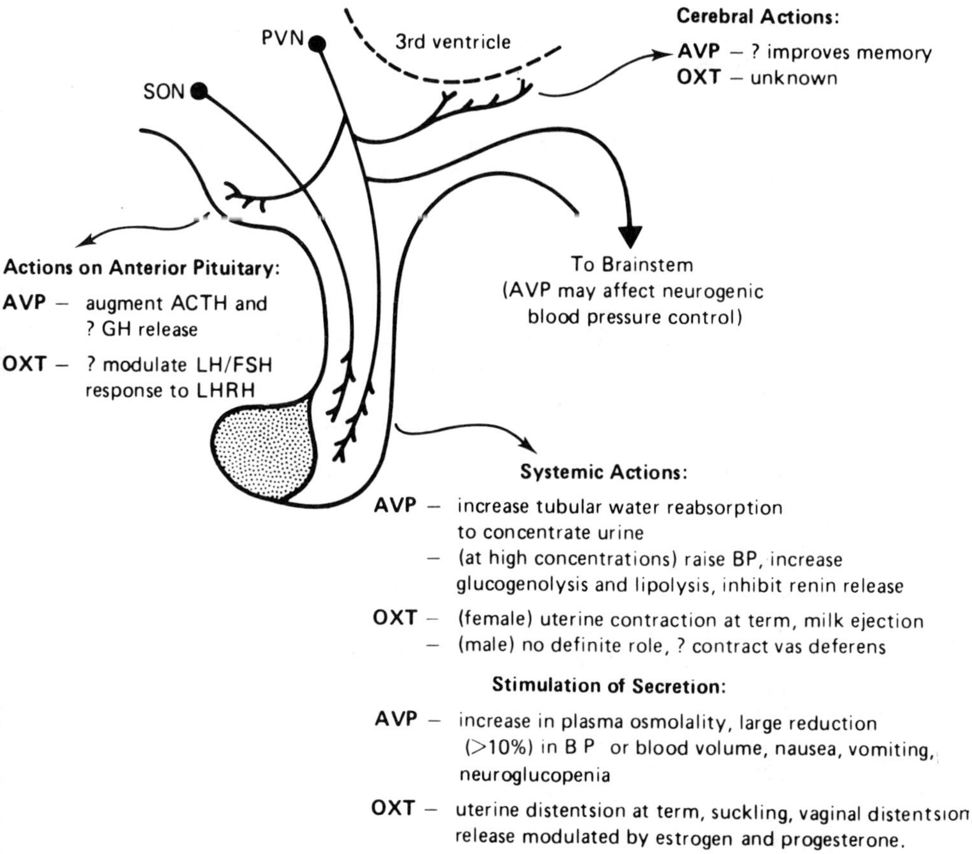

Figure 2 Summary of factors involved in secretion of vasopressin (AVP) and oxytocin (OXT) with their major functions.

AVP (cranial diabetes insipidus, CDI); (2) renal resistance to the action of AVP (nephrogenic diabetes insipidus, NDI); or (3) excessive water intake (primary polydipsia, PP). Acquired NDI (e.g., diabetes mellitus or hypercalcemia) accounts for the majority of cases of polyuria. Thirst is a common associated symptom. Each defect may result from a number of different causes which are summarized in Table 1.

Table 1 Causes of Polyuria

1. Cranial diabetes insipidus
    - Familial
        - Dominant or recessive inheritance
        - Syndrome including diabetes mellitus, optic atrophy, nerve deafness, atonia of bladder
    - Acquired
        - Idiopathic
        - Trauma (neurosurgery, head injury)
        - Tumors (large pituitary tumor, metastases, craniopharyngioma)
        - Granuloma (sarcoidosis, histiocytosis)
        - Infections (meningitis, encephalitis)
        - Vascular (Sheehan's syndrome, sickle cell disease, aneurysms)
2. Nephrogenic diabetes insipidus
    - Familial
        - Sex-linked recessive
    - Acquired
        - Metabolic (hypercalcemia, hypokalemia)
        - Postobstructive uropathy (prostatic, ureteral)
        - Infectious (pyelonephritis)
        - Toxic (lithium, demeclocycline)
        - Solute overload (glycosuria)
        - Chronic renal disease (polycystic disease, amyloid, sickle cell disease, sarcoid)
3. Primary polydipsia
    - Acquired
        - Idiopathic
        - Psychotic states

1. Cranial Diabetes Insipidus

Symptoms of CDI develop after destruction of at least 80% of the AVP-synthesizing neurones. Idiopathic CDI accounts for approximately half of the cases (Table 1). In most patients hypertonic dehydration occurs secondarily to the polyuria, which stimulates the thirst mechanism. Rarely, the thirst sensation is lost. The combination of CDI and adipsia is potentially lethal because of progressive dehydration. Such patients require constant monitoring of fluid balance and plasma osmolality. A similar serious situation occurs in CDI patients with normal thirst who are denied access to water.

Once CDI has become established it rarely improves spontaneously. Trauma to the hypothalamus or the pituitary stalk from surgery or head injury may result in a fluctuating release of AVP. Transient polyuria lasting between 24 hr and a few weeks may develop after trauma. Although the majority of these patients will then retain normal water balance, a few will revert to persistent CDI (10). Occasionally, patients continue to drink water in excess despite their posterior pituitary function returning to normal, suggesting that CDI has been converted to primary polydipsia (11).

Adrenocortical insufficiency is associated with impaired water excretion (12). Consequently, CDI may be masked in hypoadrenal patients, and it will only become apparent after steroid replacement. Thus it is wise to check the pituitary-adrenal axis before formally testing water excretion.

The investigation of CDI may be divided into two aspects: (1) defining the functional abnormality and (2) discovering the underlying cause.

The basis of establishing the diagnosis of CDI rests on stimulating the posterior pituitary gland with an adequate osmotic stimulus. This may be achieved by either dehydration or infusion of hypertonic saline. Fluid restriction is probably more physiological than saline infusion. Dashe and co-workers (13) described a 6½-hr fluid deprivation test. They investigated healthy individuals, hospitalized controls, and patients with polyuria (urine volume > 21-24 hr). None of the normals had increases of plasma osmolality greater than 6 mmol/kg and the final value was less than 300 mmol/kg. The ratio of urine to plasma osmolalities of the final samples was always greater than 1.9 and urine osmolality was greater than 630 mmol/kg in normal subjects. The patients with presumed CDI had a ratio of 1.23 ± 0.53 (mean ± SD) and the majority of final urine osmolalities was less than 630 mmol/kg, but a number of results overlapped with the normal range. A major problem occurred in differentiating partial CDI from primary polydipsia (PP). The dehydration test has been refined by Miller et al. (14). These workers continued dehydrating patients until urine osmolality, measured at hourly intervals, became constant. This required, on occasions, dehydration up to 18 hr. Patients with CDI failed to achieve urine osmolalities greater than 740 mmol/kg.

After the period of fluid deprivation, exogenous vasopressin must be administered to observe whether the polyuria is vasopressin sensitive. Now that the synthetic AVP analog desmopressin (DDAVP) is available, the problems associated with the administration of Pitressin have been overcome. Desmopressin given in the dose 40 μg intranasally or 2 μg intramuscularly will increase the urine osmolality above 650 mmol/kg in CDI, but there will be little or no response in patients with NDI or PP (15).

Dehydration tests can be most unpleasant for the patients and are bedevilled with pitfalls. Patients should be fasted, but allowed *only* water to drink before fluid restriction. Tea, coffee, and tobacco taken immediately before the test can all cause spurious results. Supervision of the patient is necessary at all times to avoid surreptitious drinking. Patients must be able to empty their bladders completely. The test should stop if weight loss is greater than 5% of the initial body weight. Although the results of urine and plasma osmolalities may distinguish severe abnormalities, there is considerable overlap between normal values and mild cases of CDI, NDI, and PP (13, 14).

Direct measurement of plasma AVP following osmotic stimulation is able to overcome some of these difficulties. Unfortunately, the AVP immunoassay is difficult to establish and perform, and is readily available only in a few centers. The test is based on the infusion of hypertonic saline which has been advocated by Moses and Streeten (16) to differentiate polyuric states, but plasma AVP is measured at regular intervals during the infusion. Patients with CDI often have detectable plasma AVP (4, 17), which is subnormal relative to plasma osmolality (Fig. 3a). This test readily differentiates PP from even the mildest form of CDI, but fails to distinguish between PP and NDI. It possesses the potential hazard of inducing congestive cardiac failure but is more pleasant for most patients since it lasts only 2 hr. Furthermore, there is usually an abrupt onset of thirst during the test which enables investigators to examine this important aspect of water regulation.

Recent work comparing the efficacy of dehydration tests to saline infusion tests with plasma AVP measurements in diagnosing CDI showed alarming discrepancies (18). There were numerous false negatives and a few false positives in diagnosing CDI using fluid deprivation tests.

Nonosmotic stimulation of AVP by nicotine or hypotension has been advocated by some investigators. A systematic investigation of 18 polyuric patients clearly indicated that none of the three nonosmotic stimuli (hypotension, nausea, hypoglycemia) were of use in differentiating the cause of polyuria (19).

The second aspect of the investigation of CDI is the diagnosis of the underlying cause. Although 50% of cases are idiopathic, it is important to exclude underlying pathology. A comprehensive history and examination may give important clues about trauma, the congenital form of the disease, or vascular incidents (Table 1). It is essential that x-rays of the skull are taken followed by CT scanning of the head if there is any suspicion of a pituitary tumor or a mass in the suprasellar region. Plotting of visual fields by perimetry may also be necessary. A hypothalamic lesion may be suspected if serum prolactin is elevated in the absence of a pituitary tumor.

2. Nephrogenic Diabetes Insipidus

The acquired form of NDI is the commonest cause of polyuria. The hallmark of the disorder is vasopressin-resistant polyuria. Almost any form of chronic renal disease may result in NDI. The various causes listed in Table 1 produce NDI by

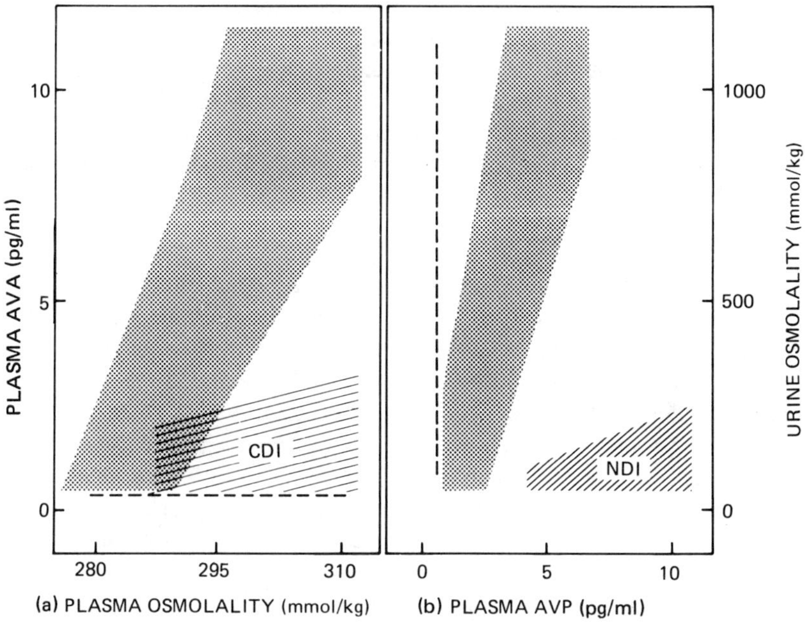

Figure 3 (a) Relationship of plasma AVP to plasma osmolality during infusion of 5% saline in normals (stippled area) and patients with CDI (shaded area). (b) Relationship of urine osmolality to plasma AVP after overnight dehydration in normals and patients with NDI. (From Ref. 28.)

many different mechanisms which have been reviewed in detail by Epstein (20). Familial NDI is very rare, presents early in life at about 6-8 weeks after birth, and may be associated with other tubular defects in the kidney.

Patients with NDI develop hypertonic dehydration and rely on their thirst mechanism to maintain plasma tonicity. In response to fluid restriction, the patients fail to achieve maximally concentrated urine (i.e., urine osmolality <630 mmol/kg) and the administration of desmopressin (DDAVP) fails to increase urine osmolality further. However, rather like the results in CDI, there is a large area of overlap between normal responses and the various types of NDI. A quick and easy method of confirming NDI is to relate plasma AVP to urine osmolality after a period of dehydration (Fig. 3b). Urine osmolality will always be inappropriately low in relation to plasma AVP. Osmoregulation of AVP remains normal in NDI, so that infusion of hypertonic saline will cause a satisfactory rise in plasma AVP. The Dashe type of dehydration test was recently compared to the direct measurement of plasma AVP in a group of hypercalcemic patients (21).

There was good correlation between the tests, and normal osmoregulation was also confirmed in this group of NDI patients.

To determine the cause of acquired NDI simple measurements of serum calcium, glucose, urea, and potassium are essential. Investigation of the renal tract by intravenous pyelography or ultrasound may be necessary. Withdrawal of toxic drugs and correction of electrolyte disturbances often restores vasopressin sensitivity (21).

3. Primary Polydipsia

Excessive fluid intake from any cause will suppress AVP secretion to allow polyuria. Plasma osmolality does not fall below 284 mmol/kg until the fluid intake exceeds 15-20 liters per day. However, patients with PP rarely develop hyponatremia. The chronic fluid load results in a decrease in the tonicity of the interstitial renal medulla so that, even, in the presence of adequate AVP, maximally concentrated urine cannot be excreted because the osmotic gradient across the collecting duct is reduced. This abnormality has been recognized for many years (22) and explains why the patients fail to respond normally to dehydration tests.

The causes of PP have not been well delineated (Table 1). It is presumed that the patients have some abnormality of their thirst mechanism. A few patients show subtle abnormalities of AVP secretion on dynamic testing, but osmoregulation of AVP appears to be normal (19). Consequently, there may be a more diffuse hypothalamic disorder rather than one affecting thirst alone. It is always important to check that patients who complain of thirst are not taking drugs known to dry the mouth (e.g., psychotropic agents)! Some patients have personality or psychiatric disorders.

As has already been indicated, fluid deprivation tests are difficult to interpret in this group of patients. Unless they have been closely supervised during the test, there is always an uncertainty that they may have drunk during the study. The classic response to dehydration is a submaximal urine concentration ($<$ 630 mmol/kg) combined with failure to respond further after exogenous vasopressin administration (13, 14, 23). But, as demonstrated by Zerbe and Robertson (18), there is a wide margin of error. Therefore, an infusion of hypertonic saline with plasma AVP measurement should be performed, together with a dehydration test to relate urine osmolality to plasma AVP. Both sets of results should fall within the normal distribution shown in Figure 3.

B. Syndrome of Inappropriate Antidiuresis

Excessive secretion of AVP was reintroduced as a cause of hyponatremia by Schwartz et al. in 1957 (23). They argued that persistent AVP release together with ingestion of normal quantities of fluid would lead to a hypotonic, normovolemic patient. The authors recognized that AVP might be released by non-

Table 2 Disorders Associated with the Syndrome of Inappropriate Antidiuresis

1. Tumors
   - Carcinoma (bronchus, duodenum, pancreas, prostate, bladder)
   - Lymphoma
   - Leukemia
   - Thymoma
   - Sarcoma
   - Carcinoid (bronchus)
2. Pulmonary disease
   - Pneumonia
   - Tuberculosis
   - Empyema
   - Pneumothorax
   - Positive-pressure ventilation
3. Neurological disorders
   - Meningitis
   - Encephalitis
   - Brain abscess
   - Guillain-Baré syndrome
   - Acute intermittent porphyria
   - Subarachnoid hemorrhage
   - Cerebellar and cerebral atrophy
   - Cavernous sinus thrombosis
   - Shy-Drager syndrome
4. Drugs
   - Vasopressin
   - Oxytocin
   - Vincristine, vinblastine, cyclophosphamide
   - Chlorpropamide
   - Thiazide diuretics
   - Phenothiazines
   - Tricyclic antidepressants
   - Monoamine oxidase inhibitors
   - Carbamazepine
   - Clofibrate
   - Nicotine
5. Miscellaneous
   - Acute psychosis
   - Hypothyroidism
   - Glucocorticoid deficiency
   - Trauma
   - Idiopathic

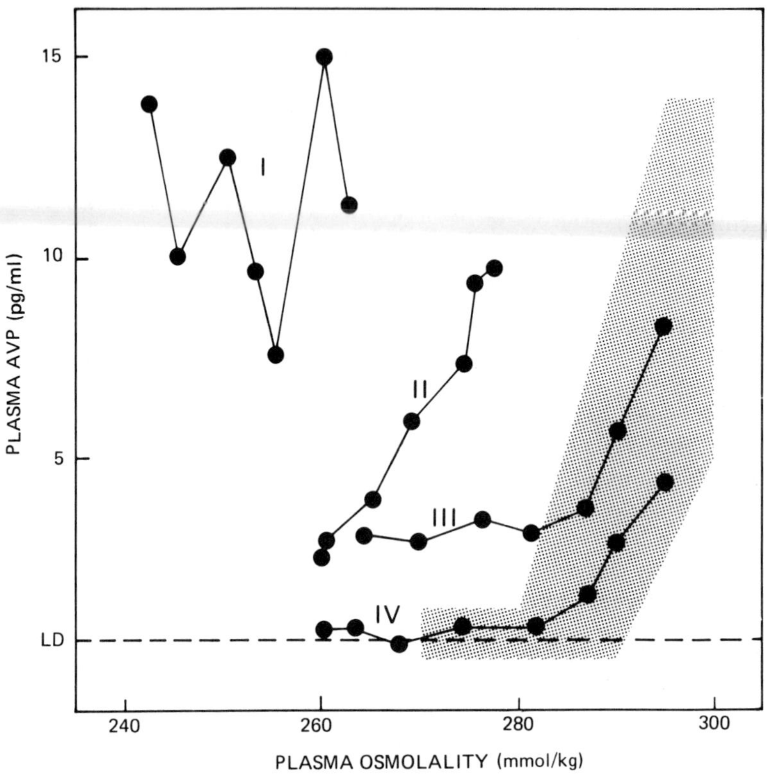

Figure 4 Types of plasma AVP response to hypertonic saline infusion in patients with SIAD. (From Ref. 24. Reproduced, with permission, from the Annual Review of Medicine, vol 31. © 1980 by Annual Reviews Inc.)

osmotic stimuli, so they carefully defined a set of criteria which excluded some of these stimuli and which would characterize the syndrome of inappropriate antidiuresis (SIAD). Hypotonic hyponatremia should be associated with a urine osmolality greater than that of plasma, persistent urinary sodium excretion, normal blood pressure and blood volume, and normal renal and adrenal function (24).

A large number of disorders associated with hyponatremia which are believed to be due to SIAD have been described (Table 2). Unfortunately, the criteria for SIAD have not been fulfilled in some of the reported associations, and are therefore open to strong criticism.

Direct measurement of plasma AVP has confirmed the "inappropriate" AVP levels in some diseases associated with SIAD. An extensive study of 79 patients with SIAD revealed that there appear to be at least four patterns of AVP secretion in this disorder (24). They are described in Figure 4. Patients with type I show erratic AVP secretion completely unrelated to plasma osmolality. A second group demonstrate resetting of the osmoregulatory system at lower osmolalities. Some patients (type III) have normal osmoregulation at high plasma osmolality but fail to suppress AVP secretion at lower levels. Finally, a few patients have normal osmoregulation, yet fulfill the criteria for SIAD. None of these patterns is associated with any particular cause of SIAD (24, 25). Bronchogenic carcinoma with SIAD may have any one of the four types (26), but type I is most common. Thus, although defining the functional disorder in AVP secretion does not aid diagnosis of the cause of SIAD, it does confirm that the hyponatremia is due to SIAD.

The majority of patients with SIAD do not have specific clinical features. Rarely, if hyponatremia is severe (pNa $<$ 110 mmol/liter) or rapid in onset, cerebral symptoms of confusion, nausea, irritability, or fits may develop.

Investigation of the hyponatremic patient has been recently reviewed (26, 27). Clearly, patients with suspected SIAD should fulfil Schwartz's criteria. They should have a dilutional hyponatremia, urine sodium excretion $>$ 20 mmol/liter, normal renal function defined by creatinine clearance, and satisfactory adrenal function (plasma cortisol $>$ 800 nmol/liter 1 hr after 0.25 mg of Synacthen, i.v.). Confirmation of the diagnosis is made by measuring plasma AVP during infusion of hypertonic saline, which will also define the type of SIAD. Administration of a water load (20 ml/kg) will not give further information and will only demonstrate failure of water excretion. One hour after water ingestion patients with SIAD show the normal reduction in plasma osmolality of 8-12 mmol/kg, but their urine osmolality will not fall below 150 mmol/kg at any time. Healthy adults excrete 80-120% of the water load by 4 hr.

The underlying cause of SIAD must be investigated. Often the diagnosis is obvious, but due attention should be given to the many drugs apparently associated with SIAD (Table 2). Chest x-ray must be performed and neurological investigations may be necessary. However, tumors responsible for SIAD may be extremely small and may take years to be clinically manifest.

C. Oxytocin

No disorders of OXT secretion have yet been described. Although OXT has been isolated from some nonendocrine tumors, it appears to be clinically insignificant. Patients with severe CDI do not suffer from delayed onset of labor or from difficulty breast feeding. There are no tests of OXT secretion or function in clinical practice.

Diagnostic Summary 1 Diabetes Insipidus

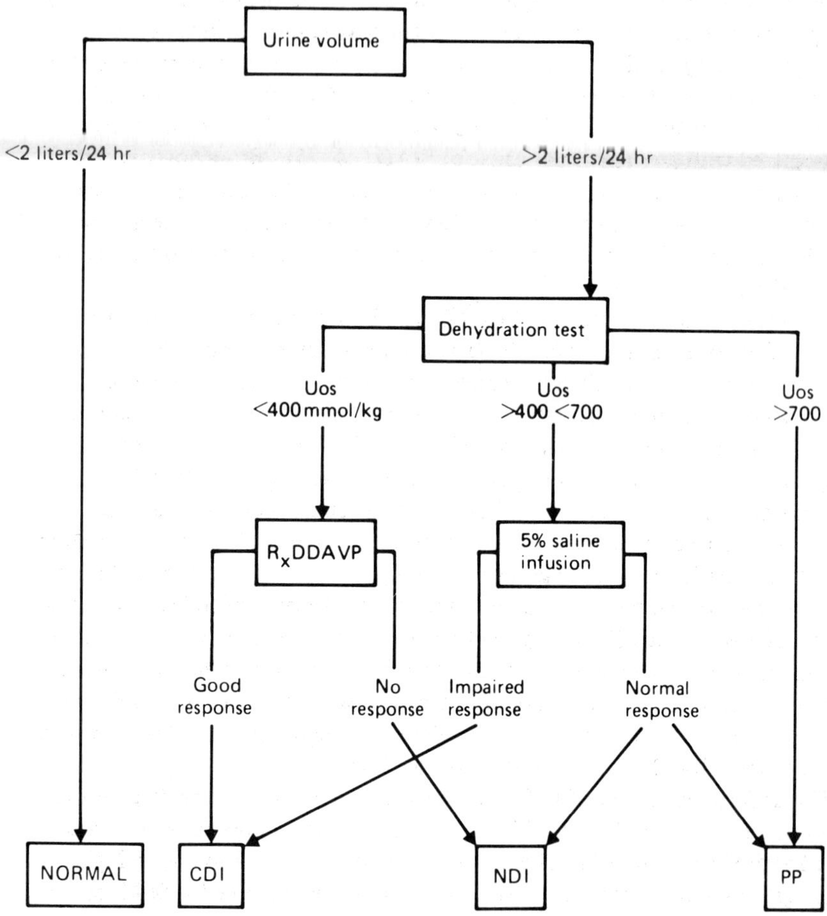

Diagnostic Summary 2 Hyponatremia

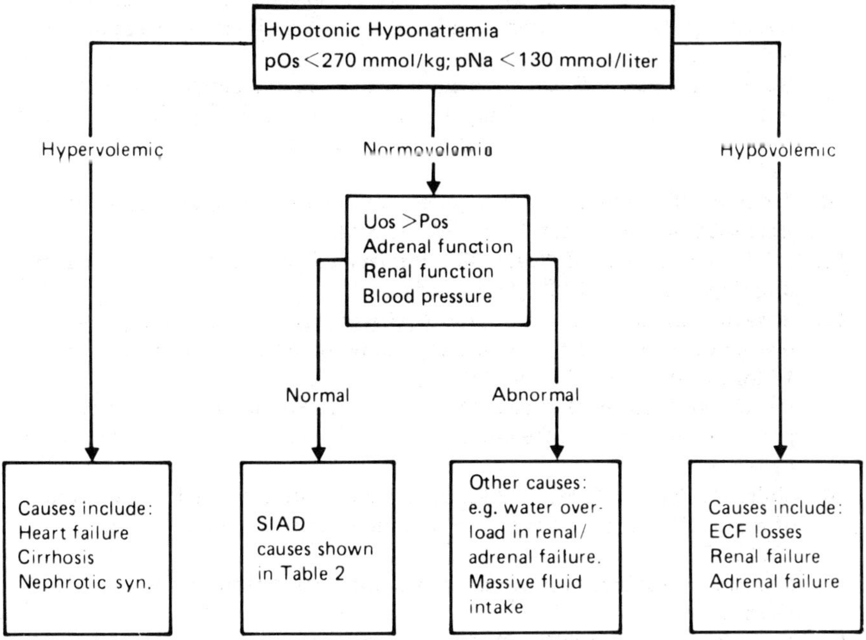

REFERENCES

1. Russell JT, Brownstein MJ, Gainer H. Biosynthesis of vasopressin, oxytocin, and neurophysins: isolation and characterization of two common precursors (propressophysin and prooxyphysin). Endocrinology 1980; 107: 1880-1891.
2. Bie P. Osmoreceptors, vasopressin, and control of renal water excretion. Physiol Rev 1980; 60:961-1048.
3. Robertson GL, Shelton RL, Athar S. The osmoregulation of vasopressin. Kidney Int 1976; 10:25-37.
4. Robertson GL. The regulation of vasopressin function in health and disease. Recent Prog Horm Res 1977; 33:333-385.
5. Lauson HD. Metabolism of the neurohyphysial hormones. In Knobil E, Sawyer WH (eds). *Handbook of Physiology,* sec 7, *Endocrinology,* vol 4, pt 1. American Physiology Society, Washington, DC, 1974, pp 287-393.
6. Aisenbrey GA, Handelman WA, Arnold P, Manning M, Schrier RW. Vascular effects of arginine vasopressin during fluid deprivation in the rat. J Clin Invest 1981; 67:961-968.

7. Roberts JS. Oxytocin. In *Annual Research Reviews,* Horrobin DR (ed). Churchill Livingstone, Edinburgh, 1977, pp 1-78.
8. Prilusky J, Deis RP. Inhibitory effect of prostaglandin F2α on oxytocin release and on milk ejection in lactating rats. J Endocrinol 1976; 69:395-399.
9. Ressler C, Popenoe EA. Oxytocin. Purification and biochemical characterization. In *Methods in Investigative and Diagnostic Endocrinology,* Berson EA, Yalow RS (eds). North-Holland, Amsterdam, 1973, vol 2A, pp 681-691.
10. Timmons RL, Dugger GS. Water and salt metabolism following pituitary stalk section. Neurology 1969; 19:790-800.
11. Stevko RM, Balsley M, Segan WE. Primary polydipsia—compulsive water drinking. J Pediatr 1968; 73:845-851.
12. Boykin J, deTorrente A, Erickson A, Robertson G, Schrier RW. Role of plasma vasopressin in impaired water excretion of glucocorticoid deficiency. J Clin Invest 1978; 62:738-744.
13. Dashe AM, Cramm RE, Crist CA, Habener JF, Solomon DH. A water deprivation test for the differential diagnosis of polyuria. JAMA 1963; 185: 699-703.
14. Miller M, Dalakos T, Moses AM, Fellerman H, Streeten DHP. Recognition of partial defects in antidiuretic hormone secretion. Ann Intern Med 1970; 73:721-729.
15. Monson JP, Richards P. Desmopressin urine concentration test. Br Med J 1978; 1:24.
16. Moses AM, Streeten DHP. Differentiation of polyuric states by measurement of responses to changes in plasma osmolality induced by hypertonic saline infusions. Am J Med 1967; 42:368-377.
17. Baylis PH, Robertson GL. Vasopressin response to hypertonic saline infusion to assess posterior pituitary function. J R Soc Med 1980; 73:255-260.
18. Zerbe RL, Robertson GL. Comparison of direct and indirect tests of vasopressin function. Clin Res 1980; 28:271A.
19. Baylis PH, Gaskill MB, Robertson GL. Vasopressin secretion in primary polydipsia and cranial diabetes insipidus. Q J Med 1981; 50:345-358.
20. Epstein FH. Disturbances of Renal Concentrating Ability. In *Disturbances in Body Fluid Osmolality,* Andreoli TE, Grantham JJ, Rector FC Jr (eds). American Physiological Society, Bethesda, Md, 1977, pp 251-265.
21. Baylis PH, Milles JJ, Wilkinson R, Heath DA. Vasopressin secretion in hypercalcaemia. Clin Endocrinol (Oxf) 1981; 15:343-351.
22. de Wardener HE, Herxheimer A. The effect of a high water intake on the kidneys ability to concentrate the urine in man. J. Physiol (Lond) 1957; 139:42-52.
23. Schwartz WB, Bennett W, Curelop S, Bartter FC. A syndrome of renal sodium loss and hyponatremia probably resulting from inappropriate secretion of antidiuretic hormone. Am J Med 1957; 23:529-542.

24. Zerbe R, Stropes L, Robertson G. Vasopressin function in the syndrome of inappropriate antidiuresis. Annu Rev Med 1980; 31:315-327.
25. Robertson GL. The physiopathology of ADH secretion. In *Clinical Neuroendocrinology,* Tolis G, Labrie F, Martin JB, Naftolin F (eds). Raven, New York, 1979, pp 247-260.
26. Baylis PH. Hyponatraemia and hypernatraemia. Clin Endocrinol Metab 1980; 9:625-637.
27. Mitchell DM, Kennedy PGE. Hyponatraemia and its management. Hosp Update 1979; 5:755-771.
28. Baylis PH. Disorders of antidiuretic hormone secretion. Med Int 1981; 1:249-252.

ADRENAL DISORDERS

25
Androgens and Glucocorticoids

A. Wayne Meikle and Don H. Nelson
University of Utah School of Medicine, Salt Lake City, Utah

As shown in Figure 1, four major products or classes of steroid hormones are produced by the adrenal cortex: mineralocorticoid (mainly aldosterone), glucocorticoids (cortisol and corticosterone), androgens (androstenedione, dehydroepiandrosterone, and dehydroepiandrosterone sulfate), and small quantities of estrogens (estradiol and estrone) (1-6). The quantity of adrenal androgens produced by the adrenal cortex relative to cortisol is summarized in Table 1. Aldosterone is produced predominantly in the zona glomerulosa, and its synthesis is under complex control by many factors, but the renin-angiotensin system is predominant. Cortisol is secreted mainly by the zona fasiculata with a small proportion by the zona reticularis, and secretion is controlled by adrenocorticotrophic hormone (ACTH). Adrenal androgens are produced mainly in the zona reticularis, but some synthesis also occurs in the zona fasciculata. Current knowledge of the control of adrenal androgen secretion is incomplete. ACTH has profound influences, but there is evidence that pituitary factors other than ACTH also have major effects on adrenal androgen production, particularly during the prepubertal period (1).

Testosterone and its potent 5α-reduced metabolite, 5α-dihydrotestosterone (DHT), are important in normal sexual differentiation (7). Testosterone is responsible for virilization of the male internal genital tract and DHT causes development of the male external genitalia. In normal males, at puberty, testosterone is responsible for growth of the phallus, scrotum, skeletal muscle, and larynx. Sexual orientation also appears to be influenced by testosterone or an estrogenic metabolite. DHT produces virilization of the prostate and skin, including male-pattern hair growth, acne, and temporal hair recession (7). The adrenals secrete

Cholesterol						
↓ (1)						
Δ^5 pregnenolone	(2 & 7) →	17-OH pregnenolone	(8) →	Dehydroepiandrosterone		
↓ (2)		↓ (2)		↓ (2)		
Progesterone	(7) →	17-OH progesterone	(8) →	Androstenedione	(9) ↔	Testosterone
↓ (3)		↓ (3)		↓ (10)		↓ (10)
Deoxycorticosterone (DOC)	→	Deoxycortisol (S)		Estrone	(9) ↔	Estradiol
↓ (4)		↓ (4)				
Corticosterone (B)		Cortisol (F)				
↓ (5, 6)						
Aldosterone						

20-hydroxylase
22-hydroxylase (1)
20-22 desmolase
3β-hydroxysteroid dehydrogenase (2)
21-hydroxylase (3)
11β-hydroxylase (4)
18-hydroxylase (5)
and
18-dehydrogenase (6)

17α-hydroxylase (7)
17,20-desmolase (8)
17-hydroxysteroid oxidoreductase (9)
aromatase (10)

Figure 1 Adrenal cortical steroid biosynthesis.

Table 1 Human Adrenal Androgen Production Rates and Plasma Content[a]

Steroid	Abbreviation	Rate (%)	Plasma content (%)
Cortisol	F	100	100
Dehydroepiandrosterone sulfate	DHAS	125	2000
Dehydroepiandosterone	DHA	8	4
Androstenedione	Δ4	3	2
Testosterone	T	0.06	0.5 (female) 0.5 (male)

[a]Relative to cortisol.

very limited quantities of 5α-reduced metabolites of testosterone, but major secretory products of the adrenal cortex may be metabolized to 5α-reduced androgens in peripheral tissues.

The major androgens secreted by the adrenal cortex are weak androgens when tested in bioassay systems. If they are produced in large quantities, however, a sufficient amount may be converted to more potent androgens and produce masculinization of the external genitalia in a female fetus. Overproduction during childhood produces rapid skeletal maturation, premature epiphyseal closure, and virilization in both sexes. Excessive androgen production in postpubertal women results in virilization (7a).

I. CONGENITAL ADRENAL HYPERPLASIA

An inherited enzyme defect in cortisol biosynthesis results in a compensatory increase in ACTH-stimulated androgen secretion and produces congenital adrenal hyperplasia (Table 2). The specific enzyme deficiencies, which are inherited as autosomal recessive, result in characteristic forms of the andrenogenital syndrome (Table 3). Some enzyme systems for steroid biosynthesis are common to both the adrenal cortex and gonads and produce abnormal steroid secretion from both glands.

A. 21-Hydroxylase Deficiency

Of the various forms of congenital adrenal hyperplasia, 21-hydroxylase deficiency is the most common. It is inherited as an autosomal recessive (8). The incidence of the salt-losing form of 21-hydroxylase deficiency varies considerably among populations (8-10). The incidence of the deficiency is 1 in 4000 to

Table 2 Types of Congenital Adrenal Hyperplasia, Enzyme Deficiencies, and Effects Produced

Congenital adrenal hyperplasia enzyme deficiency	Ambiguity of genitalia		Enzyme deficiency and effects			Puberty	
	Male	Female	Frequency	Salt loss	Hypertension	Induction required	Precocious
Partial 21-hydroxylase	−	+	95%	±	−	−	+
More complete 21-hydroxylase	−	+		+	−	−	+
11β-Hydroxylase	−	+	4%	−	±	−	±
17α-Hydroxylase	−	+	Rare	−	+	+	−
3β-ol-Dehydrogenase	+	±	Rare	+	−	+	−
Prior to Δ^5-pregnenolone	+	−	Rare	+	−	+	−
Virilizing adrenal tumor	−	±	Rare	−	±	−	+

Table 3 Diagnostic Tests Laboratory Confirmation of Congenital Adrenal Hyperplasia

Enzyme defect	ACTH	Plasma cortisol	Steroid precursor	17-Ketosteroids	Elevated metabolite
Partial 21-hydroxylase	↑	N or ↓	17-Hydroxyprogesterone	↑	Pregnanetriol
Complete 21-hydroxylase	↑	↓	17-Hydroxyprogesterone	↑	Pregnanetriol
11β-Hydroxylase	↑	↓	DOC or S	↑	THS, THDOC
17α-Hydroxylase	↑	↓	Progesterone	↓	Pregnanediol
3β-ol-dehydrogenase	↑	↓	Pregnenolone	↓	Pregnenediol
Prior to Δ^5-pregnenolone	↑	↓	None	↓	None

N, normal; ↑, increased; ↓, decreased.

1 in 15,000 births in Europe and in the United States, with a gene frequency of 1 in 35 to 1 in 128. It is even more common (1 in 490) in Yupik Eskimos of Alaska (11). The incidence of various forms of congenital adrenal hyperplasia may be underestimated; the diagnosis may be unrecognized in neonates who die from unexplained causes such as acute adrenal crisis and the salt-losing form of 21-hydroxylase deficiency. The 21-hydroxylation gene is located on the short arm of chromosome 6 in close association to the locus for the histocompatibility gene HLA-B (12). HLA typing has been used to detect heterozygotes and cryptic homozygotes in families of known affected individuals (12).

Excessive secretion of adrenal androgens in the female fetus produces masculinization of the external genitalia, enlargement of the clitoris, and various degrees of labioscrotal fusion (13, 14). With marked fusion, the neonates are mistaken for cryptorchid males with or without hypospadias. The internal sexual structures and gonads remain normal. Slight enlargement of the phallus and scrotal pigmentation at birth may occur in males, whereas others have no detectable abnormalities of the external genitalia. Progressive virilization occurs in both sexes during childhood. Early appearance of pubic and axillary hair is observed; and somewhat later, facial hair, increased body hair, and acne are noted. Deepening of the voice, phallic enlargement with erections, and rapid somatic bone and muscle growth are present. These children are taller than normal, but short adult stature results from early closure of the epiphyses. Menses are absent in most girls and the testes are small in the majority of boys due to negative feedback on pituitary gonadotropin secretion by the excess adrenal androgens. Only a few untreated male or female patients are fertile.

In the simple virilizing form, plasma cortisol levels and production rates of cortisol are normal, but plasma 17-hydroxyprogesterone values are markedly elevated in both forms of 21-hydroxylase deficiency (15–18). ACTH stimulation, which should be performed with caution in those with the salt-losing form, produces a subnormal increment in the plasma level of cortisol (Table 3). Plasma aldosterone and plasma renin activity are moderately elevated due to hypersecretion of mineralocorticoid antagonists which produce a salt-losing tendency (14). In the salt-losing form, cortisol production rates are markedly reduced, aldosterone secretion rates are normal to subnormal, and plasma renin activity is markedly elevated (19–21).

B. 11β-Hydroxylase Deficiency

About 4% of patients with congenital adrenal hyperplasia have a defect of the 11β-hydroxylase enzyme(s) and prenatal diagnosis of the deficiency is feasible (22). This produces a deficient secretion of cortisol and hypersecretion of ACTH (23). The precursors of both corticosterone [11-desoxycorticosterone (DOC)], and cortisol [11-desoxycortisol (substance S)] are secreted in excessive quantities, are elevated in blood, and their tetrahydro derivatives are increased in the urine. Hypertension, which is usually moderate but can be markedly elevated, is largely due to the hypersecretion of DOC in untreated patients.

Female patients with this type of defect show varying degrees of masculinization of the external genitalia at birth. Virilization progresses through childhood with the presence of hypertension. In male patients, the external genitalia are normal at birth, but precocious puberty and hypertension should suggest the diagnosis of 11β-hydroxylase deficiency (13, 14).

These patients characteristically have low or normal plasma levels of cortisol, but secretion of cortisol in response to ACTH is limited (23). Plasma levels and secretion rates of both DOC and S are elevated. Plasma renin activity and plasma aldosterone levels are low. Treatment with glucocorticoids may produce neonatal salt loss in these patients as a result of inhibition of ACTH and DOC secretion before the suppressed renin-angiotensin system has recovered (24).

C. Deficiency of 3β-ol-Dehydrogenase

This enzyme deficit impairs the formation of both cortisol and aldosterone. Untreated patients fail to retain urinary sodium chloride and develop adrenal crisis. Hypersecretion of ACTH in the presence of this enzyme defect results in marked secretion of dehydroepiandrosterone and its derivatives (25, 26). Both sexes may have ambiguous external genitalia. The androgenic potency of dehydroepiandrosterone is insufficient to produce normal male sexual differentiation, but it is sufficient to cause ambiguous genitalia in the female fetus. Thus the testes of the affected males must also have a similar enzyme defect. Many patients with a complete deficiency of 3β-ol-dehydrogenase have died due to cortisol insufficiency, but an increasing number of these patients have survived infancy. Patients surviving to puberty have a partial deficiency of the enzyme and present with ambiguous external genitalia and gynecomastia (27-31).

D. Lipoid Hyperplasia (Defect Prior to Δ^5-Pregnenolone)

In this disorder, no steroid secretion occurs, so that patients are deficient in all classes of steroids (32). Adrenal crisis develops in early life; and despite treatment with glucocorticoid and mineralocorticoids, most patients have not survived. The external genitalia of both male and female patients is completely female. Cortisol administration at birth is required for survival if the defect is complete (32-34).

E. 17-Hydroxylase Deficiency

Cortisol synthesis is decreased due to deficient 17-hydroxylation in these patients. ACTH secretion is increased and stimulates excessive secretion of both corticosterone and DOC by the zona fasciculata and reticularis (35, 36). Corticosterone partially compensates for the cortisol deficit, but DOC produces hypertension by excessive retention of salt and decreases the secretion of both renin and aldosterone. Androgen secretion is absent or blunted by the enzyme defect and males have inadequate differentiation of the external genitalia. Male and female patients fail to secrete gonadal steroids and pubertal development fails to occur in the absence of exogenous hormone therapy.

II. DIAGNOSIS OF CONGENITAL ADRENAL HYPERPLASIA

The most rapid and accurate test for the diagnosis of 21-hydroxylase deficiency is assay of the plasma level of 17-hydroxyprogesterone. In salt losers and non-salt losers with the defect, plasma levels of this steroid are greater than 10 times the upper limit of normal (200 ng/dl). Plasma 17-hydroxyprogesterone values are useful in determining the adequacy of glucocorticoid therapy and plasma renin activity is an excellent index for assessing the adequacy of mineralocorticoid replacement. Plasma 17-hydroxyprogesterone is also increased in patients with 11β-hydroxylase deficiency, but it usually is not as high as it is in those with 21-hydroxylase deficiency. In 11-hydroxylase deficiency, plasma levels of S and DOC are elevated, whereas these steroids are normal or decreased in patients with 21-hydroxylase deficiency. Thus some care must be taken in interpreting plasma 17-hydroxyprogesterone values in the two most common forms of congenital adrenal hyperplasia. In all patients with congenital adrenal hyperplasia, it is important to establish the genetic sex.

The plasma level of pregnenolone is elevated and cortisol is markedly reduced in patients with 3β-hydroxysteroid dehydrogenase deficiency. Patients with 17-hydroxylase deficiency have elevated plasma levels of progesterone, DOC, and corticosterone and subnormal levels of cortisol. In those with defects in steroid synthesis prior to pregnenolone, all classes of adrenal steroids are subnormal when assayed in plasma or urine.

Clinical observation suggesting congenital adrenal hyperplasia:

1. Incomplete differentiation of external genitalia in either genotypic sex.
2. Adrenal or salt-losing crisis
3. Hypertension
4. Precocious puberty with masculinization
5. Bilateral undescended testes
6. Hirsutism or virilization in females, particularly those with primary amenorrhea
7. Family history of unexplained neonatal death.
8. Family history of documented congenital adrenal hyperplasia.

III. MILD CONGENITAL ADRENAL HYPERPLASIA

The classical congenital errors in steroidogenesis are categorized as congenital adrenal hyperplasia. The degree of enzyme deficiency is moderate to marked in these patients. Mild deficiencies of some of the enzymes, however, have been described later in life (37, 38). Various terms have been assigned to these disorders (acquired, adult onset, late onset, mild, or attenuated congenital adrenal hyperplasia). This group of disorders represents inborn errors of steroidogenesis with mild or partial deficits in enzyme activity. The defects are unrecognized until later in life and more commonly in women than in men. The enzyme deficiency usually does not produce sufficient reduction in mineralocorticoids, glucocorticoids, or sex-steroid synthesis to cause clinical signs or symptoms during fetal development or childhood. During or after puberty, virilization and menstrual irregularity of variable degrees occur. Hypertension is present in those with a mild deficiency of 11β-hydroxylase. Only three defects that can impair steroidogenesis have been associated with excessive production of androgen in later life: 21-hydroxylase, 11β-hydroxylase, and 3β-hydroxysteroid dehydrogenase. Many of these patients are initially diagnosed as having polycystic ovary disease or idiopathic hirsutism. 21-Hydroxylase and 11β-hydroxylase deficiencies are present in the adrenal cortex but may secondarily affect ovarian function because of excess androgen secretion. In contrast, the hydroxysteroid dehydrogenase affects steroidogenesis in the gonads and adrenal cortices.

A. Mild 21-Hydroxylase Deficiency

These patients exhibit no abnormalities of the external genitalia at birth. At the time of puberty, or subsequently, virilization which ranges from mild hirsutism to clitoral enlargement and menstrual irregularity is common. Although urinary 17-ketosteroid and pregnanetriol excretion rates are usually moderately elevated, an incremental increase in 17-hydroxyprogesterone (and progesterone) in response to ACTH stimulation is the most sensitive test for identification of patients with partial 21-hydroxylase deficiency. Rosenwaks et al. (39) and Migeon et al. (40) reported that a 17-hydroxyprogesterone plus progesterone of greater than 6.5 ng/dl during the first 30 min of an intravenous ACTH stimulation test was diagnostic of partial or mild 21-hydroxylase deficiency. Mauseth et al. (41) used a similar test procedure and found an increase of 9.94 ng/dl per minute in obligate heterozygotes.

B. Mild 11β-Hydroxylase Deficiency

There are reports of partial or mild 11β-hydroxylase deficiency in pubertal or postpubertal females (42, 43). Hypertension, hirsutism, and menstrual irregularity are commonly observed. Baseline urinary 17-ketosteroids, plasma 11-deoxycortisol, and 11-deoxycorticosterone are elevated. Supranormal increases in plasma content of 11-deoxycortisol and 11-deoxycorticosterone in response to ACTH stimulation are diagnostic of the disorder.

C. Mild 3β-Hydroxysteroid Dehydrogenase Deficiency

Heterogeneity in the presentation of hydroxysteroid dehydrogenase deficiency is well documented (27–31, 37, 38). The deficiency may involve various degrees of deficiency in the adrenal and/or gonad. In males, various degrees of hypospadias have been observed at birth. In those who survive to puberty, most have male sexual development, but gynecomastia is relatively common. It is important to measure Δ^5 steroids in blood or their urinary metabolites. Some of these cases are misdiagnosed as having 21-hydroxylase defects because only urinary pregnanetriol is measured and found to be elevated. These patients have abnormally high urinary excretion rates of Δ^5-pregnenetriol. Plasma levels of Δ^5-androstenediol or 17-hydroxypregnenolone have also been higher than normal in these patients (27–31).

This is being diagnosed with increased frequency in women. The adolescent females present with various degrees of virilization and irregular menses. The precise incidence of the disorder is unknown, but recent studies suggest that at least 3% of hirsute and oligomenorrheic women have the disorder (37). An elevated basal level of DHEAS with relatively normal values of testosterone and androstenedione (Δ^4 steroids) have been used as criteria for careful search for the partial enzyme defect. When these criteria are used together with hirsutism and oligomenorrhea, about 15% of such women have an apparent mild or partial deficiency of hydroxysteroid dehydrogenase. Patients suspected of the disorder receive a 1-mg dose of dexamethasone at midnight followed by a single intravenous bolus of 0.25 mg of cortrosyn at 8 A.M. the next morning. Blood specimens are collected before and for up to 3 hr after the ACTH injection. Elevated blood levels of pairs of Δ^5/Δ^4 steroids are consistent with the diagnosis of hydroxysteroid dehydrogenase deficiency. The defect appears to affect both the adrenal glands and gonads, and the ACTH stimulation test appears to be valid for identification of the disorder.

IV. VIRILIZING ADRENAL TUMORS

Androgen-secreting adrenal cortical benign adenomas or carcinomas are rare (14, 44–52). The virilizing tumors can develop at any period of life including the first year, but they are more common in children than in adults (14, 44). None has been observed as arising during fetal life, and this is helpful in differentiating them from congenital adrenal hyperplasia. The clinical signs are more apparent in women and prepubertal children than in men.

In prepubertal boys, pseudoprecocious puberty is observed. The penis and prostate enlarge and pubic and axillary hair growth mature. The muscle and osseous growth are marked. The testes remain small and immature. Virilizing adrenal tumors in prepubertal girls produce pubic and axillary hair growth and clitoral enlargement but labial fusion is not observed, which contrasts with patients with congenital adrenal hyperplasia. Breast development and menses are usually not observed. Rapid statural growth with marked osseous maturation also occurs. In adult women, amenorrhea is a common and an early symptom. This is usually followed or accompanied by other signs of virilization, including clitoral hypertrophy, increased musculature, increased libido, deepening of the voice, and uterine and breast atrophy. Rarely, hirsutism may be the only manifestation of the tumor. In the adult male, virilism may not attract attention, but he may have infertility with azo- or oligospermia and a decrease in size of the testes.

A high plasma content of some androgens is highly suspicious of an androgen-producing tumor of the adrenal cortex or ovary: testosterone (in females) greater than 200 ng/dl, androstenedione over 300 ng/dl, or dehydroepiandrosterone sulfate greater than 700 μg/dl (47-52). Adenomas of the adrenal cortex usually secrete increased DHEA and DHEAS, which markedly elevate the 17-ketosteroids. In some cases only androstenedione and testosterone are increased and in those cases urinary 17-ketosteroid excretion is usually normal or moderately increased. Luteinizing hormone (LH) responsiveness is sometimes present and estrogen administration may result, in these cases, in marked reduction in androgen secretion. This gonadotropin dependency of some of these tumors suggests a gonadal origin (50). With rare exception, dexamethasone fails to suppress secretion.

Adrenal cortical carcinomas that cause virilization without producing Cushing's syndrome secrete mainly dehydroepiandrosterone and its sulfate as well as other Δ^5 steroids. In some, secretion of testosterone and androstenedione is also increased. Because of the excessive production of dehydroepiandrosterone sulfate, urinary 17-ketosteroids are usually markedly elevated. Dexamethasone is ineffective in reducing androgen secretion by adrenal cortical carcinomas.

V. ADRENAL GLUCOCORTICOID DISORDERS

A. Adrenal Cortical Failure

Adrenal cortical deficiency may be divided into two major categories: primary failure, in which there is intrinsic disease of adrenal gland (Addison's disease),

Table 4 Causes of Primary Adrenal Cortical Failure

A. Destruction or impaired development of adrenal cortical tissue
   1. Idiopathic atrophy (autoimmune)
   2. Infections
      a. Tuberculosis
      b. Histoplasmosis and other fungi
      c. Fulminating infections
   3. Hemorrhage
      a. In the newborn
      b. Anticoagulants
      c. Adrenal venography
      d. Trauma
      e. Stress
   4. Post adrenalectomy
   5. Infiltration
   6. Adrenal agenesis

B. Impaired steroidogenesis
   1. Adrenogenital syndrome
   2. Isolated glucocorticoid deficiency

C. Glucocorticoid resistance

and secondary failure due to absent or low plasma levels of ACTH (53-59). The causes of adrenal insufficiency are listed in Table 4. Adrenal cortical diseases that cause Addison's disease produce a deficiency of all classes of adrenocortical hormones: mineralocorticoid, glucocorticoid, androgens, and estrogens. In contrast, most but not all patients with secondary adrenal insufficiency have near-normal secretion of aldosterone. Thus hyponatremia and salt loss is more pronounced in patients with primary adrenal cortical failure than in those with secondary disease.

Adrenocortical failure, either primary or secondary, may develop acutely or chronically, and its clinical presentation may be either as an acute catastrophic emergency or as a chronic disease. Acute adrenal crisis may occur coincident with the development of acute adrenal cortical failure or be superimposed on chronic failure. Idiopathic adrenal-cortical failure caused by organ-specific autoimmunity is the most common disorder resulting in Addison's disease (60-65). Estimates indicate that the idiopathic disorder occurs in about 25 persons per million population. It affects women more commonly than men, whereas tuberculosis and other causes affect the sexes with about equal frequency. Addison's disease is rare before age 10 except in the patient with adrenoleukodystrophy.

Acute loss of adrenocortical function may result in Addisonian crisis. Fortunately, this is a rare occurrence. The acute state is rapidly progressive over a few days or hours. The symptoms and signs are nonspecific: vomiting, abdominal pain, muscular weakness, dehydration, hypotension, confusion, and eventually coma. If adrenal failure develops over a short period of time, typical Addisonian pigmentation is absent. Nonspecific symptoms are observed in those with a chronic and insidious onset: tiredness, anorexia, weight loss, abdominal pain, vomiting, weakness, and dizziness. Typical Addisonian pigmentation which is of recent onset is more significant than pigmentation of long duration. The increased pigmentation develops in sunexposed areas of the body, areas exposed to friction or pressure, scars which heal after the onset of the disease, and mucous membranes (buccal mucosa and vagina). Elevated plasma ACTH and β-lipotropin (β-LPH) or its metabolic products stimulate melanin formation in melanocytes. Depigmentation (vitiligo) may occur in pigmented or nonpigmented areas secondary to destruction of melanocytes. Postural hypotension with associated dizziness is caused by fluid and sodium chloride depletion as a result of mineralocorticoid deficiency. A low plasma cortisol content may also contribute because of its role in maintaining normal vascular tone. Fasting hypoglycemia with confusion may be observed. Women may have a loss of body hair in either primary or secondary adrenal insufficiency because of absent or diminished adrenal androgens, but it is usually more pronounced in those with hypopituitarism. Amenorrhea is a common in those with pituitary failure; and if menstruation fails to resume in those treated for primary adrenal insufficiency, autoimmune ovarian failure should be suspected.

Patients with Addison's disease may have a low plasma sodium content with high blood urea and potassium levels, but none of these abnormalities may be observed in patients with partial failure. Electrolyte alterations are less common in patients with hypopituitarism than in those with Addison's disease. There are several satisfactory tests that may document low cortisol secretion by the adrenal cortex. In Addison's disease, impairment of cortisol secretion may be demonstrable only by stimulation with exogenous ACTH. The failure of a low basal cortisol to rise substantially after ACTH administration is regarded as diagnostic of Addison's disease in patients with signs and symptoms suggestive of the disease.

Various protocols for administration of ACTH have been successful in the diagnosis of adrenal insufficiency (see Chap. 23 for details). Because of convenience the short ACTH stimulation tests have gained popularity. A subnormal cortisol response does not differentiate between primary and secondary adrenal insufficiency. A prolonged stimulation test is then indicated (54) and a subnormal response documents primary adrenal cortical insufficiency.

An alternative test of adrenocortical function is the simultaneous measurement of both cortisol and ACTH or β-LPH in blood samples collected between 8 and 10 A.M. A low plasma cortisol level and a high plasma ACTH or β-LPH indicate primary adrenal cortisol insufficiency (66, 67). A low plasma content of both ACTH and cortisol suggests secondary adrenocortical deficiency but may be seen in normal subjects. Local circumstances dictate which test is preferable based on the availability of adequate plasma ACTH and β-LPH measurements.

The single (or multiple)-dose overnight metyrapone test is a most useful, simple, and relatively safe procedure for the diagnosis of secondary adrenal insufficiency (68, 69). If performed in patients with Addison's disease, plasma ACTH content is elevated and plasma 11-desoxycortisol is subnormal. The plasma content of 11-desoxycortisol is determined to indicate whether metyrapone produces adequate inhibition of 11β-hydroxylase. The investigation procedure for adrenal insufficiency is outlined in Diagnostic Summary 1.

B. Cushing's Syndrome Caused by Adrenocortical Adenoma, Carcinoma, and Nodular Hyperplasia

Excess secretion of cortisol of adrenal origin produces the characteristic signs and symptoms of Cushing's syndrome. Spontaneous hypercortisolism is produced by both benign and malignant adrenal cortical tumors, and the clinical presentation is generally indistinguishable from that caused by ACTH secretion from the pituitary or from nonendocrine tumors. Ten to fifteen percent of adults with Cushing's syndrome will have either autonomous adrenal cortical adenomas or carcinomas. Adenomas and carcinomas occur with equal frequency. In contrast, adrenal cortical carcinoma is the most common cause of the syndrome in children (44, 45). It is well documented that the histologic distinction between adenomas and carcinomas is frequently in error. Tumors over 100 g in weight are more likely to be malignant and those less than 40 g are usually benign (70). Patients with adrenal tumors causing Cushing's syndrome usually fail to respond to dexamethasone suppression tests, metyrapone responsiveness is subnormal, plasma ACTH is undetectable, and secretory response to ACTH is variable.

Nodular adrenal disease is an uncommon cause of Cushing's syndrome. Micronodular and macronodular adrenal cortical disease variants have been described (48, 70-73). These probably represent distinct clinical disorders, as there are recognized differences. Micronodular disease is observed in patients who are less than 21 years of age, and the Cushing's syndrome may be familial (73). Plasma ACTH is low or undetectable. None has responded to metyrapone or dexamethasone and most exhibit no response to the ACTH stimulation test (48, 71, 73). Two features of the adrenal pathology are quite characteristic. The weights of the adrenal glands were normal or subnormal, and brown or black pigment is

Diagnostic Summary 1 Adrenal Insufficiency

Test and results			Probable diagnosis
1. Plasma cortisol and ACTH (or β-lipotropin)			
Cortisol → ↓ (<10 μg/dl) ↑ ACTH (>150 pg/ml)			Primary adrenal insufficiency
Cortisol → ↓ (<10 μg/dl) ↓ ACTH (<20 pg/ml)			Secondary adrenal insufficiency (hypopituitary)
2. Metyrapone (overnight test)			
Cortisol	Sub S	ACTH	
Normal to low	<7 μg/dl	Normal to low	Inadequate test or pituitary ACTH deficiency
Low	>7 μg/dl	>150	Normal response
Low	Low	High	Primary adrenal insufficiency
3. Acute ACTH stimulation (25-unit bolus)			
Cortisol elevated			Normal response
Cortisol stays low			Pituitary or adrenal insufficiency
4. Chronic ACTH stimulation			
Cortisol elevated			Normal response
Cortisol stays low			Primary adrenal disease
Cortisol increases slowly			Insufficient secondary to pituitary disease or suppression

Note: Renin and aldosterone measurements are also of value (see Chap. 26).

described on microscopic sections. The nodules are small, usually less than 3 mm in diameter. Lymphocytic infiltration and atrophy of the surrounding adrenal tissue are commonly observed. These tumors appear to be autonomous multiple nodules secreting cortisol without ACTH stimulation.

Patients with macronodular disease of the adrenal cortex may be older, have more severe Cushing's syndrome, and the nodules may be hyperresponsive to ACTH stimulation (71). Most often, the adrenal cortex has large macroscopic adenomas as well as hyperplasia. Most patients with this condition have measurable plasma levels of ACTH but are unresponsive to metyrapone or dexamethasone. This disorder may be influenced by chronic ACTH stimulation but pituitary tumors are not found and there does not appear to be autonomous adrenal function which suppresses plasma ACTH. Adrenal cortical carcinoma has been described in one patient with this disorder (48).

The preoperative diagnosis of an adrenal tumor or nodular hyperplasia is supported by observing unresponsiveness to dexamethasone suppression and low plasma ACTH levels before and following metyrapone. CT scans are helpful in localizing an adrenal tumor, and selective adrenal venous catheterization may be useful in identifying the source of excess cortisol production.

REFERENCES

1. Harding BW. Synthesis of adrenal cortical steroids and mechanism of ACTH effects. In *Endocrinology*, DeGroot Leslie J (ed). Grune & Stratton, New York, 1979, vol II, pp 1131-1137.
2. Sandor T. Fazekas AG, Robinson BH. The biosynthesis of corticosteroids throughout the vertebrates. In *General, Comparative and Clinical Endocrinology of the Adrenal Cortex*, Jones IC, Henderson IW (eds). Academic, New York, 1976, vol I, pp 25-142.
3. Saez JM, Morera AM, Cazord A, Bertrand J. Adrenal and testicular contribution to plasma oestrogens. J Endocrinol Metab 1972; 55:41-49.
4. Baird DT, Uno A, Melby JC. Adrenal secretion of androgens and oestrogens. J Endocrinol 1969; 45:135-136.
5. Keymolen V, Dor P, Borkowski A. Output of oestrogens, testosterone and precursors by isolated human adrenal cells as compared with that of glucocorticoids. J Endocrinol 1976; 71:219-229.
6. Neischlag E, Loriaux DL, Ruder HJ, Zucker IR, Kirschner MA, Lipsett MB. The secretion of dehydroepiandrosterone and dehydroepiandrosterone sulphate in man. J Endocrinol Metab 1973; 57:123-134.
7. Wilson JD, George FW, Griffin JE. The hormonal control of sexual development. Science 1981; 211:1278-1294.

7a. Meikle AW, Stringham JD, Wilson DE, Dolman LI. Plasma 5α-reduced androgens in men and hirsute women: role of adrenals and gonads. J Clin Endocrinol Metab 1979; 48:969-975.

8. Childs B, Grumbach MM, Van Wyk JJ. Virilizing adrenal hyperplasia: a genetic and hormonal study. J Clin Invest 1956; 35:213-222.
9. Prader A. Die Häufigkeit des kongenitalen andrenogenitalen Syndroms. Helv Paediatr Acta 1958; 13:426.
10. New MI, DuPont B, Pang S, Pollack M, Levine LS. An update of congenital adrenal hyperplasia. Recent Prog Horm Res 1981; 37:105-181.
11. Hirschfeld AJ, Fleshman JK. An unusually high incidence of salt-losing congenital adrenal hyperplasia in the Alaskan Eskimo. J Pediatr 1969; 75:492-494.
12. Levine LS, Zachmann M, New MI, Prader A, Pollack MS, O'Neill GJ, Yang SY, Oberfield SE, DuPont B. Genetic mapping of the 21 hydroxylase

deficiency gene within the HLA linkage group. N Engl J Med 1978; 299: 911–915.

13. Bongiovanni AM. Congenital adrenal hyperplasia and related conditions. In *Metabolic Basis of Inherited Disease*, 4th ed, Stanbury JB, Wyngaarden JB (eds). McGraw-Hill, New York, 1977.
14. Migeon CJ. Diagnosis and treatment of adrenogenital disorders. In *Endocrinology*, DeGroot LJ (ed). Grune and Stratton, New York, 1979, vol II, pp 1203–1237.
15. Youssefnejadian E, David R. Diagnosis of congenital adrenal hyperplasia by measurement of 17α-OH-progesterone. Clin Endocrinol 1975; 4:451.
16. Hughes IA, Winter JSD. The application of a serum 17-OH progesterone radioimmunoassay to the diagnosis and management of congenital adrenal hyperplasia. J Pediatr 1976; 88:766–773.
17. Lippe BM, La Franchi SH, Lavin N, Parlow A, Coyotupa J, Kaplan SA. Serum 17-hydroxyprogesterone, progesterone, estradiol and testosterone in the diagnosis and management of congenital adrenal hyperplasia. J Pediatr 1974; 85:782–787.
18. Pang S, Hotchkiss J, Drash AL, Levin LS, New MI. Microfilter paper method for 17α-hydroxyprogesterone radioimmunoassay. Its application for rapid screening for congenital adrenal hyperplasia. J Clin Endocrinol Metab 1977; 45:1003–1008.
19. Migeon CJ, Kenny FM. Cortisol production rate. V. Congenital virilizing adrenal hyperplasia. J Pediatr 1966; 69:779–786.
20. Kowarski A, Finkelstein JW, Spaulding JS, Holman GM, Migeon CJ. Aldosterone secretion rate in congenital adrenal hyperplasia: a discussion of theories on the pathogenesis of the salt-losing form of the syndrome. J Clin Invest 1965; 44:1505–1513.
21. New MI, Seaman MP. Secretion rates of cortisol and aldosterone precursors in various forms of congenital adrenal hyperplasia. J Clin Endocrinol Metab 1970; 30:361–371.
22. Rosler A, Leiberman E, Rosenmann A, Ben-Uzilio R, Weidenfeld J. Prenatal diagnosis of 11β-hydroxylase deficiency congenital adrenal hyperplasia. J Clin Endocrinol Metab 1979; 49:546–551.
23. Kowarski A, Russell A, Migeon CJ. Aldosterone secretion rate in the hypertensive form of congenital adrenal hyperplasia. J Clin Endocrinol Metab 1968; 28:1445–1449.
24. Holcombe JA, Keenan BS, Nichols BL, Kirkland RT, Clayton GW. Neonatal salt loss in the hypertensive form of congenital adrenal hyperplasia. Pediatrics 1980; 65:777–781.
25. Bongiovanni AM. Adrenogenital syndrome with deficiency of 3β-hydroxysteroid dehydrogenase. J Clin Invest 1962; 41:2086–2092.
26. Bongiovanni AM. Urinary steroid pattern of infants with congenital hyperplasia due to 3-beta hydroxysteroid dehydrogenase deficiency. J Steroid Biochem 1980; 13:809-811.
27. Zachman M, Vallmin JA, Mürset G, Curtius H, Prader A. Unusual type of adrenal hyperplasia due to deficiency of 3β-hydroxysteroid dehydrogenase. J Clin Endocrinol Metab 1970; 30:719–726.

28. Janne O, Perheentupa J and Vikho R. Plasma and urinary steroids in an eight year old boy with 3 beta-hydroxysteroid dehydrogenase deficiency. J Clin Endocrinol Metab 1970; 31:162–165.
29. Kenny FM, Reynolds JW, Green OC. Partial 3β-hydroxylase deficiency in a family with congenital adrenal hyperplasia with evidence for increasing 3-beta-hydroxysteroid dehydrogenase activities with age. Pediatrics 1971; 48:756–765.
30. Parks GA, New MI, Bermudez JA, Anast CS, Bongiovanni AM. A pubertal boy with a 3β-hydroxysteroid dehydrogenase defect. J Clin Endocrinol Metab 1971; 33:269–278.
31. Rosenfield RL, de Niepomniszsze AB, Kenny FM, Genel M. The response to human chorionic gonadotropin (HCG) administration in boys with and without 3-beta-hydroxysteroid dehydrogenase deficiency. J Clin Endocrinol Metab 1974; 39:370–374.
32. Prader A, Gurtner HP. Das Snydrom des Pseudohermaphroditismus masculinus bei rongenitaler Nebennierenrinden-hyperplasia ohne Androgenüberproduktion (Adrenaler Pseudohermaphroditismus masculinus) Helv Paediatr Acta 1955; 10:397.
33. Dogenhart HJ, Visser HKA, Boon H, O'Doherty NJ. Evidence for deficient 20-cholesterol hydroxylase activity in adrenal tissue of a patient with lipoid adrenal hyperplasia. Acta Endocrinol (Copenh) 1971; 71:512–518.
34. Comacho AM, Kowarski A, Migeon CJ, Brough AJ. Congenital adrenal hyperplasia due to a deficiency of one of the enzymes involved in biosynthesis of pregnenolone. J Clin Endocrinol Metab 1968; 28:153–161.
35. Biglieri EG, Herron MA, Brust N. 17-Hydroxylation deficiency in man. J Clin Invest 1966; 45:1946–1954.
36. Goldsmith O, Solomon DH, Horton R. Hypogonadism and mineralocorticoid excess: the 17-hydroxylase syndrome. N Engl J Med 1967; 277: 673–677.
37. Lobo RA, Goebelsmann U. Evidence for reduced 3β-ol-hydroxysteroid dehydrogenase activity in some hirsute women thought to have polycystic ovary syndrome. J Clin Endocrinol Metab 1981; 53:394–400.
38. Bongiovanni AM. Acquired adrenal hyperplasia with special reference to 3β-hydroxysteroid dehydrogenase. Fertil Steril 1981; 35:599–608.
39. Rosenwaks Z, Lee PA, Jones GS, Migeon CJ, Wantz AC. An attenuated form of congenital virilizing adrenal hyperplasia. J Clin Endocrinol Metab 1979; 49:355
40. Migeon CJ, Rosenwaks Z, Lee PA, Urban MD, Bian WB. The attenuated form of congenital adrenal hyperplasia as an allelic form of 21-hydroxylase deficiency. J Clin Endocrinol Metab 1980; 51:647.
41. Mauseth RS, Hansen JA, Smith EK, Giblett ER, Kelley BC. Detection of heterozygotes for congenital adrenal hyperplasia: 21-hydroxylase deficiency, a comparison of HLA typing and 17-OH progesterone response to ACTH infusion. J Pediatr 1980; 97:749–753.

42. Gabrilove JL, Sharma EC, Dorfman RI. Adrenocortical 11-β-hydroxylase deficiency and virilism first manifest in the adult women. N Engl J Med 1965;272:1189–1194.
43. Cathelineau G, Brerault J, Fiet J, Julien R, Dreux C, Canivet J. Adrenocortical 11-β-hydroxylation defect in adult women with postmenarchial onset of symptoms. J Clin Endocrinol Metab 1980;51:287–291.
44. Hutter AM Jr, Kayhoe DE. Adrenal cortical carcinoma clinical features of 138 patients. Am J Med 1966;41:572–580.
45. Hajjer RA, Hickey RC, Samaan NA. Adrenal cortical carcinoma: a study of 32 patients. Cancer 1975;35:549–554.
46. Scott HW Jr, Foster JH, Liddle GW, Davidson ET. Cushing's syndrome due to adrenocortical tumor: 11-year review of 15 patients. Ann Surg 1965;162:505–516.
47. Lipsett MB, Migeon CJ, Kirschner MA, Bardin CW. Physiological basis of disorders of androgen metabolism. Ann Intern Med 1968;68:1327.
48. Anderson DC, Child DF, Sutcliff CH, Buckley CH, Davies D, Longson D. Cushing's syndrome, nodular adrenal hyperplasia and virilizing carcinoma. Clin Endocrinol 1978;9:1–14.
49. Schteingart DE, Woodbury MC, Tsao HS, McKenzie AK. Virilizing syndrome associated with an adrenal cortical adenoma secreting predominantly testosterone. Am J Med 1979;67:140–146.
50. Larson BA, van der Laan WP, Judd HL, McCullough DL. A testosterone-producing adrenal cortical adenoma in an elderly woman. J Clin Endocrinol Metab 1976;42:882–887.
51. Costiu G, Goebelsmann U, Kogut MD. Sexual precocity due to a testosterone producing adrenal tumor. J Clin Endocrinol Metab 1977;45:912–919.
52. Check JH, Rakoff AE, Roy BK. A testosterone-secreting adrenal adenoma. Obstet Gynecol 1978;51:465–475.
53. Nelson DH. Diagnosis and treatment of Addison's disease. In *Endocrinology*, DeGroot LJ (ed). Grune & Stratton, New York, 1979, vol II, pp 1192–1201.
54. West CD, Meikle AW. Laboratory tests for the diagnosis of Cushing's syndrome and adrenal insufficiency and factors affecting those tests. In *Endocrinology*, DeGroot LJ (ed). Grune & Stratton, New York, 1979, vol II, pp 1157–1177.
55. Nerup J. Addison's disease—clinical studies. A report of 108 cases. Acta Endocrinol (Copenh) 1974; 76:127–141.
56. Thistlethwaite D, Darling JAB, Fraser R, Mason PA, Rees LH, Harkness RA. Familial glucocorticoid deficiency. Studies of diagnosis and pathogenesis. Arch Dis Child 1975;50:291–297.
57. Kelch RP, Kaplan SL, Biglieri EG, Daniels GH, Epstein CJ, Grumbach MM. Hereditary adrenocortical unresponsiveness to adrenocorticotropic hormone. J Pediatr 1972;81:726–736.

58. Sperling MA, Wolfsen AR, Fisher DA. Congenital adrenal hypoplasia: an isolated defect of organogenesis. J Pediatr 1973; 82:444–449.
59. O'Connell TX, Aston SJ. Acute adrenal hemorrhage complicating anticoagulant therapy. Surg Gynecol Obstet 1974; 139:355–358.
60. Hubay CA, Weckesser EC, Levy RP. Occult adrenal insufficiency in surgical patients. Ann Surg 1975; 181:325-332.
61. Blizzard RM, Chee D, Davis W. The incidence of adrenal and other antibodies in sera of patients with idiopathic adrenal insufficiency (Addison's disease). Clin Exp Immunol 1967; 2:19–30.
62. Irvine WJ. Endocrine diseases. In *Medical Immunology*, Irvine WJ (ed). Tevist, Edinburgh, 1979.
63. Irvine WJ, Barnes EW. Adrenocortical insufficiency. Clin Endocrinol 1972; 1:549–594.
64. Maisey MN, Lessof MH. Addison's disease: a clinical study. Guys Hosp Rep 1969; 118:363-372.
65. Nerup J. Addison's disease—serological studies. Acta Endocrinol (Copenh) 1974; 76:142–158.
66. Besser GM, Cullen DR, Irvine WJ, Ratcliffe JG, Landon J. Immunoreactive corticotropin levels in adrenocortical insufficiency. Br Med J 1971; 1:374–376.
67. Jeffcoate GH, Todd JE, Sleisenger MH. A specific radioimmunoassay for human β-lipotropin. J Clin Endocrinol Metab 1978; 47:160–167.
68. Spiger M, Jubiz W, Meikle AW, West CD, Tyler FH. Single dose metyrapone test. Review of a four-year experience. Arch Intern Med 1975; 135:698–700.
69. Liddle GW, Estep HL, Kendall JW Jr, Williams WC Jr, Townes AW. Clinical application of a new test of pituitary reserve. J Clin Endocrinol Metab 1959; 19:875–894.
70. Neville AM, Symington T. The pathology of the adrenal gland in Cushing's syndrome. J Pathol Bacteriol 1967; 93:19–35.
71. Ruder HJ, Loriaux DL, Lipsett MB. Severe osteoporosis in young adults associated with Cushing's syndrome due to micronodular adrenal disease. J Clin Endocrinol Metab 1974; 39:1138–1147.
72. Meador CK, Bowdoin B, Owen WC, Farmer TA. Primary adrenocortical nodular hyperplasia. a rare cause of Cushing's syndrome. J Clin Endocrinol Metab 1967; 27:1255-1263.
73. Schweizer-Cagianut A, Froesch ER, Hedinger C. Familial Cushing's syndrome with primary adrenocortical microadenomatosis (primary adrenocortical nodular dysplasia). Acta Endocrinol (Copenh) 1980; 94:529-535.
74. Nelson, DH. The Adrenal Cortex: Physiological Function and Disease. WB Saunders, Philadelphia and London, 1980.

26
Mineralocorticoids

Eric A. Espiner
Christchurch Clinical School of Medicine and Princess Margaret Hospital, Christchurch, New Zealand

Corticosteroids that promote sodium absorption in exchange for potassium or hydrogen ion have been loosely classified as mineralocorticoids. The most potent mineralocorticoid, and also the first to be isolated and chemically identified—aldosterone—has a unique chemical structure and is synthesized solely by the zona glomerulosa of the adrenal cortex. Other corticosteroids with sodium-retaining activity include 11-desoxycorticosterone (DOC), corticosterone (compound B), 11 desoxycortisol (compound S) 18-hydroxy-DOC, and 18-hydroxycorticosterone, but aldosterone is by far the most important. The relative potencies of these mineralocorticoids and others used in clinical practice are listed in Table 1. Most of the steroids with mineralocorticoid action have slight or negligible glucocorticoid activity, but it should be noted that cortisol—the most important naturally occurring glucocorticoid—has some mineralocorticoid action which may be relevant in some clinical situations. Patients consistently secreting more than 50 mg of cortisol daily (or receiving hydrocortisone therapy in equivalent amounts) may be prone to disorders of sodium retention and potassium depletion. The distal tubule of the nephron is the best known site of aldosterone action but other tissues, including the gut (1), sweat glands (2), and salivary glands (3), are also responsive tissues. Whether a tissue is responsive probably depends on the presence, number, and occupancy of specific mineralocorticoid receptors (4). The ensuing sodium retention plays a major part in sodium conservation and, in concert with other hormonal and renal mechanisms, serves to maintain the extracellular fluid volume. Therefore, it is not surprising that the main control of mineralocorticoid secretion should be vested in the kidney. Unlike cortisol secretion, which is solely influenced by the pituitary secretion of

Table 1 Biological Activity of Corticosteroids

Steroid	Estimated potencies[a] Glucocorticoid	Mineralocorticoid
Cortisol	1	1
Corticosterone	0.3	15
Desoxycorticosterone	0	25
Aldosterone	b	200–400
Prednisone	4	0.5
Dexamethasone	25–50	(?) 0
9α-Fluorohydrocortisone	10–25	100

[a]Compared to cortisol, which is given a value of unity for both gluco- and mineralocorticoid effects.
[b]Small effect.
Source: Maxwell MH, Kleeman CR, *Clinical Disorders of Fluid and Electrolyte Metabolism*, 3rd ed, 1980, p 1296. Copyright © 1980 McGraw-Hill. Used with the permission of McGraw-Hill Book Company.

ACTH, aldosterone is regulated by at least three different factors: the renin-angiotensin system, adrenocorticotropic hormone (ACTH), and the plasma concentration of potassium. The relative importance of these stimuli varies depending on the clinical circumstances. The renin-angiotensin system appears to be dominant in hypovolemic states, whereas ACTH and potassium may predominate in hyporeninemic states (such as primary aldosteronism) and in anephric patients (see page 378).

I. CONTROL OF MINERALOCORTICOID SECRETION

A. Renin-Angiotensin System

Renin is an enzyme with a molecular weight of approximately 40,000. It is synthesized, stored, and secreted by the juxtaglomerular granules in the wall of the renal afferent arterioles. Big renin or prorenin is probably an inactive precursor (5). Renin is secreted in response to a drop in renal perfusion pressure (see below) and acts on a specific protein substrate (angiotensinogen) to produce the decapeptide (angiotensin I) by hydrolytic cleavage between the two leucine groups (Fig. 1). Angiotensin I has little or no biological activity itself and requires conversion to the octapeptide (angiotensin II) before the peptide can act to increase aldosterone secretion. The conversion of angiotensin II is carried out in the capillary vascular bed, particularly of the lung, the endo-

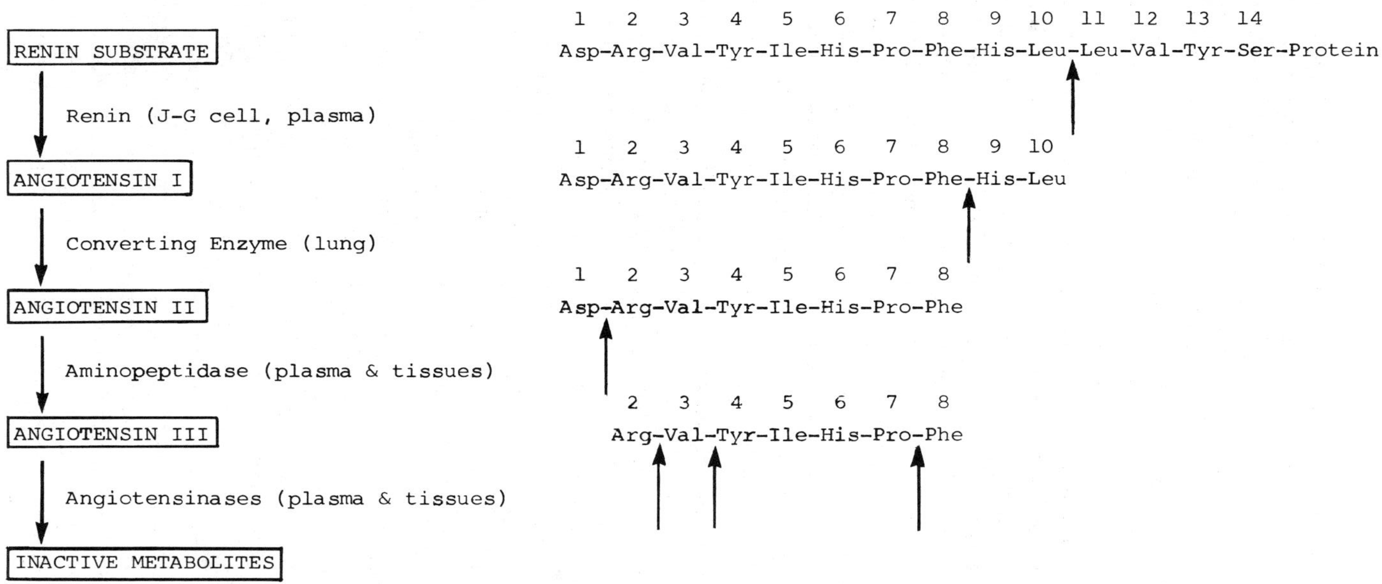

Figure 1 Formation and metabolism of angiotensins.

thelium of which is rich in converting enzyme (CE). Converting enzyme cleaves the histidyl-leucine group from the C terminus of angiotensin I. Further metabolism and degradation of angiotensin peptides occurs in blood by way of carboxy and other peptidases ("angiotensinases") which cleave the N-terminus amino acids to yield smaller fragments. One of these angiotensin III (2,8-heptapeptide) has similar biological activity to angiotensin II itself, but smaller metabolites are inactive. The site of action of angiotensin II on aldosterone synthesis is still debated, but the peptide appears to stimulate the conversion of cholesterol to pregnenolone within the glomerulosa cell. The aldosterone response continues with chronically maintained elevated levels of angiotensin II (6), and it appears that other mineralocorticoids such as 18-hydroxycorticosterone (secreted from the fasciculata) and 18-hydroxy-DOC (secreted by both the fasciculata and glomerulosa) are also stimulated by high levels of angiotensin II (6). In addition to increasing aldosterone, angiotensin II has other actions, the most important of which is its vasoconstrictor or "pressor" effect to increase blood pressure. Other actions may include stimulation of antidiuretic hormone and thirst as well as increasing catecholamine release from the adrenal medulla. All of these actions will support the maintenance of blood pressure and extracellular fluid volume.

Control of Renin Release. Renin secretion is increased in response to diminished renal blood flow (baroreceptor hypothesis) and distal tubular sodium loading (the so-called macular densa effect). In many clinical situations (e.g., salt deficiency, hypovolemia, etc.) both stimuli would act together to increase renin secretion. An intact sympathetic renal innervation is necessary for a normal response. There is increasing evidence that prostaglandins are also involved and may increase renin secretion directly, although the precise mechanism is unclear. Intriguing analogies and interrelationships exist between the renin-angiotensin (vasoconstrictor) and kinin-prostaglandin (vasodilator) systems. Thus kallikrien activates prorenin in vitro and converting enzyme is responsible for inactivating the main circulating kinin-bradykinin. Further, intrarenal infusions of bradykinin increase prostaglandin production and renin secretion (7). Readers are referred to recent summaries for details of these interrelationships (5, 8).

The increased aldosterone secretion brought about by the renin-angiotensin system promotes sodium reabsorption and eventually extracellular fluid (ECF) volume expansion, which will tend to reduce renin and close the feedback loop. Other modulating effects on renin secretion include the concentration of plasma angiotensin II (which has a direct inhibitory effect on renin release), hypothalamic activity (presumably through sympathetic innervation) and potassium status. Hypokalemia will increase renin and high levels of potassium will reduce it, but the importance of potassium's effect in humans is not settled. The same can be said for antidiuretic hormone (ADH), which inhibits renin (9).

B. ACTH and Potassium

It was once thought that ACTH had little effect on aldosterone secretion. However, recent studies confirm that physiological fluctuations in ACTH concentration result in corresponding changes in aldosterone (and 18-hydroxycorticosterone) comparable in magnitude with those of cortisol (10). ACTH stimulates aldosterone and other corticosteroids within 1-2 min chiefly by converting cholesterol to pregnenolone. However, the sustained stimulation of the adrenal cortex by ACTH has quite different effects on mineralocorticoids and glucocorticoids. After several hours of constant ACTH stimulation, the aldosterone response begins to wane, so that "normal" or even low levels of secretion are found after 24 hr (11). The same pattern is seen in 18-hydroxy-DOC, and 18-hydroxy-B secretion. Other mineralocorticoids (desoxycorticosterone, and 11-desoxycortisol), and of course cortisol itself, are well maintained during chronic ACTH stimulation. Although the mechanism is unclear, these findings explain the absence of hyperaldosteronism in patients with ACTH-dependent Cushing's syndrome. Chronic lack of ACTH, as seen in some hypopituitary states, reduces the glomerulosa's response to stimulation (e.g., sodium deficiency), but basal secretion of aldosterone continues near normally—presumably because of an intact renin-angiotensin-aldosterone axis (12). This is in marked contrast to states of primary adrenocortical insufficiency where aldosterone deficiency—and hypovolemia—may be profound.

The role of potassium in the minute-to-minute control of aldosterone in health is still uncertain, although there is no doubt that increments in plasma potassium may be associated with increased aldosterone levels (13). The effect is a direct one (14), presumably on the "late pathway" of aldosterone synthesis, and is specific to the glomerulosa.

While ACTH, angiotensin II, and potassium are believed to be the major controllers of aldosterone secretion, there are other important modulating influences. Sodium deficiency will amplify the effect of both ACTH and angiotensin on aldosterone secretion (10, 15) as will the dietary intake of potassium, which increases the aldosterone response to ACTH (16) and also to angiotensin (17). The possible modulating influence of dopamine and dopaminergic activity has yet to be clarified (18), and the same is true for other so-called "unidentified factors" (19, 20) which may be important in aldosterone control.

The aldosterone secretion rate in health varies from 50 to 200 μg/per day, increasing to over 1000 μg daily in states of sodium deficiency. Secretion rates of 18-hydroxy-DOC, DOC, and 18-hydroxycorticosterone are similar. Plasma levels will be determined by the rates of secretion and the rate of metabolic clearance, which is chiefly determined by the liver. Reduction in hepatic function or blood flow will reduce clearance and increase plasma concentration and therefore biological activity. Plasma aldosterone is only weakly protein bound

(21) and in health the concentration ranges between 150 and 550 pmol/liter (5-18 ng/per 100 ml) in subjects taking normal sodium intakes. There is a prominent diurnal variation largely in tune with plasma ACTH and renin concentration (see below). Fluctuations in plasma aldosterone concentration may be rapid since not only are the regulating factors quickly metabolized (ACTH half-life 5-10 min; renin 30 min; angiotensin 1-2 min), but aldosterone itself is cleared promptly (half-time 30 min). Conversion to the tetrahydro metabolites by the liver and the renal production of an 18-glucuronide (so-called acid labile metabolite) are the principal routes of metabolism and excretion.

II. PATHOPHYSIOLOGY

A. Mineralocorticoid Excess

The hallmark of a primary excess of mineralocorticoid is hypokalemic hypertension with an associated metabolic alkalosis. Isolated cases of primary aldosteronism in the absence of hypertension have been reported (22) but must be distinctly rare. The variability of blood pressure in individual patients with hypermineralocorticoidism has to be remembered and the factors controlling the pressor effects in individuals are largely unknown. Similarly, normokalemic hypertension, while popularized in the mid-1960s, is also unusual and probably occurs only when there is a dietary or other cause of salt restriction. The pathophysiology of this syndrome of mineralocorticoid excess is outlined in Figure 2, using the example of primary aldosteronism. Increased salt and water reabsorption at the level of the distal tubule causes an expansion in both total body sodium, extracellular fluid, and plasma volume—events which in time lead to a hyperdynamic form of hypertension (23). Concomitant with the increased plasma volume there is depression of renin secretion, an increase in glomerular filtration rate, and a reduction in the percentage of proximal tubular sodium reabsorption. This is thought to be the mechanism of "escape" from the sodium-retaining action of aldosterone whereby the rate of sodium excretion returns to a new steady state. It also explains why sodium retention sufficient to cause edema does not usually occur in primary aldosteronism. As a result of this "escape" relatively more sodium is passed to distal exchange sites, where aldosterone-dependent potassium secretion continues. The end result is hypokalemic hypertension with inappropriately high urinary potassium excretion rates. That all of these effects are mediated by mineralocorticoid excess alone is shown by the reversal of the syndrome by the antialdosterone drug spironolactone (24), or the potassium-conserving diuretic amiloride (25). Excess of other mineralocorticoids will induce the same abnormalities.

The situation is quite different in states of "secondary aldosteronism," such as cirrhosis and congestive heart failure, where diminished renal perfusion results in increased renin secretion. Here there is enhanced salt and water reabsorption

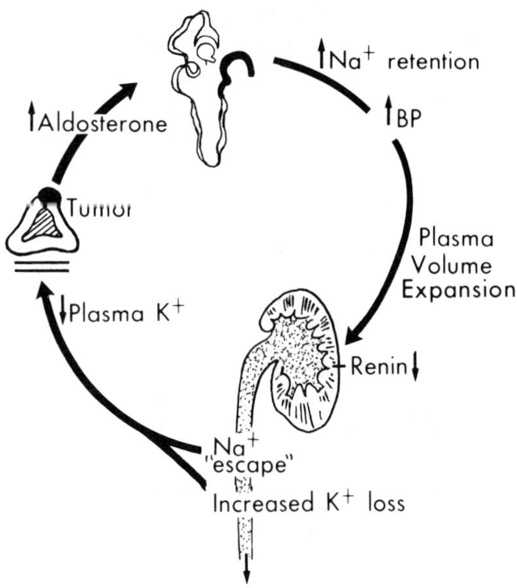

Figure 2 Pathophysiology of mineralocorticoid excess syndromes as exemplified by primary aldosteronism.

at the level of the proximal convoluted tubule in response to a drop in renal perfusion pressure. Because of some primary deficiency in the circulation or plasma proteins, the reabsorbate is not retained within the plasma compartment and increase in "effective arterial volume"—with closure of the renin feed back loop—does not occur. Sodium retention continues as long as sodium is ingested and eventually edema develops. Because proximal sodium reabsorption remains increased in these hypovolemic states, less sodium is available for potassium exchange at distal sites (irrespective of the plasma concentration of aldosterone), so hypokalemia is not severe unless diuretic drugs are given. Despite the massive increase in sodium retention, and often markedly raised levels of angiotensin II, hypertension does not develop, presumably because the pressor effect of angiotensin II is largely determined by the effective arterial blood volume or related factors (26). Secondary hyperaldosteronism is also seen in other volume depletion states, such as severe sodium depletion dehydration and hemorrhage (see Sect. IV.A.1). Such patients will not usually be edematous but the mechanism of the secondary hyperaldosteronism, namely increased renin release in response to hypovolemia, is similar.

While the forms of hyperaldosteronism discussed above are usually easily distinguished, hyperaldosteronism occurring in *hypertensive* patients secondary to increased renin secretion needs to be considered. Clinical examples include the syndrome of renal artery ischemia, accelerated or malignant phase hypertension, and a primary excess of renin as seen in patients with "reninoma" (27). In these situations, high levels of angiotensin II stimulate aldosterone production but again escape from continued sodium retention usually occurs if the unaffected kidney can compensate. Hypokalemia may occur, and there will be the important additional pressor effect from raised levels of angiotensin II. Paradoxically, the pressor effect of angiotensin II may be greater in some salt-depleted patients with severe unilateral renal ischemia and in these circumstances blood pressure may only respond when angiotensin is reduced by converting enzyme inhibitors and normovolemia is restored by salt repletion (28). In addition to plasma renin levels, an important difference between primary mineralocorticoid excess and both normol- and hypertensive forms of secondary hyperaldosteronism is the level of plasma sodium concentration. Plasma sodium is normal or slightly increased in primary states of mineralocorticoid excess and generally lower in secondary forms of the syndrome. The difference may be due to angiotensin II, which stimulates ADH and thirst, thereby lowering plasma sodium in states of secondary hyperaldosteronism.

B. Mineralocorticoid Deficiency

These states are characterized by hyperkalemia, salt wasting, metabolic acidosis, and hypovolemia if severe. The classical presentation is seen in primary adrenocortical insufficiency (Addison's disease) and in neonates with biosynthetic abnormalities of aldosterone synthesis. Plasma sodium falls, urinary sodium excretion is inappropriately high, and the tubular secretion of potassium and/or hydrogen ion is reduced. Plasma renin and angiotensin II increase markedly but to no avail if the end organ (glomerulosa) is unable to respond. Death from metabolic acidosis and renal failure occurs in the absence of specific treatment. This picture is especially likely to occur if cortisol deficiency is also present. However, mineralocorticoid deficiency *alone* may be asymptomatic and although defects in hydrogen and potassium secretion are common, salt wasting and hypovolemia do not usually occur. Presumably, the differences are dependent on a satisfactory level of cortisol, illustrating the important permissive effect of this hormone in mineralocorticoid action.

C. Regulation of Mineralocorticoid Secretion in Disease States

While changes in aldosterone secretion are explicable in most clinical states by concomitant changes in renin (angiotensin), ACTH, or potassium, in practice it is often difficult to say which of these regulators is predominant. Generally, there is a good overall correlation between renin-angiotensin activity and aldosterone in volume-depleted states (29) but poor correlation in normovolemia or in patients with presumed essential hypertension (30). The picture is made more complex by the finding of altered aldosterone sensitivity to angiotensin, for instance in subtypes of the hypertensive population. Increased sensitivity of aldosterone to angiotensin has been reported in low-renin hypertension and in idiopathic hyperaldosteronism (19), whereas a reduction in sensitivity occurs in patients with primary aldosteronism due to an adrenal adenoma (31). Primary aldosteronism is a good example of the subtle shift in aldosterone regulation that may occur in disease states. In this syndrome, the renin-angiotensin system is well suppressed and volume-dependent stimuli have little effect on aldosterone secretion. However, the adrenal tumor remains fully sensitive to potassium and may show enhanced sensitivity to ACTH (32), so that the normal diurnal rhythmicity is amplified. As a complete contrast, in patients with hyporeninemic hypoaldosteronism (where the activity of the renin-angiotensin system is also markedly diminished) the glomerulosa's ability to respond to potassium or ACTH may be lost (33). These clinical examples serve to highlight the complexities of aldosterone regulation in different disease states and emphasize the need to interpret aldosterone results on the basis of several different parameters, including ACTH, potassium, and renin whenever possible.

III. LABORATORY ASSESSMENT OF MINERALOCORTICOID STATUS

As mentioned in Section II, plasma electrolyte status and renal and "volume" status may suggest an abnormality of mineralocorticoid secretion. While biological assays have contributed in the past (e.g., salivary sodium/potassium ratios, and rectal mucosa potential difference), more precise chemical measurements are now available and should be used. Inappropriate kaliuresis in the setting of hypokalemia remains an important marker of mineralocorticoid excess. Aldosterone status can be assessed by measuring the urine excretion rate of the acid-labile metabolite, which is usually a constant portion of the daily aldosterone production rate except in patients with hepatic or renal disease. Plasma aldosterone can be readily measured by radioimmunoassay techniques, but it is important to realize that values may change rapidly and are markedly influenced by salt intake, posture, diurnal factors, and stress (see below). The secretion rate of aldosterone can be measured by the isotope dilution technique, but the advent of reliable plasma aldosterone assays has reduced the need for secretion rate measurements in clinical diagnosis. Other mineralocorticoids can be measured directly in plasma or by measuring the appropriate urinary metabolite.

Components of the renin-angiotensin system may be assessed in a variety of ways. Renin concentration, while not yet measurable by specific radioimmunoassay, can be measured indirectly by the generation of angiotensin I under standardized conditions in the presence of excess renin substrate. Plasma renin

Table 2 Physiological Factors Affecting Renin and Aldosterone

	Renin secretion	Aldosterone secretion
Age	Raised in infancy Low in aged	Higher in infancy
Menstrual cycle	Higher in luteal phase	
Sodium intake	Increased by salt restriction Decreased by salt loading	
Potassium status	Increased by K depletion	Decreased by K depletion
Posture	Increased with erect posture	
Sympathetic nervous stimulation	Increased by catecholamines	?
Time of sampling	Highest in forenoon Low in evening	Diurnal rhythm as for ACTH

activity (PRA), the more commonly measured parameter, measures the rate of angiotensin I generated from plasma incubated in vitro without added renin substrate. Techniques are available for measurement of renin substrate, angiotensin I, angiotensin II, and converting enzyme (see reviews in Refs. 34 and 35 for details). Although there is still debate concerning the most appropriate measurement, particularly with the recognition of big or inactive renin (36), PRA assays have provided a great deal of useful clinical diagnostic information (37). This is especially true if renin and aldosterone (or other mineralocorticoid) assays are measured together, preferably in the same plasma sample and interpreted in the light of the patient's clinical status. Thus high plasma renin activity with normal or low aldosterone strongly suggests glomerulosa deficiency (as may occur in Addison's disease), high aldosterone and low plasma renin activity suggests primary aldosteronism, and so on. The value of results is strengthened by simultaneous assessments of plasma and urinary electrolytes and, in some cases, by measurement of cortisol and plasma ACTH.

Interpretation of renin and aldosterone measurements is made more difficult by the variety of factors known to affect results (Table 2). Thus plasma renin activity is higher in infants (38), falls in the aged (39), is subject to prominent diurnal (40) and menstrual rhythm (41), and is strongly influenced by dietary sodium intake (42), posture (43), and sympathetic nervous activity (44). Aldosterone is similarly influenced, and in addition is reduced by potassium depletion and may vary with short-term changes in ACTH secretion. Finally, a variety of drugs (Table 3), particularly diuretics, which increase plasma renin activity, and β-adrenoreceptor blocking drugs, which reduce it, add to the interpretative difficulties.

In clinical practice it is impossible to control all the variables affecting the renin-angiotensin-aldosterone axis. However, it should be possible to standardize time of sampling, posture, and approximate sodium intake. In the author's laboratory, for screening purposes samples are taken from ambulant patients whenever possible between 8 and 10 A.M., the patients being off all drugs for 2 weeks and consuming a "normal" sodium intake. A 24-hr urine collection for sodium, potassium, and aldosterone excretion on the same day will assist interpretation (see Chap. 46). When hypertension is severe, some drug therapy may be essential but β-blocker drugs and diuretics should be avoided whenever possible. In agreement with others, in our experience prazosin (45) and methyldopa (46) cause little change in the activity of the renin-angiotensin system and are preferred when hypotensive treatment is essential. For definitive diagnosis the patient may require samples to be taken under strict conditions of metabolic balance and standardized posture (see below). Occasionally, for instance in the patient presenting with possible acute adrenal insufficiency, urgent sampling has to be performed irrespective of the conditions specified above.

A. Special Tests of the Renin-Angiotensin-Adrenal Status

Basal tests may be diagnostic, but in many cases, manipulations are required to assess the integrity of the axis. In general, stimulation tests are most valuable when hypofunction is suspected, and suppressive tests are indicated in those

Table 3 Effect of Drugs on PRA

Increase	Decrease
Diuretics	β-Adrenoreceptor blocking drugs
Vasodilators: nitroprusside, minoxidil, hydralazine, phenyoxybenzamine, prazosin[a]	Central depressants (e.g., clonidine)
Estrogens[b]	Methyldopa[a]
Sympathomimetics	Mineralocorticoids
Angiotensin II blockers: captopril, saralasin	Prostaglandin inhibitors
Cortisol blockers (e.g., o,p′-DDD, etc.)	Cyproheptadine
High-dose glucocorticoids[b]	

[a]Small effect.
[b]Raise renin substrate.

with hyperfunction. Thus in primary aldosteronism, failure to suppress aldosterone secretion by salt-loading maneuver or mineralocorticoid treatment is an important part of the diagnostic process. Because renin is suppressed in this disorder, attempts to stimulate PRA (e.g., low-salt diets, volume depletion, etc.) are necessary to confirm renin suppression. In mineralocorticoid hypofunction (as in primary adrenal insufficiency or hyporeninemia) stimulation tests employing upright posture, salt depletion, or ACTH testing may be invaluable. Finally, localizing procedures, such as renal vein renin measurements or adrenal vein hormone sampling techniques, can give definitive information once the hyperfunctioning state has been proven.

IV. CLINICAL PRESENTATION, DIFFERENTIAL DIAGNOSIS, AND DIAGNOSTIC TESTING

A. Mineralocorticoid Excess

Disorders characterized by excessive mineralocorticoid activity are conveniently separated into two classes, depending on the presence or absence of hypertension.

1. With Hypertension

An approach to the problem of hypokalemic hypertension is shown in Diagnostic Summary 1. These patients will be demonstrably hypokalemic, provided that standardized techniques for blood collection (47) are used and several estimations of plasma potassium are made (48). Occasionally, the syndrome is masked by diet or drug therapy (e.g., potassium conserving diuretics or sodium-deficient diets). From the clinicians viewpoint these patients present with hypertension and spontaneous hypokalemia which is associated with inappropriately increased potassium loss in the urine. Urine potassium of more than 30 mmol/per day of diuretic drugs when plasma potassium is 3.3 mmol/liter or less is abnormal and requires investigation. Note that salt restriction may mask this important finding, so urinary sodium excretion should exceed 40 mmol/per day in the same urine sample before dismissing the potassium loss as nonhormonal. Occasionally, a low intake of potassium can also lead to false negative results. Patients are often asymptomatic, although symptoms of potassium depletion are likely if plasma potassium is less than 2.8 mmol/liter. Most helpful in differential diagnosis is the plasma renin status (Table 4). Renin is depressed in primary mineralocorticoid excess states and plasma sodium is usually normal or slightly raised. Rarely, plasma renin may be in the normal range because of excessive diuretic use or volume depletion from other causes. On the other hand, in patients with hypokalemic hypertension due to activation of the renin-angiotensin system, peripheral plasma renin is normal or elevated and the plasma sodium concentration is frequently lower set. The severity of the hypertension is not generally helpful in separating these conditions (49).

Table 4 Hypertension and Hypokalemia

Depressed PRA		Normal or raised PRA
Primary aldosteronism		Renal ischemia
Adenoma		
Hyperplasia	Aldosterone ↑	
Dexa methasone suppressible		
		Drug induced
		Diuretic
		Estrogen
Licorice ingestion		
18-OH-DOC		Reninoma
DOC Excess		
Corticosterone		
	Aldosterone ↓	
17-Hydroxylase defect		
11-Hydroxylase defect		
Liddle's syndrome		
Dexa methasone-responsive forms		
	Cushing's syndrome[a]	

[a] Adrenal carcinoma and ectopic ACTH syndromes may present with hypokalemic hypertension. PRA and aldosterone levels are variable.

Patients with Normal or Raised PRA.

Renal Artery Stenosis. It is important to note that only a small percentage of patients with renal ischemia show obvious features of mineralocorticoid excess. Diagnosis will depend on demonstrating localized ischemia by arteriography. Peripheral plasma renin may be normal but generally responds excessively to upright posture or volume-depleting maneuvers. Renal vein sampling for PRA (see Chap. 46 for details) is necessary to confirm (1) excessive secretion from the affected kidney and (2) suppression of the contralateral renin secretion when compared to peripheral blood renin measurements. Ratios greater than 1.5 (affected renal vein/unaffected renal vein renin) (50) and ratios of contralateral renal vein renin/peripheral renin closer to 1 auger well for surgical cure of hypertension (51). In most patients blood pressure responds well to angiotensin II inhibitors such as saralasin or captopril as well as beta-blocking treatment, but these tests are not decisive in diagnosis.

Accelerated or Malignant Phase Hypertension. There will be clear-cut evidence of severe hypertensive retinopathy and often impairment in glomerular function PRA and aldosterone are usually elevated. Secondary hyperaldosteronism will usually regress once arterial pressure is reduced by hypotensive drugs unless there is some underlying disorder such as renal artery stenosis. It has to be remembered, of course, that the drugs used to treat the blood pressure may themselves reduce hyperaldosteronism independent of any effect on blood pressure per se.

Drug Induced. The commonest cause of hypokalemia in hypertensive patients is thiazide or other diuretic use. Long-term diuretic use also may lead to secondary hyperaldosteronism because of salt depletion. Diuretics should be stopped for at least 1 week and potassium status reassessed. It is important that the patient receive a normal sodium intake without potassium supplements during this period. If inappropriate urinary loss of potassium is still present, the patient should be further investigated for syndromes of mineralocorticoid excess. Other patients may require a longer period of follow-up, during which time diuretics should be avoided. Estrogen therapy (as in oral contraceptive drugs) may stimulate a renin-dependent form of hypertension, but in our experience these drugs do not greatly increase aldosterone nor do they produce hypokalemia unless an accelerated hypertensive phase develops. Estrogens should be stopped and the renin-angiotensin-aldosterone status reassessed some 6 weeks later.

Reninoma is rare but may mimic primary aldosteronism. Peripheral PRA is elevated and does not change with variations in sodium intake (27). Arteriography may be normal, but renal vein renin levels should localize the abnormality.

Other causes, such as Cushing's syndrome (particularly ectopic ACTH secretion), may present with hypokalemic hypertension. Plasma renin activity is not always suppressed in this syndrome presumably because excess cortisol secretion increases renin substrate levels and may raise PRA into the normal range. Rarely, renal tubular acidosis, producing a potassium-losing state and secondary hyperaldosteronism, may present diagnostic difficulties, since such patients are often hypertensive. Hyperchloremic acidosis and failure to acidify the urine should differentiate these patients from other forms of hypokalemic hypertension. Patients with essential hypertension may occasionally develop transient hypokalemia for reasons such as poor intake or excessive bowel loss. In these instances urinary potassium loss is usually less than 30 mmol/per day unless alkalosis is prominent (e.g., from vomiting) (52). Continued follow-up of such patients is necessary to determine the cause of the potassium deficiency.

Patients with Depressed PRA

Primary Aldosteronism. At least three distinct forms of the disease are now recognized: a solitary cortical adenoma (80% of cases), bilateral hyperplasia

("idiopathic hyperplasia," 10-20% of cases), and a rare fam
suppressible by dexamethasone. The clinical features are sir
kalemic hypertension without edema. Potassium depletion
severe in adenoma cases. The etiology of the hyperplastic an
suppressible forms is unknown. The criteria for the diagnosis
primary aldosteronism are (1) inappropriate kaliuresis which i ... load dependent (2) suppressed renin activity despite stimulation using maneuvers of volume depletion, and (3) sustained and excessive aldosterone secretion (when potassium replete) despite high sodium intakes. Patients should also be shown to have normal and not increased levels of cortisol secretion. Inappropriate kaliuresis may be shown by urine collections while ingesting a normal or high-salt diet, or by sodium loading procedures (53). Suppressed PRA is shown by restricting salt intake (10 mmol sodium intake/per day) for at least 4 days and should be combined with the stimulation of 2 hours of upright posture (54). An alternative test employs frusemide-induced volume depletion (55). Autonomy of aldosterone secretion is shown by tests requiring salt loading or 9α-fluorohydrocortisone. In the former, the change in plasma aldosterone after 2 liters of isotonic saline given over a 4-hr period is examined (56). The prominent diurnal rhythm in plasma aldosterone must be kept in mind when interpreting these results since plasma aldosterone is usually considerably lower after noon, compared to 8 A.M. values both in Conn's syndrome (54) and in normal subjects. A convenient protocol combining salt restriction to assess PRA suppression followed by saline infusions for two successive days to assess aldosterone autonomy is employed in the author's laboratory (54). The administration of 400 μg of 9α-fluorohydrocortisone for 3 days to subjects taking a normal sodium diet can also be used since this maneuver fails to suppress plasma or urine aldosterone secretion in patients with primary aldosteroneism (57), whereas it will suppress the hormone in most other forms of hypertension. Potassium depletion itself may reduce aldosterone secretion (see Fig. 3) and results must be interpreted in relation to the prevailing plasma potassium concentration.

While the biochemical and hormonal abnormalities are usually more severe in adenoma patients, the tests described above do not distinguish the cause of the hyperaldosteronism. It must be remembered that as many as 20% of patients with essential hypertension may show resistance of aldosterone to supression by salt loading (58). Since low plasma renin activity is also commonly found in the hypertensive population (59), confusion can arise if careful appraisal of potassium status is not made (see Diagnostic Summary 1).

Once a diagnosis of primary aldosteronism is established it is necessary to determine the cause. This is important since the blood pressure response to therapy is different—adenoma cases being much more responsive. The more florid features of adenoma cases have been used to develop an index [quadric analysis (60)] which may help to separate adenoma from bilateral hyperplasia patients. Plasma 18-hydroxycorticosterone is raised in primary

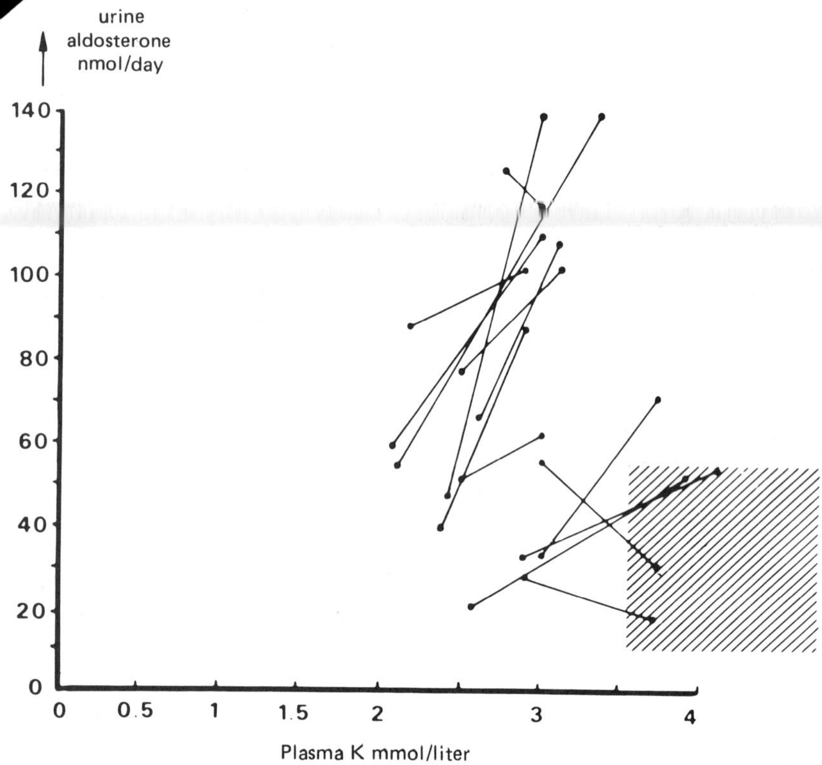

Figure 3 Effect of plasma potassium on aldosterone excretion in 14 patients with primary aldosteronism. The hatched area indicates the normal range.

aldosteronism and separates adenoma from hyperplasia according to Biglieri and Schambelan (61). The most useful discriminatory tests, however, are the plasma aldosterone response to prolonged upright posture (62) and localizing techniques employing adrenal venography and in particular adrenal venous sampling and/or adrenal scanning procedures.

Four-hour upright posture test. The test makes use of the finding that a prominent aldosterone diurnal rhythm exists in primary aldosteronism, but both the renin response to posture [and the aldosterone response to angiotensin (63)] are greater in patients with idiopathic hyperplasia. In patients with adenoma or dexamethasone-suppressible aldosteronism, plasma aldosterone falls or changes little, whereas in hyperplasia there is a distinct rise after prolonged upright posture. Plasma cortisol should also be checked since a stress effect may invalidate the test.

Adrenal scanning. Results may be difficult to interpret when isotope uptake is asymmetrical, as may happen in normal adrenals (64) and in patients with nodular or asymmetrical adrenal hyperplasia. The reliability of current tracer techniques for separating types of primary aldosteronism is therefore still in doubt, although it seems likely that improved techniques giving more discriminating data on adrenal function will be developed within the next few years.

Computerized axial tomographic (CAT) adrenal scanning. CAT scanning is easier and more generally available in most main centers (see Chap. 16). It must be remembered that small nonfunctioning adrenal cortical adenomas are common in hypertensive patients and it is imperative that the diagnostic process be logically pursued (as mentioned above, see also Diagnostic Summary 1) before acting on the strictly anatomical data given by CAT scanning. Again errors may be made in patients with macronodular or asymmetrical adrenal hyperplasia.

Adrenal venography and venous sampling. While invasive, this test is the most valuable for localizing adenomas (see Chap. 46).

Dexamethasone suppressability. A rare form of primary aldosteronism characterized by hypertension which is normalized by dexamethasone in low dose has been reported (65). Patients are likely to be in the younger age groups. Unlike normal subjects or patients with other forms of primary aldosteronism, chronic ACTH stimulation produces a sustained increase in aldosterone secretion (66) similar to the cortisol response to sustained ACTH stimulation. Dexamethasone 2.0 mg/per day normalizes potassium balance, aldosterone, renin, and blood pressure abnormalities over a 2- to 3-week period. While dexamethasone causes a temporary reduction in aldosterone in patients with other forms of primary aldosteronism (54), it is not sustained (67) and no change in potassium or blood pressure occurs.

Predictive response to surgery. The administration of the competitive inhibitor of aldosterone, spironolactone 400 mg daily for 3 weeks, will reduce blood pressure significantly in most patients with primary aldosteronism. Those not responding are said to be unlikely to respond to surgical removal of an aldosterone-secreting tumor. Since patients with hyperplasia and adenoma appear to be equally responsive to spironolactone (68) the test does not necessarily distinguish between these two entities. Further, patients with essential hypertension may respond, so a positive result is in no way a diagnostic test for primary aldosteronism.

In summary. Provided that criteria for primary aldosteronism are fulfilled, florid cases can be finally categorized by a 4-hr posture test and a scanning procedure. Where there is less certainty or ambiguous results are obtained, adrenal venous sampling with venography is recommended before surgery is contemplated. Because aldosterone-secreting tumors are often inconspicuous even at operation, there is no place these days for the "let's have a look and see" approach, and some preoperative localizing procedures are always necessary.

Iatragenic causes. Obviously, excessive use of potent sodium-retaining drugs such as 9α-fluorohydrocortisone or hydrocortisone may induce hypokalemic hypertension. A nasal spray containing the steroid 9α-fluoroprednisolone was found to produce a similar picture (69).

Pseudohyperaldosteronism due to licorice ingestion. Chronic consumption of licorice will result in hypokalemic hypertension which closely mimics primary aldosteronism. Licorice contains glycyrrhizic acid. A substance that promotes sodium retention and potassium secretion into the distal tubular urine. This effect can be reversed by spironolactone. As in primary aldosteronism, profound suppression of PRA occurs (70) but can be readily distinguished from this disorder by low and subnormal levels of plasma aldosterone or aldosterone excretion. Prompt natriuresis occurs on cessation of the drug and the renin-angiotensin-aldosterone axis returns to normal within a few months of stopping licorice ingestion. A similar syndrome may occur in peptic ulcer patients taking carbeonoxolone, which contains derivatives of glycyrrhizic acid. Licorice also increases urinary cortisol excretion (71), which could give rise to further diagnostic confusion. These conditions should be readily detected by careful history taking and specific questioning directed to licorice ingestion (taken as confectionery, drinks, or in cough medicine or other proprietary medicines) in all patients presenting with hypokalemia.

Disorders of "isolated mineralocorticoid excess" (other than aldosterone). Isolated hypersection of DOC, corticosterone, and 18-hydroxy-DOC has been described (72).* These disorders mimic primary aldosteronism except that aldosterone secretion is normal or low. Renin is not always suppressed (see Ref. 68 for a review).

17- and 11-hydroxylase deficiency syndrome. These are rare but important causes of hypokalemic hypertension. 17-hydroxylase deficiency affects both adrenocortical and gonadal steroid biosynthesis, so deficient sex steroid production is an associated feature (73). Females present with hypogonadism and primary amenorrhea, whereas the affected male shows inadequate virilization (male pseudohermaphroditism) (74). Urinary 17-keto and ketogenic steroid metabolites are low, in keeping with 17-hydroxylase deficiency. Corticosterone and 11-desoxycorticosterone and their metabolites are increased and are responsible for the mineralocorticoid hypertension and suppression of renin and aldosterone. The hypersecretion of ACTH (which is consequent upon reduced cortisol production) further stimulates mineralocorticoids, including 18-hydroxycorticosterone (75) but not aldosterone. Treatment with low-dose dexamethasone corrects the blood pressure and restores potassium and plasma renin activity to normal.

---

*A similar picture has been described in a family with primary cortisol resistance (Chrousos G. P., J. Clin Invest 1982; 69, 1261–1269).

11β-Hydroxylase deficiency affects only adrenal cortical biosynthesis. Here increased DOC and 11-desoxycortisol cause hypertension and hypokalemia with suppression of renin (76). Because of the excessive precursor steroid secretion with androgen effect, female patients will show virilizing features which are associated with other forms of congenital adrenal hyperplasia, such as 21-hydroxylase deficiency. Unlike 17-hydroxylase deficiency, urinary 17-hydroxysteroids and ketogenic steroids will be increased because of the excessive output of 11-desoxycortisol metabolites (tetrahydro S, etc.). Again, glucocorticoid treatment restores blood pressure, potassium, and renin status to normal levels.

Dexamethasone responsive mineralocorticoid hypertensions. A form of hypokalemic hypertension with suppressed renin and suppressed aldosterone and normal DOC and 18-hydroxy-DOC levels have been described in young women (77). Blood pressure, renin, and aldosterone return to normal with dexamethasone treatment. The cause of the syndrome is unknown. It should be distinguished from dexamethasone-suppressible primary aldosteronism where aldosterone secretion is increased.

Liddle's syndrome. This is a familial disorder characterized by excessive renal sodium reabsorption, the precise cause of which is unknown. Patients will present with hypokalemic hypertension and depression of renin and aldosterone. The syndrome is unresponsive to spironolactone, but is reversed by triamterine or amiloride. More recent evidence suggests that the disorder of sodium transport may be more generalized and not simply confined to the renal tubules, as originally conceived (78).

Cushing's syndrome. While hypertension is common in Cushing's syndrome, spontaneous hypokalemia is unusual except in the setting of the ectopic ACTH syndrome (79). The very high ACTH levels sometimes observed in this disorder may be associated with increased output of corticosterone and DOC (80) as well as cortisol. Aldosterone secretion is not always low and PRA is not necessarily suppressed (81) possibly because of an effect of high glucocorticoids on renin substrate levels. These disorders should be readily diagnosed by the clinical features of glucocorticoid excess and the characteristic abnormalities in cortisol secretion.

Adrenal carcinoma may present with hypokalemic hypertension. Usually, but not always, there will be hypersecretion of other corticosteroids. An ovarian tumor has been associated with hyperaldosteronism (see Ref. 68).

Low-renin essential hypertension. Controversy still surrounds the significance and definition of hypertensive patients with low renin (82). Despite an enormous research effort there is no convincing evidence that "low-renin hypertension" represents a distinct disorder of mineralocorticoid secretion. Patients with low-renin hypertension can be readily recognized from mineralocorticoid hypertension by careful evaluation of potassium status.

Table 5 Causes of Secondary Hyperaldosteronism (Nonhypertensive Forms)

With edema	Without edema
Congestive heart failure	Pregnancy
Nephrotic syndrome	Chronic sodium deficiency (e.g., ileostomy)
Cirrhosis	
Some forms of localized edema	Sodium losing nephritis
	Bartters syndrome
	Compensated congenital adrenal hyperplasia

2. Mineralocorticoid Excess without Hypertension

As described under pathophysiology, increase in aldosterone secretion is one of the body's defense mechanisms against hypovolemia. Hyperaldosteronism is therefore to be expected whenever salt deficiency or fall in "effective arterial blood volume" develops–and in such cases is a response to increased renin secretion. For reasons already given, increased kaliuresis and severe potassium depletion are not usually seen (unless diuretic drugs are given) and blood pressure is not increased despite very high levels of circulating angiotensin. Edema will be present when a chronic circulatory or protein abnormality exists. A list of common causes of nonhypertensive hyperaldosteronism is given in Table 5.

Hyperaldosteronism with Edema. Readers are referred to previous studies of patients with heart failure (83), nephrotic syndrome (84), and cirrhosis (85). The role of the renin-angiotensin-aldosterone system in idiopathic edema is disputed, and many patients show quite normal levels.

Hyperaldosteronism Without Edema

Pregnancy. Plasma levels of aldosterone increase during normal pregnancy, as do PRA and levels of renin substrate. The pressor response to exogenous angiotensin II is reduced. Some of the secondary aldosteronism may be a compensatory response to the massive rise in progesterone secretion, which has some antialdosterone activity and promotes natriuresis.

Salt-Losing States. Abnormal salt loss may occur in renal tubular disease, patients with ileostomy and diarrheal states, and other disorders. Anorexia nervosa patients may be severely volume depleted by chronic starvation. Patients using purgatives and diuretics–often surreptitiously–may also show severe secondary hyperaldosteronism (86).

21-Hydroxylase Deficiency, Congenital Adrenal Hyperplasia. While a proportion of patients with 21-hydroxylase deficiency present with salt loss and adrenal crisis (see below), many patients with less severe defects show no obvious abnormality in sodium handling. Rather than deficiency, studies in these patients have demonstrated increased circulating levels of both renin and aldosterone, particularly when the disorder in adrenal biosynthesis is less than fully controlled by glucocorticoid therapy. It is possible that in patients with mild or incomplete forms of the syndrome, hyperaldosteronism is secondary to increased production of natriuretic steroids such as progesterone and 17-hydroxyprogesterone. These patients do not generally show clinical abnormalities in blood pressure, salt handling, or in plasma electrolytes and separation from other forms of secondary aldosteronism should not be difficult.

Bartter's syndrome was described in 1962 (87) in two patients demonstrating spontaneous severe hypokalemia associated with excessive urinary loss of potassium, normotension, and raised levels of renin and aldosterone. The patients showed increased juxtaglomerular cell numbers on renal biopsy without any obvious abnormality in glomerular or tubular function. While a defect in vascular responsiveness to angiotensin II was suspected, subsequent studies in patients with Bartter's syndrome indicate that the disorder is more complex than a simple vascular receptor defect, as originally proposed. The disorder, which may be familial, can present at any age, usually with symptoms related to potassium depletion. Tetany, fatigue, and parasthesiae are common. Clinical examination is usually otherwise unremarkable and shows normotension. Laboratory findings show hypokalemic metabolic alkalosis, normal or lowish plasma sodium, raised renin and angiotensin, and normal or raised aldosterone levels. There is inappropriate urinary loss of potassium which is only partly reversed by spironolactone. Excessive magnesium excretion may also occur, but patients usually show a normal ability to conserve sodium when placed on a low-salt diet. Recent studies (88) have shown increased urinary prostaglandin E and Kallikrein excretion together with high levels of plasma bradykinin. Treatment with prostaglandin inhibitors (such as indomethacin) not only restores prostaglandin E (PGE), kallikrein, and PRA to near-normal values, but also reduces the abnormality in renal potassium handling. The basic defect in Bartter's syndrome is still unclear, but it has been suggested that a defect in chloride reabsorption in the ascending limb of Henle's loop is the primary abnormality. The resulting increase in distal tubular urine flow will also promote potassium secretion and increase prostaglandins, which may be responsible for activation of the renin-angiotensin-aldosterone axis. Presumably, severe hypokalemia is the reason for the minimal increase in aldosterone observed in some patients with Bartter's syndrome. The disorder is readily distinguished from primary aldosteronism because of the normal or lowish blood pressure (or in difficult cases by the raised plasma renin activity) but may be closely mimicked by chronic diuretic abusers, who present an exactly similar picture (89). Evidence for diuretic drug use or abuse should therefore be carefully sought in all patients presenting with "Bartter's syndrome."

Table 6 Disorders of Mineralocorticoid Deficiency

1. *Primary deficiency*	
Addison's disease Adrenal enzyme deficiency states Chronic drug therapy: heparin, o,p′-DDD, aminoglutethamide	Low aldesterone, high PRA
2. *Secondary deficiency*	
Hyporeninemic (idiopathic) Postadrenalectomy in Conn's syndrome	Low aldosterone, low PRA
3. *Tissue unresponsiveness to aldosterone*	
Pseudohypoaldosteronism	High aldosterone, high PRA

B. Mineralocorticoid Deficiency

Deficiency of mineralocorticoids may be due to diminished renin secretion, diminished glomerulosa response, or diminished tissue response to circulating mineralocorticoids (see Table 6). Disorders characterized by diminished renin secretion generally give rise to subtle abnormalities in hydrogen and potassium homeostasis and do not usually present with hyponatremic hypovolemic syndrome characteristic of the other types of deficiency. However, hyperchloremic metabolic acidosis may be a feature of all types of mineralocorticoid deficiency.

1. Primary Deficiency States

Primary deficiency of mineralocorticoid hormones occurs classically in Addison's disease, where cortisol secretion is usually also reduced. The combination of both chronic cortisol and aldosterone deficiency is particularly lethal. Lack of mineralocorticoid is responsible for chronic sodium wasting, hypovolemia leading to prerenal failure, hyponatremia, hyperkalemia, and associated metabolic acidosis. Diagnosis is established by showing a low or normal aldosterone level despite marked elevation in plasma renin activity in conjunction with raised plasma ACTH, normal or low cortisol levels, and absent responses to exogenous ACTH. While most patients with Addison's disease show both cortisol and aldosterone deficiency, it is important to note that mineralocorticoid deficiency may predominate in some patients (90). Thus skin pigmentation and extreme elevation in plasma ACTH may not always be present and early in the course of the disease some cortisol response to ACTH may still persist. Plasma electrolytes need not be abnormal, particularly if high salt intake is maintained. Whenever possible, blood for PRA and aldosterone should be obtained, preferably between 8 and 10 A.M. with the patient ambulant for at least 15 min, since some stimulation of the renin-angiotensin axis is helpful in bringing out the defect (37).

Using this approach it is generally not necessary to challenge the volume status further by employing, for example, a low-salt diet, which could be hazardous. While renin substrate is reduced in cortisol deficiency states (91), in our experience this is not sufficient to mask the PRA increase characteristic of Addison's disease (37). However, it may be part of the explanation for the low renin values encountered in ACTH deficiency states. In any event, ambulant PRA is most helpful in the differential diagnosis of patients presenting with cortisol deficiency. A short ACTH stimulation test (92) to assess aldosterone response can also aid in the diagnosis and help to separate patients with ACTH deficiency whose increment in plasma aldosterone should be near normal ($>$10 ng/per 100 ml or 300 pmol/liter). Absent responses are typical of a primary glomerulosa defect.

Adrenalectomized subjects will be prone to mineralocorticoid deficiency unless they are treated with salt-retaining steroids. Not all patients require this treatment, however, presumably because of the mineralocorticoid activity of hydrocortisone treatment. Renin status helps to assess these requirements (37).

Disorders of mineralocorticoid biosynthesis may present with mineralocorticoid deficiency. The best known examples are salt-wasting forms of congenital adrenal hyperplasia (e.g., C-21 hydroxylase deficiency or earlier defect), which usually present as acute adrenal crisis within 2 weeks of birth. Rarely, such infants present later in life. Diagnosis can be made by employing tests as mentioned above, in conjunction with assays for specific precursor corticosteroids, which will usually disclose the nature of the enzyme deficiency. The higher range of values for renin and aldosterone in normal infants (38) must be remembered when interpreting results. Mineralocorticoid deficiency is not seen in all neonatal cases of severe adrenocortical insufficiency: for instance, neonates with familial insensitivity to ACTH will show normal aldosterone secretion. Infants with congenital adrenal hypoplasia will show combined glucocorticoid and mineralocorticoid deficiency.

Isolated defects in aldosterone biosynthesis may occur (e.g., defective conversion of corticosterone to aldosterone) which may be familial. Infants show failure to thrive, growth failure, and salt wasting despite hyponatremia and hyperkalemia. A metabolic acidosis is common. Plasma renin activity is markedly elevated, aldosterone low, and the appropriate precursor steroids (18-hydroxy-DOC and 18-hydroxycorticosterone metabolites) are elevated (93). The ACTH-cortisol axis is intact. The condition responds to mineralocorticoid replacement or a high-salt diet. Some neonates show a temporary salt-wasting syndrome which spontaneously remits with age.

Certain drugs will reduce aldosterone secretion and mimic primary deficiency states. Long-term heparin, spironolactone, captopril (and other converting enzyme inhibitors), and aminoglutethimide are examples.

Diagnostic Summary 1 Hypokalemic Hypertension

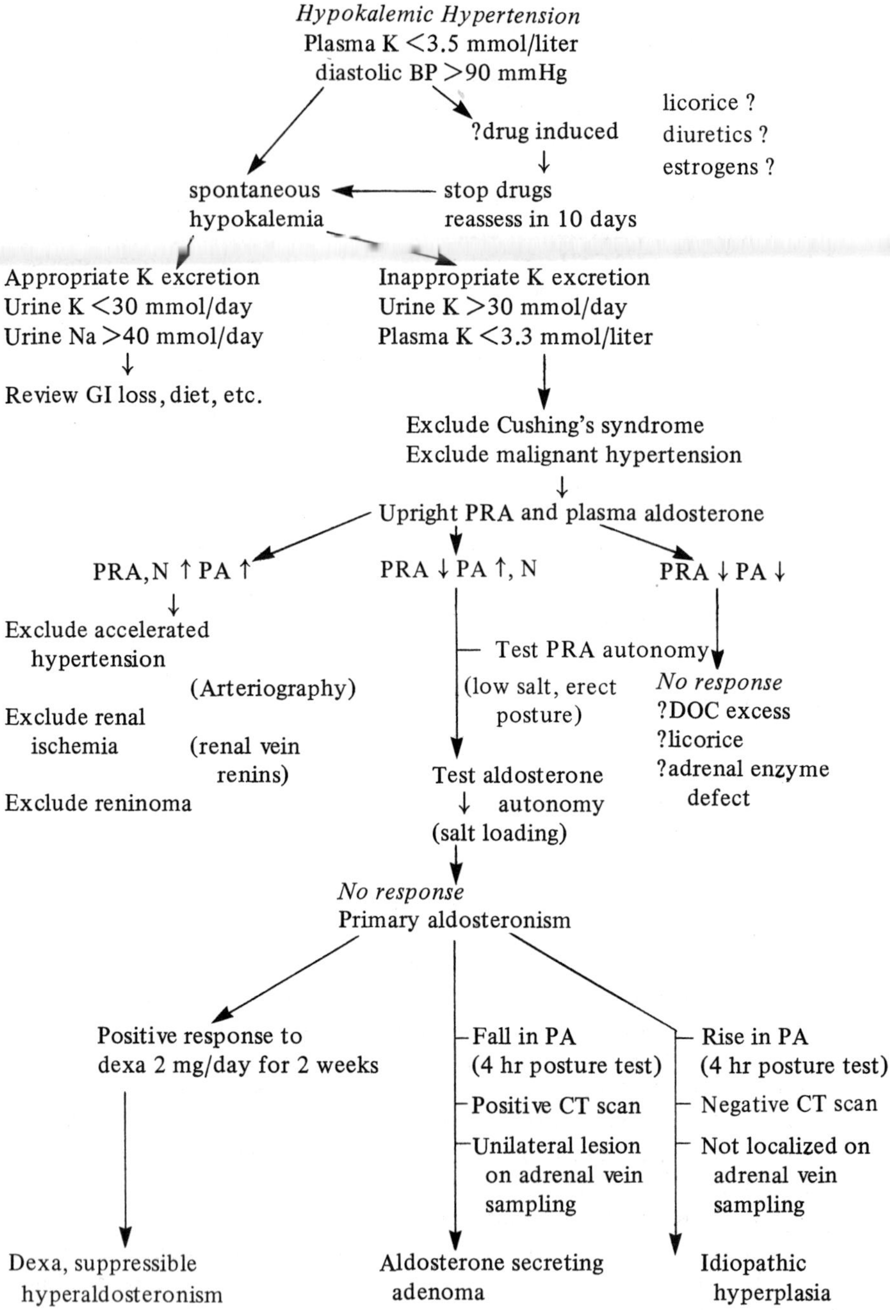

Note: ↑ increased; ↓ decreased; PRA plasma renin activity; PA plasma aldosterone; N normal.

2. Secondary Deficiency

Impaired renin secretion associated with persistent mild hyperkalemia and lowish aldosterone secretion has recently been reported with increasing frequency in elderly patients (94). Hypertensive patients with reduced carbohydrate tolerance seem particularly prone and mild renal failure (serum creatinine 2–3 mg/per 100 ml) is commonly also present. Patients are usually asymptomatic, but cardiac arrhythmias from hyperkalemia may occur. Laboratory studies show raised serum potassium, usually normal plasma sodium, mild metabolic acidosis, and reduced potassium clearance. PRA and aldosterone are low and do not respond to standard volume-depleting maneuvers. The aldosterone response to infused angiotensin or ACTH may be subnormal or blunted. Reduced renal production of prostaglandin E has been reported and the syndrome may be induced (or aggravated) by prostaglandin inhibitors such as indomethacin (95). Autonomic insuffiency may reduce renin responsiveness and contribute to the syndrome in diabetes mellitus (96), but in many patients the cause of the hyporeninemia is unclear (97).

Hyporeninemic hypoaldosteronism is expected after removal of an aldosterone-secreting adenoma or sudden cessation of mineralocorticoid therapy, licorice, and so on.

A rare hyperkalemic syndrome associated with hypertension, low PRA, and aldosterone and metabolic acidosis has been described by Gordon et al. (98). The disorder appears to be the antithesis of Bartter's syndrome and a primary renal defect causing enhanced proximal sodium reabsorption has been proposed as a basis for this syndrome. Patients respond to a low-salt diet or thiazide diuretic treatment.

3. Resistance to Mineralocorticoids

A resistance to mineralocorticoid action, resulting in a salt-wasting disorder and hyponatremia and hyperkalemia, has been described (99). Both PRA and aldosterone are elevated, and there is no or little response to exogenous mineralocorticoid (100). An abnormality in mineralocorticoid receptors is the likely basis for the syndrome. Reduced response to mineralocorticoid has also been described in adults with renal disease, particularly salt-wasting renal tubular acidosis, chronic interstitial nephritis, and some patients with hyporeninemic hypoaldosteronism (97). The antialdosterone effects of progesterone and related steroids have already been mentioned.

REFERENCES

1. Edmonds, CJ. Effect of aldosterone, on mammalian intestine. J Steroid Biochem 1972;3:143–149.
2. Collins KJ. The action of exogenous aldosterone on the secretion and composition of drug-induced sweat. Clin Sci 1966;30:207–221.

3. Coghlan JP, Denton DA, Goding JR, Wright RD. The control of aldosterone secretion. Post Grad Med J 1960; 36:76–102.
4. Funder JW, Feldman D, Edelman IS. Roles of plasma binding in rat kidney and parotid. Endocrinology 1973; 92:994–1004.
5. Schalecamp MADH, Derkx FHM. Plasma kallikrein and plasmin as activators of prorenin: links between the renin-angiotensin system and other proteolytic systems in plasma. Clin Sci 1981; 61:15–21.
6. Schoneshofer M, Oelkers W. Effect of prolonged infusions of angiotensin II on eight serum corticosteroids in man on different sodium diets. Horm Metab Res 1980; 12:614–620.
7. Flamenbaum W, Gagnon J, Ramwell P. Bradykinin-induced renal hemodynamic alterations: renin and prostaglandin relationships. Am J Physiol 1979; 237:F433–440.
8. Carretero OA, Scicli AG. Possible role of kinins in circulatory homeostasis. Hypertension 1981; 3(suppl I):I-4 to I-12.
9. Tagawa H, Vander AJ, Bonjour JP, Malvin RL. Inhibition of renin secretion by vasopressin in unanesthetized sodium deprived dogs. Am J Physiol 1971; 220:949–957.
10. Kem DC, Gomez-Sanchez C, Kramer NJ, Holland OB, Higgins JR. Plasma aldosterone and renin activity response to ACTH infusion in dexamethasone suppressed normal and sodium-depleted man. J Clin Endocrinol Metab 1975; 40:116–124.
11. Biglieri EG, Schambelan M, Slaton PE. Effect of adrenocorticotropin on desoxycorticosterone, corticosterone and aldosterone excretion. J Clin Endocrinol Metab 1969; 29:1090–1101.
12. Birkhäuser M, Riondel AM, Gaillard R, Mantero F, Vallotton B. Plasma aldosterone response to acute stimulation in panhypopituitarism. Acta Endocrinol (Copenh) 1981; 97:514–521.
13. Himathongkam T, Dluhy RG, Williams GH. Potassium-aldosterone-renin interrelationships. J Clin Endocrinol Metab 1975; 41:153–159.
14. Lun S, Espiner EA, Hart S. Effect of ACTH on the aldosterone response to potassium in sheep with adrenal transplants. Am J Physiol 1979; 237: E500–E503.
15. Oelkers W, Brown JJ, Fraser R, Lever AF, Morton JJ, Robertson JIS. Sensitization of the adrenal cortex to angiotension II in sodium-deplete man. Circ Res 1974; 34:69–77.
16. Williams GH, Dluhy RG, Underwood RH. The relationship of dietary potassium intake to the aldosterone stimulating properties of ACTH. Clin Sci 1970; 39:489–496.
17. Linde R, Winn S, Latta D Hollifield J. Graded dose effects of angiotensin II on aldosterone production in man during various levels of potassium intake. Metabolism 1981; 30:549–553.
18. Whitfield L, Sowers JR, Tuck ML, Golub MS. Dopaminergic control of plasma catecholamine and aldosterone responses to acute stimuli in normal man. J Clin Endocrinol Metab 1980; 51:724–729.

19. Brown RD, Wisgerhof M, Carpenter PC, Brown G, Jiang NS, Kao P, Hegstad R. Adrenal sensitivity to angiotensin II and undiscovered aldosterone stimulating factors in hypertension. J Steroid Biochem 1979; 11:1043–1050.
20. Mulrow PJ. Editorial. N Engl J Med 1981; 305:1012.
21. Zipser RD, Meidav V, Horton R. Characteristics of aldosterone binding in human plasma. 1980; 50:158–162.
22. Kono T, Ikeda F, Oseko F, Imura H, Tanimura H. Normotensive primary aldosteronism: report of a case. J Clin Endocrinol Metab 1981; 52: 1009–1013.
23. Tarazi RC, Ibrahim MM, Bravo EL, Dustan HP. Hemodynamic characteristics of primary aldosteronism. N Engl J Med 1973; 289:1330–1335.
24. Ferriss JB, Brown JJ, Fraser R, Haywood E, Davies DL, Kay AW, Lever AF, Robertson JIS, Owen K, Peart WS. Results of adrenal surgery in patients with hypertension, aldosterone excess and low plasma renin concentration. Br Med J 1975; 1:135–138.
25. Kremer D, Boddy K, Brown JJ, Davies DL, Fraser R, Lever AF, Morton JJ, Robertson JIS. Amiloride in the treatment of primary hyperaldosteronism and essential hypertension. Clin Endocrinol 1977; 7:151–157.
26. Hollenberg NK, Chenitz WR, Adams DF, Williams GH. Reciprocal influence of salt intake on adrenal glomerulosa and renal vascular responses to angiotensin II in normal man. J. Clin Invest 1974; 54:34–42.
27. Conn JW, Cohen EL, Lucas CP, McDonald WJ, Mayor GH, Blough WM, Eveland WC, Bookstein JJ, Lapides J. Primary reninism. Arch Intern Med 1972; 130:682–696.
28. Atkinson AB, Brown JJ, Davies DL. Hyponatraemic hypertensive syndrome with renal-artery occlusion corrected by captopril. Lancet 1979; 2:606–609.
29. Rosei EA, Brown JJ, Cumming AMM, Fraser R, Semple PF, Lever AF, Morton JJ, Robertson AS, Robertson JIS, Tree M. Is the sodium index a useful way of expressing clinical plasma renin, angiotensin and aldosterone values? Clin Endocrinol 1978; 8:141–147.
30. McDonald RH, Corder CN, Vagnucci AH, Shuman J. Multiple factors affecting plasma renin activity in essential hypertension. Arch Intern Med 1978; 138:557–561.
31. Fraser R, Beretta-Piccoli C, Brown JJ, Cumming AMM, Lever AF, Mason PA, Morton JJ, Robertson JIS. Response of aldosterone and 18-hydroxy corticosterone to angiotensin II in normal subjects and patients with essential hypertension, Conn's syndrome, nontumerous hyperaldosteronism. Hypertension 1981; 3(suppl I):I-87 to I-92.
32. Kem DC, Weinberger MH, Higgins JR. Plasma aldosterone response to ACTH in primary aldosteronism and in patients with low renin hypertension. J Clin Endocrinol Metab 1978; 46:552–560.
33. Brown JJ, Chinn RH, Fraser R, Lever AF, Morton JJ, Robertson JIS, Tree M, Waite MA, Park DM. Recurrent hyperkalemia due to selective aldosterone deficiency: correction by angiotensin infusion. Br Med J 1973; 1: 650–654.

34. Oparil S, Haber E. The renin-angiotensin system. N Engl J Med 1974; 291(8):389–401; 291(9):446–457.
35. Oparil S. Theoretical approaches to estimation of plasma renin activity: a review and some original observations. Clin Chem 1976:22:583–593.
36. Derkx FHM, V Gool JMG, Wenting GJ. Inactive renin in human plasma. Lancet 1976; 2:496–498.
37. Espiner EA, Donald RA, Miles K. Clinical use of plasma renin assays. NZ Med J 1978;87:92–96.
38. Stalker HP, Holland NH, Kotchen JM, Kotchen TA. Plasma renin activity in healthy children. J Pediatr 1976; 89:256–258.
39. Weidmann MJ, De Myttenaere Bursztein S, Maxwell MH. Effect on aging of plasma renin and aldosterone in normal man. Kidney Int 1975; 8: 325–333.
40. Modlinger RS, Sharif-Zadeh K, Entel NH, Gutkin M. The circadian rhythm of renin. J Clin Endocrinol Metab 1976; 43:1276–1282.
41. Michelakis AM, Yoshida H, Dormois JC. Plasma renin activity and plasma aldosterone during the normal menstrual cycle. Am J Obstet Gynecol 1975; 123:724–726.
42. Brown JJ, Davies DL, Lever AF, Robertson JIS. Influence of sodium deprivation and loading on the plasma-renin in man. J Physiol 1964; 173: 408–419.
43. Sassard J, Vincent M, Annat G. A kinetic study of plasma renin and aldosterone during changes of posture in man. J Clin Endocrinol Metab 1976; 42:20–27.
44. Gordon RD, Kuchel O, Liddle GW. Role of the sympathetic nervous system in regulating renin and aldosterone production in man. J Clin Invest 1967; 46:599–605.
45. Falch CK, Paulsen AQ, Ødegaard AE, Norman N. Central and renal circulation, renin and aldosterone in plasma during prazosin treatment in essential hypertension. Acta Med Scand 1979; 206:489–494.
46. Lowder SC, Liddle GW. Effects of guanethidine and methyldopa on a standardized test for renin responsiveness. Ann Intern Med 1975; 82: 757–60.
47. Brown JJ, Chinn RH, Davies DL, Fraser R, Lever AF, Rae RJ, Robertson JIS. Falsely high plasma potassium values in patients with hyperaldosteronism, Br Med J 1970; 2:18–20.
48. Brown JJ, Davies DL, Chinn RH. Plasma electrolytes renin and aldosterone in the diagnosis of primary hyperaldosteronism. Lancet 1968; 2:55–59.
49. Ferriss JB, Beevers DG, Brown JJ. Clinical, biochemical and pathological features of low-renin "primary" hyperaldosteronism. Am Heart J 1978; 95:375–388.
50. Stockigt JR, Collins RD, Noakes CA. Renal-vein renin in various forms of renal hypertension. Lancet 1972; 1:1194–1198.

51. Stanley JC, Gewertz BL, Fry WJ. Renal systemic renin indices and renal vein ratios and prognostic indicators in remedial renovascular hypertension. J Surg Res 1976; 20:149-156.
52. Schwartz WB, Van Ypersele de Strihou C, Kassirer JP. Role of anions in metabolic alkalosis and potassium deficiency. N Engl J Med 1968; 279: 630-639.
53. Christlieb AR, Espiner EA, Amsterdam EA. The pattern of electrolyte excretion in normal and hypertensive subjects before and after saline infusions. Am J Cardiol 1971; 27:595-601.
54. Espiner EA, Donald RA. Aldosterone regulation in primary aldosteronism; influence of salt balance, posture and ACTH. Clin Endocrinol 1980; 12:277-286.
55. Kaplan NM, Kem DC, Holland OB. The intravenous furosemide test: a simple way to evaluate renin responsiveness. Ann Intern Med 1976; 84: 639-645.
56. Kem DC, Weinberger MH, Mayes DM. Saline suppression of plasma aldosterone in hypertension. Arch Intern Med 1971; 128:380-386.
57. Biglieri EG, Stockigt JR, Schambelen M. A preliminary evaluation for primary aldosteronism. Arch Intern Med 1970; 126:1004-1007.
58. Weinberger MH, Dowdy AJ, Nokes GW. Plasma renin activity and aldosterone secretion in hypertensive patients during high and low sodium intake and administration of diuretic. J Clin Endocrinol Metab 1968; 28:359-371.
59. Espiner EA, Christlieb AR, Amsterdam EA. The pattern of plasma renin activity and aldosterone secretion in normal and hypertensive subjects before and after saline infusions. Am J Cardiol 1971; 27:585-594.
60. Aitchison J, Brown JJ, Ferriss JB, Fraser R, Kay AW, Lever AF, Neville AM, Symington T, Robertson JIS. Quadric analysis in the pre-operative distinction between patients with or without adrenocortical tumours in hypertension with aldosterone excess and low plasma renin. Am Heart J 1971; 82:660-671.
61. Biglieri EG, Schambelan. The significance of elevated levels of plasma 18-hydroxycorticosterone in patients with primary aldosteronism. J Clin Endocrinol Metab 1979; 49:87-91.
62. Ganguly A, Melada GA, Luetscher JA, Dowdy AJ. Control of plasma aldosterone in primary aldosteronism: distinction between adenoma and hyperplasia. J Clin Endocrinol Metab 1973; 37:765-775.
63. Wisgerhof M, Brown RD, Hogan MJ. The plasma aldosterone response to angiotensin II infusion in aldosterone-producing adenoma and idiopathic hyperaldosteronism. J Clin Endocrinol Metab 1981; 52:195-198.
64. Freitas JE, Thrall JH, Swanson DP, Rifae A, Beierwaltes WH. Normal adrenal asymmetry explanation and interpretation. J Nucl Med 1978; 19:149-153.
65. Sutherland DJA, Ruse JL, Laidlaw JC. Hypertension, increased aldosterone secretion and low plasma renin activity relieved by dexamethasone. Can Med Assoc J 1966; 95:1109-1119.

66. Gill JR, Bartter FC. overproduction of sodium-retaining steroids by the zona glomerulosa is adrenocorticotropin-dependent and mediates hypertension in dexamethasone-suppressible aldosteronism. J Clin Endocrinol 1981; 53:331-337.
67. Ganguly A, Chavarri M, Leutscher JA. Transient fall and subsequent return of high aldosterone secretion by adrenal adenoma during continued dexamethasone administration. J Clin Endocrinol Metab 1977;44:775-779.
68. Beevers DG, Brown JJ. Low renin ("primary") hyperaldosteronism. Am Heart J 1978;95:641-657.
69. Funder JW, Adam WR, Mantero F. The etiology of a syndrome of facitious mineralocorticoid excess: a steroid-containing nasal spray. J Clin Endocrinol Metab 1979;49:842-846.
70. Epstein MT, Espiner EA, Donald RA, Hughes H. Liquorice toxicity and the renin-angiotensin-aldosterone axis in man. Br Med J 1977; 1:209-210.
71. Epstein MT, Espiner EA, Donald RA. Licorice raises urinary cortisol in man. J Clin Endocrinol Metab 1978;47:397-400.
72. Melby JC, DAle SL, Wilson TE. 18-Hydroxy-deoxycorticosterone in human hypertension. Circ Res 1971;28, 29 (suppl 2):143-152.
73. Biglieri EG, Herron MA, Brust N. 17-Hydroxylation deficiency in man. J Clin Invest 1966;45:1946-1954.
74. New MI. Male pseudohermaphroditism due to 17α-hydroxylase deficiency. J Clin Invest 1970;49:1930-1941.
75. Biglieri EG. Mechanisms establishing the mineralcorticoid hormone patterns in the 17-α-hydroxylase deficiency syndrome. J Steroid Biochem 1979;11:653-657.
76. New MI, Seaman MP. Secretion rates of cortisol and aldosterone precursor in various forms of congenital adrenal hyperplasia. J Clin Endocrinol Metab 1970;30:361.
77. Hoefnagels WHL, Drayer JIM, Hofman JA, Kloppenborg PWC, Smals AGH, Benraad ThJ. Dexamethasone-responsive hypertension in young women with suppressed renin and aldosterone. Lancet 1978;1:741-43.
78. Gardner JD, Lapey A, Simopoulos AP, Bravo EL. Abnormal membrane sodium transport in Liddle's syndrome. J Clin Invest 1971;50:2253-2258.
79. Rees LH, Bloomfield GA, Gilkes JJH, Jeffcoate WJ, Beser GM. ACTH as a tumor marker. Ann NY Acad Sci 1977; 297:603-620.
80. Schambelam, Slaton PE, Biglieri EG. Mineralocorticoid production in hyperadrenocorticism. Am J Med 1971; 51(Sept):299-303.
81. Mantero F, Armanini D, Boscaro M. Plasma renin activity and urinary aldosterone in Cusing's syndrome. Hormone Metab Res 1978; 10:65-71.
82. Kotchen TA, Guthrie GP. Renin-angiotensin aldosterone and hypertension. Endocr rev 1980 1:78-99.
83. Nicholls, MG, Espiner EA, Donald RA, Hughes H. Aldosterone and its regulation during diuresis in patients with gross congestive heart failure. Clin Sci Mol Med 1974;47:301-315.
84. Medina A, Davies DL, Brown JJ, Fraser R, Lever AL, Mallick NP, Morton JJ, Robertson JIS, Tree M. A study of the renin-angiotensin system in the nephrotic syndrome. Nephron 1974: 12:233-240.

85. Epstein M, Levinson R, Sancho J, Haber E, Re R. Characterization of the renin-aldosterone system in decompensated cirrhosis. Circ Res 1977;41: 818–829.
86. Wolff HP, Vecsei P, Kruck F, Roscher S, Brown JJ, Düsterdieck GO, Lever AF, Robertson JIS. Psychiatric disturbance leading to potassium depletion, sodium depletion, raised plasma-renin concentration, and secondary hyperaldosteronism. Lancet 1968;1:257–261.
87. Bartter FC, Pronove P, Gill JR, MacCardle RC. Hyperplasia of juxtaglomerular complex with hyperaldosteronism and hypokalemic alkalosis. Am J Med 1962;33:811–828.
88. Vinci JM, Gill JR, Bowden, RE, Pisano JJ, Izzo JL Jr, Raafar N, Taylor AA, Zusman RM, Bartter FC, Keiser HR. The kallikreinkinin system in Bartter's syndrome and its response to prostaglandin synthetase inhibition. J Clin Invest 1978;61:1671–1682.
89. Rosenblum M, Simpson DP, Evenson M. Factitious Bartter's syndrome. Arch Intern Med 1977;137:1244–1245.
90. Nicholls MG, Espiner EA, Donald RA. Schmidt's syndrome presenting as hypopituitarism. Ann Intern Med 1974;80:505–509.
91. Stockigt JR, Hewett MJ, Topliss DJ. Renin and renin substrate in primary adrenal insufficiency. Am J Med 1979;66:915–922.
92. Dluhy RG, Himathongkam TH, Greenfield M. Rapid ACTH test with plasma aldosterone levels. Ann Intern Med 1974;80:693–696.
93. Veldhuis JD, Kulin HE, Santen RJ. Inborn error in the terminal step of aldosterone biosynthesis. N Engl J Med 1980;303:117–121.
94. Schambelan M, Stockigt JR, Biglieri EG. Isolated hypoaldosteronism in adults: a renin deficiency syndrome. N Engl J Med 1972;287:573–578.
95. Tan SY, Shapiro R, Franco R, Stockard H, Mulrow PJ. Indomethacin-induced prostaglandin inhibition with hyperkalaemia; a reversible cause of hyporeninemic hypoaldosteronism. Ann Intern Med 1979;90:783–785.
96. Tuck ML, Sambhi MP, Levin L. Hyporeninemic hypoaldosteronism in diabetes mellitus. Studies of the autonomic nervous system control of renin release. Diabetes 1979;28:237–241.
97. Vaamonde CA, Perez GO, Oster JR, Syndromes of aldosterone deficiency. Miner Electrolyte Metab 1981;5:121–134.
98. Gordon RD, Geddes RA, Pawsey CGK, O'Halloran MW. Hypertension and severe hyperkalaemia associated with suppression of renin and aldosterone and completely reversed by dietary sodium restriction. Australas Ann Med 1970;19:287–294.
99. Cheek DB, Perry JW. A salt waste syndrome in infancy. Arch Dis Child 1958;33:252–256.
100. Oberfield SE, Levine LS, Carey RM. Pseudohypoaldosteronism: multiple target organ unresponsiveness to mineralcorticoid hormones. J Clin Endocrinol Metab 1979;48:228–234.

27
Pheochromocytoma

M. Gary Nicholls
Princess Margaret Hospital, Christchurch, New Zealand

Although rare (0.1-0.2% of the hypertensive population), pheochromocytoma is important because it is frequently fatal if undiagnosed, yet is eminently curable when diagnosed and managed with care. [A text by Manger and Gifford (1) covers most aspects of pheochromocytoma in great detail up to the time of its publication in 1977.] In many cases, pheochromocytomas which have contributed to or caused death, are discovered unexpectedly at postmortem (2). The tumor is of neuroectodermal origin arising from cells with an affinity for chromium salts (chromaffin cells). While the majority arise within the adrenal medulla, the right more commonly than the left (3), approximately 10% are extraadrenal, and in about 10% of patients the tumors are multiple. Malignancy, which in the absence of characteristic cytological features can be diagnosed only "in the presence of secondary tumor deposits in sites where chromaffin tissue is not found normally" (4), affects 10% of patients, predominantly females (5). Pheochromocytoma in children differs from that in adults in its greater incidence in males than females, the increased frequency of multiple tumors, and the predominance of sustained rather than paroxysmal hypertension (1).

I. CLINICAL PRESENTATION

The clinical manifestations of pheochromocytoma are protean, earning it the title of the "great mimic." Most clinical features can be readily explained by the pharmacological effects of high circulating catecholamine levels on α- and

β-adrenergic receptors (6). The most frequent symptoms are headache, excessive sweating, palpitations, nervousness, chest or abdominal pain, weakness or fatigue, weight loss, dyspnea, heat intolerance, and constipation (1). These and many other symptoms may occur spontaneously or be precipitated by a variety of factors, including physical manuvers (bending, exercise, intubation), eating, drinking, smoking, and medications [opiates, metoclopramide, tricyclic antidepressents, glucagon, adrenocorticotropic hormone (ACTH), saralasin, and butyrophenones]. Beta-blocker therapy can exacerbate the hypertension or precipitate pulmonary edema (7). Most patients have hypertension, either paroxysmal or sustained, although a small minority are normotensive (8), or present with cardiomyopathy, or in shock following trauma, surgery, or parturition (1). Hyperglycemia or frank diabetes mellitus is common and presumably results from catecholamine effects to reduce glucose clearance, accelerate glycogenolysis and gluconeogenesis, and impair insulin release (9, 10). Although hypertension is common in the diabetic population (11, 12), this combination in any patient should raise the possibility of pheochromocytoma.

Physical signs include postural hypotension (due arguably to reduced plasma volume, or to down-regulation of receptors), hyperhydrosis, a cool periphery sometimes with Raynaud's phenomenon or livedo reticularis, arrhythmias, pallor (occasionally flushing), anxiety and tremulousness, mild intermittent fever, and a palpable abdominal mass in patients with a large tumor (1).

Pheochromocytoma may be one manifestation of a familial disorder, of which there are two broad categories.

(a) *Multiple endocrine adenoma (MEA) type II or Sipple's syndrome* (13). Inherited as an autosomal dominant disorder, it is characterized by multicentric hyperplastic involvement of the thyroid C cells (resulting in medullary carcinoma of the thyroid), parathyroids (causing hyperparathyroidism), and adrenal medullae (leading ultimately to bilateral pheochromocytomas). A variant form (MEA type IIB or type III) has in addition characteristic features of marfanoid habitus, acromegalic facies, and neuromas of skin and mucosal surfaces. To screen the patient with pheochromocytoma for MEA type II, plasma thyrocalcitonin should be measured, and adrenal medullary tissue separate from the pheochromocytoma must be studied for evidence of hyperplasia (14). When pheochromocytoma is part of the MEA syndrome, bilateral adrenalectomy is advised before surgery to the thyroid or parathyroids (15).

(b) *Pheochromocytoma associations*. Neurofibromatosis, retinal angiomatosis, or hemangioblastoma of the cerebellum or spinal cord are well-known associates of pheochromocytoma.

Other reported associations which do not have a familial basis are cholelithiasis, Cushing's syndrome, acromegaly, Addison's disease, and renal artery stenosis.

II. DIAGNOSTIC TESTS

A. Routine Tests

The hematocrit may be high, possibly because of a decreased plasma volume, or because an erythropoiesis-stimulating factor is secreted by the tumor (16). A leukocytosis is not rare, and increased plasma glucose and free fatty acids are common. Hypokalemia is occasionally reported and can relate to catecholamine-induced renin secretion and thence hyperaldosteronism (17), or to the concurrence of renal artery stenosis, ACTH secretion by the pheochromocytoma (18), or to an aldosterone-secreting adrenal tumor (19, 20). Hypercalcemia, corrected by tumor removal (21), is rare. A variety of nonspecific electrocardiogram (ECG) abnormalities may be observed.

B. Specific Biochemical Diagnosis

Urine metanephrines, vanillylmandellic acid (VMA), or catecholamines are elevated in almost all patients, and are accepted as satisfactory screening tests. If only one of these is to be measured, metanephrines are preferred by most authorities (5, 22, 23). Normally, a complete 24-hr urine collection is made. Alternatively, urine passed over some hours after a symptomatic episode, or collected through the night, may establish the diagnosis when 24-hr excretion levels are equivocal (24, 25).

Plasma catecholamines, drawn with the patient resting in the supine position and measured by radioenzymatic assay (see Chap. 9), may be more useful than determinations of urine metabolites (26). Since normal plasma catecholamine levels have been reported (27), it is advisable to draw a number of samples. Blood drawn during a hypertensive-symptomatic episode should secure the diagnosis. In equivocal cases, a suppression test using measurements of plasma catecholamines before and after clonidine or pentolinium (28) has appeal, but widespread experience is lacking.

C. Tumor Localization

Accurate preoperative localization of the catecholamine-secreting tumor is essential. Increased plasma or urinary epinephrine levels strongly suggest that the tumor is sited in an adrenal gland, although rare exceptions do occur (29). Since 99% of tumors are intra-abdominal, and 85–90% arise within an adrenal gland, localization techniques should initially be focused at the adrenal areas. A plain abdominal radiograph will detect tumor calcification in a few patients (30, 31). Nephrotomography, with or without an intravenous urogram, carries little risk and may be rewarding (5). Aortography detects almost all pheochromocytomas, since in most cases the tumor is highly vascular. For small or

Diagnostic Summary 1 Pheochromocytoma

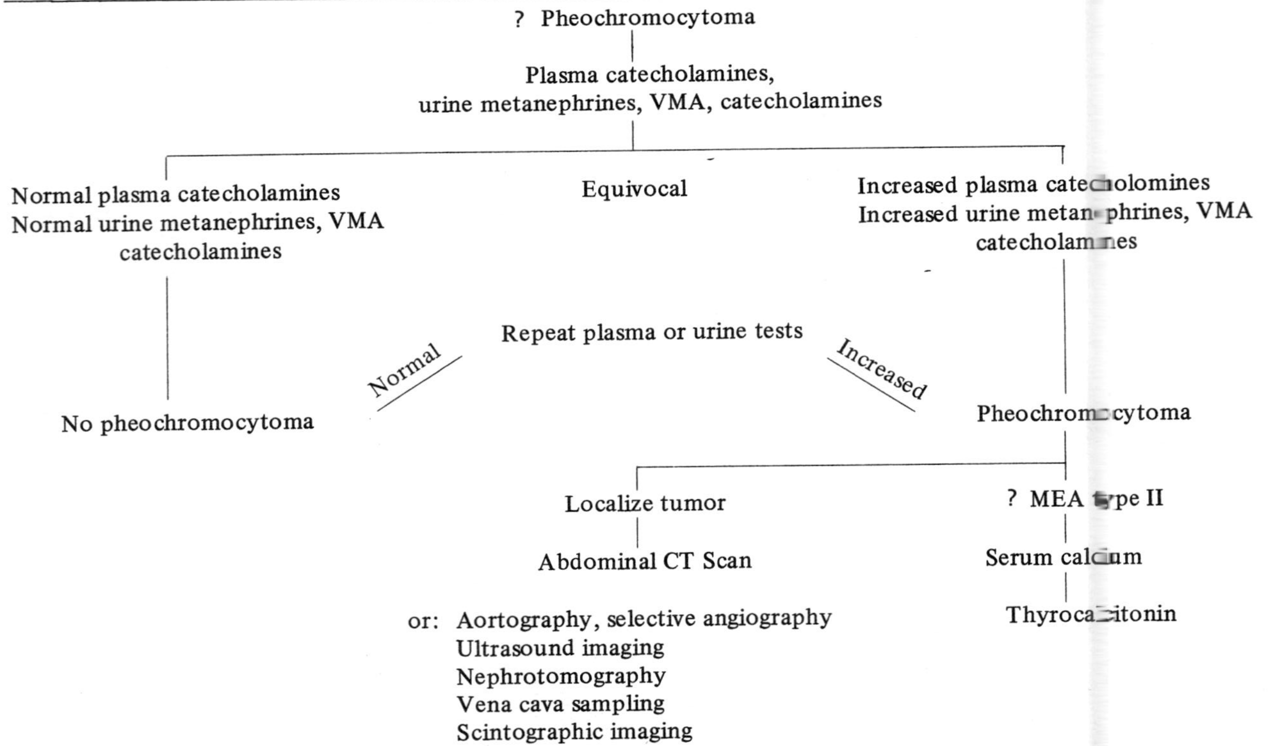

less vascular tumors, selective arteriography may be required. Since aortography can precipitate a hypertensive crisis, the patient should be treated with an alpha-blocking agent before the procedure, and all facilities required to deal with hypertension, hypotension, or arrhythmia must be readily available. Ultrasound imaging will locate large, but not small tumors. A major advance is the use of computerized tomography (CT). Since most tumors are greater than 2 cm in diameter, they will be readily detected by CT scanning even when they are relatively avascular (32), and without risk to the patient (33). Where the foregoing methods have failed, vena cava catheterization with multiple-site sampling for plasma catecholamine measurements may assist localization (34, 35). The technique is particularly useful when tumors are small, multiple, or metastatic. Retrograde injection of dye into the adrenal vein can outline the tumor but must be performed with caution in case a sudden release of catecholamines is provoked. The future holds the exciting possibility of scintigraphic imaging of pheochromocytomas, whether single (36) or multiple (37), using radiolabeled agents which are concentrated in adrenergic neurotransmitter vesicles.

D. Differential Diagnosis

The list of conditions that can be mimicked by pheochromocytoma is long (1). More common conditions include essential hypertension, particularly if paroxysmal or with associated symptoms, anxiety states, hyperthyroidism, diabetes mellitus, the menopause, paroxysmal tachycardia, and migraine headache. In the final analysis, pheochromocytoma patients have elevated catecholamines or metabolite levels, whereas they are normal or only marginally increased in the disorders above. Two conditions may prove unusually difficult to differentiate from pheochromocytoma. The first is surreptitious self-administration of catecholamines (38, 39), or covert manipulation of urine collections (40). Equally confusing can be patients with severe cardiac failure, since catecholamine levels are elevated in most patients in gross cardiac failure (41), and pheochromocytoma occasionally presents as heart failure. Improvement in cardiac performance with conventional therapy for heart failure should ultimately lower catecholamine levels, but if a pheochromocytoma is present the catecholamines will remain grossly elevated.

REFERENCES

1. Manger WM, Gifford RW, *Pheochromocytoma.* Springer-Verlag, New York, 1977.
2. Modlin IM, Farndon JR, Shepherd A, Johnston IDA, Kennedy TL, Montgomery DAD, Welbourn RB. Phaeochromocytomas in 72 patients: clinical and diagnositc features, treatment and long term results. Br J Surg 1979; 66:456-465.

3. Melicow MM. One hundred cases of pheochromocytoma (107 tumors) at the Columbia-Presbyterian Medical Center, 1926-1976. A clinicopathological analysis. Cancer 1977; 40:1987–2004.
4. Symington T, The adrenal medulla. In *Functional Pathology of the Human Adrenal Gland*. Williams & Wilkins, Baltimore, 1969, pp 246–324.
5. Remine WH, Chong GC, Van Heerden JA, Sheps SG, Harrison EG Jr. Current Management of pheochromocytoma. Ann Surg 1974; 179:740–747.
6. Weiner N. In *The Pharmacological Basis of Therapeutics*, 6th ed, Goodman LS, Gillman A (eds). Macmillan, New York, 1980, pp 138–175.
7. Wark JD, Larkins RG. Pulmonary oedema after propranolol therapy in two cases of phaeochromocytoma. Br Med J 1978; 1:1395–1396.
8. Ho AD, Feurle G, Gless K-H. Normotensive familial phaeochromocytoma with predominant noradrenaline secretion. Br Med J 1978; 1:81–82.
9. Clutter WE, Bier DM, Shah SD, Cryer PE. Epinephrine plasma metabolic clearance rates and physiological thresholds for metabolic hemodynamic actions in man. J Clin Invest 1980; 66:94-101.
10. Vance JE, Buchanan KE, O'Hara D, Williams RH, Porte D Jr. Insulin and glucagon responses in subjects with pheochromocytoma: effects of alpha adrenergic blockade. J Clin Endocrinol 1969; 29:911–916.
11. Pell S, D'Alonzo CA. Some aspects of hypertension in diabetes millitus. JAMA 1967; 202:104–111.
12. Garcia MJ, McNamara PM, Gordon T, Kannell WB. Morbidity and mortality in diabetics in the Framingham population. Sixteen year follow-up study. Diabetes 1974; 23:105–111.
13. Sizemore GW, Heath H, Carney JA. Multiple endocrine neoplasia type 2. Clin Endocrinol Metab 1980; 9:299–315.
14. Webb TA, Sheps SG, Carney JA. Differences between sporadic pheochromocytoma and pheochromocytoma in multiple endocrine neoplasia, type 2. Am J Surg Pathol 1980; 4:121-126.
15. Lips KJM, Van Der Sluys Veer J. Struyvenberg A, Alleman A, Leo JR, Wittebol P, Minder WH, Kodiker CJ, Geerdink RA, Van Waes PFG, Hackeng WHL. Bilateral occurrence of pheochromocytoma in patients with the multiple endocrine neoplasia syndrome type 2A (Sipple's syndrome). Am J Med 1981; 70:1051-1060.
16. Waldmann TA, Bradley JE. Polycythemia secondary to a pheochromocytoma with production of an erythropoiesis stimulating factor by the tumor. Proc Soc Exp Biol Med 1961; 108:425–427.
17. Vetter H. Vetter W, Warnholz C, Bazer J-M, Käser H, Vielhaber K, Krück F. Renin and aldosterone secretion in pheochromocytoma. Effects of chronic alpha-adrenergic receptor blockage. Am J Med 1976; 60:866-871.
18. Spark RF, Connolly PB, Gluckin DS, White R, Sacks B, Landsberg L. ACTH secretion from a functioning pheochromocytoma. N Engl J Med 1979; 301:416-418.
19. Wilson RJ, Craig GM, Mills IH. Metabolic studies in a patient with phaeochromocytoma associated with hypokalaemia and hyperaldosteronism. J Endocrinol 1973; 56:69-78.

20. Wilkins GE, Schmidt N, Lee-Son L. Coexistence of pheochromocytoma, adrenal adenoma and hypokalemia. Can Med Assoc J 1977; 116:360–362.
21. Gray RS, Gillon J. Normotensive phaeochromocytoma with hypercalcaemia: correction after adrenalectomy. Br Med J 1976; 1:378.
22. Crout JR, Pisano JJ, Sjoerdsma A. Urinary execretion of catecholamines and their metabolites in pheochromocytoma. Am Heart J 1961; 61: 375–381.
23. Gitlow SE, Mendlowitz M, Bertani LM. The biochemical techniques for detecting and establishing the presence of a pheochromocytoma. A review of ten years' experience. Am J Cardiol 1970; 26:270–279.
24. Sullivan JM, Solomon HS. The diagnosis of pheochromocytoma. Overnight excretion of catecholamine metabolites. JAMA 1975; 231:618–619.
25. Ganguly A, Henry DP, Yune HY, Pratt JH, Grim CE, Donohue JP, Weinberger MH. Diagnosis and localization of pheochromocytoma. Detection by measurement of urinary norepinephrine excretion during sleep, plasma norepinephrine concentration and computerized axial tomography (CT-scan). Am J Med 1979; 67:21-26.
26. Bravo EL, Tarazi RC, Gifford RW, Steward BH. Circulating and urinary catecholamines in pheochromocytoma. New Engl J Med 1979; 301: 682-686.
27. Jones DH, Reid JL, Hamilton CA, Allison DJ, Welbourne RB, Dollery CT. The biochemical diagnosis, localization and follow up of phaeochromocytoma: the role of plasma and urinary catecholamine measurements. Q J Med 1980; 49:341–361.
28. Brown MJ, Allison DJ, Jenner DA, Lewis PJ, Dollery CT. Increased sensitivity and accuracy of phaeochromocytoma diagnosis achieved by use of plasma-adrenaline estimations and pentolinium-suppression test. Lancet 1981; 1:174–177.
29. Engelman K, Hammond WG. Adrenaline production by an intrathoracic phaeochromocytoma. Lancet 1968; 1:609–611.
30. Grainger RG, Lloyd GAS, Williams JL. Egg-shell calcification: a sign of phaeochromocytoma. Clin Radiol 1967; 18:282–286.
31. Mori Y, Kiyohara H, Miki T, Kotake T. Pheochromocytoma with prominent calcification and associated pancreatic islet cell tumor. J Urol 1977; 118:843-844.
32. Hahn LC, Nadel NS, Bernstein NM, Staya KL. Localization of pheochromocytoma by computerized axial tomography. J Urol 1978; 120: 349–351.
33. Stewart BH, Bravo EL, Haaga J, Meaney TF, Tarazi R. Localization of pheochromocytoma by computed tomography. N Engl J Med 1978; 299:460–461.
34. Davies RA, Patt NL, Sole MJ. Localization of pheochromocytoma by selective venous catheterization and assay of plasma catecholamines. Can Med Assoc J 1979; 120:539–542.

35. Jones DH, Allison DJ, Hamilton CA, Reid JL. Selective venous sampling in the diagnosis and localization of phaeochromocytoma. Clin Endocrinol 1979; 10:179–186.
36. Sisson JC, Frager MS, Valk TW, Gross MD, Swanson DP, Wieland DM, Tobes MC, Beierwaltes WH, Thompson NW. Scintigraphic localization of pheochromocytoma. N Engl J Med 1981; 305:12-16.
37. Valk TW, Frager MS, Gross MD, Sisson JC, Wieland DM, Swanson DP, Mangner TJ, Beierwaltes WH. Spectrum of pheochromocytoma in multiple endocrine neoplasia. Ann Intern Med 1981; 94:762-767.
38. Lurvey A, Yusin A, DeQuattro v. Pseudopheochromocytoma after self-administered isoproterenol. J Clin Endocrinol Metab 1973; 36:766–769.
39. To LB, Sangster JF, Rampling D, Cammens I. Ephedrine-induced cardiomyopathy. Med J Aust 1980; 2:35–36.
40. Brandenburg RO, Gutnik LM, Nelson RL, Abboud CF, Edis AJ, Sheps SG, Factitial epinephrine-only secreting pheochromocytoma. Ann Intern Med 1979; 90:795–796.
41. Thomas JA, Marks BH. Plasma norepinephrine in congestive heart failure. Am J. Cardiol 1978; 41:233-243.

28
Enkephalins

Lesley H. Rees
St. Bartholomew's Hospital Medical College, London, England

Speculation that the source of circulating met-enkephalin in humans might be from the adrenal medulla has been given credence by the findings of high concentrations of immunoreactive met-enkephalin in the adrenal veins, high levels in adrenal medullary tissue, and even higher levels in pheochromocytoma tissues (1,2). Indeed, one pheochromocytoma contained enough material to allow purification and amino acid sequence determination confirming the identity of this met-enkephalin with that originally isolated from porcine brain by Hughes and colleagues (3,4). However, adrenal medullary tissue also contains several higher molecular weight materials, some of which contain both met- and leu-enkephalin immunoreactivities and which may be putative precursors of the smaller opiate pentapeptides (3,5).*

Furthermore, met-enkephalin has been localized to the catecholamine-containing chromaffin cells, and concomitant release of the enkephalin-related peptides and catecholamines has been reported both from isolated perfused adrenal glands (6) and cultured adrenal medullary cells (7) as well as from superfused cat adrenal gland after nicotinic-cholinergic stimulation (8). However, despite these observations, evidence for in vivo release is sparse. Thus a variety of stimuli known to be associated with catecholamine secretion in vivo, such as insulin-induced hypolycemia (9), posture changes, histamine infusion, and operative stress, have all so far failed to significantly alter circulating immunoreactive met-enkephalin (R. Smith, personal communication, 1981). Furthermore, the adrenal medulla cannot be the only source of circulating met-enkephalin since

*Since the preparation of this manuscript the amino acid sequence of a human adrenal enkephalin precursor has been predicted (13).

bilateral adrenalectomy fails to alter basal met-enkephalin levels (9), and since met-enkephalin immunoreactivity has been demonstrated in the carotid body, kidney, liver, atria, skin, retina, and throughout the gut, these may be alternative sources. In fact, the only stimulus that so far reproducibly results in changes in circulating met-enkephalin immunoreactivity has been the administration of oral ethanol after pretreatment with oral chlorpropamide (10).

Unfortunately, the clinical relevance of the presence of high enkephalin levels in the adrenal medulla remains unknown, and at the present time it is even unclear whether met-enkephalin is actively secreted from pheochromocytomas in vivo. Furthermore, the situation is made much more complex by the presence in the adrenal medulla of other novel leu-enkephalin-related peptides such as α-neoendorphin and dynorphin, which are also potent opiate agonists. If all of these are released into the circulation, it is of course possible that they may subserve as yet unknown hormonal roles. However, it is important to remember that local neurotransmitter or neuromodulatory roles may be more important. Such a local modulatory role is suggested by several observations. Thus splanchnic nerve terminals located in the adrenal medulla also contain enkephalin-like materials (11); furthermore, not only do adrenal chromaffin cells possess opiate receptors, but opiates themselves can inhibit nicotine-stimulated catecholamine release from chromaffin cells (12). Hopefully, the next decade will reveal the answers to the many questions regarding the function(s) of the adrenal medullary enkephalins.

REFERENCES

1. Clement-Jones V, Lowry PJ, Rees LH, Besser GM. Methionine enkephalin circulates in human plasma. Nature 1980; 283:295–297.
2. Clement-Jones V, Lowry PJ, Rees LH, Besser GM. Development of a specific extracted radioimmunoassay for methionine-enkephalin in human plasma and cerebrospinal fluid. J Endocrinol 1980; 86:231–243.
3. Clement-Jones V, Corder R, Lowry PJ. Isolation of human met-enkephalin and two groups of putative precursors (2K pro-met-enkephalin) from an adrenal medullary tumour. Biochem Biophys Res Commun 1980; 95: 665–673.
4. Hughes J, Smith TW, Kosterlitz HW, Fothergill LA, Morgan BA, Morris HR. Identification of two related pentapeptides from the brain with potent opiate agonist activity. Nature 1975; 258:577–579.
5. Lewis RV, Stern AS, Kimura S, Rossier J, Stern S, Udenfriend S. An about 50,000 dalton protein in adrenal medulla: a common precursor of (met) and (leu) enkephalin. Science 1980; 208:287–292.
6. Viveros OH, Diliberto EJ, Hazum E, Chang K–J. Opiate-like materials in the adrenal medulla: evidence for storage and secretion with catecholamines. Mol Pharmacol 1979; 16:1101–1108.

7. Corder R, Mason DFJ, Clement-Jones V, Besser GM, Rees LH. Simultaneous release of somatostatin and met-enkephalin from perfused cat adrenal gland. 164th Meeting of the Society for Endocrinology, 1981, Abstract 7.
8. Smith R, Grossman A, Gaillard R, Clement-Jones V, Ratter S, Mallinson J, Lowry PJ, Besser GM, Rees LH. Studies on circulating met-enkephalin and β-endorphin: normal subjects and patients with renal and adrenal disease. Clin Endocrinol 1981; 15:291–300.
9. Medbak S, Wass JAH, Clement-Jones V, Cooke ED, Bowcook SA, Cudworth AG, Reese LH. Chlorpropamide alcohol flush and circulating met-enkephalin: a positive link. Br Med J 1981; 283:937-939.
10. Schultzberg M, Lundberg JM, Hökfelt T, Terenius J, Brandt J, Elde RP, Goldstein M. Enkephalin-like immunoreactivity in gland cells and nerve terminals in the adrenal medulla. Neuroscience 1978; 3:1169–1186.
11. Kumukura K, Karoum F, Guidotti A, Costa E. Modulation of nicotinic receptors by opiate receptor agonists in cultured adrenal chromaffin cells. Nature 1980; 283:489-492.
12. Comb M, Seeburg PH, Adelman J, Eiden L, Herbert E. Primary structure of the human net- and leu-entrephalin precursor and its MRNA. Nature 1982; 295:206-209.

THYROID AND PARATHYROID DISORDERS

29
Thyroid Disorders

H. K. Ibbertson
University of Auckland School of Medicine, Auckland, New Zealand

I. DISORDERS OF THYROID FUNCTION

The initial step in the diagnosis of functional abnormality of the thyroid gland is the recognition of the clinical manifestations of thyroid hormone deficiency or excess. Diagnostic emphasis has shifted to the detection of minor clinical abnormalities and the interpretation of unexpected serum thyroid hormone deviation in patients with nonspecific symptoms (Fig. 1). In this brief account particular attention is paid to minor or less common manifestations of thyroid disease.

A. Thyroid Hormone Excess

The clinical features of overt thyrotoxicosis are well known. The diagnostic process involves the recognition of peripheral manifestations of thyroid hormone excess, changes in size or quality of the thyroid gland, and certain clinical associations which may indicate the underlying etiology.

1. Symptoms and Signs

The anxious patient with slight lid retraction who complains of shakiness "inside" merits study particularly if the hands are warm. Demonstration of mild lid lag may help but is seen in euthyroid anxiety, cor pulmonale, and in myopic patients. The characteristic accentuation of the (10 per second) physiological tremor of the hands is best felt. Visible tremor is likely to be nonspecific. Breathlessness may merely reflect increased oxygen requirement but also left ventricular failure or intercostal muscle weakness when muscle wasting is marked (1). Weakness can be proximal from thyrotoxic myopathy and (rarely)

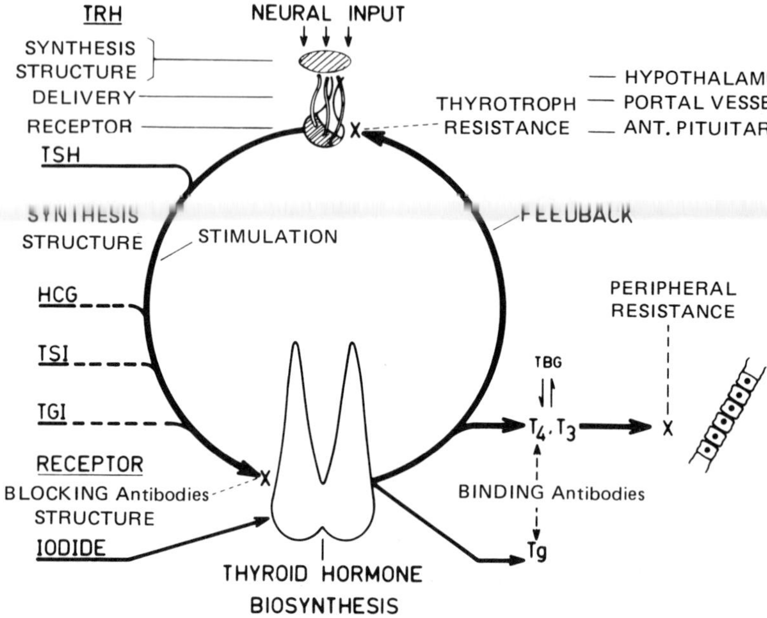

Figure 1 Levels of (thyroid) abnormality. The biosynthesis of thyroid hormones is modulated by extrinsic and intrinsic mechanisms. Variations in thyrotroph and peripheral tissue sensitivity can modify their metabolic effects independently of serum hormone levels.

fatigable from associated myasthenia gravis (2) or episodic from periodic paralysis (3). Increased thirst and polyuria are not uncommon but may indicate diabetes mellitus or hypercalcemia. Onycholysis with separation of the distal fingernail from its bed is an important sign most frequently seen in the ring finger and indicates long-standing thyrotoxicosis. Thyroid enlargement is almost the rule in the female but may be absent in the male. In Graves' disease this could reflect a difference in serum levels of thyroid growth stimulating immunoglobulins (TGI) (4), although evidence of this is lacking. The thyroid may be tender in uncomplicated Graves' disease, but this sign should suggest the possibility of subacute thyroiditis. An arterial systolic thyroid bruit may be diagnostic and is present in about 60% of diffuse toxic goiters. It is usually bilateral, may have a diastolic component, and should be distinguished from other murmers heard in the neck (Table 1).

In children the diagnosis may be difficult and hyperkinesis the only symptom. Slight lid retraction, thyroid swelling (and bruit), and shoulder girdle muscle wasting may give a clue. Acceleration of growth (with increased bone maturation) is sometimes seen, although the reverse is recorded. The establishment of the cause of thyrotoxicosis is important and has therapeutic and prognostic implications.

2. Syndromes (See Table 2)

Graves' Disease. This disorder classically occurs in young women and is 20 times more common in the female than in the male. It also accounts for about half of all thyrotoxicosis diagnosed in older patients. The thyroid is diffusely enlarged, although multiple cold nodules are occasionally present. These obviously respond poorly to thyroid stimulating immunoglobulins (TSI) but may concentrate ^{131}I normally under the influence of thyroid stimulating hormone (TSH) after ^{131}I ablation of internodular tissue. This phenomenon (the Marine-Lenhart syndrome) has been attributed to a difference in TSH and TSI receptors in the nodular tissue (5). The clinical diagnosis of Graves' disease is supported by the presence of one or more extrathyroidal manifestations. The eye signs are characteristic, but lid lag is not in itself diagnostic and may be present in toxic nodular goiter. Infiltrative features such as chemosis, lid swelling, and ophthalamoplegia are more specific and are fully developed in opthalmic Graves' disease. In this condition most patients are euthyroid or even hypothyroid. In about

Table 1 Neck Bruits

Origin	Characteristics	Cause
Venous hum	Continuous variable pitch, lateral Silence by light pressure distal to stethoscope bell	Venous return Often normal in young Increased incidence in thyrotoxicosis
Arterial murmers		
Thyroid related	Bilateral systolic and often diastolic: maximal upper poles	Increased vascularity Diffuse toxic goiter (60%) TSI-mediated TSH-mediated in over-treatment
	Unilateral systolic: increase by lateral thyroid pressure	Local distortion thyroid arteries Multinodular goiter
Extrinsic	Unilateral systolic Bilateral systolic	Carotid atherosclerosis Conducted from aortic valve or flow murmer (e.g., pregnancy)

Table 2 Syndromes of Thyrotoxicosis

Graves' disease	Toxic diffuse goiter (includes hashitoxicosis)
Plummer's disease	Toxic nodular goiter
Chemical varients	T_3-toxicosis
	T_4-toxicosis
Transient	Subacute thyroiditis (de Quervain's giant cell)
	Painless thyroiditis (lymphocytic thyroiditis)
	Transient Graves' in the adult
	Neonatal Graves'
Rare	hCG-mediated
	Trophoblastic disease
	Chorioncarcinoma
	Hydatidiform mole
	Embryonal testicular carcinoma
	TSH-mediated
	Thyrotrope tumor
	Thyrotrope resistance
	Extrathyroidal
	Struma ovarii
	Metastic thyroid carcinoma
Iatrogenic	T_4/T_3 therapy
	Post-^{131}I therapy (uncommon and transient)
	Post-^{131}I administration (Jodbasedow)

two-thirds there is partial or complete suppression of the TSH response to thyroid releasing hormone (TRH), indicating variable autonomy of thyroid function (6). The test is normal in the remainder, confirming independence of the ocular and thyroidal manifestations of the disease. Localized myxedema rarely occurs in the absence of eye signs. Although typically pretibial it may occur elsewhere and even on the face and neck. It develops particularly after treatment of the hyperthyroidism and is associated with high serum LATS levels. Finger clubbing may indicate thyroid acropachy, a rare complication identified in x-rays by bubblelike subperiosteal bone formation. Other autoimmune disorders may be present, and vitiligo, insulin-dependent diabetes mellitus, pernicious anemia, adrenocortical failure, and thrombocytopenic purpura are all specific although uncommon associations.

Positive hemagglutination tests for thyroglobulin (TgHA) and microsomal (MCHA) antibodies occur in 60% and 90% of patients, respectively. The syndrome of Graves' disease is determined by a balance between a variety of circulating immunoglobulins. These include thyroid stimulating (TSI), thyroid blocking (TSI-block) (7), thyroid growth and growth blocking (TGI and

TGI-block) (4), and cytotoxic immunoglobulins. Although the opthalmopathy has features of an autoimmune process, attempts to demonstrate antibodies to orbital contents have generally been unsuccessful (8).

The thyroid stimulating immonoglobulins (TSI) are elevated in the majority but fall with pregnancy, during antithyroid drug medication (9, 10) and with spontaneous remissions. Blocking immunoglobulins modulate the effect of TSI on the thyroid receptor and by transplacental passage may cause temporary neonatal hypothyroidism (11) in the same way that TSI causes neonatal thyrotoxicosis (12). In a minority (10%) of patients remission comes through autoimmune destruction of the gland and hypothyroidism may ensue (hypothyroid Graves'). Occasionally, thyrotoxicosis may replace hypothyroidism in established Hashimoto's thyroiditis [hashitoxicosis (13)]. Thyroglobulin (TgHA) and microsomal (MCHA) titers are high and TSI are present.

Plummer's Disease. The prevalence of multinodular goiter probably reflects the severity of preexisting iodine deficiency and its legacy of nodular thyroid disease. Its expression depends on the availability of substrate (iodine) and the level of thyroid autonomy. It occurs particularly in older patients and lacks the autoimmune features of Graves' disease. Weakness and lethargy may be prominent, and this together with skeletal and smooth muscle (dysphagia) wasting may combine to give the clinical picture of "apathetic" thyrotoxicosis.

The thyroid contains one or more nodules which concentrate technetium (^{99m}Tc) or radioiodine (^{131}I). The internodular tissue which is suppressed (via TSH) fails to concentrate therapeutic radioiodine, hence the low incidence of hypothyroidism.

Biochemical Variants. Elevated serum thyroxine (T_4) and triiodothyronine (T_3) levels are present in most patients with clinical hyperthyroidism through the serum T_3 may be normal in as many as on-third (14). With increasing severity there is a disproportionate elevation of T_3 and a rise in the T_3/T_4 ratio, the T_3 being derived from preferential T_3 synthesis and peripheral T_4 conversion.

In *T_3-toxicosis*, however, the clinical manifestations of hyperthyroidism result solely from the elevated T_3 and the serum T_4 is normal (although not suppressed as with T_3 administration) (15). This condition occurs both in Graves' disease and in toxic nodular goiter. Its incidence varies from approximately 5 to 15% and is more common in areas of endemic iodine deficiency. The radioiodine uptake is normal or increased but nonsuppressible and the TSH response to TRH is absent. Isolated serum T_3 elevation sometimes occurs as an *early* manifestation of Graves' hyperthyroidism particularly during relapse (16). T_3-toxicosis may merely represent a variant of this usual phenomenon.

In *T_4-toxicosis* the serum T_4 is increased and the T_3 normal or low (17). This condition is less well defined than its T_3 counterpart and the pattern usually reflects the reduction in T_4 to T_3 conversion in sick patients (18). This is further suggested by the facts that the serum T_3 often rises to above normal when the intercurrent illness is treated and the TRH-stimulated TSH response is absent. This pattern must be distinguished from that in nonthyroidal systemic illness (19, 20), in which the high serum T_4 and low T_3 return to normal with treatment and the TRH response is normal or blunted. The latter finding can often be explained by the common presence of occult autonomous thyroid nodules (21).

Other Causes of Thyrotoxicosis

Subacute (de Quervain's) Thyroiditis (22). High serum thyroid hormones and thyroglobulin levels characterize this inflammatory disorder, which is often attended by symptoms suggestive of a viral illness. A number of viruses, including mumps and coxsackievirus, have been implicated. The thyroid is often "hard" and the histology is characteristic with clusters of histiocycles around masses of colloid, giving an appearance of "giant cells." the disease runs a variable course and in the acute phase thyroid pain radiating to the ears with weight loss and other symptoms of thyrotoxicosis are common. The illness is sometimes more chronic and local tenderness is minimal. It may then persist for months and mimic malignant disease or conditions such as temporal arteritis or polymyalgia rheumatica. Fine needle biopsy may supply diagnostic cytology. The blood sedimentation rate is elevated often to high levels in 70% of patients, but it may be normal in more chronic disease. The leukocyte count is normal and only minimal titers of serum thyroid antibodies are observed. During the acute phase the release of performed T_4 and T_3 from damaged follicles leads to suppression of TSH, radionuclide uptake, and hormonal synthesis. Serum T_4 is elevated but T_3 levels are less than those seen in Graves' disease in which T_3 synthesis is relatively increased. This biochemical pattern must be distinguished from that in a number of nonthyroidal systemic illnesses in which the serum T_4 is spuriously elevated. During the recovery phase transient hypothyroidism is common and may last for months, but permanent thyroid deficiency is rare. Both radionuclide uptake and ESR may return to normal before recovery of hormonal synthesis.

Painless (benign) Lymphocytic Thyroiditis (23). This disorder, which seems to be relatively common in North America, causes a disturbance in thyroid function similar to that of subacute thyroiditis. The gland is however nontender and infiltrated with lymphocytes, although the typical germinal centers of autoimmune thyroiditis are absent. Thyroid antibodies can be detected but only by highly sensitive techniques. The illness presents as mild thyrotoxicosis of short duration (2-6 months) with absent eye signs and only slight or moderate (painless) enlargement of the thyroid gland. A number of patients have developed symptoms during the postpartum period (24) and in this respect are similar to classical autoimmune thyroiditis with hypothyroidism (25). As with subacute thyroiditis, serum T_4 and T_3 are raised and radionuclide uptake is suppressed. The blood sedimentation rate is however often normal.

The basis of this disorder is still uncertain but its time course is relatively short and complete resolution of the histological changes can be expected (26). Failure to make the diagnosis (by thyroid-uptake measurement) may lead to needless antithyroid drug treatment.

Iatrogenic Thyrotoxicosis. (a) *Thyroxine overdosage* is a common cause of reversible thyrotoxicosis. As judged by TSH suppression, the optimal average daily dose for the treatment of hypothyroidism is 160 μg and the requirement is seldom higher than 200 μg (27). Such recommendations assume a normal servo-mechanism and these doses may prove excessive when there is partial thyroid autonomy, as in nodular goiter or following surgical or radioiodine therapy for Graves' disease. A higher mean dose ($>$200 μg/per day) is necessary to suppress the TSH response in patients with thyroid carcinoma receiving replacement thyroxine. At this dose level the serum thyroxine is elevated in about 40% of patients (28).

(b) *Iodide-induced thyrotoxicosis* may complicate the administration of iodide to iodine-deficiency subjects (jodbasedow thyrotoxicosis) and the serum T_3/T_4 ratio may be reduced (30). It can also occur in the absence of iodine deficiency when thyroid autonomy is present from either TSI or more usually in nodular thyroid disease (31). Symptoms may continue despite withdrawal of iodine. This phenomenon may dictate the prevalence of thyrotoxicosis in Western societies such as the United States, where the average daily intake of iodine is over 500 μg (32).

Uncommon Causes. (a) *Molar thyrotoxicosis* occurs in pregnant women with chorionepithelioma or hydatidiform mole and is thought to result from stimulation by high levels of human chorionic gonadotropin (hCG) (33). The normal placenta produces two other thyroid stimulating factors, human chorionic thyrotropin (hCT) and human molar thyrotropin (hMT), but these have not been implicated. The disorder is often latent and high serum levels of T_4 or (more often) T_3 may be present without symptoms. The thyrotoxicosis is cured by control of the trophoblastic disease by chemotherapy or surgery.

(b) *TSH-mediated thyrotoxicosis* may result from a pituitary thyrotrope tumor (34, 35) or selective thyrotrope resistance to thyroid hormone feedback (36). In the tumor cases the pituitary fossa is usually enlarged with poor TRH-stimulated TSH response but an increased α subunit/TSH ratio. In the resistance syndromes TRH responsiveness is usually normal with appropriate ratios of α subunits to TSH. This topic is discussed further on pages 324 and 325.

(c) *Unusual extrathyroidal sources* of excess thyroid hormone include struma ovarii (37) and metastatic follicular thyroid carcinoma. In the latter condition the thyrotoxicosis usually reflects the large bulk of functioning metastatic tissue (38) but in one patient who developed Graves' disease functioning pulmonary metastases were shown to be dependent on a high titer of thyroid stimulating immunoglobulins (TSI) (39). In these patients with extrinsic sources of thyroid hormones, radionuclide thyroid uptake is suppressed and the ectopic source can be identified by scintiscanning.

B. Laboratory Diagnosis of Thyrotoxicosis

In suspected hyperthyroidism measurement of serum T_4 and T_3 provides confirmation of increased thyroid hormone levels. The presence of thyroid autonomy can be checked by the TSH response to TRH. Thyroid radionuclide measurements have been relegated to a secondary (though still important) role and other dynamic tests such as the T_3 suppression test now have little place in routine diagnosis. Although confirming thyrotoxicosis with great efficiency the routine use of the TRH test as a primary diagnostic procedure can hardly be justified on a cost-benefit basis. Current strategy concentrates on maximizing the information to be obtained from basal serum thyroid hormone measurement and dynamic testing is required in fewer than 20% of patients (see Diagnostic Summary 1).

1. Serum Thyroid Hormones

The *serum T_4*, measured by competitive binding radioassay (40) radioimmunoassay (RIA) (41), or enzyme assay (emit) is widely used as the first line investigation. Since serum T_4 is almost totally bound (99.9%) to thyroxine binding globulin (TBG) and to a lesser extent albumin and prealbumin, it is necessary to correct for changes in TBG levels. This is commonly performed using a variety of techniques, all of which measure the occupancy of T_3 binding sites on TBG; albumin and prealbumin binding usually being inhibited by barbitone buffer. They include T_3 resin uptake (42), Sephadex column separation (43), and T_4/TBG ratio (44) and the results are expressed as a free thyroxine index (FTI) or adjusted thyroxine (T_4 adj) (45). The latter has a conceptual advantage in that the normal range is close to the normal range of serum T_4. The effective thyroxine ratio (ETR) (46) combines the thyroxine measurement and its correction in a single assay. All of these methods correlate well with the free T_4 (fT_4) measured by equilibrium dialysis, which is usually regarded as a reference method (47), although it possibly overestimates fT_4 (69). Some advantage is claimed for the T_4/TBG ratio at extremes of TBG abnormality (44) when TBG levels are markedly decreased, as occurs in hereditary TBG deficiency, but even this may give false low values. fT_4 can now be measured with more convenience and equal accuracy (at least in uncomplicated thyroid disease) with equilibrium (Amerlex fT_4) (48) and kinetic (Corning Immophase fT_4) (49) assays, which along with several similar methods promise to replace existing indirect techniques.

The *serum T_3* is disproportionately increased in thyrotoxicosis (14) and measurement by radioimmunoassay (RIA) (50) provides an early index of hyperthyroidism. A reduction of T_4 to T_3 conversion detracts from its value in patients with associated systemic illness, when serum T_3 may be normal or low, despite unequivocal thyrotoxicosis, a situation not always clarified by measurement of reverse T_3 (rT_3) by RIA (51). Changes in binding proteins alter T_3 levels and as with T_4, correction can be made to give a free T_3 index (fT_3I) or adjusted T_3 (T_3adj) (52). This may be inaccurate when T_3 and T_4 levels are widely divergent. Direct measurement of fT_3 is now possible and kits are available.

Serum T_4 and T_3 Deviations (Table 3). The serum T_4 and T_3 can be increased in euthyroid patients from drug administration, intrinsic alterations in binding protein, and in systemic nonthyroidal illness. RIA may also give misleading results in rare patients with circulating antibodies to thyroid hormones (53). Here the level may be falsely low with nonspecific separation methods (e.g., charcoal) and high when solid phase or second antibody is used (54).

Drug Administrations. A variety of pharmacologic agents cause an increase in serum T_4 (and T_3) (55). Best known is the estrogen-mediated increase in TBG synthesis which occurs even with low-dose oral contraceptives (56). The FTI usually gives a valid index of free thyroxine, but because of nonlinearity between TBG and fT_3 uptake it may sometimes be erroneously elevated, an effect which can be avoided by the use of the T_4/TBG ratio (44) or by direct measurement of fT_4 (48, 49). Increased TBG is thought to be the cause of heroin-induced increase in T_4 and T_3 and the elevated levels reported during medication with the hypolipemic agent clofibrate and the cytostatic compound 5-fluorouracil (55). With all these drugs TBG changes cannot be predicted and there is a marked individual variation.

Displacement from binding sites accounts for temporary T_4 and T_3 elevation during salicylate (57) and phenylbutazone (58) therapy. This is also the case following various iodine-containing contrast agents such as iopodate (Telepaque) which displace T_4 from intrahepatic sites and cause transient increase in serum T_4 which may last for 1-2 weeks (59). There is an associated inhibition of T_4 to T_3 conversion with a fall in serum T_3, giving a pattern which mimics T_4 thyrotoxicosis, although the TSH response to TRH is normal or exaggerated. The situation is further complicated by the liability of these compounds by virtue of their iodide content to precipitate thyrotoxicosis (with normal or low T_3), but here the response to TRH is suppressed.

A *reduction* in TBG binding is a more common sequel of drug administration and the resultant fall in T_4 and T_3 may mask the biochemical pattern of thyrotoxicosis. This is discussed further later.

Intrinsic Protein Binding Abnormalities. An increase in TBG concentration and both total T_4 and T_3 occurs during normal pregnancy and with hydatidiform mole- and estrogen-producing tumors (60). It also complicates systemic diseases such as infectious hepatitis, collagen disease, myelomatosis, and acute

Table 3 Serum T_3/T_4 Relationships[a]

Serum free T_4 index	(Low)	Serum Free T_3 Index	(High)
(High)	T_4-*toxicosis*[b] Iodide–induced toxicosis Nonthyroidal illness[b]	T_4-toxicosis *Iodide radiocontrast media* *Familial euthyroid T_4 excess syndrome*	*Thyrotoxicosis* *Subacute thyroiditis* *Painless thyroiditis* T_4 *Administration* Genetic TBG excess[b]
	Nonthyroidal illness[b]	*Normal euthyroid*	T_3-*toxicosis*
(Low)	*Central hypothyroidism* Primary hypothyroidism *Critical nonthyroidal illness*[b] *Genetic TBG deficiency*[b]	*Primary hypothyroidism* (includes iodine deficiency)	T_3 *Administration*

[a]Titles in italic indicate the most common pattern.

[b]Disorders in which fT_4 and T_3 indices can be at variance with free hormone measurement by equilibrium dialysis.

intermittent porphyria (61). It is increased in hypothyroidism and usually reduced in thyrotoxicosis, although it may be high (62). Failure to recognize this variant may lead to overtreatment. Inherited TBG abnormalities occur with a frequency of 1 in 2000 and increased TBG is the least common accounting for less than one-third (63). The inheritance is X-linked and other serum proteins, including TBPA, are normal. The serum T_4 and FTI can both be elevated, although the fT_4 is normal and the subject euthyroid.

Familial Euthyroid T_4 Excess. Changes in TBPA concentration have relatively little effect on serum T_3 and T_3 and no genetic abnormalities have been described. On the other hand, a genetic defect in which T_4 is bound to an albumin-like protein is the basis of this syndrome, with high T_4 and fT_4I in euthyroid subjects. The serum T_3 and fT_3I are normal (64). The inheritance is autosomal dominant and many patients have received inappropriate treatment before the correct diagnosis is made. The conventional T_3 resin uptake fails to correct the high T_4 because T_3 has low affinity for the abnormal binding sites, which are inhibited by the barbitone buffer usually present. Correct assessment of thyroid status is made by avoidance of barbitone use of $[^{125}I]$ T_4 rather than T_3 and by the addition of excess unlabeled T_4. fT_4 levels which are normal (equilibrium dialysis) in this condition may be falsely elevated when measured by the amerlex free T_4 method since the labeled inert analog used in the assay interacts with the abnormal albumin binding sites (65).

Nonthyroidal Illness (NTI). The serum T_3 and fT_3I are reduced in various acute and chronic systemic illnesses (66), in starvation (67), and following medical and surgical stress. The serum T_4 and fT_4I can also be reduced but are often elevated (21, 68), and this must be distinguished from T_4 thyrotoxicosis. The serum fT_4 is usually normal by equilibrium dialysis, but other methods have shown elevated levels. Most evidence indicates that these patients are euthyroid. The reason for the inadequate correction of T_4 by the T_3 resin uptake is uncertain but cannot be attributed to the small changes in TBG (69) or to a circulating inhibitor which has been identified in the *low*-T_4 syndrome of critical illness (149, 150). Whatever the basis of these changes, the TSH response to TRH is normal or blunted (but not absent) and the abnormalities disappear as the patient's condition improves (70).

2. TRH Simulation Test

This test finds its greatest use in suspected thyrotoxicosis and with few exceptions gives excellent discrimination between normal and thyrotoxic subjects (71). The response can be defined on the basis of the baseline and peak TSH value on serum samples at 0 and +20 min (21). An absent response with peak and increment values at 20 min equal to or less than 1.5 and 0.5 μU/ml, respectively, confirms thyrotoxicosis when the serum T_4 and T_3 are elevated. Such a response is also seen in the absence of thyrotoxicosis in solitary hot thyroid nodules and in some patients with ophthalmic Graves' disease (72). Here the sensitive servomechanism recognizes free hormone elevation, which in insufficient to cause clinical effects.

A blunted TSH response indicates only partial thyroid autonomy and excludes thyrotoxicosis. It is common in multinodular goiter (73) and can occur in chronic renal failure (74) and in any severe illness (75). In elderly subjects it may indicate occult nodularity of the thyroid gland, which can be demonstrated only by scintiscanning. A blunted TSH response can also reflect persisting abnormality of TSH release following withdrawal of antithyroid drugs in thyrotoxic patients and of thyroid hormone replacement in hypothyroidism. Also during treatment with a variety of therapeutic agents, which include glucocorticoids, growth hormone, somatostatin, L-dopa, bromocryptine, thioridazine, and many others (55). None of these influences inhibit the TRH response completely and seldom cause diagnostic difficulty.

In thyrotoxicosis caused by thyrotrope adenomas or in the selective thyrotroph resistance syndrome the TRH-stimulated TSH response may be absent, blunted, or normal (see page 628).

3. Other Tests

To answer the question "Is this patient thyrotoxic?" the clinician can rely on the combination of serum thyroid hormone measurement and TRH test with a high degree of confidence. Refinements in hormone measurement technique can elucidate mechanisms but seldom increase the diagnostic yield, and older tests of thyroid autonomy (T_3 suppression) are now superceded.

Supplementary tests give etiological information. The radionuclide thyroid uptake is no longer a first-line investigation but is reserved for patients in whom subacute or painless thyroiditis is suspected. The scan can also assist the classification of cause and provide a guide to subsequent therapeutic radioiodine dosage.

Graves' disease is associated with presence of serum thyroid stimulating immunoglobulins (TSI) (76). There is considerable variation in specificity and sensitivity of assay systems. These include the bioassays; long-acting thyroid stimulator (LATS) and LATS protector (LATS-P) (77); the in vitro thyroid stimulator assays, which utilize cyclic AMP or T_3 as the end point (78, 79); and the receptor assay or thyrotropin binding inhibitor immunoglublin assay (TBII), which measures inhibition of [^{125}I] TSH binding to thyroid receptors (80). The latter assay has the advantage of simplicity but is positive in only 70% of Graves' patients and occasionally in multinodular goiter and autoimmune thyroiditis. It may still have utility in the prediction of relapse (103) or of neonatal thyrotoxicosis, although discrepancies occur (81). A better yield is claimed for both LATS-P and TSI (cyclic AMP) and over 90% of Graves' patients are identified (76). Both predict neonatal thyrotoxicosis better than TBII, although TSI (cyclic AMP) appears superior. In terms of accuracy and practicability, neither method can be recommended as a routine procedure.

Diagnostic Strategy. In overt thyrotoxicosis, minimal confirmatory testing is required and the free thyroxine (fT_4I) or its equivalent will establish the diagnosis in over 90% of patients. In less obvious disease the success rate is only about 70% and additional tests are required. In many patients with nonthyroidal illness an initial elevation of fT_4I will prove to be normal in a second sample when the patient's condition has improved, and this will obviate the need for supplementary tests (21). If fT_4I is used as the screen, the serum T_4 is corrected to minimize discrepancies from alterations in TBG binding. This involves a second test which is relatively time consuming and expensive. An alternative approach is to use the *uncorrected* serum T_4 as the basic screen and to measure FTI and other supplementary tests when the result lies outside carefully defined "action limits." In an analysis of 860 samples the decision on the need for supplementary testing differed by less than 3% when T_4 instead of fT_4I was used as the initial screen (82). This difference could be eliminated by widening the indications for additional tests such as the serum fTI, T_3, or TRH stimulation.

Notwithstanding the logic of this approach, it is difficult to deny the attraction of the comparatively simple recent techniques for free T_4 measurement which are designed to measure the biological active moiety in a single-step assay (48, 49). This appears to be the case in uncomplicated hypo- and hyperthyroidism, and good correlation is reported between the various methods and the fTI (47). As with the fTI, however, discrepancies occur, particularly in low-TBG states (65) and in nonthyroidal illness. In one study (83) only three of six methods used were judged to give a correct assessment of the fT_4.

Reliance on a measurement of free thyroxine as the definitive screen may thus for methodological reasons give the clinician unwarranted confidence in the end product. The "gray area" is still a problem and the need for supplementary testing remains. The ultimate decision on which screening test may ultimately be made on financial grounds and the fT_4 assay can now be automated at a reagent cost of only U.S. \$1.45 (84).

It is apparent that much effort has been expended on improving the diagnostic efficiency of the initial serum sample. However, nothing can eliminate intrinsic biological and assay variation and the inherent limitation of "population" ranges when applied to the patient whose personal normal range is tighter by a factor of at least 50% (85). Because of these limitations there is an increasing tendency to cut short the diagnostic cascade and to resort to dynamic (TRH) testing when the initial serum sample is borderline or discrepant. With this test thyrotoxicosis can be excluded with certainty, but an absent TSH response requires the backup of increased serum T_4 or T_3 before antithyroid therapy is indicated.

Having confirmed autonomous overproduction of thyroid hormones, the clinician must establish its cause (Table 2). In the absence of autoimmune stigmata a distinction between Graves' and Plummer's disease can be aided by a ^{99m}Tc or ^{131}I scan and by serum thyroid antibody (MCHA, TGHA) measurement. Demonstration of hyperfunctioning thyroid nodules has implications for radioiodine therapy (see later), while diffuse uptake may, on the other hand, indicate subacute thyroiditis [with erythrocyte sedimentation rate (ESR) elevation] or painless (lymphocytic) thyroiditis in which the ESR is often normal. Fine needle biopsy may help distinguish these two conditions. Absence of Graves' features in a relatively young patient should also raise the possibility of a rare cause of thyrotoxicosis, such as thyrotrope adenoma or resistance. In the presence of clinical and biochemical hyperthyroidism an unsuppressed or elevated TSH justifies further investigation, which should include a TRH test and lateral skull x-ray. Measurement of thyroid stimulating immunoglobulins (TSI) has little primary diagnostic value.

Assessment of Therapy. For the treatment of Graves' disease with antithyroid drugs the initial dosage is dependent on the size of the thyroid enlargement and the severity of the disease. This is normally obvious but can also be assessed by measurement of serum T_3 (14) and the carbimazole dosage adjusted accordingly; doses above 10 mg every 8 hr being reserved for patients with large goiters or T_3 levels more than three times the upper limit of normal. Improvement in the clinical manifestations of thyrotoxicosis often lag behind changes in biochemical indices, although body weight measurement is an important (and cheap) index of response. Regular measurement of serum T_4 provides a useful guide to dose adequacy and also of overtreatment since the TSH response is often delayed. Measurement of serum methimazole levels (the active metabolite of carbimazole) during therapy shows wide variation with little relation to therapeutic response (86). Selective intrathyroidal concentration of methimazole may be a more important determination of its antithyroid action (87).

Prognosis in Thyrotoxicosis. The prediction of outcome during antithyroid drug treatment has proved an elusive goal. The two main methods involve measurement of either ^{131}I or ^{99m}Tc uptake 20 min after a tracer dose (88, 89) or measurement of thyroid stimulating immunoglobulins (TSI) by LATS protector (LATS-P) assay (90), human thyroid adenyl cyclase stimulation activity (hTACS) (78), or receptor assay (TBII) (80). Failure to suppress 20-min [^{131}I] thyroid uptake was shown to predict relapse following antithyroid drug therapy with 70% accuracy, but recurrence also occurred when the uptake was fully suppressed (91, 92). This was partially explained by the demonstration that carbimazole influenced the organic binding of iodine within the 20-min period (93). Measurement of ^{131}I 0- to 5-min clearance allowed better prediction, but discrepancies still occurred even with technetium (89), which measures only the trapping mechanism and is uninfluenced by carbimazole.

Similar results are obtained with tests measuring serum thyroid stimulators. Relapse occurred in 83% of 52 patients with positive LATS-P levels at the end of anythyroid drug treatment but also in 29 patients who were LATS-P negative (94). Similar results were reported for hTACS (90) and TBII (95) and a direct comparison between these two indices showed little correlation (96).

Neither the TBII or LATS-P assay directly measures thyroid stimulatory activity and both TBII and LATS-P have been detected in patients who are euthyroid. Alternative approaches to prediction of outcome include measurement of serum antimicrosomal or antithyroglobulin antibodies (97) or thyroglobulin (Tg) itself (98), but neither method has proved useful. Serum Tg levels are higher and fail to fall with antithyroid drug treatment in patients whose disease subsequently relapses. Interference with Tg RIA by circulating anti-Tg antibodies has limited the use of this technique, but a recent modification of the standard RIA promises to overcome these difficulties.

The factors that determine recurrence or persistence of thyrotoxicosis in Graves' disease include its initial severity, iodide availability (99), and spontaneous fluctuations in the autoimmune disease process (100). The fall in TSI that occurs in many patients treated with carbimazole can be attributed to its immunosuppressive action (101, 102) but also in some patients to a spontaneous resolution of the disease process. Whether short-term immunosuppression really influences long-term remission is still unproven and prediction based on short-term changes must of necessity be of limited value.

More recent evidence implicates the patient's HLA antigen status and increased frequency of HLA-DRW3 antigen has been reported in Graves' disease in Caucasians (103) but not in Chinese (104). Nevertheless, in both racial groups this antigen has almost invariably been present when relapse has occurred. The presence of both TBII and HLA antigen DRW3 allowed prediction of short-term relapse in 90% of patients studied by MacGregor et al. (103). At best (with the possible exception of tissue typing) most of these prognostic indices provide an expensive and relatively inaccurate forecast of the future. In practical terms a large goiter makes long-term remission following antithyroid drug treatment unlikely and definitive therapy is indicated. For the remainder, long-term single-dose antithyroid drug treatment with periodic (annual withdrawal) provides a reasonable alternative. Patients can be told to report for a blood sample at any time that they sense a return of symptoms or notice a fall in weight. By this means relapse can be detected early and drug therapy reinstituted automatically with minimal morbidity and doctor intervention.

C. Thyroid Hormone Deficiency

In primary hypothyroidism the availability of a radioimmunoassay for serum TSH (105) provides a convenient and precise yardstick against which to measure the clinical diagnosis. By this criterion the clinical method has been found wanting and minor degrees of hypothyroidism are often undetected. Recent evidence indicates, however, that TSH elevation occurs before peripheral tissue hypothyroidism (106) and the final arbiter, a sensitive test of peripheral thyroid hormone action, awaits development.

1. Symptoms and Signs

Lassitude, lack of drive, and mild cold intolerance may be the only overt symptoms of mild hypothyroidism. Minimal periorbital puffiness, slight chemosis (the silver sign), and carotenemia can provide clues and slow relaxation of the ankle reflex may be diagnostic. This sign, which must be elicited with the patient kneeling (without shoes), may be absent in mild hypothyroidism but is often abnormal in patients in whom other clinical evidence of thyroid hormone deficiency is minimal. These remarks are particularly true of patients with central hypothyroidism in whom the manifestations of TSH deficiency are mild and conditioned by the lack of other trophic hormones.

2. Syndromes

Symptoms and signs of thyroid hormone deficiency (Table 4) may arise as a result of intrinsic thyroid abnormality or disease of the pituitary or hypothalamus (i.e., primary, secondary, and tertiary hypothyroidism). The term "central hypothyroidism" indicates an abnormality at either hypothalamic or pituitary level.

Other rarer peripheral causes include congenital thyroid unresponsiveness to thyrotropin (107) and blocking immunoglobulins to the thyroid TSH receptor (11). Antibodies to the circulating thyroid hormones themselves interfere with RIA measurements but are not believed to alter thyroid status (108). Peripheral tissue unresponsiveness to normal serum T_4 and T_3 levels is also described in a number of rare syndromes (109–111), but minor degrees of tissue insensitivity may be more common than presently recognized.

Primary (Thyroid) Hypothyroidism. By far the most common causes of hypothyroidism are endemic iodine deficiency and autoimmune thyroiditis. Previous radioiodine or surgical treatment of thyrotoxicosis now accounts for as many as one-third of overt cases in nonendemic areas. This may reflect the relative prevalence of thyrotoxicosis, which is almost twice that of spontaneous hypothyroidism.

Iodine Deficiency. In severe endemic areas with urine iodide content of less than 25 μg per day, TSH elevation occurs in more than 50% of the population (112). In children the manifestations of hypothyroidism are most obvious in the myxedematous cretin with intellectual defect, deaf mutism, neuromuscular disorder, and growth failure. Goiter may or may not be present. In adults the severity of hypothyroidism increases with goiter size and elderly women with massive multinodular goiters are most obviously affected. In such areas despite low serum T_4 and T_3 levels are normal or elevated in more than 80%. A proportion of these individuals are euthyroid, the high TSH reflecting the unsaturation of T_3 thyrotroph receptors, which normally depend on the ambient thyroxine level as a substrate for T_3 (106).

Table 4 Syndromes of Hypothyroidism

Primary (thyroid) hypothyroidism
Loss of functional tissue
Dysgenesis
Autoimmune thyroiditis (Hashimoto's disease)
Radioiodine therapy and thyroidectomy
Infiltrations
Defects in thyroid hormone biosynthesis
Inherited defects (dyshormonogenesis)
Iodine deficiency or excess
Antithyroid compounds
Central hypothyroidism
Pituitary (secondary hypothyroidism)
Hypothalamic (tertiary hypothyroidism)
Peripheral hypothyroidism
Peripheral tissue resistance to thyroid hormones
Binding antibodies to thyroid hormones[a]
Low T_3 syndrome

[a]These usually cause little functional disturbance.

Autoimmune Thyroiditis (113). A survey in the village of Wickham in north-east England (114) showed significant titers of thyroid microsomal antibodies (MCHA) in 7% of the population. The serum TSH was also raised in 3% of these and when both were present clinical hypothyroidism appeared at a rate of about 4% per year. The annual incidence was much higher (26%) in another study, which included patients with initial TSH elevation and *high* titer antibodies (115). This condition should be considered in any patient with a personal or family history of organ-specific autoimmune disease, such as insulin-dependent diabetes mellitus, Graves' disease, pernicious anaemia, and myasthenia gravis.

It presents as either goitrous (Hashimoto's) thyroiditis with or without hypothyroidism or atrophic autoimmune thyroiditis with severe hypothyroidism (myxedema) and an impalpable thyroid gland. HLA typing suggests a genetic distinction since DR5 predominates in goitrous thyroiditis, whereas the atrophic variety is associated with an excess of DR3 (116).

There are three main histological variants (Table 5)—focal, oxyphil, and fibrous—each with its own associated antibody pattern and clinical course. The clinical picture also depends on the interaction of stimulating (TSI and TGI) and blocking (TSI-block and TGI-block) immunoglobulins; the latter being absent in goitrous thyroiditis (117). Proportional variation in these opposing influences probably determines the characteristic fluctuation of the natural

Table 5 Comparison of Main Features in Three Histological Variants of Hashimoto's Thyroiditis

Features	Focal lymphocytic thyroiditis	Oxyphil variant	Fibrous variant
Sex ratio	Children 5F:1M	20F:1M	5F:1M
	Young adults 20F:1M		
Prevalence	40% of nontoxic goiters	Fairly common	Rare
Age at presentation	11-13	30-60	Middle-aged and elderly
Thyroid function at presentation	Euthyroid	Euthyroid	Often hypothyroid
Goiter			
Size	Small	Moderate; occasionally rapid growth	Moderate or small, a few very large
Consistency	Moderately soft	Moderately firm	Very firm
Shape	Diffuse thyroid-shaped	Horseshoe shaped; sometimes irregular	Horseshoe shaped or asymmetrical
Surface	Smooth	Smooth or finely granular	Bosselated or granular
Pain/tenderness	Painless	Occasionally attacks of pain, sometimes persistent	Painless

Response to T_4	Good	Rapid loss of pressure symptoms; slow reduction; 10–20% no response	Mostly rapid shrinking, a few resistant
Ultimate outcome	Remissions and exacerbations	More than 50% lose thyroid reserve	Complete disappearance of goitre and loss of thyroid reserve
Histology	Moderate lymphocytic infiltrate marked colloidophagy, no Askenazy cells, some focal thyroid cell hyperplasia	Dense lymphocytic infiltrate with germinal centers, extensive oxyphil metaplasia, some giant cells, minimal fibrosis; in large goiters active growth of new thyroid acini	Predominantly plasma cell infiltrate. Askenazy cells, marked fibrosis, loss of normal lobular architecture
Immunology			
Microsomal antibodies (MCHA)	Low or moderate titers	Moderate to high titers	Mostly high titers
Thyroglobulin			
TGHA	Trace or absent	Negative in 30% cases	High titers
Precipitin	Negative	4% positive	96% positive

Source: Ref. 113.

history of the disorder. Thus spontaneous remission occurs particularly in adolescent girls with focal thyroiditis (118) and with pregnancy, when a rebound in antibody titers during the puerperium may be accompanied by a recurrence of hypothyroidism (25). Treatment with corticosteroids may also reverse hypothyroidism in autoimmune Addison's disease with associated thyroiditis (Schmidt's syndrome) (119).

Diagnosis. The onset of autoimmune thyroiditis is usually insidious but occasionally thyroid enlargement is relatively rapid and sometimes painful (120). This syndrome can be distinguished from subacute (viral) thyroiditis by a normal or elevated radionuclide uptake and the presence of thyroid antibodies. It may sometimes present as a hot or cold thyroid nodule and the diagnosis can be confirmed by fine needle biopsy. It is occasionally an unsuspected accompaniment of multinodular goiter or other pathology, such as thyroid carcinoma or lymphoma. The serum T_4 is normal or low and T_3 usually normal. Serum TSH is normal or elevated and radionuclide uptake is usually increased. Despite increased iodide trapping there is an associated organification defect which can be revealed by the perchlorate discharge test (page 361) in as many as 80%. Thyroglobulin (TgHA) and microsomal (MCHA) antibodies are present in moderate or high titers. In about 15% of patients thyroid atrophy is present and antibody titers are low.

In Graves' disease focal thyroiditis is common and MCHA titers are increased in 85% of patients. Occasionally, spontaneous hypothyroidism develops in patients with firm goiters and high titers (hypothyroid Graves'). In this situation thyroid stimulating immunoglobulins (TSI) are denied functional expression by the reduction in thyroid capacity from autoimmune destruction, although blocking antibodies may also be implicated (121). A reverse situation is seen in hashitoxicosis when thyrotoxicosis appears in a patient with well-established primary hypothyroidism from autoimmune thyroiditis (13). This transition can also follow steroid administration and becomes apparent when the usual T_4 replacement dose seems suddenly to become excessive.

Destructive Therapy. Between 5 and 70% of patients with Graves' disease develop hypothyroidism within 12 months of therapy. This is attributable to radionecrosis and is dose related. Transient hypothyroidism is common within the first 3 months (122) and recovery is possible up to 6 months. This may be related to the rise in TSI which occurs following therapy (123). Late-onset hypothyroidism appears at a rate of 1-3% per year and results from failure of replication of ^{131}I-damaged cells.

Hypothyroidism is uncommon in nodular goiter since the suppressed normal internodular tissue tends to escape the radiation dose. External radiation to the neck for malignant diseases such as carcinoma of the larynx or lymphoma may cause hypothyroidism in as many as 25% (124).

Following subtotal thyroidectomy the reported incidence of hypothyroidis varies from 5 to 40%. The lower figure reflects short follow-up and as with radioiodine therapy, late hypothyroidism appears at a rate of 1-2% per year. The total incidence is dependent on the size of the thyroid remnant (125), the presence and severity of thyroiditis (126), and the residual level of thyroid stimulating immunoglobulins (123).

Drugs. Clinical hypothyroidism may complicate treatment with any goitrogenic drug provided that it is taken for long enough and in sufficient quantities.

Minor degrees of unrecognized hypothyroidism are common during antithyroid drug treatment of thyrotoxicosis, and secondary elevation of TSH may increase the size and vascularity (bruit) of the gland, giving a false impression of continuing hyperthyroidism.

The antithyroid effects of most other drugs are relatively slight and not clinically important, although there are some exceptions. Aminoglutethemide, which is used to inhibit cortisol synthesis in Cushing's syndrome and metastatic breast carcinoma, blocks thyroid iodine organification and frequently causes hypothyroidism (127). Routine T_4 replacement is warranted. Lithium may cause transient elevation of serum TSH in as many as 30% of treated patients (128) and this may persist particularly when thyroid antibodies are positive. Routine T_4 therapy is unnecessary but the patient should be checked for hypothyroidism, which may secondarily slow excretion of the drug.

Of more general importance is the liability of iodide to cause goiter and hypothyroidism by direct inhibition of organic binding and thyroid hormone release (Woolf-Chaikoff effect) (129). This is relatively uncommon and occurs usually when there is preexisting thyroid damage from autoimmune thyroiditis, surgery, or radioiodine (130). An apparent exception is the *normal* fetal thyroid, which appears particularly susceptible to this effect. Over half the subjects with iodine goiter are hypothyroid and this reverses completely within a few weeks of iodine withdrawal. The diagnosis can be confirmed by a history of iodide administration. The thyroid ^{131}I uptake is normal or increased in the presence of high serum and urine ^{127}I levels, reflecting greatly increased absolute iodide turnover.

Uncommon Causes. *Dyshormonogenesis.* Detailed consideration of these rare inherited syndromes is beyond the scope of this chapter and excellent accounts are available (131). They have in common the presence of goiter, varying degrees of hypothyroidism, and often a family history. They include:

Iodide trapping defect. This rare condition is recognized by the combination of goiter with low or absent radioiodine uptake and biochemical evidence of hypothyroidism. Salivary/serum iodide ratios and thyroid iodide content are low. Consanguinity has been described and the defect is inherited as an autosomal recessive. Treatment with potassium iodide increases thyroidal iodide content by passive diffusion and allows normal iodothyroinine biosynthesis.

Organification defect. Relative or absolute failure of binding of iodide with thyroglobulin characterizes this heterogeneous group of disorders. The abnormality can be demonstrated by the perchlorate discharge test (see page 631), which causes release of unbound inorganic iodide from the thyroid gland. Defects include deficiency or absence of peroxidase and defective H_2O_2 formation with failure of iodine generation, an essential step in the organification process. The exact nature of the defect is uncertain in Pendred's syndrome. In this autosomal recessive condition which presents in early childhood, high-tone deafness and goiter are usual but hypothyroidism is rare.

Coupling defect. This has been less well defined as a genetically transmitted disorder. The radioiodine uptake is high and the ratio of iodotyrosine/iodothyronine in thyroglobulin is also increased. The primary abnormality could result from low iodination of tyrosyl residues in thyroglobulin, but there is often an associated iodoprotein abnormality and iodoalbumin can be identified.

Dehalogenase defect. Conservation of body iodine stores is normally dependent on recycling of iodide by deiodination of MIT and DIT in the thyroid and peripheral tissues. In this genetic disorder the dehalogenase enzyme is usually absent from both sites, but the abnormality may be restricted to the thyroid alone. Goitrous hypothyroidism is usual and the condition can be identified by the presence of iodotryosines in the urine or by the excretion of administered labeled MIT or DIT. Like the trapping defect, hypothyroidism can be corrected by the administration of potassium iodide.

All these conditions are rare but should be suspected in children with a family history of goiter or in sporadic cases when goiter is associated with high radionuclide uptake or negative thyroid antibodies, with or without clinical evidence of hypothyroidism.

Thyroid infiltrations. This heterogeneous group of disorders includes sarcoidosis (132), amyloidosis (133), histiocytosis (134), and lymphoma (135), particularly postirradiation). Autoimmune thyroiditis may be associated and this can also impair thyroid function. In cystinosis (136), a rare metabolic disorder with recessive inheritance, intrathyroidal deposits of the amono acid cause hypothyroidism in about 25% of cases.

Central Hypothyroidism. The causes, clinical features, and diagnosis of secondary and tertiary hypothyroidism are discussed in Chapter 23.

D. Laboratory Diagnosis of Hypothyroidism

The laboratory diagnosis of hypothyroidism is reviewed in Diagnostic Summary 2. The availability of the TSH radioimmunoassay has made possible the certain exclusion of primary hypothyroidism in untreated patients with nonspecific symptoms or borderline serum T_4 levels. TSH elevation is invariable in overt primary hypothyroidism and reflects a reduction in negative feedback by circulating T_4 and T_3. Minor TSH elevation can occur following administration of dopamine antagonists such as metaclopromide (137), but this does not present a problem in practice.

The exquisite sensitivity of the servomechanism has to some extent been a source of diagnostic embarrassment since the serum TSH may be elevated in the presence of *normal* T_4 and T_3 levels. Such a pattern has been variously described as "subclinical hypothyroidism," "compensated hypothyroidism," or "compensated euthyroidism" (138), the differing emphasis reflecting doubts about the true significance of the phenomenon. Resolution of this dilemma is important since TSH elevation is claimed to be a risk factor for coronary artery disease and minor electrocardiogram (ECG) changes have been demonstrated (139). Recent evidence from Larsen and his co-workers has clarified the mechanisms involved (106). Preferential generation of T_3 from T_4 in the pituitary thyrotrope normally modulates TSH synthesis and secretion. A minimal decrement in serum T_4 from a reduction in thyroid biosynthesis results in a fall in T_3 generation and reduced T_3 occupancy of thyrotrope receptors. A consequent increase in TSH secretion stimulates thyroidal T_3 synthesis, which by virtue of its greater biological potency ensures a euthyroid periphery. TSH elevation may persist for many years without any obvious decline in thyroid function (140). Any reduction in T_4 is balanced by a proportionate rise in serum T_3, which remains normal in 80% of patients with overt hypothyroidism. The point (or TSH level) at which compensation fails and peripheral tissues become hypothyroid is still uncertain. Hypothyroidism can be confirmed in some patients by measurement of ankle reflex time (141) or ventricular function (142) before and after T_3 administration. However, this is not practicable in clinical practice and the dilemma will remain unresolved until a more sensitive test of thyroid hormone action is available. Even a modest elevation of serum TSH indicates a significant reduction in thyroid functional capacity and the rate of appearance of clinical hypothyroidism in this group is about 4% per year. Most clinicians favor replacement of thyroxine to prevent insidious hypothyroidism and to allow shrinkage of thyroid enlargement in goitrous thyroiditis. A case can be made for "no treatment" in patients under regular supervision (e.g., following radioiodine therapy) (140).

Neither TRH nor TSH stimulation has any real place in the confirmation of primary hypothyroidism. The TRH-stimulated TSH response is exaggerated, but the peak level correlates with the baseline value. Following TSH there is a normal rise in ^{131}I uptake or serum T_4 and T_3 in at least half of patients with serum TSH elevation (143), a testimony to the sensitivity of the intrinsic servomechanism.

In central hypothyroidism there is a proportionate reduction in serum T_4 and T_3 (67). The serum TSH is usually normal with conventional RIA, but with sensitive methods levels can be shown to be low, although usually still detectable. In about 25% of patients immunoreactive TSH is mildly elevated and this may cause diagnostic difficulty. The material is, however, biologically inactive, as indicated by the failure of serum T_3 to rise after TRH stimulation. The presence of other evidence of pituitary dysfunction and the absence of serum thyroid antibodies confirms a central origin for the hypothyroidism.

An absent TSH response to TRH confirms thyrotrope failure, but a normal or prolonged response is consistent with hypothalamic *or* pituitary abnormality. This is discussed further in Chapter 39, page 630.

1. Assessment of Therapy

In primary hypothyroidism the serum TSH can be used to monitor T_4 dosage and the aim is to reduce TSH into the normal range. In elderly patients ECG monitoring is also essential and suboptimal replacement may be desirable when ischemia is detected. The serum T_4 defines the upper limit of dosage and more precise information can be obtained from the TRH test, but this is seldom indicated. Surveys indicate a substantial drop-out from therapy and long-term surveillance is essential (27).

2. Screening for Hypothyroidism

Screening programs have provided important data on the prevalence of hypothyroidism in the newborn (144). Permanent primary hypothyroidism occurs in 1 in 4300 live births (compared with 1 in 16,000 births for phenylketonuria). Thyroid dysgenesis of varying degree accounts for most cases and genetic dyshormonogenesis for about one-tenth. The prevalence of ectopic thyroids (by scintiscan) varies and is higher in European centers (60%) than in North America and Australia (35%). There is also a geographical variation in the prevalence of transient hypothyroidism and the permanent/transient ratio in Europe is 2.4:1, compared with 10:1 in North America and Australia. It appears to be more common in areas of iodine deficiency, although a *high* iodine intake may be implicated in Japan. Pituitary-hypothalamic hypothyroidism (central hypothyroidism) is much less common (1 in 110,000 live births), although not all programs screen for this.

The benefits of early treatment are now undoubted, yet very few hypothyroid babies are recognized clinically before 3 months (145). Treatment before this time results in a normal development quotient at 1.5-3 years and almost 80% achieve an IQ of above 85% (146). With late treatment one-third of children require special schooling and one-fourth have an IQ of less than 70% (145). On a cost-benefit basis such figures amply justify the widespread introduction of screening programs and there are now at least 80 such programs in operation. Most centers use capillary serum T_4 followed by supplemental TSH measurement on samples with the lowest 3-10% of T_4 results. The sample is taken by heel prick at 2-7 days and the dried blood filter paper spot is the preferred collection method. Serum T_4 levels tend to be less reduced in infants with ectopic thyroid tissue and the higher cutoff point is required to detect such cases. Routine T_4 and TSH on all samples avoids this difficulty but is much more expensive. Screening with TSH alone is cost effective but fails to detect infants with central hypothyroidism, delayed TSH elevation, transient functional abnormality, or TBG deficiency. Although not a primary goal, the identification of such abnormalities may have important immediate and long-term implications. In this respect the TBG assay (44) may be helpful.

A thyroid scintiscan with ^{99m}Tc or ^{123}I is recommended in all infants with congenital hypothyroidism, demonstrable uptake in the thyroid bed or in an ectopic site being suggestive of dyshormonogenesis. Guidelines for the organization of screening programs and the evaluation, therapy, and developmental assessment of affected infants were formulated recently at an International Conference on Neonatal Thyroid Screening (144).

Screening for hypothyroidism in adults is much less well validated. TSH elevation occurs in about 3% of the population (144), although often the rise is small and not all such subjects are hypothyroid (106). The influence of therapy on long-term longevity in this group has yet to be demonstrated. The detection of thyrotoxicosis is an additional bonus from a screening program and the prevalence is twice that of hypothyroidism. Here again, however, many patients are asymptomatic and the inconvenience and potential complications of therapy (including permanent hypothyroidism) may outweight the theoretical benefits.

The diagnostic yield from wholesale "admission multiphasic (biochemical) screening" (AMS) is low (147), and there are difficulties in the interpretation of serum T_4 in sick patients. Nevertheless, the inclusion of serum T_4 in a screening program has been claimed to be both efficient and cost effective (148). Current opinion favors a "case-finding" approach, with serum T_4 ± TSH being measured in susceptible subjects. These include patients receiving goitrogenic drugs, those with goiter or autoimmune diseases, and elderly patients with nonspecific symptoms, cardiac failure, or unexplained wasting.

3. Serum T_4 and T_3 Deviations

A number of nonthyroidal influences cause a reduction in serum T_4 and T_3, and since the TSH is usually normal, this must be distinguished from central hypothyroidism.

(a) In critical nonthyroidal illness the serum T_4 and T_3 are often very low, and recent studies have sought to clarify the mechanisms involved (83). In these patients the fT_4 (by equilibrium dialysis) and the T_4 production rate are in fact normal and the TSH response to TRH is normal, although often blunted. Despite this apparent normality and notwithstanding normal TBG levels, the free thyroxine index (T_4I) is reduced. Such findings indicate defective serum T_4 binding to the carrier protein, and a nondialyzable circulating inhibitor with characteristics of IgM (149) or another macromolecule (150) has been implicated. The situation is not always clarified by measurement of serum reverse T_3 (rT_3), which may be normal or elevated (151). Measurement of the serum fT_4 also by either the equilibrium (Amerlex) free T_4 method (48) or the kinetic (Corning Immunophase) T_4 method (49) concurs with the free T_4 index more closely than with the free T_4 concentration by equilibrium dialysis. A better indication of the true T_4 level is claimed for an antibody-coated tube (Clinical Assays) method and an enzyme (Abbott) immunoassay (83). These studies suggest that such patients are euthyroid and the T_4 therapy is inappropriate.

(b) Inherited TBG abnormalities occur with a frequency of about 1 in 2000 and absent or low TBG is the most common defect (152). The inheritance is X-linked. Serum total T_4 is low and serum FTI may also be low because of nonlinearity of the T_3 resin uptake at very low TBG levels. The diagnosis can be confirmed by direct measurement of serum TBG (44). Direct T_4 measurement by equilibrium or kinetic methods may underestimate T_4. The subjects with this disorder are euthyroid.

(c) Drugs may cause a fall in serum T_4 and T_3 without blocking their synthesis by reducing TBG (androgens, high-dose glucocorticoids) by competing with TBG (diphenylhydantoin, diazepam) by enzyme induction (diphenylhydantoin, carbamazepine) and by increasing conversion of T_4 to T_3 growth hormone therapy (55). As with TBG abnormalities, the normal servomechanism ensures euthyroidism and the serum TSH is normal.

II. DISORDERS OF THYROID MORPHOLOGY

When goiter occurs in association with overt hyper- or hypothyroidism its presence is incidental to the functional disturbance and seldom a cause for investigation in its own right. When it occurs in isolation it merits attention either because of local pressure effects or its malignant potential.

Mechanisms of thyroid enlargement are multiple and early growth at least is often TSH dependent. In autoimmune disease other external stimulators, such as TSI or TGI, may be important, while intrinsic factors determine the development of the solitary nodule. Subtle genetic enzyme defects which modify iodide utilization may be the basis of "simple" goiter, which continues to appear in iodide-replete communities. Disorders of thyroid morphology are reviewed in Diagnostic Summary 3.

A. Varieties of Goiter

1. Diffuse and Multinodular Euthyroid Goiter

In Western societies thyroid antibodies are detectable in almost 10% of the population (113) and autoimmune thyroiditis is now the commonest cause of diffuse thyroid enlargement in the adolescent. In the absence of antibodies, there is often a strong family history and minor enzyme defects are probably implicated, although they are usually unmeasurable. Definable enzyme defects are much less common and can sometimes be suspected by the presence of hypothyroidism, the association of deafness (Pendred's syndrome), or by the family history. Other etiological factors include goitrogenic drugs and iodide excess, which is more often a problem in older patients with preexisting thyroid damage from autoimmune thyroiditis, surgery, or radioiodine. A reduction in the use of therapeutic iodine-containing preparations is offset by the current fad for natural foodstuffs, which include kelp and other seaweed products with a high iodine content.

Chronic TSH (or TSI) stimulation leads to cellular hyperplasia and hypertrophy with ultimate nodule formation. In such goiters a spectrum of functional autonomy has been described, but this represents the end result of chronic stimulation rather than a primary defect (153).

Investigation. A careful history is essential and this must include inquiry into family and drug history and previous irradiation of the neck. Hoarseness, or local pain, dyspnea or dysphagia, the consistency of the gland, and the presence of palpable lymph nodes may give etiological information. The woody firmness of autoimmune thyroiditis is characteristic and the stony hard gland is malignant in over 50%. This is likely to be confused only with subacute thyroiditis (particularly if painless) or rarely with massive calcification of the gland.

Measurement of serum thyroid hormones, TSH and thyroid antibodies may indicate hyper- or hypothyroidism, which usually but not invariably indicates a benign lesion. The serum thyroglobulin is often raised but this is of little diagnostic value (154). Tracheal deviation or compression can be demonstrated by an x-ray of the thoracic inlet, and laryngoscopy allows visualization of the vocal cords, although cord paresis is rare in the absence of malignant infiltration. A dominant nodule may be cystic and this can be demonstrated by ultrasound examination. Recent local pain may indicate hemorrhage into a nodule and this can be confirmed by diagnostic aspiration, which can incidentally relieve local discomfort and pressure effects. The radionuclide scan is rarely contributory and merely confirms heterogeneous uptake with multiple "cold" areas throughout the gland. Malignant potential is minimal and thyroid biopsy or surgical exploration is not usually indicated unless there has been recent enlargement or suspicious findings on examination (155).

2. The Solitary Nodule

The diagnostic approach to the solitary nodule is determined less by the risk of functional or pressure effects than by its malignant potential. The incidence of thyroid carcinoma is variously reported as between 2.5% (156) and 29% (157) and such figures could justify removal of all solitary nodules. However, the data are biased by prior selection and only one-fourth of all solitary nodules achieve clinical recognition (156). The high-risk group can be identified by clinical examination, and radionuclide scanning can reveal impalpable multiple nodules, which presage a better prognosis (158). Judicious use of these and other screening techniques allows a selective approach without demonstrable increase in morbidity.

Benign Nodules. Most benign thyroid nodules are follicular adenomata and papillary, and atypical types are much less common. Scintiscanning allows functional classification into hot, warm, or cold nodules. More than half are cold and a specific abnormality of the iodide transport mechanism has been demonstrated (159). Such nodules are usually benign, but most carcinomas are of this type. A solitary cold nodule may represent cyst formation in a benign adenoma or sometimes an area of subacute or autoimmune thyroiditis. Ultrasound examination and fine needle biopsy will usually distinguish these benign conditions. About 20% of nodules are hot, and half of these are associated with thyrotoxicosis. The remainder are autonomous and the TRH response is suppressed but serum fT_4 is normal. Thyroid carcinoma is rare. The warm nodule is also usually benign, although occasional cold nodules appear warm in the anterio-posterior (AP) scan when there is overlying (or underlying) functioning tissue. In one study, 25% of warm nodules were cold on oblique scanning (160).

Malignant Nodules. Thyroid carcinoma is a protean disorder which involves most age groups. It differs from other thyroid disease in that the female preponderance is less than that from other carcinomas and the prognosis is better in younger patients.

Its prevalence is related to genetic factors, iodide availability (TSH stimulation), and exposure to ionizing radiation. As many as 80% of children with thyroid carcinoma have previously received x-ray treatment to the head and neck (162) and almost 10% of irradiated glands develop thyroid carcinoma (162). This topic has been reviewed recently (163).

There are four basic histologic types of thyroid carcinoma and these usually present as a solitary cold nodule or a dominant "cold" area in a preexisting goiter.

Papillary Adenocarcinoma. This is the commonest of the thyroid carcinomas and occurs typically in younger women (F/M 3:1), with a peak incidence in the late teens and early twenties. It is relatively infrequent in endemic goiter areas and more common in iodide-rich regions (164). It is the commonest thyroid carcinoma following irradiation to the neck in childhood and a history of this should always be sought (163). The distribution is often multicentric and the tumor spreads via lymphatic channels to the jugular chain, superclavicular nodes, and trachea. Microscopic calcification (psammoma bodies) occurs in the more differentiated tumors and aggregations of these may be visible as fine stippling in radiographs of the neck. Occasional lymph node deposits concentrate ^{131}I despite the presence of normally functioning tissue. Blood spread occurs relatively late and the lungs are particularly involved. The prognosis is better in the young patient.

Follicular Adenocarcinoma. This is less common than papillary carcinoma. It comprises about 30% of all malignant thyroid tumors. It occurs in an older age group and typically in women in the fifties. In contrast to papillary carcinoma, it is more common in endemic goiter areas and this and other evidence indicates its dependence on TSH stimulation. The distinction between low-grade carcinoma and follicular adenoma is often difficult and made easier when capsular and vascular invasion has occurred and certain when there is spread to local lymph nodes, lungs, or skeleton. Almost half the patients have metastases by the time the diagnosis is made. Prognosis is again better in younger patients, in whom radioiodine uptake (hence radioiodine therapy) can be stimulated by ablation of normal thyroid tissue. In both these differentiated carcinomas thyroglobulin production is increased but only very high levels are diagnostic since moderate elevation is common in benign nodular goiter (154).

Anaplastic Carcinoma. This typically occurs in older women with preexisting goiter. Areas of differentiated carcinoma can usually be found, indicating an anaplastic change in a previously differentiated lesion. In contrast to the other carcinomas, the tempo of the disease is rapid. Recent enlargement of a known goiter with hoarseness, positional dyspnea, and maybe dysphagia are characteristic. Stridor is sometimes marked and made worse by extending the neck. The thyroid mass is stony hard and often involves adjacent lymph nodes. Lymphatic and bloodstream spread is characteristic. Spindle cell, giant cell, and small cell types are described. Small-cell carcinomas are probably mostly lymphomas, which have a better prognosis. The diagnosis can be easily confirmed by fine needle biopsy. The serum thyroglobulin is normal.

Medullary Carcinoma. These tumors, which are derived from the calcitonin-secreting parafollicular cells (C cells), are responsible for fewer than 10% of all thyroid carcinomas. They occur sporadically but also in about 20% as part of the genetic syndrome of multiple endocrine adenoma type II (MEA II) (also known as MEA IIa, or Sipple's syndrome). In this disorder medullary carcinoma is associated with pheochromocytoma (bilateral in 70%) and chief cell hyperplasia of the parathyroid glands. The thyroid tumor presents as a hard local cold nodule, often with evidence of spread to local lymph nodes and upper mediastinum. Blood-borne spread is late and favors lung, liver, adrenal, and bone (165). The histology is characteristic, with sheets of cells with granular cytoplasm and abundant stromal amyloid. These cells, which belong to the amine precursor uptake and decarboxylation (APUD) system, regularly secrete calcitonin and measurement of this hormone is basal and stimulated samples provides valuable clues to the diagnosis. Carcinoembryonic antigen (CEA) is another hormonal marker which is consistently present (166). Other humoral secretions may have clinical consequences. Watery diarrhea is present in 20% and prostaglandins have been implicated (167) although not consistently demonstrated. As in the carcinoid syndrome, the diarrhea may be associated with flushing in about one-third of patients. Cushing's syndrome occurs in about 5% and both ACTH and calcitonin production have been demonstrated in the same tumor (168). Other associations include gynecomastia and galactorrhea. Parathyroid hyperplasia leads to increased production of PTH, but the incidence of hypercalcemia is variable. It is uncommon in the genetic syndrome and this contrasts with the other humoral abnormalities, which are shared equally with sporadic cases. Genetic syndromes comprise about 20% of the total and medullary carcinoma may be inherited alone or in association with pheochromocytoma and/or multiple mucosal neuromas and ganglioneuromatosis of the gastrointestinal tract. These features give the patient a characteristic appearance with Marfanoid habitus and a characteristic facies with thickened and sometimes nodular lips and small polypoid tumors on the eyelid margins and anterior third of the tongue. This syndrome has been labeled MEA IIb (or MEA III).

Other Neoplasmas. Many of the small-cell carcinomas of the thyroid previously reported were probably lymphomas, which have a much better prognosis. Associated autoimmune thyroiditis is common but not invariable. Rarer turmors include sarcoma, hemangioendotheliomas, and squamous carcinoma. Metastatic disease of the thyroid is relatively common and recorded in 25% of patients dying with nonthyroidal carcinoma (169). The commonest primary tumors are hypernephromas, melanomas, bronchogenic carcinomas, and carcinoma of the breast and colon. The serum Tg is usually normal.

B. Diagnostic Strategy

Among patients with a solitary thyroid nodule, a minority high-risk group can be isolated by history and clinical examination, although most present without distinguishing features. Particular attention is directed to younger patients, males of any age, and those with a history of neck irradiation in childhood (163). Larger nodules (greater than 4 cm) are more likely to be malignant, but many carcinomas are smaller. Tracheal distortion can be assessed by x-ray, which may incidentally reveal the fine-stippled calcification of papillary carcinoma, which contrasts with the flecks or "signet ring" patterns of benign lesions. The majority (70%) of benign nodules are nonfunctioning (cold) on scintiscan and cannot be distinguished from carcinomas or cysts. However, the risk of malignancy is more than halved by the finding of a warm nodule and is insignificant in hot nodules. Care is needed since about one-fourth of warm nodules may in fact be cold on oblique scanning (160) and a lesion which is correctly identified by ^{133}I scan as a cold carcinoma may appear hot with ^{99m}Tc (170). A scan diagnosis of multiple nodules favors a benign lesion, although a dominant mass must be evaluated independently (155). Almost 20% of cold nodules are cysts. This can be simply confirmed by ultrasound examination, which may show a unilocular cyst or cystic generation within a solid lesion. Less than 2% of small cysts (less than 4 cm) are malignant (171) and confirmation of a benign lesion can be obtained by diagnostic aspiration, which yields a clear yellow fluid. Degenerate blood or brownish aspirate may indicate malignancy, particularly in large nodules, and this can be confirmed by cytological examination of the aspirate.

Needle biopsy (see page 633) of solid lesions is a useful procedure and risks of spreading carcinoma have been overstressed. Fine needle biopsy (FNB) is a lesser procedure than core biopsy (CNB) (Trucut) and provides similar diagnostic information (172). The availability of both techniques is helpful, with FNB as the primary procedure and CNB reserved for nodules greater than 2 cm. These techniques may confirm subacute or immune thyroiditis, although the latter can be confused with lymphoma. It can also distinguish a predominantly papillary from a follicular lesion but cannot diagnose follicular carcinoma with any certainty. A planometric method which measures nuclear area shows promise of doing this, measurements of below 90 μm^2 strongly indicating a benign lesion (173).

The serum thyroglobulin is elevated in most patients with follicular or papillary thyroid carcinoma. Exceptions occur, but these are usually very small localized lesions (154). The levels are also normal in medullary anaplastic or metastatic carcinoma. The serum Tg is increased in more than 70% of patients with benign single or multiple thyroid nodules, and for this reason its

Diagnostic Summary 1 Thyrotoxicosis

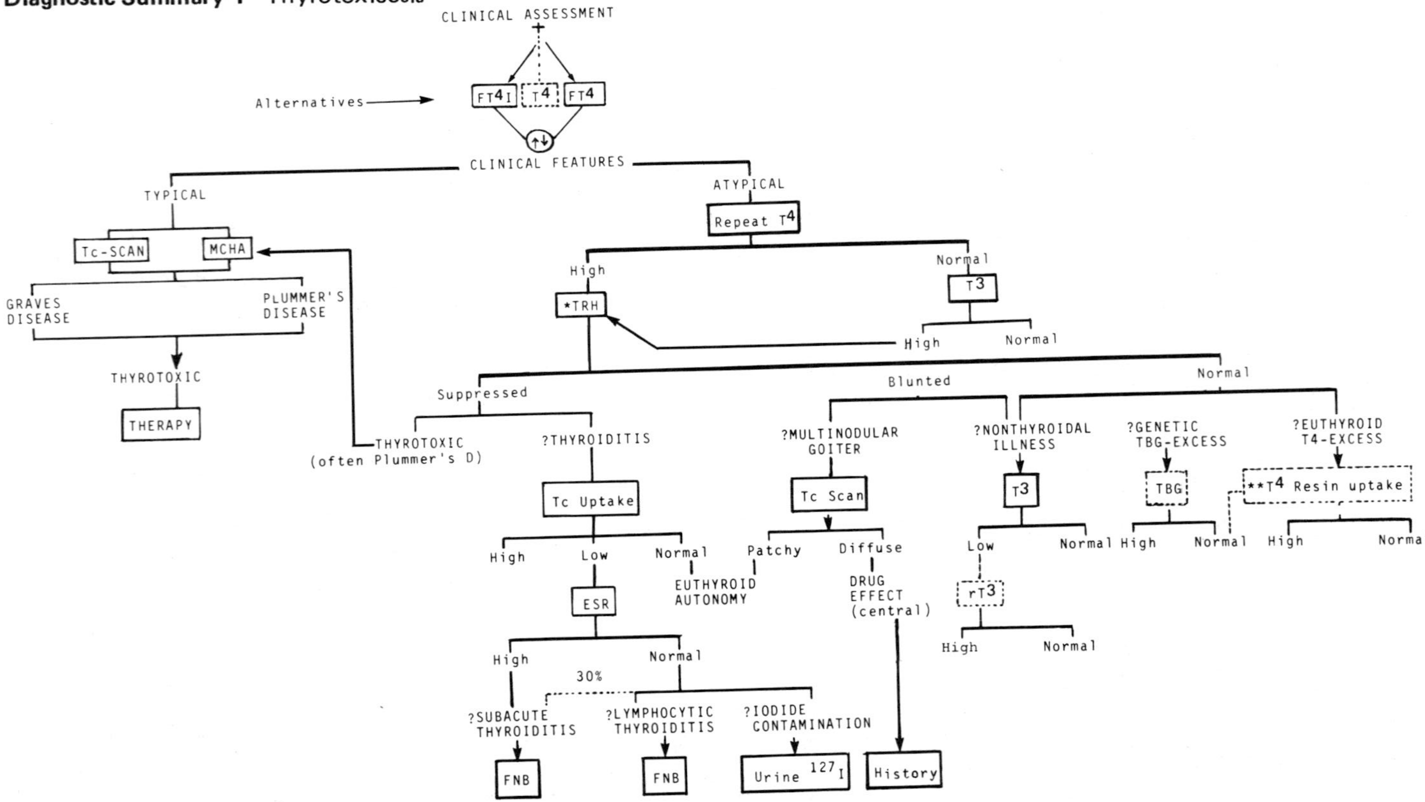

In typical overt thyrotoxicosis a high serum T_4 (or equivalent) is confirmatory and additional tests are required only to elucidate cause. When the serum T_4 or clinical picture is equivocal (and particularly when systemic illness is present) a repeat estimation will be normal in approximately half and serum T_3 will be elevated in a further 10% (T_3-toxicosis). Persistent T_4 elevation is an indication for TRH testing and thyrotoxicosis is confirmed only when the TSH response is suppressed. Dashed lines indicate procedures which elucidate mechanisms without influencing management decisions.

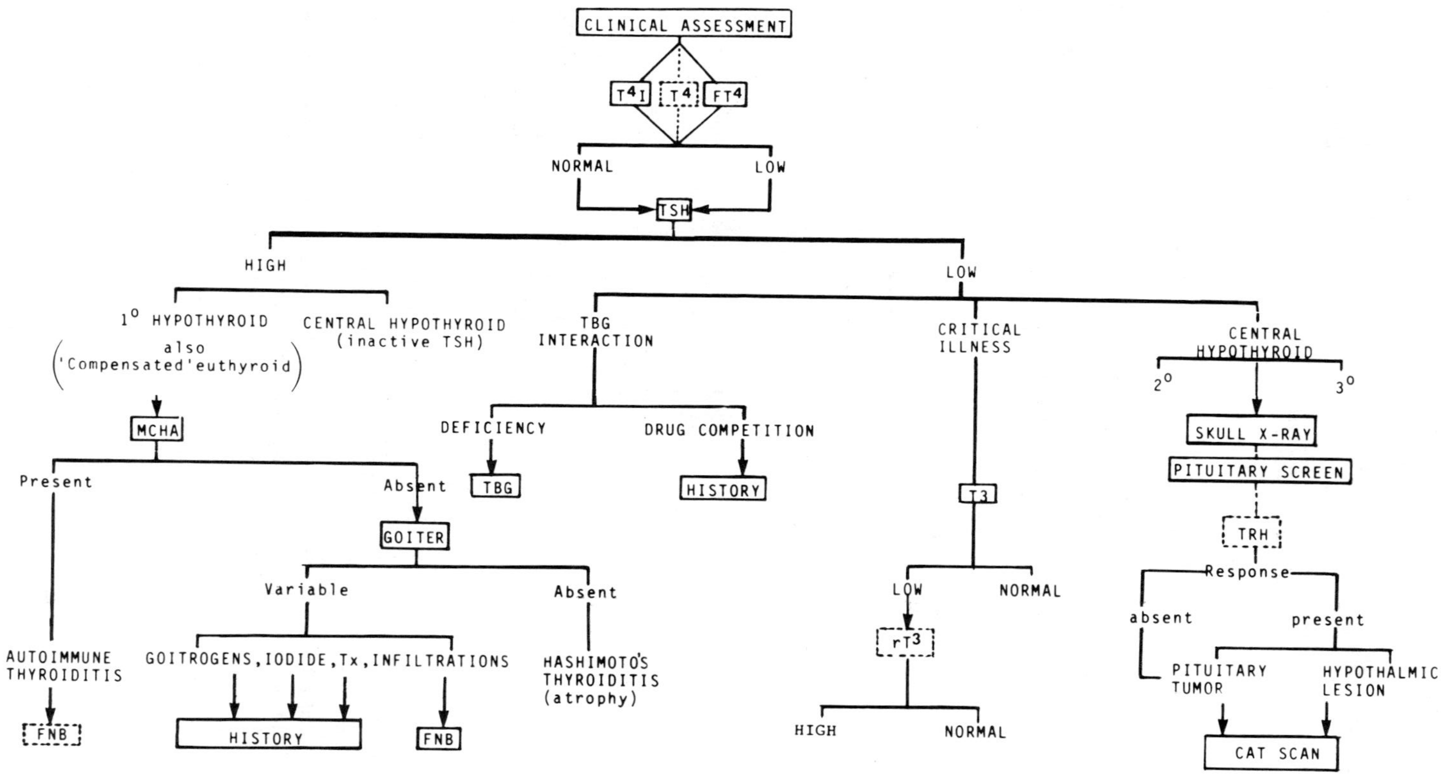

Serum TSH may be inappropriately high in central hypothyroidism when "inactive" TSH is present or low in primary hypothyroidism following withdrawal of T_4 replacement. Dashed lines indicate procedures which elucidate mechanisms but seldom influence management decisions.

Diagnostic Summary 3 Goiter

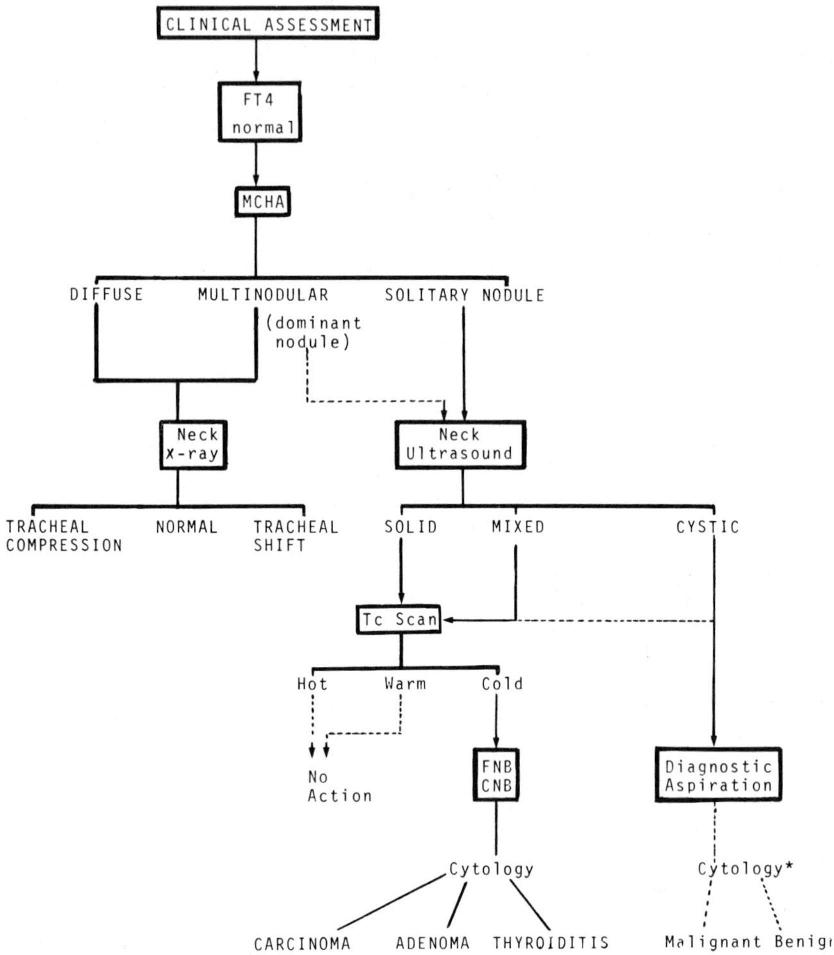

*The diagnostic yield from "pure" cysts is low. Occasionally, positive cytology is obtained in fluid from "mixed" solid-cystic lesions as defined by ultrasound.

measurement is of little value as a primary diagnostic procedure. It finds its greatest use in patients with differentiated thyroid carcinoma following radioiodine ablation of thyroid tissue, when a rise in previously undetectable levels may then signal a recurrence of the tumor. Care must be taken in evaluating serum Tg in patients maintained on thyroxine since the levels rise when the medication is withdrawn (174).

By judicious use of these diagnostic tests, approximately one-third of patients presenting with a solitary nodule can be managed conservatively. In the remainder, particularly in the high-risk group, surgical excision and frozen section is the logical management.

REFERENCES

1. Ayers J, Rees J, Clark TJH, Maisey MN. Thyrotoxicosis and dyspnoea. Clin Endocrinol 1982; 16:65–71.
2. Weickhardt GD, Redmond AJ. Myasthenia gravis and hyperthyroidism; report of two cases and review of the literature. Ann Intern Med 1960; 52:1246–1257.
3. Cheah JS. Thyrotoxic periodic paralysis in Singapore. 6th Asia and Oceania Congress of Endocrinology, Singapore, 1978, vol 1, pp 282–299.
4. Drexhage HA, Bottazzo GH, Doniach D, Bitensky L, Chayen J. Evidence for thyroid-growth-stimulating immunoglobulins in some goitrous thyroid diseases. Lancet 1980; 2:287–292.
5. Park HM, Ziererink S, Ransburg RC, Yum MN, Maxon HR, Ryo UY. Marine-Lenhart syndrome (Graves' disease with poorly functioning nodules). In *Thyroid Research VIII*, Stockigt JR, Nagataki S (eds), Proceedings of the VIIIth International Congress, Sydney. Australian Academy of Science, Canberra, 1980, pp 641–644.
6. Tamai H, Nakagawa T, Ohsako N, Fukino O, Takahashi H, Matsuzuka F, Kuma K, Nagasaki S. Changes in thyroid functtions in patients with euthyroid Graves' disease. J Clin Endocrinol Metab 1980; 50:108–112.
7. Orgiazzi J, Williams DE, Chopra IJ, Solomon DH, Human thyroid adenylcyclase stimulating activity in immunoglobulin G of patients with Graves' disease. J Clin Endocrinol Metab 1976; 42:341–348.
8. Henderson J, Wall JR. Failure of haemagglutination and immunofluorescence methods to detect serum orbital antibodies in patients with Graves' opthalmopathy. Clin Endocrinol 1981; 14:153–158.
9. Bech K, Nistrup Madsen S. Influence of treatment with radioiodine and propylthiouracil on thyroid stimulating immunoglobulins in Graves' disease. Clin Endocrinol 1980; 13:417–424.
10. McGregor AM, Peterson M, McLachlan SM, Rooke P, Smith BR, Hall R. Carbimazole and the autoimmune response in Graves' disease. N Engl J Med 1980; 303:302–307.

11. Matsuura N, Yamada Y, Nohara Y, Konishi J, Kasagi K, Endo K, Kojima H, Wataya K. Familial neonatal transient hypothyroidism due to maternal TSH-binding inhibitor immunoglobulins. N Engl J Med 1980; 303: 738–741.
12. Munro DS, Dirmikis SM, Humphries H, Smith T, Bonahead GD. The role of thyroid stimulating immunoglobulins of Graves' disease in neonatal thyrotoxicosis. Br J Obstet Gynaecol 1978; 85:837–843.
13. Irvine WJ, Lambert B-A, Cullen DR, Gordin R. Primary hypothyroidism preceding thyrotoxicosis: a report of two cases and a review of the literature. J Clin Lab Immunol 1979; 2:349–352.
14. Fragu P, Alperovitch A, Tubiana M, Ekins R, Faglia G, Francesco A (eds). A procedure for thyroid investigation in clinical practice: value of a computer programme. In *Free Thyroid Hormones.* Exerpta Medica, Amsterdam, 1979, pp 130–136.
15. Hollander CS, Mitsuma T, Nihei N, Shenkman L, Bunday SZ, Blum M. Clinical and laboratory observations in cases of triiodothyronine toxicosis confirmed by radioimmunoassay. Lancet 1972; 1:609–611.
16. Marsden P, Howorth PJN, Chalkley S, Acosta M, Leatherdale B, McKerron CG. Hormonal pattern of relapse in hyperthyroidism. Lancet 1975; 1: 944–947.
17. Birkhäuser M, Bussett R, Burger TH, Burger A. Diagnosis hyperthyroidism when serum-thyroxine alone is raised. Lancet 1977; 2:53–56.
18. Burger A, Suter P, Nicod P, Valloton MB, Vagenakis A, Braverman L. Reduced active thyroid hormone levels in acute illness. Lancet 1976; 1: 653–655.
19. Carter JN, Corcoran JM, Eastman CH, Lazarus L. The effect of severe, chronic illness on thyroid function. Lancet 1974; 3:971.
20. Burrows AW, Shakespear RA, Hesch RD, Cooper E, Aicken CM, Burke CW. Thyroid hormones in the elderly sick: "T4 euthyroidism." Br Med J 1975; 4:437–439.
21. Croxson MS, Wilson TM, Ballantyne GH. TRH testing, T4 thyrotoxicosis and the aging thyroid gland. NZ Med J 1981; 93:417–420.
22. Volpe R, Subacute (de Quervain's) thyroiditis. In *Clinics in Endocrinology and Metabolism*, Evered D, Hall R (eds). Saunders, Philadelphia 1979, vol 8, pp 81–95.
23. Nikolai TF, Brosseau J, Kettrick MA, Roberts R, Belataos E. Lymphocytic thyroiditis with spontaneously resolving thyroiditis (silent thyroiditis). Arch Intern Med 1980; 140:478–482.
24. EeKel RH, Green WL. Post partum thyrotoxicosis in a patient with Graves' disease, association with low radioactive iodine uptake. JAMA 1980; 243: 1454–1456.
25. Amino N, Miyai K, Kuro R, Tanizawa O, Azokizawa M, Taka S, Tanaka F, Nishi K, Kawashima M, Kumamara Y. Transient post partum hypothyroidism; fourteen cases with autoimmune thyroiditis. Ann Intern Med 1977; 87:155–159.

26. Inada M, Nishikawa M, Naito K, Ishii H, Tanaka K, Imura H. Reversible changes in the histological abnormalities of the thyroid in patients with painless thyroiditis. J Clin Endocrinol Metab 1981;52:431–435.
27. Scottish automated follow-up register group. Thyroxine replacement therapy: prescribing patterns and problems in 2710 patients. Br Med J 1980;281:969–971.
28. Lamberg B-A, Rantanen M, Sarrinen P, Liewendahl Sivula A. Suppression of the TSH response to TRH by thyroxine therapy in differentiated thyroid carcinoma patients. Acta Endocrinol (Copenh) 1979;91:248–256.
29. Croxson MS, Gluckman PD, Ibbertson HK. The acute thyroidal response to iodised oil in severe endemic goitre. J Clin Endocrinol Metab 1976;42: 926–930.
30. Haberman J, Leisner B, Witte A, Pickardt CR, Scribe PC. Iodine contamination as a cause of hyperthyroidism or lack of TSH response to TRH stimulation. (Results based on a screening investigation.) J Endocrinol Invest 1982;5:153–1560.
31. Veganakis AG, Wang CA, Burger A, Maloof F, Braverman CE, Ingbar SH. Iodine-induced thyrotoxicosis in Boston. N Engl J Med 1972;287: 523–527.
32. Park YK, Hortand BF, Vanderween JE, Shank FR, Prosky L. Estimation of dietary iodine intake of Americans in recent years. Research 1981; 79:17–23.
33. Chan V, Wang C, Ho PC, Yeung RTT, Ma HK. Biochemical thyroid hyperfunction in trophoblastic diseases. In *Thyroid Research VIII*, Stockigt JR, Nagataki S (eds), Proceedings of the VIIIth International Thyroid Congress, Sydney. Australian Academy of Science, Canberra, 1980, pp 598–600.
34. Sato T, Suzuki Y, Ishiguro K, Masuyama T, Takata I, Sano M, Kanashima H, Koizumi S, Nakajima H. Enhanced peripheral conversion of thyroxine to triiodothyronine during HGH therapy in GH deficient children. J Clin Endocrinol Metab 1977;45:324–329.
35. Bevoit R, Pearson-Murphy BE, Roberts F, Marcovitz S, Hardy J, Tsokas G, Gardiner RJ. Hyperthyroidism due to a pituitary TSH secreting tumour with amenorrhoea-galactorrhoea. Clin Endocrinol 1980;12:11–19.
36. Gershengkorn MC, Weintraub BD. Thyrotropin-induced hyperthyroidism caused by selective pituitary resistance to thyroid hormone. A new syndrome of "inappropriate" secretion of TSH. J Clin Invest 1975;56: 633–642.
37. Lempers TD, Dokerty MB, Hoffman DL, Bartholomew LG. Struma ovarii-ascitic, hyperthyroid and asymptomatic syndromes. Ann Intern Med 1970;72:883–893.
38. Baumann K, Weitzel M, Burgi H. Hormone producing thyroid carcinoma with hyperthyroidism. Schweiz Med Wochenschr 1979; 109:309–314.

39. Snow MH, Davies T, Smith BR, Ross WM, Evans RG, Teng CS, Hall R. Thyroid stimulating antibodies and metastatic thyroid carcinoma. Clin Endocrinol 1979; 10;413–418.
40. Murphy BEP, Jachon C. The determination of thyroxine by competitive protein binding analysis employing an anion-exchange and radiothyroxine. J Lab Clin Med 1965; 66:161–167.
41. Chopra IJ. A radioimmunoassay for measurement of thyroxine in unextracted serum. J Clin Endocrinol Mctab 1972; 34:938–947.
42. Mitchell ML, Harden AB, O'Rourke ME. The in vitro resin sponge uptake of triiodothyronine ^{131}I from serum in thyroid disease and pregnancy. J Clin Endocr Metab 1960; 20:1475–1483.
43. Gimlette TMD. Sephadex column chromotography in the assessment of thyroid status. J Clin Pathol 1967; 20:170–174.
44. Burr WA, Evans SE, Lee J, Prince HP, Ramsden DB. The ratio of thyroxine to thyroxine-binding globulin in the assessment of thyroid function. Clin Endocrinol 1979; 11:333–342.
45. Stein RB, Price L. Evaluation of adjusted total thyroxine (free thyroxine index) as a measure of thyroid function. J Clin Endocrinol Metab 1972; 34:225–228.
46. Mincey EK, Thorson SC, Brown JL. A new in vitro blood test for determining thyroid status–the effective thyroxine ratio. Clin Biochem 1971; 4:216–221.
47. Fyffe JA, Ayanb L, Cohen HN, Turner JG, Thomson JA, Ratcliffe JG. Clinical and laboratory evaluation of four methods of assessing free thyroxine status in thyroid clinic patients. Ann Clin Biochem 1980; 17: 334–338.
48. Wellby ML, Guthrie L, Reilly CP. Evaluation of a new assay for free thyroxine. J Clin Biochem 1981; Abstr 19.
49. Braverman L, Abreau CM, Brock P, Kleinman R, Fournier L, Odstrchel G, Schoemaker, HS. Measurement of serum thyroxine by RIA in various clinical states. J Nucl Med 1980; 21:233-239.
50. Chopra IJ, Solomon DH, Beall GN. Radioimmunoassay for measurement of triiodothyronine in human serum. J Clin Invest 1971; 50:2033–2041.
51. Chopra I, Solomon DH, Hepner GW, Morgenstein AA. Misleading low free thyroxine index and usefulness of reverse triiodothyronine measurement in nonthyroidal illness. Ann Intern Med 1979; 90:905–912.
52. Snyder SM, Cavalieri RR, Ingbar SH. Simultaneous measurement of percentage free thyroxine: comparison of equilibrium dialysis and sephadex chromatography. J Nucl Med 1976; 17:660–664.
53. Geola FL, Hershman JM, Reed AW, Premachandra BN. Circulating thyroid hormone autoantibodies in a hypothyroid patient: effect on thyroxine metabolic clearance rate. J Clin Endocrinol Metab 1981: 53:580–586.
54. Heyma P, Harrison LL, Peluso I, Martin FIR. Antibodies to thyroid hormones. Proc Endocr Soc Australia 1981; 24:Abstract 22.

55. Wensel KW. Pharmacological interference with in vitro tests of thyroid function. Metabolism 1981; 30:717–732.
56. Barsivala V, Vikkar K, Kulkarni RD. Thyroid functions of women taking oral contraceptives. Contraception 1974; 9:305–314.
57. Langer P, Földes O, Michailovskij N, et al. Short term effect of acetyl salicylic acid analogue on pituitary-thyroid axis and plasma cortisol level in healthy human volunteers. Acta Endocrinol (Copenh) 1978; 88:698–702.
58. Abiodun MO, Bird R, Havard CWH, Sood NK. The effects of pnenylbutazone on thyroid function. Acta Endocrinol (Copehn 1973; 7: 257–264.
59. Beng CL, Wellby ML, Symons RL, Stuart S, Marshall J. The effects of iopodate on the serum iodothyronine pattern in normal subjects. Acta Endocrinol (Copehn) 1980; 93:175–178.
60. Galton VA, Ingham SH, Jiminez-Fonseca J, Hershman JM. Alterations in thyroid hormone economy in patients with hydatidiform mole. J Clin Invest 1971; 50:1345–1354.
61. Hollander CS, Scott RL, Tschendy DP, Perlroth M, Waxman A, Sterling K. Increased protein bound iodine and thyroxine binding globulin in acute intermittent porphyria. N Engl J Med 1967; 277:995–1000.
62. Yabu Y, Amino N, Nakatami K, Ichihara K, Azukizawa M, Miyaik K. Graves' disease associated with elevated serum thyroxine-binding globulin concentrations. J Clin Endocrinol Metab 1980; 514:325–333.
63. Refetoff S, Hagan SR, Selenkow HA. Estimation of the T4 binding capacity of serum TBG and TBPA by a single load-ion exchange resin method. J Nucl Med 1972; 13:2–12.
64. Stockigt JR, Topliss DJ, Barlow JW, White EL, Hurley DM, Taft P. Familial euthyroid thyroxine excess: an appropriate response to abnormal thyroxine binding associated with albumin. J Clin Endocrinol Metab 1981; 53:353–359.
65. Stockigt JR, De Garis M, Csicsmann J, Barlow JW, White EL, Hurley DM. Limitations of a new free thyroxine assay (Amerlex free T4). Clin Endocrinol 1981; 15:313–318.
66. Cavalieri RR, Rapoport B. Impaired peripheral conversion of thyroxine to to triiodothyronine. Annu Rev Med 1977; 28:57–65.
67. Croxson MS, Ibbertson HK. Low serum triiodothyronine (T3) and hypothyroidism in anorexia nervosa. J Clin Endocrinol Metab 1977; 44: 167–174.
68. Gavin LB, Rosenthal M, Cavalieri RR. Diagnostic dilemma of isolated hyperthyroxinemia in acute illness. JAMA 1979; 242:242–251.
69. Helenius T, Liewendahl K. Abnormal thyroid function tests in severe nonthyroidal illness diagnostic and pathophysiologic aspects. Scand J Clin Lab Invest 1979; 39:389–397.
70. Birkhäuser M., Busset R, Burer TH, Burger A. Diagnosis of hyperthyroid-

ism when serum-thyroxine alone is raised. Lancet 1977; 2:53–56.

71. Ormston BJ, Garry R, Cryer RJ, Besser GM, Hall R. Thyrotropin-releasing hormone as a thyroid function test. Lancet 1971; 2:10–14.
72. Ormston BJ, Alexander L, Evered DC, Clark E, Bird T, Appleton D, Hale R. Thyrotropin response to releasing hormone in ophthalamic Graves' disease: correlation with other aspects of thyroid function, thyroid suppressibility and activity of eye signs. Clin Endocrinol 1973; 2:369–376.
73. Utiger RD. Tests of the hypothalamic-pituitary-thyroid axis. In *The Thyroid*, 4th ed, Werner SC, Ingbar SH (eds). Harper & Row, New York, 1978, pp 367–374.
74. Gomez-Pan A, Alverez-Ude F, Yeo PPB, Hall R, Evered DC, Kerr DNS. Function of the hypothalamo-hypophysial thyroid axis in chronic renal failure. Clin Endocrinol 1979; 11:567–574.
75. Burrows AW, Cooper E, Shakespear RA, Aicken CM, Fraser S, Hesch R-D, Burke CN. Low serum T3 levels in the elderly sick: protein binding, thyroid and pituitary responsiveness and reverse T3 concentrations. Clin Endocrinol 1977; 7:289–300.
76. Luttrell BM, Hales IB. Thyroid stimulating immunoglobulins in Graves' disease. Aust NZ J Med 1981; 11:293–298.
77. Adams DD, Kennedy TH. Evidence to suggest that LATS protector stimulates the human thyroid gland. J Clin Endocrinol Metab 1971; 33:47–51.
78. McKenzie JM, Zakarija M, Sato A. Humoral immunity in Graves' disease. Clin Endocrinol Metab 1978; 7:31–45.
79. Atkinson S, Kendall-Taylor P. The stimualtion of thyroid hormone secretion in vitro by thyroid-stimulating antibodies. J Clin Endocrinol Metab 1981; 53:1263–1266.
80. Smith BR, Hall R. Thyroid stimulating immunoglobulins in Graves' disease. Lancet 1974; 2:427–431.
81. Croxson MS, Lim TMT, Graham FM, Ibbertson HK. Thyrotropin displacement activity of serum immunoglobulins in health and disease. Aust NZ J Med 1980; 10:151–156.
82. Goldie DJ, Jones SR, Thomas MJ. A reappraisal of the free thyroxine index. Lancet 1981; 11:572–573.
83. Kaptein EM, Grieb DA, Spencer CA, Wheeler WS, Nicoloff JT. Thyroxine metabolism in the low thyroxine state of critical nonthyroidal illnesses. J Clin Endocrinol Metab 1981; 53:764–771.
84. Kadury S, John R, Woodhead SS, Kurtz AB. Automated radioimmunoassay of total and free thyroxine in human serum. Ann Clin Biochem 1981; 18:97–101.
85. Ibbertson HK. Hypothyroidism. In *The Thyroid: Physiology and Treatment of Disease*, Hershman JM, Bray GA (eds). Pergamon Press, Oxford, 1979, pp 329–348.

86. Dahlberg PA, Karlsson FA, Lindstrom B, Wide L. Studies of thyroid hormone and methimazole levels in patients with Graves' disease on a standardised anti-thyroid drug regimen. Clin Endocrinol 1981; 14:555–562.
87. Marchant B, Lees J, Alexander WD. Antithyroid drugs. Pharmacol Ther 1978;(b), 3:305–348.
88. Alexander WD, McLarty DG, Horton P, Pharmakiotis AD. Sequential assessment during drug treatment of thyrotoxicosis. Clin Endocrinol 1973;2:43–50.
89. Vant Hoff W, Paver GG, Drury P. Technetium uptake in the management of thyrotoxicosis. Clin Endocrinol 1978;8:327–333.
90. Hardisty CA, Hanford CA, Munro DS. The prediction of relapse after drug treatment of Graves' disease by assay of long acting thyroid stimulator-protector (LATS-P). Clin Endocrinol 1981; 14:509–517.
91. Alexander WD, McLarty DG, Robertson J, Shimmins J, Brownlie BEW, Harden McGR, Datel AR. Prediction of the long term results of anti-thyroid drug therapy for thyrotoxicosis. J Clin Metab 1970;30:540–543.
92. Wilkin TJ, Isles TE, Crooks J, Gunn A, Swanson Beck J. Patterns of change in the early (20 minute) radioiodine uptake during carbimazole treatment for Graves' disease and their relationships to outcome. J Clin Endocrinol Metab 1981;52:1067–1072.
93. Ibbertson HK, Hunton RB, White B, McL , Gluckman P. Early thyroid clearance measurement for the assessment of carbimazole therapy in thyrotoxicosis. In *Further Advances in Thyroid Research*, Fellinger K, Hoefer R (eds). Wein Verlag der Weiner Medzinischen Akademia, Vienna, 1971, pp 653–662.
94. Hardisty CA, Hanford L, Monro DS. The prediction of relapse after drug treatment of Graves' disease by assay of long acting thyroid stimulator-protector (LATS-P). Clin Endocrinol 1981; 14:509–517.
95. Docter R, Bos G, Visser TJ, Hennemann G. Thyrotrophin binding inhibiting immunoglobulins in Graves' disease before, during and after antithyroid therapy and its relation to long acting thyroid stimulator. Clin Endocrinol 1980;12:143–153.
96. Macchia E, Fenzi GF, Monzani F, Lippi F, Vitti P, Grasso K, Bartalena L, Baschieri L, Pinchera A. Comparison between thyroid stimulating and TSH-binding inhibiting immunoglobulins of Graves' disease. Clin Endocrinol 1981; 15:175–182.
97. Wilkin TJ, Beck JS, Gunn A, Moussah MA, Isles TE, Crooks J. Autoantibodies in thyrotoxicosis; a quantitative study of their behaviour in relation to the course and outcome of treatment. J Endocrinol Invest 1980; 3:5–14.
98. Gardiner DF, Rothman J, Utiger RD. Serum thyroglobulin in normal subjects and patients with hyperthyroidism due to Graves' disease: effects of T3, iodide, ^{131}I and antithyroid drugs. Clin Endocrinol 1979; 11: 585–594.

99. Alexander WD, Harden RMcG, Koutras DA, Wayne E. Influence of iodine intake after treatment with antithyroid drugs. Lancet 1965; 2: 866–868.
100. Wilkin TJ, Swanson Beck J, Crooks J, Isles TE, Gunn A. Time and tide in Graves' disease: their implications in predicting outcome of treatment. Br Med J 1979; 1:88–89.
101. McGregor AM, Petersen MM, McLachlan SM, Rooke P, Smith BR, Hall R. Carbimazole and the autoimmune response in Graves' disease. N Engl J Med 1980; 303:302–307.
102. McGregor AM, Ibbertson HK, Rees-Smith B, Hall R. Carbimazole and autoantibody synthesis in Hashimoto's thyroiditis. Br Med J 1980; 281: 168–969.
103. McGregor AM, Smith BR, Hall R, Petersen MM, Miller M, Dewer PJ. Prediction of relapse in hyperthyroid Graves' disease. Lancet 1980; 1:1101–1103.
104. Teng CS, Yeung RTT, Kawa A, Nakamura S, Nomoto K, Arima N, Koreeda N, Tsuji K, Ho PWM. Thyrotrophin-binding inhibitory immunoglobulins and HLA-DRW3—two prognostic factors in Graves' disease. Aust NZ J Med 1981; 11:383–385.
105. Odell WD, Wilber JF, Paul WE. Radioimmunossay of thyrotropin in human serum. J Clin Endocrinol Metab 1965; 15:1179–1183.
106. Larsen PR, Enrique Silva J, Kaplan MM. Relationship between circulating and intracellular thyroid hormones: physiological and clinical implications. Endocr Rev 1981; 2:87–102.
107. Cadaccioni JL, Carayon P, Michel-Bechet M, Foucault F, Lefort G, Piernon H. Congenital hypothyroidism associated with thyrotropin unresponsiveness and thyroid cell membrane alterations. J Clin Endocrinol Metab 1980; 50:932–937.
108. Pearce CJ, Byfield PG, Edmonds CJ, Lalloz MRA, Himsworth RL. Autoantibodies to thyroglobulin cross reacting with iodothyronines. Clin Endocrinol 1981; 15:1–10.
109. Refetoff S, De Wind LT, De Groot LJ. Familial syndrome combining deaf mutism, stippled epiphyses, goitre and abnormally high PBI: possible target-organ refractoriness to thyroid hormone. J Clin Endocrinol Metab 1967; 27:279–283.
110. Refetoff S, De Groot LJ, Barsano LP. Defective thyroid hormone feedback regulation in syndrome of peripheral resistance to thyroid hormone. J Clin Endocrinol Metab 1980; 51:41–45.
111. Lamberg BA. Congenital euthyroid goitre and partial peripheral resistance to thyroid hormones. Lancet 1973; 1:854.
112. Ibbertson HK. Endemic goitre and cretinism. Clin Endocrinol Metabol 1979; 8:97–128.

113. Doniach D, Bottazzo GF, Russell RCG. Goitrous autoimmune thyroiditis (Hashimoto's disease). Clin Endocrinol Metab 1979; 8:63-80.
114. Turnbridge WMG, Evered DC, Hall R, et al. The spectrum of thyroid disease in a community: the Whickham survey. Clin Endocrinol 1977; 7: 481-493.
115. Gordin A, Lamberg B-A. Spontaneous hypothyroidism in symptomless autoimmune thyroiditis. A long-term follow up study. Clin Endocrinol 1981; 15:537-543.
116. Weissel M, Hoffer R, Zameta H, Mayr WR. HLA-DR and Hashimoto's thyroiditis. Tissue Antigens 1980; 16:256-257.
117. Drexhage HA, Bottazzo GF, Bitensky L, Chayen J, Doniach D. Thyroid growth-blocking antibodies in primary myxoedema. Nature 1981: 289: 594-596.
118. Rolhson ML, Debyns BM, Keating FR, Rall JE, Tyler FH. Occurrence and natural history of chronic lymphocytic thyroiditis in childhood. J Paediatr 1975; 86:675-682.
119. Gharib H, Hodgson SF, Gastineau CF, Schlolz DA, Smith LA. Reversible hypothyroidism in Addison's disease. Lancet 1972; 2:734-736.
120. El Kabir DJ, Doniach D, Turner-Warwick R. Serum content of thyrotrophic hormone in human thyroiditis: low TSH levels with high radioiodine uptake in autoimmune thyroiditis. J Clin Endocrinol Metab 1963; 25:514-520.
121. Endo K, Kasagi K, Konishi J. Detection and properties of TSH-binding inhibitor immunoglobulins in patients with Graves' disease and Hashimoto's thyroiditis. J Clin Endocrinol Metab 1978; 46:734-739.
122. Sawers JSA, Toft AD, Irvine WJ, Brown NS, Seth J. Transient hypothyroidism after iodine-I^{131} treatment of thyrotoxicosis. J Clin Endocrinol Metab 1980; 50:226-229.
123. Teng CS, Yeung RTT, Khoo RKK, Alaganatham TT. A prospective study of the changes in thyrotropin binding inhibitory immunoglobulins in Graves' disease treated by subtotal thyroidectomy or radioactive iodine. J Clin Endocrinol Metab 1980; 50:1005-1010.
124. Prager D, Sembot JT, Southlard M. Cobalt-60 therapy of Hodgkin's disease and the subsequent development of hypothyroidism. Cancer 1972; 29:458-460.
125. Toft AD, Irvine WJ, Sinclair I, McIntosh D, Seth J, Cameron EHD. Thyroid function after surgical treatment of thyrotoxicosis—a report of 100 cases treated with propranolol before operation. N Engl J Med 1978; 298:643-647.
126. Whitsell FB Jr, Black BM. A statistical study of the clinical significance of lymphocytic and fibrocytic replacements in the hyperplastic thyroid gland. J Clin Endocrinol Metab 1949; 9:1202-1215.

127. Rallinson ML, Kumagai LF, Tyler FIH. Goitrous hypothyroidism induced by aminoglutethamide anticonvulsant drug. J Clin Endocrinol Metab 1967;27:265–272.
128. Emerson CH, Dyson WL, Utiger RD. Serum thyrotropin and thyroxine concentrations in patients receiving lithium carbonate. J Clin Endocrinol Metab 1973;36:338–346.
129. Wolfe J. Iodide goitre and the pharmacologic effects of excess iodide. Ann J Med 1969;47:101–124.
130. Braverman CE, Ingbar SH, Vagenakis AG, Adams L, Maloof F. Enhanced susceptibility to iodide myxoedema in patients with Hashimoto's disease. J Clin Endocrinol Metab 1971; 32:515–521.
131. Barsano CP, De Groot LJ. Dyshormonogenetic goitre. Clin Endocrinol Metab 1979;8:145–165.
132. Karlish AJ, MacGregor GA. Sarcoidosis, thyroiditis and Addison's disease. Lancet 1970; 2:330–333.
133. Danovitch GM, Le Roith D, Sobel R, Sikuler E, Straus R. Amyloid goitre in familial Mediterranean fever. Clin Endocrinol 1979; 11:595–601.
134. Turief J. Adult X histiocytosis with pulmonary, thyroid, meningoencephalic and thalamohypophyseal locations. Sem Hop Paris 1971; 47: 2923–2932.
135. Burke JS, Butler JJ, Fuller LM. Malignant lymphomas of the thyroid: a clinical pathologic study of 35 patients including ultrastructural observations. Cancer 1976;39:1587–1602.
136. Chan AM, Lynch MJG, Bailey JD, Ezrin C, Fraser D. Hypothyroidism in cystinosis. Ann J Med 1970;48:678–692.
137. Healy DL, Burger HG. Increased prolactin and thyrotrophin secretion following oral metaclopromide dose response relationships. Clin Endocrinol 1977;7:195–201.
138. Evered DC, Ormston BJ, Smith PA, Hall R, Rind T. Grades of hypothyroidism. Br Med J 1973;1:657–662.
139. Turnbridge WMG, Evered DC, Hall R, Appleton D, Brewis M, Clark J, Grimley Evans J, Young E, Bird T, Smith PA. Lipid profiles and cardiovascular disease in the Whickham area with particular reference to thyroid failure. Clin Endocrinol 1977;7:495–508.
140. Toft AD, Seth J, Irvine WJ, Hunger WM, Cameron EHD. Thyroid function in the long-term follow up of patients treated with iodine 131 for thyrotoxicosis. Lancet 1975;2:576–590.
141. Croxson MS, Ibbertson HK. Subclinical hypothyroidism. NZ Med J 1980;91:89–91.
142. Davies HA, Dawdle RJ, Lazarus JH, Davies CJ. Do peripheral thyroid indicators reflect response to treatment in latent hypothyroidism. In *Thyroid Research VIII*, Stockigt JR, Nagataki S (eds), Proceedings of the VIIIth International Thyroid Congress, Sydney. Australian Academy of Science, Canberra, 1980, pp 529–532.

143. Irvine WJ, Toft AD, Hunter WM, Kirkham KE. An assessment of plasma TSH radioimmunoassay and of the TSH stimulation test in the diagnosis of 100 consecutive patients with suspected hypothyroidism. Clin Endocrinol 1973; 2:135–139.
144. Fisher DA. Status of neonatal hypothyroid screening. Reprint from the Quebec International Conference on Neonatal Thyroid Screening. Proceedings of the VIIIth International Thyroid Congress, Sydney 1980; 1980:1A (abstract).
145. Hulse JA, Grant DB, Clayton BE, Lilly P, Jackson D, Speacklan A, Edwards RWH, Narse D. Population screening for congenital hypothyroidism. Br Med J 1980; 280:675–678.
146. Kein AH, Meltzer S, Kenny FM. Improved prognosis in congenital hypothyroidism treated before age three months. G Pediatr 1972; 81: 912–915.
147. Durbridge TC, Edwards F, Edmonds RG, Atkinson M. Evaluation of benefits of screening tests done immediately on admission to hospital. Clin Chem 1976; 22:968–971.
148. Epstein KA, Schneiderman LJ, Bush JW, Zettner A. The 'abnormal' screening serum thyroxine (T4): analysis of physician response, outcome, cost and health effectiveness. J Chron Dis 1981; 34;175–190.
149. Chopra IJ, Teco GN, Nguyen AH, Solomon DH. In search of an inhibitor of thyroid hormone binding to serum proteins in nonthyroidal illnesses. J Clin Endocrinol Metab 1979; 49:63–69.
150. Oppenheimer JH, Schwartz HL, Kaiser FE, Marish CN. A nondialyzable inhibitor in sera of patients with nonthyroidal illness inhibits binding of iodothyronines by charcoal plasma proteins and cells. Clin Res 1981; 29: 566A.
151. Chopra IJ, Chopra U, Smith SR, Reza M, Solomon D. Reciprocal changes in serum concentrations of 3,3′5′-triiodothyronine (reverse T_3) and 3,3′5′ triiodothyronine in systemic illness. J Clin Endocrinol Metab 1975; 41:1043–1049.
152. Nusynowitz ML, Clark RF, Strader WJ, Estrin HM, Seal US. Thyroxine-binding globulin deficiency in three families and total deficiency in a normal woman. Am J Med 1971; 50:458–464.
153. Smeulers R, Docter TJ, Visser TJ, Hennemann G. Response to TRH and triiodothyronine suppressibility in euthyroid multinodular goitre. Clin Endocrinol 1977; 7:389–397.
154. Schlossberg AH, Jacobson JC, Ibbertson HK. Serum thyroglobulin in the diagnosis and management of thyroid carcinoma. Clin Endocrinol 1979; 10:17–27.
155. Thomas CG, Buckwater JA, Staab ES, Kerr CY. Evaluation of dominant thyroid masses. Ann Surg 1976; 183:463–469.
156. Mortensen JD, Woolner LB, Bennett WA. Gross and microscopic findings in clinically normal thyroid glands. J Clin Endocrinol Metab 1955; 15: 1270–1280.

157. Hoffman GL, Thompson NW, Heffron C. The solitary thyroid nodule. A reassessment. Ann Surg 1972; 105:379–385.
158. Kendall LW, London RE. Prediction of malignancy in solitary thyroid nodules. Lancet 1969; 1:1071–1073.
159. Shiroozu A, Inoue K, Nakashima T, Okamura K, Yoshinari M, Nishitani H, Omae T. Defective iodide transport and normal organification of iodide in cold nodules of the thyroid. Clin Endocrinol 1981; 15:411–416.
160. Karelitz JR, Richards JB. Necessity of oblique views in evaluating the functional status of a thyroid nodule. J Nucl Med 1974; 154:782–785.
161. Clark DE. Association of irradiation with cancer of the thyroid in children and adolescents. JAMA 1955; 159:1007–1009.
162. Favus MJ, Schneider AB, Stachura ME, Arnold JE, Ryo Yun Pinsky SM, Colman M, Arnold MJ, Frohman LA. Thyroid cancer occurring as a late consequence of head and neck irradiation. N Engl J Med 1976; 294: 1019–1025.
163. In De Groot LJ, Frohman LA, Kaplan EL, Refetoff S (eds). *Radiation Associated Thyroid Carcinoma.* Grune and Stratton, New York 1977.
164. Williams ED, Doniach I, Bjarnason O, Mitchie W. Thyroid cancer in an iodide rich area. Cancer 1977; 39:215–222.
165. Williams ED, Brauen CL, Doniach I. Pathological and clinical findings in a series of 67 cases of medullary carcinoma of the thyroid. J Clin Pathol 1966; 19:103–105.
166. Ishikawa N, Hamada S. Association of medullary carcinoma of the thyroid with carcino embryonic antigen. Br J Cancer 1976; 34:111–115.
167. Barrowman JA, Bennett A, Hillebrand P, Rolles K, Pollack DJ, Wright JT. Diarrhoea in thyroid medullary carcinoma: role of prostaglandins and therapeutic effect of nutmeg. Br Med J 1975; 3:11–15.
168. Melvin KEW, Tashjian AH Jr, Cassidy CE, Givens JR. Cushing's syndrome caused by ACTH and calcitonin-secreting medullary carcinoma of the thyroid. Metabolism 1970; 19:831–838.
169. Silverberg SG, Vidone RA. Metastatic tumor in the thyroid. Pac Med Surg 1966; 74:175–180.
170. Steinberg M, Cavalieri RR, Choy SH. Uptake of technetium 99-pertechetate in a primary thyroid carcinoma: need for caution in evaluating nodules. J Clin Endocrinol Metab 1970; 31:81–85.
171. Crile G Jr. Treatment of thyroid cysts by aspiration. Surgery 1966; 59;210–212.
172. Edis AJ, Goellner JR, Gorman CA, Kini S. An evaluation of fine-needle aspiration (FNA) and core-needle biopsy (CNB) of solitary thyroid nodules. Proceedings of 62nd Annual Meeting of the American Endocrine Society, Washington, DC, June 1980 (abstract).

173. Boon ME, Löwhagen T, Willems J-S. Planometric studies on fine-needle aspirates from follicular adenoma and follicular carcinoma of the thyroid. Acta Cytol 1980; 24:145–148.

174. Pacini F, Pinchera Giani C, Grasso L, Doveni F, Baschieri L. Serum thyroglobulin in thyroid carcinoma and other thyroid disorders. J Endocrinol Invest 1980; 3:283–292.

30

Parathyroid and Calcium Disorders

Solomon Posen
University of Sydney, Sydney, Australia

I. PRIMARY HYPERPARATHYROIDISM

A. Pathology

In this disorder (or group of disorders) there is hyperplasia or neoplasia of parathyroid tissue with hypersecretion of parathyroid hormone (1). As a rule, only one of the parathyroid glands is involved (1), and in the large majority of cases, hyperparathyroidism occurs as an isolated abnormality. In a few hyperparathyroid patients, particularly those suffering from other endocrine disorders, such as acromegaly, hypergastrinemia, and familial hyperparathyroidism, all parathyroid tissue may be involved in the hyperplastic process (2). Parathyroid carcinomas are rare (1).

B. Pathophysiology

Excessive activity by the parathyroid glands results in high blood levels of parathyroid hormone (PTH) (3,4) and in various biochemical abnormalities secondary to the effects of PTH. There is enhanced renal excretion of inorganic phosphate with hypophosphatemia (Fig. 1). Bone resorption is enhanced resulting in hypercalcemia and hypercalciuria. The associated increase in osteoblastic activity may lead to elevation in serum alkaline phosphatase (5). PTH stimulates the synthesis of cyclic AMP (6) and 1,25-dihydroxyvitamin D (7) by renal tubules so that urinary cyclic AMP and serum 1,25-dihydroxyvitamin D are increased. Hypercalcemia leads to defects in urinary concentration and acidification, so that in spite of high plasma vasopressin levels (8), urine osmolalities are relatively low. Severe hypercalcemia may result in life-threatening dehydration.

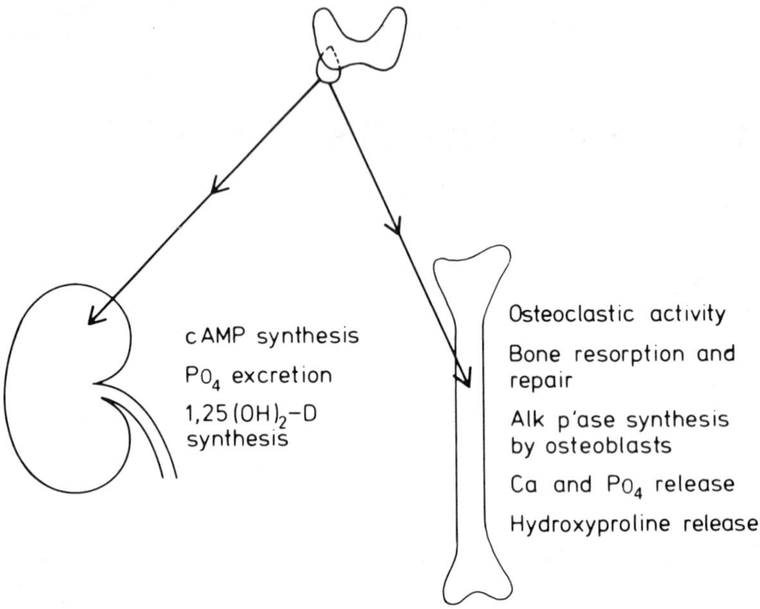

Figure 1 Effects of parathyroid hormone on its major target organs, bone and kidney.

C. Clinical Features

1. Incidence

Primary hyperparathyroidism is being detected with increasing frequency, especially among elderly females (9, 10), and constitutes the commonest cause of hypercalcemia in nonhospitalized patients. The incidence of primary hyperparathyroidism has been estimated at 28 per 100,000 per year with six times that frequency among women over 60. The majority of these patients are symptomless (9).

2. Stones

If symptomless individuals are excluded, the commonest mode of presentation consists of renal stones (11). Some 60% of patients with primary hyperparathyroidism have or have had renal calculi (11, 12), while 3% of patients with renal calculi have primary hyperparathyroidism (11, 13).

3. Bones

The prevalence of bone disease among patients with primary hyperparathyroidism varies according to the diagnostic criteria employed. Clinical bone disease (osteitis fibrosa cystica) with the formation of cystic masses was present in approximately 3% of patients seen at Sydney Hospital (12, 14). Radiological bone disease (especially subperiosteal resorption) occurred in approximately 10% of patients, while histological bone disease was present in over 50% of patients with available data (15).

4. Abdominal Symptoms

There is some controversy concerning the prevalence of peptic ulceration and pancreatitis among patients with primary hyperparathyroidism. In the older series (those not containing many symptomless individuals) the association with peptic ulcer seems firmly established (1, 12). The mechanism of this association is not entirely clear, but it appeared sufficiently strong to suggest to Betts et al. (16) that even in families with hypergastrinemia the full-blown Zollinger-Ellison syndrome does not develop unless hyperparathyroidism is present.

Pancreatitis occurs in some 3% of patients with primary hyperparathyroidism (12, 17), sometimes in the postparathyroidectomy period (15). It is probable that hyperparathyroidism causes pancreatitis rather than the reverse (1).

5. Other Associations

Other disorders that have been described in association with hyperparathyroidism include various malignancies (18), osteoporosis (19), Paget's disease (20), gout (2), and pseudogout (21). The articular complications may appear or persist after parathyroidectomy (22, 23). Previous exposure to neck irradiation predisposes to hyperparathyroidism (24, 25). Hypertension is present in a large proportion of hyperparathyroid patients, but there is no firm evidence either for an association greater than would be expected by chance (9) or for a reduction in blood pressure after parathyroidectomy (26, 27).

6. Physical Examination

Physical examination is usually not helpful in primary hyperparathyroidism except insofar as it helps exclude other causes of hypercalcemia, such as malignancy, sarcoidosis, or hyperthyroidism. Muscle weakness, described by Patten et al. (28), is rarely a clinical problem. Palpation of the neck may help to localize the lesion in a small percentage of cases.

D. Diagnostic Tests

Several types of tests are employed in hypercalcemic patients in order to answer three questions: (1) Does this patient have hyperparathyroidism? (2) What is the severity of the disease and does this patient require surgery? (3) Where is the lesion?

1. Serum Calcium

Hypercalcemia is the most important diagnostic criterion for primary hyperparathyroidism. Although it is possible, in rare instances, for hyperparathyroid patients to remain normocalcemic (29, 29a), such instances are rare and almost all patients are hypercalcemic at least on an intermittent basis.

The following questions have to be raised before the presence of hypercalcemia is accepted:

1. Might this be a "tourniquet effect" (30)? Various correction factors, such as serum albumin (31) and serum specific gravity, are used to identify hypercalcemia due to hemoconcentration. None are entirely satisfactory but a serum calcium of 2.58 mmol/liter in a patient with a serum specific gravity of 1.030 obviously means much less than the same serum calcium concentration in a patient with a serum specific gravity of 1.022.
2. How long has the serum calcium been elevated? It is useful to look through the patient's case notes for previous serum calcium determinations. If an elevated value was present some years earlier, the diagnosis of hyperparathyroidism becomes extremely likely.
3. Has the patient been taking thiazide diuretics? Normal persons taking thiazide diuretics do not usually develop hypercalcemia (32). In hyperparathyroid individuals, thiazide-induced rises in serum calcium may exceed 0.5 mmol/liter (33). Thiazide medication should therefore be withdrawn for 2 weeks and serum calcium reestimated before further investigations are performed and before any therapeutic decisions are made.

2. Exclusion of Other Causes of Hypercalcemia

Once a patient has been found to be indubitably hypercalcemic, a brief review of the history and physical examination will, as a rule, rapidly exclude nonparathyroid causes of hypercalcemia. A few simple questions rule out the consumption of vitamin D, vitamin A, or large quantities of calcium. Appropriate simple tests (such as blood pressure readings in the upright position, thyroid functions, chest x-ray, and intravenous pyelography) exclude Addisonism, hyperthyroidism, and malignancies. Ultrasonography and abdominal computerized tomography (CT) scans may occasionally be required to exclude intraabdominal or retroperitoneal lesions.

3. Parathyroid Hormone Assays

With the advent of immunoreactive iPTH assays the diagnosis of hyperparathyroidism has become relatively easy (see Diagnostic Summary 1). Many tests which used to be performed on hypercalcemic patients have now become redundant (15), and provided that a hypercalcemic patient can be shown to have elevated or even normal levels of iPTH, the diagnosis of hyperparathyroidism is virtually established. Admittedly, some patients with hypercalcemia of malignancy have elevated serum iPTH values (15, 34, 35). However, in hypercalcemia of malignancy, serum iPTH values are rarely greater than twice the upper limit of the normal range and there is no correlation between serum iPTH and serum calcium (15, 36). In addition, the large majority of patients with hypercalcemia of malignancy have clinically overt lesions and constitute no diagnostic problem.

Most iPTH assays currently in use are based on antibodies prepared against bovine parathyroid hormone and "standard curves" involving bovine material of varying degrees of purity. Moreover, most antibodies "recognize" the biologically inactive carboxy terminal end of the PTH molecule, where the biochemical differences between human and bovine materials are greatest (37). Region-specific immunoassays based on fragments of human PTH are currently becoming available, but their clinical advantages over the older assays have not yet been established.

Clinically useful bioassays for circulating parathyroid hormone are not yet available. Cytochemical assays (38, 39), although very sensitive, are currently too cumbersome for diagnostic purposes. The adenylate cyclase assay described by Nissenson et al. (40), although more cumbersome than radioimmunoassays, has the advantage of requiring a relatively short incubation period with results available on the same day. This bioassay shows some clinical promise (41).

4. Nephrogenous Cyclic AMP

Broadus et al. (6) showed that the estimation of urinary and plasma cyclic AMP gave a degree of discrimination between hyperparathyroid and nonhyperparathyroid patients as good as if not better than iPTH estimations. Cyclic AMP assays have the advantage that they involve an incubation period of hours rather than days, so that they are particularly useful when urgent decisions have to be made. Unfortunately, hypercalcemia of malignancy may also be associated with high "nephrogenous" cyclic AMP values (35, 42). The intraoperative measurement of urinary cyclic AMP (43), which may help to determine whether the operation should be terminated, is not yet in general use.

5. Bone Biopsy

We do not recommend bone biopsy as a routine investigation in suspected hyperparathyroidism (see Diagnostic Summary 1). If skeletal lesions are clinically and radiologically obvious, there is no need for skeletal histology (15). If no radiological lesions are present, even detailed dynamic histomorphometry may give negative results (44).

The greatest value of skeletal biopsies in patients with suspected hyperparathyroidism lies in the occasional diagnosis of nonhyperparathyroid lesions such as malignancies and sarcoidosis (15). Dynamic histomorphometry with tetracycline labeling is not required in this clinical situation.

6. Urine Calcium

This investigation should be performed in every patient prior to neck exploration. While high values are by no means universal (12), a value below 3 mmol/ per day should raise the possibility of familial hypocalciuric hypercalcemia (45). This "entity," whatever its mechanism, requires a different surgical approach from that adopted toward most patients with hyperparathyroidism.

7. Corticosteroid Suppression

This test was described by Dent (46) before iPTH and nephrogenous cyclic AMP assays were available. A 10-day course of corticosteroids was said to normalize serum calcium in hypercalcemia of nonhyperparathyroid origin, while serum calcium would remain elevated in hyperparathyroidism. False positive and false negative results have been reported (47). Nevertheless, this test remains useful when some doubt exists about the diagnosis (e.g., in a patient with high serum calcium and only moderately elevated serum iPTH or nephrogenous cyclic AMP).

8. Other Tests

Serum inorganic phosphate and serum magnesium are usually low, while serum chloride tends to be high in primary hyperparathyroidism. These tests, although cost effective, have only statistical value; they are not generally used to make "stop-go" types of decisions. Calcium infusion tests (48) and complex calculations of phosphate clearances (49) are not generally used for diagnostic purposes. Measurements of ionized calcium (50) have no advantage over estimations of total serum calcium.

E. Severity of the Disease

Once the diagnosis of hyperparathyroidism has been established, a decision has to be made as to whether the patient requires surgery. If serum calcium values are in excess of 3.0 mmol/liter, other tests are generally unnecessary. If serum calcium elevation is relatively mild, some ancillary investigations may be of help. X-rays of the kidneys may show the presence of stones. Pancreatic calcification may be seen on abdominal ex-rays. Both these findings constitute an indication for surgery.

Similarly, radiological signs of osteitis fibrosa, elevations of serum alkaline phosphatase, and high urine hydroxyproline values are an indication of severe skeletal involvement (5) and emphasize the need for surgical intervention. Longitudinal studies by means of osteodensitometry or neutron activation analysis (51) may show that bone is being lost at a rapid rate.

Some units adopt an aggressive policy and recommend surgery on all patients with hyperparathyroidism (9, 52). Those adopting a more conservative approach (14) usually employ longitudinal observations such as repeated measurements of serum calcium and creatinine, together with a series of arbitrary "major" and "minor" indications for surgical intervention. Repeated parathyroid hormone assays are not considered indicated as a test for the severity of the disease (53).

F. Localization of the Tumor(s)

Several tests have been described for the preoperative and intraoperative localization of parathyroid lesions. These include arteriography, venography, isotope scanning, estimation of iPTH in venous effluent, computerized tomography, ultrasound, and the use of vital stains (54, 55)

The cost/benefit ratio of these procedures is high, so that they are not used routinely prior to initial operations. However, every effort should be made to localize parathyroid lesions prior to any reexploration (56). The problem has not been satisfactorily resolved, and even in specialized units negative neck and chest explorations still occur (57).

II. HYPERCALCEMIA DUE TO CAUSES OTHER THAN HYPERPARATHYROIDISM

Hypercalcemia may occur with a variety of endocrine and nonendocrine disorders, including hyperthyroidism (58, 59), hypoadrenalism (60), and increased serum concentrations of various vitamin D metabolites. Nonendocrine disorders leading to hypercalcemia include the milk alkali syndrome and immobilization (61). Hypercalcemia of malignancy is more common than all these disorders put together and constitutes the commonest form of hypercalcemia among hospital inpatients.

Several mechanisms have been described to account for hypercalcemia occurring in patients with malignant disorders. In some patients the tumors contain parathyroid hormone-like material (34, 62). In others there is evidence that substance(s) of tumor origin different from parathyroid hormone stimulate renal adenylate cyclase (35). Osteoclast activating factor(s) have been shown to be produced by cells derived from lymphatic tumors (63). Some patients with malignancies have coexistent hyperparathyroidism (18). Skeletal metastases are present in most patients with hypercalcemia of malignancy. There is at present no single test to confirm or refute the diagnosis of hypercalcemia of malignancy. In patients with demonstrable neoplastic lesions these dominate the clinical picture and it is unnecessary to investigate the cause of hypercalcemia. Even in patients with greatly elevated serum immunoreactive PTH concentrations or elevated urinary cyclic AMP values, which constitute presumptive evidence for coexistent hyperparathyroidism (15, 18), it is rarely important to investigate (or treat) the parathyroid lesion.

The problem is different if a patient has had a malignancy in the past and is now apparently free of neoplastic disease but hypercalcemic. In such patients every effort should be made to exclude the presence of malignant disease.

A bone biopsy may be useful under these circumstances. If all tests for malignancy are negative, the patient "reenters" the flowchart shown in Diagnostic Summary 1.

III. SECONDARY HYPERPARATHYROIDISM

Patients with chronic renal failure and, to a lesser extent, patients with chronic malabsorptive states (64) develop hyperplasia of all parathyroids with hypersecretion of parathyroid hormone. Serum immunoreactive PTH is high in such patients and the skeletal effects shown in Figure 1 may be present. However, hypercalcemia is usually absent because parathyroid hyperplasia and hypersecretion is "secondary" to hypocalcemia associated with the underlying disease. In addition, patients with renal failure are resistant to the hypercalcemic action of parathyroid hormone (65).

The majority of patients with advanced renal failure have high values of serum radioimmunoassayable PTH (47) and histological evidence of hyperparathyroidism (66), with a good correlation between the two parameters (67). Urinary nephrogenous cyclic AMP (corrected for creatinine clearance) is also correlated with the severity of parathyroid osteopathy (as assessed histologically), although the correlation is not as good as that obtained between parathyroid osteopathy and serum iPTH (Chan, unpublished observations, 1983).

For reasons that are not entirely understood, secondary hyperparathyroidism is more severe in some patients than in others and occasionally leads to skeletal symptoms in patients with stable renal failure or in patients on chronic hemodialysis, although not usually in allograft recipients (68).

The clinician faced with a uremic patient who complains of diffuse pain has to decide by means of iPTH assays, skeletal radiology, and skeletal histology whether such pain is of skeletal origin, what skeletal lesions are present, and whether or not parathyroidectomy should be performed.

Some patients with secondary hyperparathyroidism respond to the administration of phosphate binding agents. In others objective improvement may occur following the administration of 1,25-$(OH)_2$-cholecalciferol (69), while others require a parathyroidectomy. It is difficult to predict, on the basis of biochemical or histological tests, which patients will report an improvement in skeletal symptoms following subtotal parathyroidectomy. In general, I am reluctant to recommend surgery unless serum PTH is greater than 10 times the reference value *and* gross radiological or histological signs of hyperparathyroidism are present. If the hypothesis that parathyroid hormone is responsible for soft tissue damage in renal failure (70, 71) is confirmed, the assay of serum iPTH in uremic patients will become a major factor in clinical decision making.

IV. SURGICAL HYPOPARATHYROIDISM

Chronic hypoparathyroidism may follow the deliberate or accidental removal or the infarction of parathyroid tissue during thyroid or parathyroid surgery. Thyrotoxic patients (72), patients with malignant disorders (73), and patients undergoing second or third thyroid explorations are particularly at risk of developing chronic postoperative hypoparathyroidism. Parathyroidectomy (for hyperparathyroidism) may lead to hypoparathyroidism if all functioning parathyroid tissue is removed (52).

A. Pathophysiology

A lack of parathyroid hormone leads to low rates of calcium release from bone and (directly or indirectly) to low rates of calcium absorption from the intestine. The patients are therefore hypocalcemic. Tubular reabsorption of phosphate is high, resulting in hyperphosphatemia. There is usually no detectable circulating immunoreactive parathyroid hormone and urinary cyclic AMP is low (although it rises promptly if the patients are given intravenous parathyroid hormone preparations).

Chronic hypocalcemia leads to "loose membranes" with a leakage of various electrolytes down their respective concentration gradients (74). This results in increased "neuromuscular irritability" with epilepsy, tetany, and extrapyramidal syndromes. In addition, the defective membranes allow the entry of sodium, water, and paradoxically, calcium into cells of the ocular lens and parts of the nervous system (Fig. 2).

Symptoms of hypocalcemia, including paresthesiae and tetany, usually occur within the first few days of surgery (75). The patients may then remain clinically well, presenting years later with cataracts (76) or fits (77). Trousseau's sign is elicited by inflating a sphygmomanometer cuff above the patient's systolic blood pressure. In the presence of hypocalcemia, carpal spasm (Fig. 3) will occur within 3 min. Chvostek's sign is elicited by percussion of branches of the facial nerve after their emergence from the stylomastoid foramen. In the presence of hypocalcemia, contractions of the facial muscles occur during this procedure. Chvostek's sign is positive in a small proportion of normocalcemic individuals.

Many patients with surgical hypoparathyroidism are also hypothyroid (78) and about one-third suffer from paralysis of one or both vocal cords (79) presumably as the result of traumatic surgery. Personality assessments with the Minnesota Multiple Personality Inventory Test showed a greater prevalence of

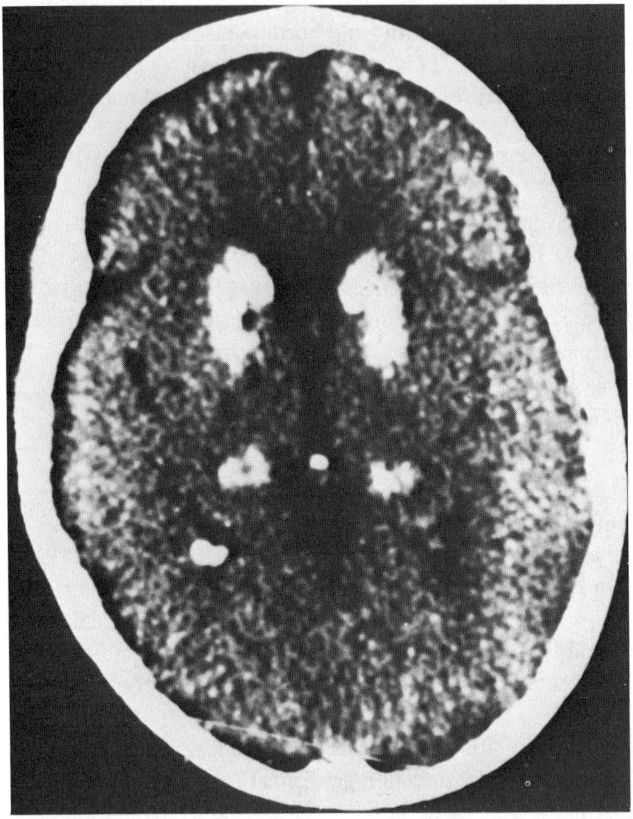

Figure 2 Calcification of parts of the nervous system is being recognized with increasing frequency in hypoparathyroidism by the use of CT scanning. The reason why some parts, such as the basal ganglia, are more prone to calcification than others is not known.

hypochondriasis, anxiety, and depression in patients with surgical hypoparathyroidism than in matched controls. However, there was no difference between patients with surgical hypoparathyroidism and an age- and sex-matched group of thyroidectomized normocalcemic women (Posen, unpublished observation, 1970).

B. Diagnostic Tests

Patients with surgical hypoparathyroidism have hypocalcemia, hyperphosphatemia, and undetectable or low serum PTH values. Several provocative tests [including ethylenediaminetetraacetic acid (EDTA) infusion] have been described for the detection of "partial" or "latent" hypoparathyroidism (72). In practice, such tests are rarely required: In overt cases they are unnecessary for diagnosis, while in mild cases they have little or no influence on clinical management.

Serum 25-hydroxyvitamin D concentrations are normal in untreated hypoparathyroidism and rise markedly when the patients are treated with pharmacological doses of vitamin D (80). We have found 25-hydroxyvitamin D measurements useful in predicting whether vitamin D-treated patients are likely to develop vitamin D intoxication (80).

Long-standing surgical hypoparathyroidism may lead to cerebral calcification. This complication, which used to be regarded as rare (81), is being diagnosed with increasing frequency by computerized tomography (82).

Characteristic lenticular opacities are seen by slit lamp examination in 25% of patients (76). The presence of cerebral calcification or early cataracts may help to make noncompliant patients more receptive to medical advice.

Electroencephalographic abnormalities are present in 50% of patients with surgical hypoparathyroidism (77). They tend to persist even after the patients' biochemical abnormalities have been corrected. Patients with electroencephalographic abnormalities are more likely to develop epileptiform seizures than are patients with normal electroencephalograms (77).

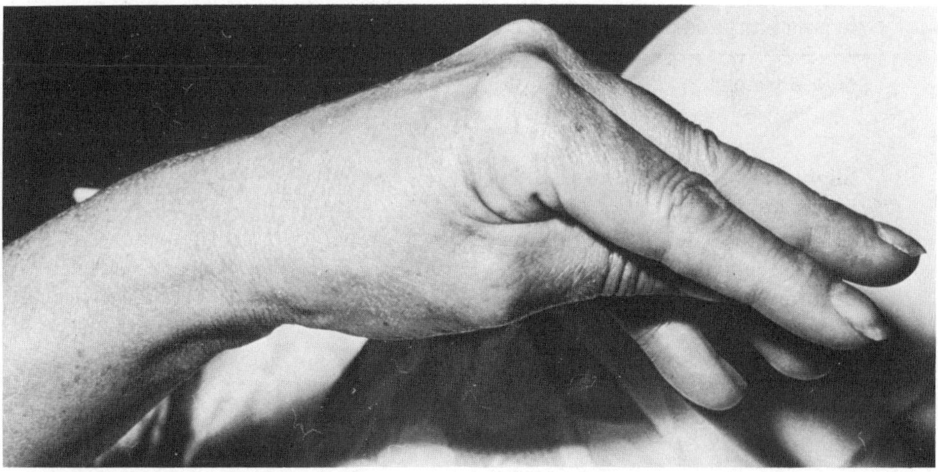

Figure 3 Classical position of the hand in tetany ("obstetrician's hand"), with adduction of the thumb, flexion of the metacarpophalangeal joints, and extension of the intraphalangeal joints.

V. NONSURGICAL HYPOPARATHYROIDISM

A. Idiopathic Hypoparathyroidism

A variety of syndromes may lead to hypocalcemia and hyperphosphatemia in patients who have not been submitted to neck surgery (Table 1). Parathyroid failure may occur as an isolated phenomenon. It may be associated with failure of other endocrine or nonendocrine organs, such as the adrenals, the thyroid, the gastric parietal cells, or the ovaries (83). We have seen patients with a "idiopathic" hypoparathyroidism and central diabetes insipidus (84).

Some patients with idiopathic hypoparathyroidism have demonstrable immunological abnormalities with B-cell or T-cell dysfunction. B-cell abnormalities manifest themselves by the presence, in many of these patients, of circulating immunoglobulins which bind to parathyroid, thyroid, or adrenal tissue. Dysfunction of T cells is demonstrable by absent or delayed hypersensitivity responses in the skin or by abnormal in vitro responses to standard stimuli (85).

Table 1 Some Syndromes Associated with Hypocalcemia and Hyperphosphatemia in the Absence of Renal Failure

Etiology of "hypoparathyroidism"	Serum immunoreactive PTH	Response to exogenous PTH	Associated features
Surgical trauma	Low	Normal	Hypothyroidism vocal cord paralysis
"Idiopathic," isolated disorder	Low	Normal	
"Idiopathic" with immunological abnormalities	Low	Normal	Other endocrinopathies; T- and B-cell abnormalities; fungal infections; alopecia
Pseudohypoparathyroidism	High	Diminished	Short metacarpals; evidence of parathyroid osteopathy
(?) Abnormal hormone	High	Normal	(?) Familial involvement

The propensity of these patients to develop fungal infections is probably associated with their immunological abnormalities (85, 86). Alopecia may be related to the production of anti-hair follicle antibodies or to hypocalcemia at a crucial stage of hair follicle development. Dental hypoplasia (72, 83) is probably due to hypocalcemia rather than to immune deficiencies (87).

B. Pseudohypoparathyroidism

This syndrome (or group of syndromes) is characterized by the usual biochemical changes of hypoparathyroidism (hypocalcemia, hyperphosphatemia) in the presence of high concentrations of immunoreactive PTH (Table 1). There is evidence (88, 89) of parathyroid hormone malfunction either because of defective parathyroid hormone receptor(s) or, more likely, because of the absence or abnormal structure of a regulatory protein linking parathyroid hormone receptors in kidney cell membranes with adenyl cyclase. Paradoxically, osteoclast stimulation is enhanced in some of these patients, with radiological and histological appearances of osteitis fibrosa (90).

Patients with pseudohypoparathyroidism tend to have round faces, short statures, and shortening of one or more metacarpals or metatarsals (72). Pseudohypoparathyroidism is not associated with immunological abnormalities. However, associated primary hypothyroidism has been repeatedly noted (89, 91, 92).

In the absence of skeletal abnormalities, pseudohypoparathyroidism has to be distinguished from other forms of hypoparathyroidism by the presence of high serum concentrations of immunoreactive or bioactive (41) parathyroid hormone and by the response of the patient to exogenous parathyroid hormone (Table 1). Patients with pseudohypoparathyroidism show none of the normal responses to the infusion of parathyroid hormone. They show no increase in urine cyclic AMP, phosphate excretion, or concentrations of serum 1,25-dihydroxy vitamin D (93, 94), at least not during the first 24 hr after the administration of PTH (95).

Drezner et al. (96) described a syndrome which they called pseudohypoparathyroidism type II. The patients suffering from this disorder are hypocalcemic and hyperphosphatemic and they have high serum concentrations of immunoreactive PTH. They differ from the usual form of pseudohypoparathyroidism because their urine cyclic AMP increases normally after PTH infusions, while phosphaturia does not occur. Drezner et al. (96) speculated that in these individuals renal adenylate cyclase is normally activated and that the cellular defect(s) are due to a postcyclic AMP event. Farfel et al. (89) also produced evidence to show that pseudohypoparathyroidism was not a single nosological entity.

There is some confusion concerning the diagnostic validity of PTH infusions in patients whose serum calcium has previously been normalized by treatment with vitamin D. Nagant de Deuxchaisnes and Krane (72) performed PTH infusions in three patients with pseudohypoparathyroidism before and after treatment with vitamin D. No increase in phosphate excretion occurred on either occasion. Many of the original pseudohypoparathyroid patients tested by Chase et al. (88) failed to raise their urinary cyclic AMP values after PTH infusion in spite of the fact that they had previously been made normocalcemic. On the other hand, Rodriguez et al. (97) and Stögmann and Fischer (98) showed that previous normalization of serum calcium enhanced some of the biological effects of infused PTH in pseudohypoparathyroidism. The reasons for these apparently discrepant findings are discussed by Potts (99).

Some patients with a past history of physical signs consistent with pseudohypoparathyroidism may be normocalcemic and normophosphatemic for long periods of time either before or after bouts of hypocalcemia (100, 101). Nagant de Deuxchaisnes and Krane (72) discuss this syndrome at length and express the view that it should not be called pseudo-pseudohypoparathyroidism unless the responses to PTH infusions are normal.

VI. VITAMIN D DEFICIENCY

Circulating vitamin D metabolites, including cholecalciferol, 25-OH-cholecalciferol, 24,25-$(OH)_2$-cholecalciferol, or 1,25-$(OH)_2$-cholecalciferol are derived from precursors synthesized in the skin under the influence of ultraviolet light. An alternative source of supply consists of foods fortified with ergocalciferol which is hydroxylated to 25-OH-ergocalciferol and to dihydroxylated metabolites of ergocalciferol.

In subjects with adequate exposure to sunlight some 80% of circulating vitamin D metabolites are derived from material synthesized in the skin (102, 103). All circulating vitamin D metabolites (whether originally derived from the skin or from food) are reabsorbed via the enterohepatic circulation so that many gastrointestinal or hepatic disorders may result in vitamin D deficiency (104).

A. Clinical Features

Vitamin D deficiency should be suspected in dark-skinned patients living in relatively sunless climates (105, 105a), especially if they are vegetarians with a low dietary intake of vitamin D (106). Other clinical scenarios leading to vitamin D deficiency include the postgastrectomy state (107), various other forms of malabsorption, inflammatory disorders of the bowel, and hepatic disorders, particularly primary biliary cirrhosis (108). In addition, chronically ill patients, regardless of the underlying cause, tend to be vitamin D deficient.

Many patients with vitamin D deficiency are symptomless. Even mild osteomalacia may not be associated with any symptoms or signs (107). When

Table 2 Some Causes of Osteomalacia

Vitamin D related	Not obviously vitamin D related
Vitamin D deficiency	Fluoride excess
Lack of 25-OH-vitamin D	Diphosphonate consumption
Lack of dihydroxylated metabolites	Heavy metals (aluminum, cadmium, ? iron)
Lack of receptors	X-linked hypophosphatemic rickets

symptoms and signs occur they tend to be vague, consisting of diffuse pain or weakness so that the patients are misdiagnosed as suffering from functional disorders (109). Patients with gross osteomalacia may complain that all movements are painful.

Physical examination of osteomalacic patients may show tibial tenderness and/or tenderness over one or several ribs. Some patients may be so weak that they cannot stand unaided. One mentally retarded patient cried out every time an attempt was made to move him. If vitamin D deficiency develops before the cartilaginous growth plates have been obliterated, the patients may show signs of rickets with swollen costochondral junctions, swollen wrists, and bowed legs.

Vitamin D deficiency is not synonymous with osteomalacia or rickets. Some patients with vitamin D deficiency do not have osteomalacia (110), while some forms of osteomalacia are totally unrelated to any abnormality of vitamin D metabolism (Table 2).

B. Diagnostic Tests

Tests for vitamin D deficiency fall into three groups: those relating to vitamin D metabolites in biological fluids (usually blood), those concerned with the examination of bone by histological or other means and, those depending on the secondary (usually nonspecific) effects of the D-deficient state.

The measurement of the serum concentrations of 25-OH-vitamin D is the most useful test for the assessment of the vitamin D status of a patient. Like other circulating vitamin D metabolites, 25-OH-vitamin D is relatively resistant to denaturation by heat or ultraviolet light (111), so that no special precautions need to be taken during collection or storage. Unlike the dihydroxylated metabolites, 25-OH-vitamin D is relatively easy to measure (112). Separation procedures into 25-OH-vitamin D_2 and 25-OH-vitamin D_3 are available (102, 103), but these are not usually required for clinical purposes.

Most important, it has been repeatedly shown (110, 113) that low serum 25-OH-vitamin D values are correlated with the presence and the severity of histological osteomalacia. Long et al. (114), who studied a group of patients with liver disorders, were unable to find a correlation between low serum 25-OH-vitamin D values and histological evidence of osteomalacia, but in other conditions there is a clear relationship between these parameters (115, 116).

The measurement of blood levels of dihydroxylated metabolites is less useful in the diagnosis of vitamin D deficiency. Blood levels of 24, 25-dihydroxy-vitamin D usually correlate well with blood levels of 25-OH-vitamin D (110, 117), so that there is no particular clinical advantage in performing the more cumbersome 24,25-$(OH)_2$-vitamin D assay. Blood levels of 1,25-$(OH)_2$-vitamin D may be low, normal, or high in vitamin D deficiency (115, 117) and give no indication of whether a patient is or is not vitamin D deficient and whether he or she does or does not have osteomalacia (110).

There is, at present, no noninvasive method for the determination of the presence or the severity of osteomalacia. Conventional radiology is too insensitive (107) for the diagnosis of any but the most severe forms. Osteodensitometry (118, 119), neutron activation analysis (51), and computerized tomographic (CT) scanning of bone (120), while capable of quantitating mineralized bone, cannot quantitate uncalcified osteoid.

Until recently, "hyperosteoidosis" as seen on biopsy was considered the sole histological criterion for the presence and severity of osteomalacia. It has since been shown (121) that not all patients with hyperosteoidosis have mineralization defects. The histological diagnosis of osteomalacia therefore requires both the presence of hyperosteoidosis and some evidence, usually based on double tetracycline labeling (122, 123), that osteoid is not being synthesized at an accelerated rate (121).

Indirect effects of vitamin D deficiency include hypocalcemia, hypophosphatemia, elevated serum iPTH concentrations, and elevated serum alkaline phosphatase values (124). Although some of these tests are cost effective, none of them are sufficiently sensitive or precise for the diagnosis or the exclusion of osteomalacia (5, 125). Hypocalcemia occurs only in very severe cases of vitamin D deficiency.

When vitamin D-deficient patients are treated with small doses of ergocalciferol, serum 25-OH-vitamin D values rise to within the normal range on or about day 10 of treatment (117). Serum alkaline phosphatase values may rise transiently after 3–4 weeks of therapy and then fall into the normal range 3 months later.

VII. ABNORMALITIES INVOLVING SPECIFIC VITAMIN D METABOLITES

There are several disorders associated with abnormal rates of formation or, possibly, degradation of vitamin D metabolites or with abnormalities of tissue receptors for these metabolites. Low values may be associated with osteomalacia, hypocalcemia, or secondary hyperparathyroidism, while high values are usually associated with hypercalcemia or hypercalciuria.

A. Diminished Serum 25-OH-Vitamin D Values

There is general (126–128) although not universal (129) agreement that patients receiving anticonvulsant drugs have low serum 25-OH-vitamin D concentrations. Some of these patients also develop osteomalacia (130, 131). Serum alkaline phosphatase (both skeletal and nonskeletal in origin) may be elevated in such patients (126). The effects of various drugs on vitamin D metabolites are reviewed by Hahn (132). Corticosteroids, in spite of their profound influence on skeletal mass, are without effect on serum concentrations of 25-OH-vitamin D (132).

Renal failure is associated with low 25-OH-vitamin D values (113, 133). Goldstein et al. (134) and Malluche et al. (135) showed that blood levels of 25-OH-vitamin D are low in patients with the nephrotic syndrome, even in the presence of normal renal function. Presumably, in the nephrotic syndrome, the loss of vitamin D binding proteins in urine leads to low plasma levels of D metabolites.

Zerwekh et al. (136) reported a single case of a patient apparently unable to synthesize 25-OH-vitamin D from vitamin D. Such cases are unusual; the 25-hydroxylation step in liver microsomes is not generally considered to be rate limiting.

B. Elevated Serum 25-OH-Vitamin D Values

Taylor et al. (137) recently claimed that hypercalcemia of infancy, also known as Williams' syndrome, may be due to the excessive synthesis of 25-OH-vitamin D from vitamin D. This hypothesis is awaiting confirmation.

The consumption of large quantities of vitamin D_2 or D_3 leads to elevated serum 25-OH-vitamin D values. If these exceed 700 nmol/liter (80) the patient is in danger of developing hypercalcemia. Serum 24,25-$(OH)_2$-vitamin D concentrations are also elevated in such patients, while 1,25-$(OH)_2$-vitamin D concentrations are low (110).

C. Low Serum Concentrations of Dihydroxylated Vitamin D Metabolites

Changes associated with vitamin D deficiency or excess were discussed in preceding sections. In general, 24,25-$(OH)_2$-vitamin D values follow those of 25-OH-vitamin D, while 1,25-$(OH)_2$-vitamin D values do not (110, 117, 138). Severe vitamin D depletion (64, 117, 139) and the nephrotic syndrome (140) may lead to low serum levels of 1,25-$(OH)_2$-vitamin D. Patients with renal failure have low or undetectable serum concentrations of 1,25-$(OH)_2$- and 24,25-$(OH)_2$-vitamin D (67).

Patients with "vitamin D dependency," an autosomal recessive disorder, have normal serum 25-OH-vitamin D concentrations but low 1,25-$(OH)_2$-vitamin D values (141, 142). It is believed that this disorder is due to a deficiency of renal 25-OH-vitamin D 1-hydroxylase.

Tumor-induced osteomalacia has been described in several patients in the presence of benign or malignant tumors. These patients have low blood levels of 1,25-$(OH)_2$-vitamin D as well as hypophosphatemia (143–145). The exact mechanism whereby tumors cause lack of 1,25-$(OH)_2$-vitamin D and hypophosphatemia is unknown.

There have been conflicting findings relating to serum vitamin D metabolites in X-linked hypophosphatemic rickets. It is generally (146, 147) although not universally (148) agreed that untreated patients suffering from this disorder have normal serum 25-OH- and 1,25-$(OH)_2$-vitamin D concentrations. Serum 24,25-$(OH)_2$-vitamin D values were found to be low by Drezner et al. (149) and Mason et al. (147). Treatment with ergocalciferol causes serum 25-OH- and 24,25-$(OH)_2$-vitamin D values to rise, while serum 1,25-$(OH)_2$ values fall (146, 147, 149, 150). Treatment with 1,25-$(OH)_2$-cholecalciferol was said by Delvin and Glorieux (148) both to raise and to lower blood levels of the metabolite, depending on the time interval between the last dose and venipuncture. Patients with X-linked hypophosphatemic rickets are apparently unable to respond to PTH infusions by a rise in serum 1,25-$(OH)_2$-vitamin D (151).

There is some controversy concerning the serum concentration of dihydroxylated vitamin D metabolites in patients treated with anticonvulsants. It is generally agreed (152, 153) that serum 24,25-$(OH)_2$-vitamin D values are diminished. Serum 1,25-$(OH)_2$-vitamin D concentrations were found to be normal or elevated by Jubiz et al. (138) but diminished by Christensen et al. (153).

Klein et al. (154) reported low serum 1,25-$(OH)_2$-vitamin D values in patients who had been receiving total parenteral nutrition for more than 3 months. The serum concentrations of two other vitamin D metabolites [24,25-$(OH)_2$-vitamin D and 25-OH-vitamin D] were normal.

D. Elevated Serum 1,25-$(OH)_2$-Vitamin D Values

Patients with abnormal receptors for 1,25-$(OH)_2$-vitamin D (155–158) tend to be rachitic, alopecic, and hypocalcemic. They have high serum concentrations of 1,25-$(OH)_2$-vitamin D and low concentrations of 24,25-$(OH)_2$-vitamin D, presumably because the target tissue (i.e., the kidney) does not "see" the high levels of 1,25-$(OH)_2$-vitamin D and fails to "switch off" the synthesis of 1,25-$(OH)_2$-vitamin D.

Patients with sarcoidosis also have high serum concentrations of 1,25-$(OH)_2$-vitamin D (159, 160), possibly because of the synthesis of this compound by sarcoid tissue (161). Corticosteroids, which normally have no influence on serum 1,25-$(OH)_2$-vitamin D values (162) reduced these values significantly in patients with this disorder (163).

Other conditions associated with "hypercalcitriolemia" include hyperparathyroidism (164–166), absorptive hypercalciuria (163, 167), and the administration of calcitriol for therapeutic purposes (146, 148, 168, 169). Because of the short pharmacological half-life of 1,25-$(OH)_2$-vitamin D (168, 170), there is not a close correlation between blood levels of this metabolite and hypercalcemia. When vitamin D-deficient patients are treated with small doses of vitamin D, serum 1,25-$(OH)_2$-vitamin D concentrations rise to supranormal values within 72 hr (117, 139).

Blood levels of three vitamin D metabolites in some clinical conditions are shown in Table 3. Infants have higher serum 1,25-$(OH)_2$-vitamin D values than do older children or adults (171). Serum 1,25-$(OH)_2$-vitamin D values rise during pregnancy (172).

Table 3 Blood Levels of Three Vitamin D Metabolites in Selected Clinical States[a]

Condition	25-OH-vitamin D	24,25-$(OH)_2$-vitamin D	1,25-$(OH)_2$-vitamin D	Reference
Vitamin D deficiency	↓	↓	Not consistent	117
Vitamin D_2 consumption	↑	↑	↓	110
Renal failure	↓	↓	↓	67
Nephrotic syndrome	↓	↓	↓	140
Anticonvulsants	↓	↓	(?) ↑	138, 152
Sarcoidosis	N		↑	159
Hypercalcemia of infancy	↑		N	137
Hyperparathyroidism	N		↑	165
Hypoparathyroidism (untreated)	N		↓	168
Hypoparathyroidism (treated)		*See* vitamin D_2 consumption		
X-linked hypophosphatemic rickets (untreated)	N	↓	N	149
X-linked hypophosphatemic rickets (treated)		*See* vitamin D_2 consumption		
1,25-$(OH)_2$-D receptor abnormalities	N	↓	↑	157
Tumor rickets	N	(?) N	↓	145
Vitamin D dependency, type I	N		↓	142
Total parenteral nutrition	N	N	↓	154

[a]N, normal; ↑, increased; ↓, decreased.

VIII. OSTEOPOROSIS

Osteoporosis is usually defined as a reduction in histological bone per unit volume of anatomic bone. Such a definition makes no distinction between cortical and cancellous bone, between the axial and the peripheral skeleton, or between "low turnover" and "high turnover" osteoporosis. It establishes histology as the main criterion for the diagnosis of osteoporosis, whereas most epidemiological studies are based on conventional radiology or osteodensitometry. Byers (44) and Avioli (173) review the diagnostic criteria of osteoporosis based on histology, radiology, and photon absorptiometry.

A. Prevalence

Regardless of the criteria employed, osteoporesis is extraordinarily common. In middle-aged and elderly females prevalence rates of 30% have been reported (174).

B. Clinical Features

The majority of patients with osteoporosis are symptomless. Some present with crush fractures of vertebrae or with peripheral fractures such as those involving the neck of the femur or the distal radius. There may also be a history of progressive loss of height.

Physical signs include thoracic kyphosis and a diminution in the distance between the lower ribs and the iliac crest. The measured height of the patient may be considerably less than a height previously recorded on a passport.

C. Diagnostic Tests

Apart from the diminution in skeletal mass (shown by radiographic techniques, neutron activation, photon absorption, CT scanning, or histology) there are no characteristic diagnostic features in osteoporosis. However, the patient who presents with skeletal pain and is found by conventional radiology to have crush fracture(s) of vertebra(e) and/or loss of mineralized bone requires a minimum number of tests before being told that he or she suffers from osteoporosis. All patients require an estimation of hemoglobin and erythrocyte sedimentation rate; multiple myeloma may present with radiological features indistinguishable from those of osteoporosis. Serum calcium, serum inorganic phosphate, and serum alkaline phosphatase should be normal; if they are not, the patient is likely to suffer from some disorder other than or in addition to osteoporosis.

Serum 25-OH-vitamin D estimations are useful in patients suspected of suffering from osteoporosis. Many geriatric individuals suffer from vitamin D deficiency-induced osteomalacia as well as from osteoporosis. If serum 25-OH-vitamin D values are low, appropriate supplements should be given.

Attempts to link osteoporosis with specific abnormalities of one or the other of the vitamin D metabolites (175, 176) have not resulted in any consistent findings. Measurements of adrenal androgens (177) and other steroids are of statistical rather than diagnostic interest.

Skeletal scans are not usually helpful except in so far that they help exclude widespread skeletal metastases. Bone biopsies have two functions: (1) they help exclude other types of bone pathology (especially osteomalacia), and (2) they subdivide osteoporotics into those with high and those with low bone turnover rates. The first is usually unnecessary. The second has not yet been found to make any difference to prognosis and management and the various histological turnover rates cannot be correlated with any other parameter (178). Hyperthyroidism [including triiodothyronine thyrotoxicosis] and hypercortisolism should be excluded (see Sec. VIII. D).

D. Osteoporosis Secondary to Endocrine Disorders

Hypercortisolism leads to osteoporosis by mechanisms which are not understood (179). Histological observations by Gallagher et al. (180) showed some diminution in bone formation and a marked increase in bone resorption. Hypercortisolism has no direct influence on vitamin D metabolites (162), and apart from the changes associated with Cushing's syndrome there are no characteristic biochemical, radiological, or histological changes associated with corticosteroid-induced osteoporosis (181).

Thyroid hormones stimulate bone resorption (182). Patients with hyperthyroidism may develop hypercalcemia (58, 59), hyperphosphatemia, and elevated serum alkaline phosphatase values (183) as well as osteoporosis.

Diabetes mellitus has been reported to lead to a diminution in bone mass (184). Heath et al. (185) showed that this association does not appear to lead to clinical problems.

The most important endocrine disorder to be associated with osteoporosis is congenital or acquired hypogonadism, especially in females. Oophorectomy leads to osteoporosis (186). The administration of estrogens to postmenopausal females prevents bone loss (187, 188) and fractures (189). Although osteoporosis has been described in men and in young women, the vast majority of osteoporotic patients are women in the postreproductive age group.

Hyperprolactinemia is associated with osteoporosis (190), presumably on the basis of diminished gonadal function in hyperprolactinemic states. Acromegaly is frequently included in lists of causes of osteoporosis, although it is difficult to find any clear evidence in support of this association. The role of the relative hypocalcitonemia of women in the pathogenesis of osteoporosis remains obscure (191).

E. Osteoporosis Secondary to Nonendocrine Causes

Garrick et al. (107) showed that gastrectomized patients develop osteoporosis as well as osteomalacia. Patients with alcoholism have a diminished bone mass compared to an age- and sex-matched control population (192).

Immobilization (193) and weightlessness (194) have been shown to lead to osteoporosis. In many patients no obvious endocrine or nonendocrine causes are identifiable.

IX. HYPER- AND HYPOCALCITONINEMIA

The pathophysiology of calcitonin was recently the subject of a detailed review (191). Conditions associated with the presence of high serum values of immunoreactive calcitonin include renal failure (195) and a variety of nonthyroidal tumors, particularly carcinoma of the lung (196). Elevated serum immunoreactive calcitonin values have been described in male patients with hyperparathyroidism (197). The most spectacular elevations of serum calcitonin occur in patients with medullary carcinomas of the thyroid (198, 199).

Medullary carcinomas of the thyroid have extraordinarily variable clinical manifestations. They may be quite symptomless or, at the other extreme, be associated with intense and disabling diarrhea or ectopic adrenocorticotropic hormone (ACTH) secretion (199). They may run a protracted course or, alternatively, be rapidly fatal. With few exceptions (200), patients with overt medullary carcinoma of the thyroid have high serum calcitonin values.

Serum calcitonin assays have their greatest use in situations involving symptomless individuals who for one reason or another are suspected of suffering from medullary thyroid carcinoma. Such persons may have a previous history of a pheochromocytoma. Alternatively, they may have a first degree relative with medullary carcinoma. In each case, an elevated serum calcitonin constitutes a clear indication for total thyroidectomy.

If basal serum calcitonin values are normal in subjects suspected of harboring a small medullary carcinoma (such as first-degree relatives of patients), a stimulation test should be performed. A variety of stimuli, including calcium, alcohol, and pentagastrin are available (201-203). There is evidence (203) that pentagastrin stimulation is a little more sensitive than calcium in detecting preclinical medullary carcinoma.

If appropriate stimulation tests fail to elevate serum calcitonin in a first-degree relative (especially a young relative) of a patient with medullary carcinoma, the test should be repeated at yearly intervals (203).

Hypercalcitoninemia persists after total thyroidectomy in patients harboring metastases. Goltzman et al. (204) performed calcitonin immunoassays on blood obtained during neck vein catheterization in order to localize metastases.

Diagnostic Summary 1 Hyperparathyroidism

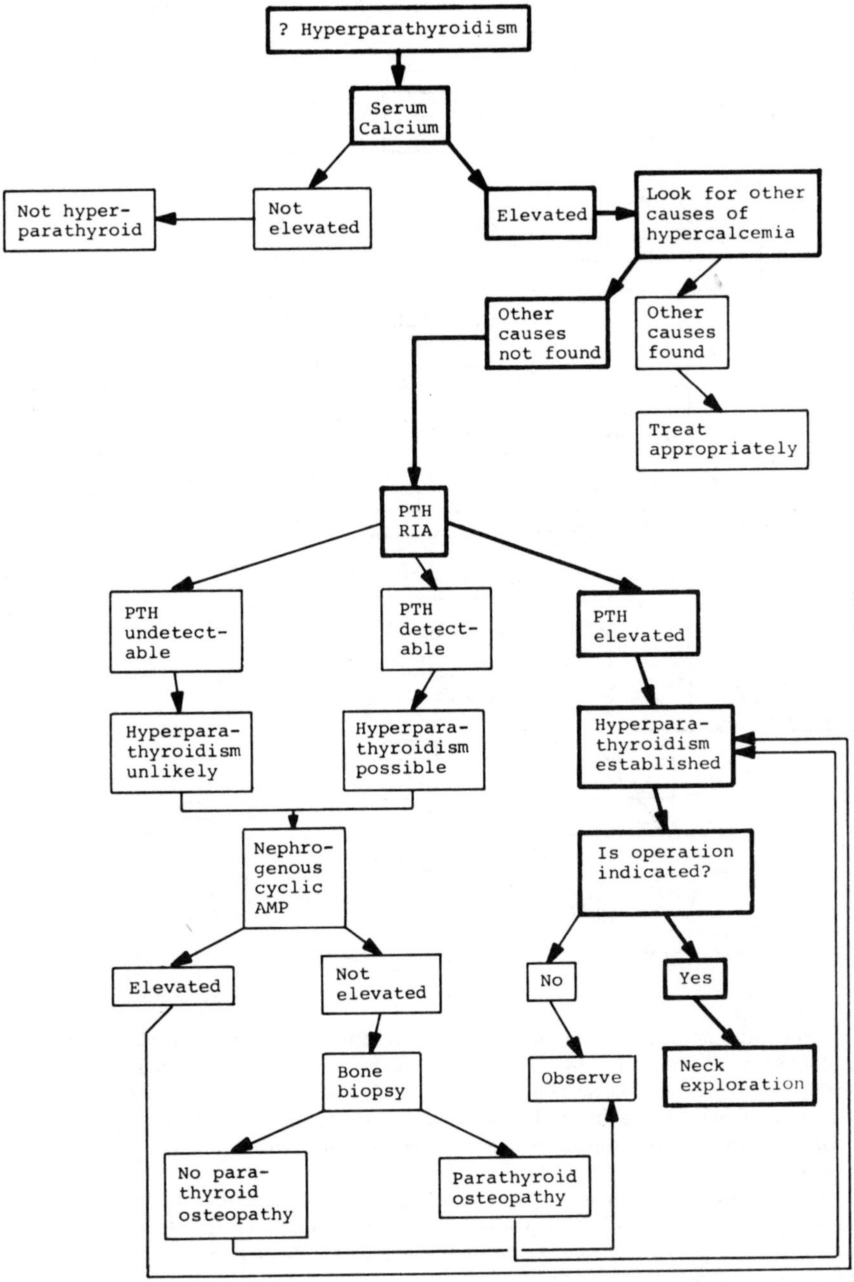

Diagnostic Summary 2 Hypocalcemia

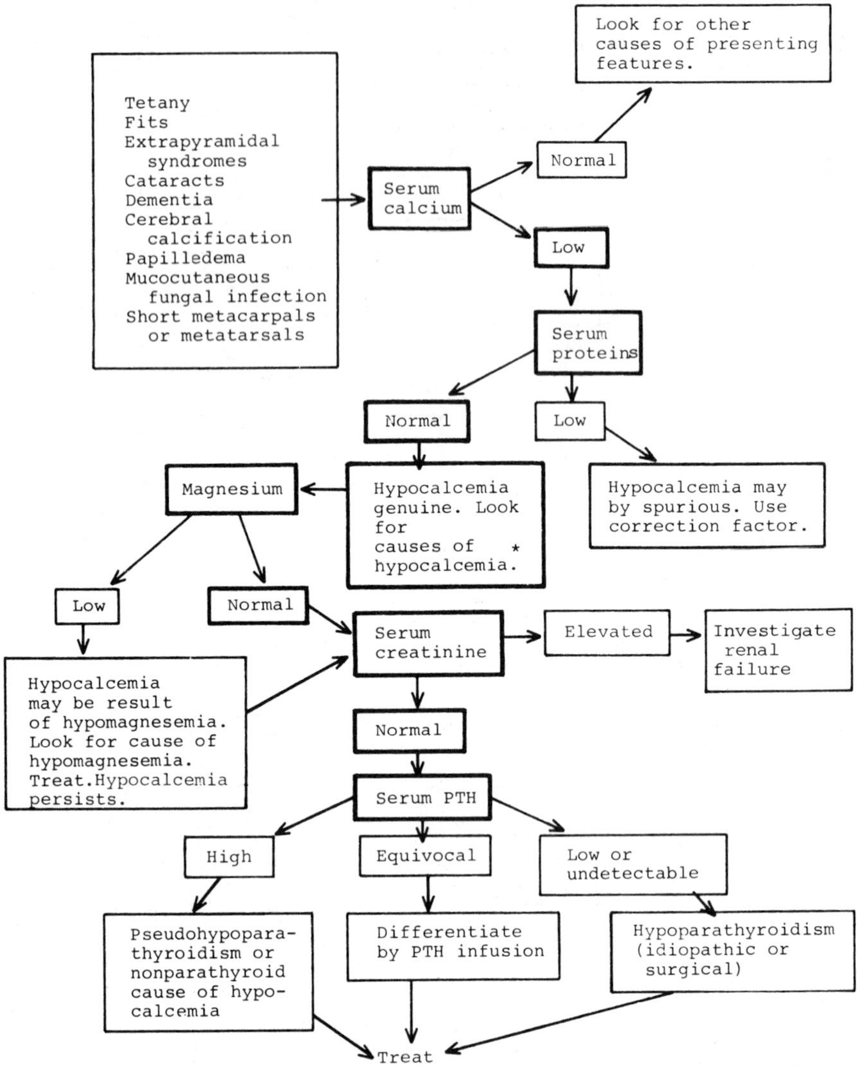

*In particular, pancreatitis (remember to reestimate serum calcium and PTH after recovery), and a history of thyroidectomy or parathyroidectomy (see Ref. 213). Other causes of hypocalcemia include malignancy (e.g., carcinoma of prostate) and cytotoxic drugs such as platinum. Serum 25-OH-vitamin D measurements may be useful in checking the compliance of hypoparathyroid patients taking vitamin D. For a general review of the investigation of hypocalcemia, see Ref. 214.

In neonates, hypocalcemia may be due to high phosphate intake, prematurity, or maternal hyperparathyroidism. There is currently no evidence that the assays of either parathyroid hormone or vitamin D metabolites are useful in decision making in neonatal hypocalcemia (see Refs. 215 and 216).

Unfortunately, such lesions are usually widespread so that surgical removal rarely leads to a cure or even to significant reductions in serum calcitonin.

Immunoreactive calcitonin has been measured in the urine of patients with medullary carcinoma of thyroid, nonthyroidal malignancies, normal subjects, and thyroidectomized subjects (205-208). The value of such measurements in clinical medicine is not established.

Relative hypocalcitoninemia has been described after thyroidectomy (205), although patients with hypothyroidism may be eucalcitoninemic (205, 209). It has also been shown that women have lower serum calcitonin levels than men do (210, 211). The relevance of this observation to the development of osteoporosis and to the relative intolerance of salmon calcitonin in females (212) is obscure.

X. SUMMARY

The principal diagnostic measures currently employed in the diagnosis of parathyroid and calcium disorders include (in addition to the older "Albrightian" tests, such as serum calcium and serum alkaline phosphatase) estimations of serum parathyroid hormone, calcitonin, and 25-OH-vitamin D. Estimations of serum levels of dihydroxylated vitamin D metabolite are currently not used in clinical decision making, although they have clarified the pathogenesis of some vitamin D-related disorders.

Newer techniques to study bone morphology (such as neutron activation analysis and CT scanning) are becoming available but a firm diagnosis of osteomalacia will continue to require, in many cases, a bone biopsy. Stimulation and suppression tests involving parathyroid hormone and vitamin D metabolites are currently as useful as dynamic tests for some other endocrine disorders. However, stimulation tests are essential in the early diagnosis of medullary thyroid carcinoma.

REFERENCES

1. Habener JE, Potts, JT. Parathyroid physiology and primary hyperparathyroidism. In *Metabolic Bone Disease*, Avioli LV, Krane SM (eds). Academic, New York, 1978, vol 2, pp 1–147.
2. Mallette LE, Bilezikian JP, Heath DA, Aurbach GD. Primary hyperparathyroidism: clinical and biochemical features. Medicine 1974; 53: 127–146.
3. Arnaud CD, Tsao HS, Littledike T. Radioimmunoassay of human parathyroid hormone in serum. J Clin Invest 1971; 50:21–34.
4. Kleerekoper M, Ingham JP, McCarthy SW, Posen S. Parathyroid hormone assay in primary hyperparathyroidism. Experiences with a radioimmunoassay based on commercially available reagents. Clin Chem 1974; 20: 369–375.

5. McComb RB, Bowers GN, Posen S. *Alkaline Phosphatase*. Plenum, New York, 1979.
6. Broadus AE, Mahaffey JE, Bartter FC, Neer RM. Nephrogenous cyclic adenosine monophosphate as a parathyroid function test. J Clin Invest 1977; 60:771–783.
7. Bone RG, Zerwekh JR, Haussler MR, Pak CYC. Effects of parathyroidectomy on serum 1α,25-dihydroxyvitamin D and intestinal calcium absorption in primary hyperparathyroidism. J Clin Endocrinol 1979; 48: 877–879.
8. Robinson BG, Clifton-Bligh P, Posen S, Morris BJ. Plasma vasopressin in hypercalcaemic states. Aust NZ J Med 1983; 13:5–7.
9. Heath H, Hodgson SF, Kennedy MA. Primary hyperparathyroidism. Incidence, morbidity and potential economic impact in a community. N Engl J Med 1980; 302:189–193.
10. Mundy GR, Cove DH, Fisher R. Primary hyperparathyroidism: changes in the pattern of clinical presentation. Lancet 1980; 1:1137–1320.
11. Broadus AE. Nephrolithiasis in primary hyperparathyroidism. In *Nephrolithiasis, Contemporary Series in Nephrology*, Coe FL, Brenner BM, Stein JH (eds). Churchill Livingstone, New York, 1980, vol 5, pp 59–85.
12. Pratley SK, Posen S, Reeve TS. Primary hyperparathyroidism. Experiences with 60 patients. Med J Aust 1973; 1:421–426.
13. Lavan JN, Neale FC, Posen S. Urinary calculi. Clinical, biochemical and radiological studies in 619 patients. Med J Aust 1971; 2:1049–1061.
14. Rohl PG, Wilkinson M, Posen S. Hyperparathyroidism. Experiences with treated and untreated patients. Med J Aust 1981; 1:519–521.
15. Posen S, Clifton-Bligh P, Mason RS. The management of primary hyperparathyroidism. Aust NZ J Med 1979; 9:17–23.
16. Betts JB, O'Malley BP, Rosenthal FD. Hyperparathyroidism: a prerequisite for Zollinger-Ellison syndrome in multiple endocrine adenomatosis type I. Report of a further family and a review of the literature. Q J Med 1980; 49: 69–76.
17. Wang CA. Surgery of the parathyroid glands. Adv Surg 1971; 5:109–127.
18. Drezner MK, Lebovitz HE. Primary hyperparathyroidism in paraneoplastic hypercalcaemia. Lancet 1978; 1:1004–1009.
19. Tougaard L, Hau C, Rodbro P, Ditzel J. Bone mineralization and bone mineral content in primary hyperparathyroidism. Acta Endocrinol 1977; 84:314–319.
20. Posen S, Clifton-Bligh P, Wilkinson M. Paget's disease of bone and hyperparathyroidism: coincidence or causal relationship? Calcif Tissue Res 1978; 26:107–109.
21. Wang CA, Miller LM, Weber AL, Krane SM. Pseudogout: a diagnostic clue to hyperparathyroidism. Am J Surg 1969; 117:558–565.
22. Kiss ZS, Neale FC, Posen S, Reed CSH. Acute arthritis and hyperuricemia following parathyroidectomy. Arch Intern Med 1967; 119:279–282.
23. Glass JS, Grahame R. Chondrocalcinosis after parathyroidectomy. Ann Rheum Dis 1976; 35:521–525.

24. Paloyan E, Lawrence AM, Prinz RA, Pickleman JR, Braithwaite S, Brooks MH. Radiation-associated hyperparathyroidism. Lancet 1977; 1:949.
25. Tisell LE, Hansson G, Lindberg S, Ragnhult I. Occurrence of previous neck radiotherapy among patients with associated non-medullary thyroid carcinoma and parathyroid adenoma or hyperplasia. Acta Chir Scand 1978; 144:7-11.
26. Madhavan T, Frame B, Block MA. Influence of surgical correction of primary hyperparathyroidism on associated hypertension. Arch Surg 1970; 100:212-214.
27. Britton DC, Thompson MH, Johnson IDA, Fleming LB. Renal function following parathyroid surgery in primary hyperparathyroidism. Lancet 1971; 2:74-75.
28. Patten BM, Bilezikian JP, Mallette LE, Prince A, Engel WK, Aurbach GD. Neuromuscular disease in primary hyperparathyroidism. Ann Intern Med 1974; 80:182-193.
29. Transbol I. On the diagnosis of so-called normocalcaemic hyperparathyroidism. Acta Med Scand 1977; 202:481-487.
29a. Case records of the Massachusetts General Hospital. Case 4–1978. N Engl J Med 1978; 298:266-274.
30. Statland BE, Bokelund H, Winkel P. Factors contributing to intra-individual variation of serum constituents. 4. Effect of posture and tourniquet application on variation of serum constituents in healthy subjects. Clin Chem 1974; 20:1513-1519.
31. Payne RB, Carver ME, Morgan DB. Interpretation of total serum calcium: effects of adjustment for albumin concentration on frequency of abnormal values and on detection of change in the individual. J Clin Pathol 1979; 32:56-60.
32. Klimiuk PS, Davies M, Adams PH. Primary hyperparathyroidism and thiazide diuretics. Postgrad Med J 1981; 57:80-83.
33. Parfitt AM. Chlorothiazide-induced hypercalcemia in juvenile osteoporosis and hyperparathyroidism. N Engl J Med 1969; 381:55-59.
34. Hirshorn JE, Vrhovsek E, Posen S. Carcinoma of the breast associated with hypercalcemia and the presence of parathyroid hormone-like substances in the tumor. J Clin Endocrinol Metab 1979; 48:217-221.
35. Stewart AF, Horst R, Deftos LJ, Cadman EC, Lang R, Broadus AE. Biochemical evaluation of patients with cancer-associated hypercalcemia. N Engl J Med 1980; 303:1377-1383.
36. Raisz LG, Yajnik CH, Bookman RS, Bower BF. Comparison of commercially available parathyroid hormone immunoassays in the differential diagnosis of hypercalcemia due to primary hyperparathyroidism or malignancy. Ann Intern Med 1979; 91:739-740.
37. Keutmann HT, Sauer MM, Hendy GN, O'Riordan JLH, Potts JT. Complete amino-acid sequence of human parathyroid hormone. Biochemistry 1978; 17:5723-5729.
38. Chambers DJ, Dunham J, Zanelli JM, Parsons JA, Bitensky L, Chayen JA. Sensitive bioassay for parathyroid hormone in plasma. Clin Endocrinol 1978; 9:375-379.

39. Boltzman D, Henderson B, Loveridge N. Cytochemical bioassay of parathyroid hormone: characteristics of the assay and analysis of circulating forms. J Clin Invest 1980; 65:1309–1317.
40. Nissenson RA, Abbott SR, Teitelbaum AP, Clark OH, Arnaud CD. Endogenous biologically active human parathyroid hormone: measurement by a guanyl nucleotide-amplified renal adenylate cyclase assay. J Clin Endocrinol Metab 1981; 52:840–846.
41. Seshadri MS, Chan YL, Wilkinson M, Mason RS, Posen S. Adenylcyclase bioassay for PTH–Some clinical experiences. American Society for Bone and Mineral Research, Abstracts of Fifth Annual Meeting, San Antonio, 1983, Abstract A51.
42. Rude RK, Sharp CF, Fredericks RS, Oldham SB, Elbaum N, Link J, Irwin L, Singer FR. Urinary and nephrogenous adenosine 3′,5′-monophosphate in the hypercalcemia of malignancy. J Clin Endocrinol 1981; 52:765–771.
43. Spiegel AM, Eastman ST, Attie MF, Downs RW, Levine MA, Marx SJ, Stock JL, Saxe AW, Brennan MG, Aurbach GD. Intraoperative measurements of urinary cyclic AMP to guide surgery for primary hyperparathyroidism. N Engl J Med 1980; 303:1457–1460.
44. Byers PD. The diagnostic value of bone biopsies. In *Metabolic Bone Disease*, Avioli LV, Krane SM (eds). Academic, New York, 1977, vol 1, pp 183–236.
45. Marx SJ, Stock JL, Attie MF, Downs RW, Gardner DG, Brown EM, Spiegel AM, Doppman JL, Brennan MF. Familial hypocalciuric hypercalcemia: recognition among patients referred after unsuccessful parathyroid exploration. Ann Intern Med 1980; 92:351–356.
46. Dent CE. Some problems of hyperparathyroidism. Br Med J 1962; 2: 1419–1425.
47. Posen S, Kleerekoper M, Ingham JP, Hirshorn JE. Parathyroid hormone assay in clinical decision making. Br Med J 1976; 1:16–19.
48. Broadus AE, Deftos LJ, Bartter FC. Effects of the intravenous administration of calcium on nephrogenous cyclic AMP. Use as a parathyroid suppression test. J Clin Endocrinol Metab 1978; 46:477–487.
49. Walker DA, Davies SJ, Siddle K, Woodhead JS. Control of renal tubular phosphate reabsorption by parathyroid hormone in man. Clin Sci Mol Med 1977; 53:431–438.
50. Ladenson JH, Lewis JW, Boyd JC. Failure of total calcium corrected for protein, albumin and pH to correctly assess free calcium status. J Clin Endocrinol Metab 1978; 46:896–993.
51. Maziere B, Kuntz D, Comar D, Ryckewaert A. In vivo analysis of bone calcium by local neutron activation of the hand: results in normal and osteoporotic subjects. J Nucl Med 1979; 20:85–91.
52. Paloyan E, Lawrence AM, Straus FH. *Hyperparathyroidism*. Grune & Stratton, New York, 1973.
53. Posen S, Clifton-Bligh P, Mason RS. Testing for disorders of calcium metabolism. Pathology 1980; 12:511–515.

54. Brennan MF, Doppman JL, Marx SJ, Spiegel AM, Brown EM, Aurbach GD. Reoperative parathyroid surgery for persistent hyperparathyroidism. Surgery 1978; 83:669–676.
55. Stock JL, Krudy AG, Doppman JL, Jones AE, Brennan MF, Attie MF, Downs RW, Levine MA, Marx SJ, Spiegel AM, Aurbach GD. Parathyroid imaging after intra-arterial injections of (^{75}Se) selenomethionine. J Clin Endocrinol Metab 1981; 52:835–839.
56. Case records of the Massachussetts General Hospital. Case 21–1981. N Engl J Med 1981; 304:1284–1291.
57. Clark OH. Parathyroid localization. Med Times 1982; 110:95–105.
58. Parfitt AM, Dent CE. Hyperthyroidism and hypercalcaemia. Q J Med 1970; 171–187.
59. Farnsworth AE, Dobyns BM. Hypercalcaemia and thyrotoxicosis. Med J Aust 1974; 2:782–784.
60. Jorgensen H. Hypercalcemia in adrenocortical insufficiency. Acta Med Scand 1973; 193:175–179.
61. Stewart AF, Adler M, Byers CM, Segre GV, Broadus AE. Calcium homeostasis in immobilization: An example of resorptive hypercalciuria. N Engl J. Med 1982; 306:1136–1140.
62. Skrabanek P, McPartlin J, Powell D. Tumor hypercalcemia and "ectopic" hyperparathyroidism. Medicine 1980; 59:262–282.
63. Mundy GR, Raisz LG, Cooper RA, Schechter GP, Salmon SE. Evidence for the secretion of an osteoclast stimulating factor in myeloma. N Engl J Med 1974; 291:1040–1046.
64. Mosekilde L, Melsen F, Hesso I, Christensen MS, Lund BJ, Lund BI, Sorensen OH. Low serum levels of 1,25-dihydroxyvitamin D and histomorphometric evidence of osteomalacia after jejunoileal bypass for obesity. Gut 1980; 21:624–631.
65. Massry SG, Tuma S, Dua S, Goldstein DA. Reversal of skeletal resistance to parathyroid hormone in uremia by vitamin D metabolites: evidence for the requirement of $1,25(OH)_2D_3$ and $24,25(OH)_2D_3$. J Lab Clin Med 1979; 94:152–157.
66. Ingham JP, Stewart JH, Posen S. Quantitative skeletal histology in untreated end-stage renal failure. Br Med J 1973; 2:745–748.
67. Mason RS, Lissner D, Wilkinson M, Posen S. Vitamin D metabolites and their relationship to azotaemic osteodystrophy. Clin Endocrinol 1980; 13:375–385.
68. Kleerekoper M, Ibels LS, Ingham JP, McCarthy SW, Mahony JF, Stewart JH, Posen S. Hyperparathyroidism after renal transplantation. Br Med J 1975; 2:680–682.
69. Memmos DE, Eastwood JB, Talner JB, Gower PE, Curtis JR, Phillips ME, Carger GD, Alaghband-Zadeh J, Roberts SP, DeWardener HE. Double blind trial of oral 1.25-dihydroxy vitamin D_3 versus placebo in asymptomatic hyperparathyroidism in patients receiving maintenance haemodialysis. Br Med J 1981; 282:1919–1924.

70. Massry SG, Goldstein DA. The search for uremic toxin(s) "X". "X" = PTH. Clin Nephrol 1979; 11:181–189.
71. Drüeke T, Fauchet M, Fleury, J, Lesourd P, Toure Y, Le Pailleur C, De Vernejoul P, Crosnier J. Effect of parathyroidectomy on left-ventricular function in haemodialysis patients. Lancet 1980; 1:112–114.
72. Nagant de Deuxchaisnes C, Krane SM. Hypoparathyroidism. In *Metabolic Bone Disease*, Avioli LV, Krane SM (eds). Academic, New York, 1978, vol 2, pp 217–445.
73. Barraclough BH, Reeve TS. Postoperative complications of thyroidectomy: a comparison of two series at an interval of ten years. Aust NZ J Surg 1975; 45:21-29.
74. Frankenhaeuser B, Hodgkin AL. The action of calcium of the electrical properties of squid axon. J Physiol (Lond.) 1957; 137:218–244.
75. Parfitt AM. Delayed recognition of postoperative hypoparathyroidism. Med J Aust 1967; 1:702–708.
76. Ireland AW, Hornbrook JW, Neale FC, Posen S. The crystalline lens in chronic surgical hypoparathyroidism. Arch Intern Med 1968; 122: 408–411.
77. Basser LS, Neale FC, Ireland AW, Posen S. Epilepsy and electroencephalographic abnormalities in chronic surgical hypoparathyroidism. Ann Intern Med 1969; 71:507–515.
78. Ireland AW, Clubb JS, Neale FC, Posen S, Reeve TS. The calciferol requirements of patients with surgical hypoparathyroidism. Ann Intern Med 1968; 69:81–89.
79. Shearman BT, Clubb JS, Neale FC, Posen S. Vocal cord paralysis and voice changes in patients with surgical hypoparathyroidism. Br Med J 1965; 2: 619–621.
80. Mason RS, Posen S. The relevance of 25-hydroxycalciferol measurements in the treatment of hypoparathyroidism. Clin Endocrinol 1979; 10: 265–269.
81. Smith KD, Geraci A, Luparello FJ. Basal ganglia calcification in postoperative hypoparathyroidism. NY State J Med 1973; 73:1087–1089.
82. Posen S, Clifton-Bligh P, Cromer T. Computerized tomography of the brain in surgical hypoparathyroidism. Ann Intern Med 1979; 92:415–417.
83. Kleerekoper M, Basten A, Penny R, Posen S. Idiopathic hypoparathyroidism with primary ovarian failure. Arch Intern Med 1974; 134:944–947.
84. Clifton-Bligh P, Lee C, Smith H, Posen S. The association of diabetes insipidus with hypoparathyroidism, Addison's disease and mucocutaneous candidiasis. Aust NZ J Med 1980; 10:548–551.
85. Arulanantham K, Dwyer JM, Genel M. Evidence for defective immunoregulation in the familial candidiasis endocrinopathy syndrome. N Engl J Med 1979; 300:164–168.
86. Sams WM, Jorizzo JL, Snyderman R, Jegosothy, BV, Ward FE, Weiner M, Wilson JG, Yount WJ, Dillard SB. Chronic mucocutaneous candidiasis. Immunological studies of three generations of a single family. Am J Med 1979; 67:948-959.

87. Stimmler L, Snodgrass GJAI, Jaffe E. Dental defects associated with neonatal symptomatic hypocalcaemia. Arch Dis Child 1973; 48: 217-220.
88. Chase LR, Nelson GL, Aurbach GD. Pseudohypoparathyroidism: defective excretion of 3,5-AMP in response to parathyroid hormone. J Clin Invest 1969; 48:1832-1844.
89. Farfel Z, Brickman AS, Kaslow HR, Brothers VM, Bourne HR. Defect of receptor-cyclase coupling protein in pseudohypoparathyroidism. N Engl J Med 1980; 303:237-242.
90. Frame B, Hanson CA, Frost HM, Block M, Arnstein AR. Renal resistance to parathyroid hormone with osteitis fibrosa. "Pseudohypohyperparathyroidism." Am J Med 1972; 52:311-321.
91. Marx SJ, Hershman JM, Aurbach GD. Thyroid dysfunction in pseudohypoparathyroidism. J Clin Endocrinol 1971; 33:822-828.
92. Werder EA, Illig R, Bernasconi S, Kind H, Prader A. Excessive thyrotropin-releasing hormone in pseudohypoparathyroidism. Pediatr Res 1975; 9:12-16.
93. Mason RS, Lissner D, Posen S. Parathyroid hormone effect on 1,25-dihydroxyvitamin D in hypoparathyroidism. Ann Intern Med 1980; 92:260.
94. Braun JJ, Birkenhäger JC, Visser TJ, Juttman JR. Lack of response of 1,25-dihydroxycholecalciferol to exogenous parathyroid hormone in a patient with treated pseudohypoparathyroidism. Clin Endocrinol 1981; 14:403-407.
95. Lawoyin S, Norman DA, Zerwekh JE, Breslau NA, Pak CYC. A patient with pseudohypoparathyroidism with increased serum calcium and 1α, 25-dihydroxyvitamin D after exogenous parathyroid hormone administration. J Clin Endocrinol Metab 1979; 49:783-786.
96. Drezner M, Neelon FA, Lebovitz HE. Pseudohypoparathyroidism type II: a possible defect in the reception of the cyclic AMP signal. N Engl J Med 1973; 289:1056-1060.
97. Rodriguez HJ, Villareal H, Klahr S, Slatopolsky E. Pseudohypoparathyroidism type II. Restoration of normal renal responsiveness to parathyroid hormone by calcium administration. J Clin Endocrinol Metab 1974; 39:693-701.
98. Stögmann W, Fisher JA. Pseudohypoparathyroidism. Disappearance of the resistance to parathyroid extract during treatment with vitamin D. Am J Med 1975; 59:140-144.
99. Potts JT Jr. Pseudohypoparathyroidism. In *Endocrinology*, DeGroot LJ, Cahill GJ, Odell WD, Martini L, Potts JT Jr, Nelson DH, Steinberger E, Winegrad AI (eds). Grune & Stratton, New York 1979, vol 2, pp 769-776.
100. Mautalen CA, Dymling JF, Horwith M. Pseudohypoparathyroidism 1942-1966. A negative progress report. Am J Med 1967; 42:977-985.
101. Dudley AW, Hawkins H. Mineralization of the central nervous system in pseudopseudo-hypoparathyroidism (PPH). J Neurol Neurosurg Psychol 1970; 33:147-152.

102. Hughes MR, Baylink DJ, Jones PG, Haussler MR. Radioligand receptor assay for 25-hydroxyvitamin D_2/D_3 and 1α,25-dihydroxyvitamin D_2/D_3. Application to hypervitaminosis D. J Clin Invest 1976; 58:61–70.
103. Arnaud SB, Matthusen M, Gilkinson JB, Goldsmith RS. Components of 25-hydroxyvitamin D in serum of young children in upper midwestern United States. Am J Clin Nutr 1977; 30:1082–1086.
104. Meredith SC, Rosenberg IH. Gastro-intestinal-hepatic disorders and osteomalacia. Clin Endocrinol Metab 1980; 9:131–150.
105. Holick MF, MacLaughlin JA, Doppelt SH. Regulation of cutaneous previtamin D_3 synthesis in man: skin pigment is not an essential regulator. Science 1981; 211:590–593.
105a. Clemens TL, Adams SL, Holick MF. Increased skin pigment reduces the capacity of skin to synthesise vitamin D_3. Lancet 1982; 1:74–76.
106. Stamp TCB, Walker PG, Perry W, Jenkins MV. Nutritional osteomalacia and late rickets in greater London 1974–1979: clinical and metabolic studies in 45 patients. Clin Endocrinol Metab 1980; 9:81–105.
107. Garrick R, Ireland AW, Posen S. Bone abnormalities after gastric surgery. A prospective histological study. Ann Intern Med 1971; 75:221–225.
108. Reed JS, Meredith SC, Nemchausky BA, Rosenberg IH, Boyer JL. Bone disease in primary biliary cirrhosis: reversal of osteomalacia with oral 25-hydroxyvitamin D. Gastroenterology 1980; 78:512–517.
109. Melick RA, Larkins RG, Greenberg PB, Wark JD. Osteomalacia due to unusual causes presenting in adults. Aust NZ J Med 1979; 9:253–257.
110. Mason RS, Lissner D, Grunstein HS, Posen S. A simplified assay for dihydroxylated vitamin D metabolites in human serum: application to hyper- and hypovitaminosis D. Clin Chem 1980; 26:444–450.
111. Lissner D, Mason RS, Posen S. The stability of vitamin D metabolites in human blood serum and plasma. Clin Chem 1981; 27:773.
112. Mason RS, Posen S. Some problems associated with assay of 25-hydroxycalciferol in human serum. Clin Chem 1977; 23:806–810.
113. Mason RS, Moddel D, McElduff A, Stewart JH, Mahony JF, Posen S. The relevance of 25-hydroxycalciferol measurements in sera of patients with renal failure. Aust NZ J Med 1979; 9:257–260.
114. Long RG, Meinhard E, Skinner RK, Varghese Z, Wills MR, Sherlock S. Clinical, biochemical and histological studies of osteomalacia, osteoporosis and parathyroid function in chronic liver disease. Gut 1978; 19:85–90.
115. Rasmussen H, Baron R, Broadus A, DeFronzo R, Lang R, Horst R. $1,25(OH)_2D_3$ is not the only D metabolite involved in the pathogenesis of osteomalacia. Am J Med 1980; 69:360–368.
116. Eastwood JB, DeWardener HE, Gray RW, Lemann J Jr. Normal plasma $1,25(OH)_2$ vitamin D concentrations in nutritional osteomalacia. Lancet 1979; 1:1377–1378.
117. Mawer EB. Clinical implications of measurements of circulating vitamin D metabolites. Clin Endocrinol Metab 1980; 9:63–79.

118. Christiansen C, Christensen MS, Transbol I. Bone mass in post-menopausal women after withdrawal of oestrogen/gestagen replacement therapy. Lancet 1981; 1:459–461.
119. Seeman E, Wahner HW, Offord KP, Kumor R, Johnson WJ, Riggs BL. Differential effects of endocrine dysfunction on the axial and the appendicular skeleton. J Clin Invest 1982; 69:1302–1309.
120. Genant HK, Cann CE, Chafetz NI, Helms CA. Advances in computed tomography of the musculoskeletal system. Radial Clin N Am 1981; 19:645–674.
121. Teitelbaum SL. Pathological manifestations of osteomalacia and rickets. Clin Endocrinol Metab 1980; 9:43–62.
122. Frost HM. Tetracycline-based histological analysis of bone remodeling. Calcif Tissue Res 1969; 3:211–237.
123. Parfitt AM. The quantitative approach to bone morphology. In *Clinical Aspects of Metabolic Bone Disease*, Frame B, Parfitt AM, Duncan H (eds). Excerpta Medica, New York, 1973, pp 86–94.
124. Preece MA, Tomlinson S, Ribot CA, Pietrek J, Korn HT, Davies DM, Ford JA, Dunnigan MG, O'Riordan JLH. Studies of vitamin D deficiency in man. Q J Med 1975; 44:575–589.
125. Posen S, Cornish C, Kleerekoper M. Alkaline phosphatase and metabolic bone disorders. In *Metabolic Bone Disease*, Avioli LV, Krane SM (eds). Academic, New York, 1977, pp 141–181.
126. Hahn TJ, Hendin BA, Scharp CR, Boisseau VC, Haddad JG Jr. Serum 25-hydroxycholecalciferol levels and bone mass in children on chronic anticonvulsant therapy. N Engl J Med 1975; 292:550–554.
127. Mosekilde L, Christensen MS, Lund B, Sorensen OH, Melson F. The interrelationships between serum 25-hydroxycholecalciferol, serum parathyroid hormone and bone changes in anticonvulsant osteomalacia. Acta Endocrinol (Copenh) 1977; 84:559–565.
128. Pylypchuk, G, Oreopoulos DG, Wilson DR, Harrison JE, McNeill KG, Meema HE, Ogilvie R, Sturtridge WC, Murray TM. Calcium metabolism in adult outpatients with epilepsy receiving long-term anti-convulsant therapy. Can Med Assoc J 1978; 118:635–638.
129. Wark JD, Larkins RG, Perry-Keene D, Peter CT, Ross DL, Sloman JG. Chronic diphenylhydantoin therapy does not reduce plasma 25-hydroxyvitamin D. Clin Endocrinol 1979; 11:267–274.
130. Tolman KG, Jubiz W, Sannella JJ, Madsen JA, Belsey RE, Goldsmith RS, Freston JW. Osteomalacia associated with anti-convulsant drug therapy in mentally retarded children. Pediatrics 1975; 56:45–51.
131. Crosley CJ, Chee C, Berman PH. Rickets associated with long-term anticonvulsant therapy in a pediatric out-patient population. Pediatrics 1975; 56:52–57.
132. Hahn JT. Drug induced disorders of vitamin D and mineral metabolism. Clin Endocrinol Metab 1980; 9:107–129.

133. Eastwood JB, Harris E, Stamp TCB, DeWardener HE. Vitamin-D deficiency in the osteomalacia of chronic renal failure. Lancet 1976; 2:1209–1211.
134. Goldstein DA, Oda Y, Kurokawa K, Massry SG. Blood levels of 25-hydroxyvitamin D in nephrotic syndrome. Studies in 26 patients. Ann Intern Med 1977; 87:664–667.
135. Malluche HH, Goldstein DA, Massry SG. Osteomalacia and hyperparathyroid bone disease in patients with nephrotic syndrome. J Clin Invest 1979; 63:494–500.
136. Zerwekh JE, Glass K, Jowsey J, Pak CYC. An unique form of osteomalacia associated with end organ refractoriness to 1,25-dihydroxyvitamin D and apparent defective synthesis of 25-hydroxyvitamin D. J Clin Endocrinol Metab 1979; 49:171–175.
137. Taylor AB, Stern PH, Bell NH. Abnormal regulation of circulating 25-hydroxyvitamin D in Williams syndrome. N Engl J Med 1982; 306: 972–975.
138. Jubiz W, Haussler MR, McCain TA, Tolman KG. Plasma 1,25-dihydroxyvitamin D levels in patients receiving anticonvulsant drugs. J Clin Endocrinol Metab 1977; 44:617-621.
139. Papapoulos SE, Clemens TL, Fraher LJ, Gleed J, O'Riordan JLH. Metabolites of vitamin D in human Vitamin D deficiency: effect of vitamin D_3 or 1,25-dihydroxycholecalciferol. Lancet 1980; 2:612–615.
140. Goldstein, DA, Haldimann B, Sherman D, Norman AW, Massry SG. Vitamin D metabolites and calcium metabolism in patients with nephrotic syndrome and normal renal function. J Clin Endocrinol Metab 1981; 52: 116–121.
141. Fraser D, Kooh SW, Kind HP. Pathogenesis of hereditary vitamin D dependent rickets. An inborn error of vitamin D metabolism involving defective conversion of 25-hydroxyvitamin D to 1α,25-dihydroxyvitamin D. N Engl J Med 1973; 289:817–822.
142. Scriver CR, Reade TM, DeLuca HF, Hamstra AJ. Serum 1, 25-$(OH)_2$D levels in normal subjects and in patients with hereditary rickets or bone disease. N Engl J Med 1978; 299:976–979.
143. Fukumoto Y, Tarui S, Tsukiyama K, Ichihara K, Moriwaki K, Nonaka K, Mizushima T, Kobayashi Y, Dokah S, Fukunaga M, Morita R. Tumor-induced vitamin D-resistant hypophosphatemic osteomalacia associated with proximal renal tubular dysfunction and 1,25-dihydroxyvitamin D deficiency. J Clin Endocrinol Metab 1979; 49:873–878.
144. Lyles KW, Berry WR, Haussler M, Harrelson JM, Drezner MK. Hypophosphatemic osteomalacia: association with prostatic carcinoma. Ann Intern Med 1980; 93:275–278.
145. Sweet RA, Males JL, Hamstra AJ, DeLuca HF. Vitamin D metabolite levels in oncogenic osteomalacia. Ann Intern Med 1980; 93:279–280.
146. Drezner MK, Lyles KW, Haussler MR, Harrelson JM. Evaluation of a role for 1,25-dihydroxyvitamin D_3 in the pathogenesis and treatment of X-linked hypophosphatemic rickets and osteomalacia. J Clin Invest 1980; 66:1020–1031.

147. Mason RS, Rohl PG, Lissner D, Posen S. Vitamin D metabolism in hypophosphatemic rickets. Am J Dis Child 1982; 136:909–913.
148. Delvin EE, Glorieux FH. Serum 1,25-dihydroxyvitamin D concentration in hypophosphatemic vitamin D-resistant rickets. Calcif Tissue Int 1981; 33:173–175.
149. Drezner MK, Lyles KW, Harrelson JM. Vitamin D resistant osteomalacias: evaluation of vitamin D metabolism and response to therapy. In *Hormonal Control of Calcium Metabolism*, Cohn DV, Talmage RV, Matthews JL (eds), Int Congr Ser 511. Excerpta Medica, Amsterdam, 1981, pp 243–251.
150. Chesney RW, Mazess RB, Rose P, Hamstra AJ, DeLuca HF. Supranormal 25-hydroxyvitamin D and subnormal 1,25-dihydroxyvitamin D. Their role in X-linked hypophosphatemic rickets. Am J Dis Child 1980; 134: 140–143.
151. Lyle KW, Drezner MK. Parathyroid hormone effects on serum 1,25-dihydroxy-vitamin D levels in patients with X-linked hypophosphatemic rickets: evidence for abnormal 25-hydroxyvitamin D-1-hydroxylase activity. Clin Res 1981; 29:413A.
152. Weisman Y, Fattal A, Eisenberg Z, Harel S, Spirer Z, Harell A. Decreased serum 24,25-dihydroxy vitamin D concentrations in children receiving chronic anticonvulsant therapy. Br Med J 1979; 2:521–523.
153. Christensen CK, Lund B, Lund BJ, Sorensen OH, Nielsen HE, Mosekilde L. Reduced 1,25-dihydroxyvitamin D and 24,25-dihydroxyvitamin D in epileptic patients receiving chronic combined anticonvulsant therapy. Metab Bone Dis Relat Res 1981; 3:17–22.
154. Klein GL, Horst RL, Norman AW, Ament ME, Slatopolsky E, Coburn JW. Reduced serum levels of 1α,25-dihydroxyvitamin D during long term total parenteral nutrition. Ann Intern Med 1981; 94:638–643.
155. Brooks MH, Bell NH, Love L, Stern PH, Orfei E, Queener SF, Hamstra AJ, DeLuca HF. Vitamin D dependent rickets type II: resistance of target organs to 1,25-dihydroxyvitamin D. N Engl J Med 1978; 298:996–999.
156. Rosen JF, Fleischman AR, Finberg L, Hamstra A, DeLuca HF. Rickets with alopecia: an inborn error of vitamin D metabolism. J Pediatr 1979; 94:729–735.
157. Liberman UA, Samuel R, Halabe A, Kauli R, Edelstein S, Weisman Y, Papapoulos SE, Clemens TL, Fraher LJ, O'Riordan JLH. End-organ resistance to 1,25-dihydroxycholecalciferol. Lancet 1980; 1:504–507.
158. Eil C, Liberman VA, Rosen JF, Marx SJ. A cellular defect in hereditary vitamin-D-dependent rickets type II: defective nuclear uptake of 1,25-dihydroxyvitamin D in cultured skin fibroblasts. N Engl J Med 1981; 304:1588–1591.
159. Bell NH, Stern PH, Pantzer E, Sinha TK, DeLuca HF. Evidence that increased circulating 1α,25-dihydroxyvitamin D is the probable cause for abnormal calcium metabolism in sarcoidosis. J Clin Invest 1979; 64: 218–225.
160. Stern PH, Olazabal JD, Bell NH. Evidence for abnormal regulation of circulating 1α,25-dihydroxyvitamin D in patients with sarcoidosis and normal calcium metabolism. J Clin Invest 1980; 66:852–855.

161. Barbour GL, Coburn JW, Slatopolsky E, Norman AW, Horst RL. Hypercalcemia in an anephric patient with Sarcoidosis: evidence for extrarenal generation of 1,25-dihydroxyvitamin D. N Engl J Med 1981; 305: 440–442.
162. Seeman E, Kumar R, Hunder GG, Scott M, Heath H, Riggs BL. Production, degradation and circulating levels of 1,25-dihydroxy-vitamin D in health and in chronic glucocorticoid excess. J Clin Invest 1980; 66: 664–669.
163. Zerwekh JE, Pak CYC, Kaplan RA, McGuire JL, Upchurch K, Breslau N, Johnson R. Pathogenetic role of 1α,25-dihydroxy vitamin D in sarcoidosis and absorptive hypercalciuria: different response to prednisolone therapy. J Clin Endocrinol Metab 1980; 51:381–386.
164. Kaplan RA, Haussler MR, Deftos LJ, Bone H, Pak CYC. The role of 1α, 25-dihydroxyvitamin D in the mediation of intestinal hyperabsorption of calcium in primary hyperparathyroidism and absorptive hypercalciuria. J Clin Invest 1977; 59:756–760.
165. Gray RW, Wilz DR, Caldas AE, Lemann J. The importance of phosphate in regulating plasma 1,25-$(OH)_2$ vitamin D levels in humans: studies in healthy subjects, in calcium-stone formers and in patients with primary hyperparathyroidism. J Clin Endocrinol Metab 1977; 45:299–306.
166. Broadus AE, Horst RL, Lang R, Littledike ET, Rasmussen H. The importance of circulating 1,25-dihydroxyvitamin D in the pathogenesis of hypercalciuria and renal stone formation in primary hyperparathyroidism. N Engl J Med 1980; 302:421–426.
167. Caldas AE, Gray RW, Lemann J. The simultaneous measurement of vitamin D metabolites in plasma: studies in healthy adults and in patients with calcium nephrolithiasis. J Lab Clin Med 1978; 91:840–849.
168. Rosen JF, Fleischman AR, Finberg L, Eisman J, DeLuca HF. 1,25-Dihydroxycholecalciferol: its use in the long-term management of idiopathic hypoparathyroidism in children. J Clin Endocrinol Metab 1977; 45:457–468.
169. Bell NH, Epstein S, Stern PH. Hypercalcemia during long term treatment with 1,25-dihydroxyvitamin D_3 in hypoparathyroidism. N Engl J Med 1979; 301:1183–1184.
170. Mason RS, Lissner D, Posen S, Norman AW. Blood concentrations of dihydroxylated vitamin D metabolites after an oral dose. Br Med J 1980; 1:449–450.
171. Lund B, Clausen N, Lund B, Anderson E, Sorensen OH. Age-dependent variations in serum 1,25-dihydroxyvitamin D in childhood. Acta Endocrinol (Copenh) 1980; 94:426–429.
172. Steichen JJ, Tsang RC, Gratton TL, Hamstra A, DeLuca HF. Vitamin D homeostasis in the perinatal period. N Engl J Med 1980; 302:315–319.
173. Avioli LV. Osteoporosis: pathogenesis and therapy. In *Metabolic Bone Disease*, Avioli LV, Krane SM (eds). Academic, New York, 1977, vol 1, pp 307-385.

174. Goldsmith NF, Johnson JO, Picetti G, Garcia C. Bone mineral in the radius and vertebral osteoporosis in an insured population: a correlative study using ^{125}I photon absorption and miniature roentgenography. J Bone Jt Surg 1973; 55A:1276–1296.
175. Gallagher JC, Riggs BL, Eisman J, Hamstra A, Arnaud SB, DeLuca HF. Intestinal calcium absorption and serum vitamin D metabolites in normal subjects and osteoporotic patients: effects of age and dietary calcium. J Clin Invest 1979; 64:729–736.
176. Slovik DM, Adams JS, Neer RM, Holick MF, Potts JT Jr. Deficient production of 1,25-dihydroxyvitamin D in elderly osteoporotic patients. N Engl J Med 1981; 305:372–374.
177. Marshall DH, Crilly RG, Nordin BEC. Plasma androstenedione and oestrone levels in normal and osteoporotic postmenopausal women. Br Med J 1977; 2:1177–1179.
178. Clinicopathologic Conference, Osteopenia. Am J Med 1980; 69:915–922.
179. Raisz LG. Effects of glucocorticosteroids on calcium metabolism. In *Hormones and the Kidney*, Stokes GS, Mahony JF (eds). Prog. Biochem. Pharmacol. (Karger, Basel) 1980; 17:212–219.
180. Gallagher JC, Aaron J, Horsman A, Wilkinson R, Nordin BEC. Corticosteroid osteoporosis. J Clin Endocrinol Metab 1973; 2:355–368.
181. Aloia JF, Roginsky M, Ellis K, Shukla K, Cohn S. Skeletal metabolism and body composition in Cushing's syndrome. J Clin Endocrinol 1974; 39:981–985.
182. Mundy GR, Shapiro JL, Bandelin JG, Canalis EM, Raisz LG. Direct stimulation of bone resorption by thyroid hormones. J Clin Invest 1976; 58: 529–534.
183. Posen S, Doherty E. The measurement of serum alkaline phosphatase in clinical medicine. Adv Clin Chem 1981; 22:163–245.
184. Levin ME, Boisseau VC, Avioli LV. Effects of diabetes mellitus on bone mass in juvenile and adult-onset diabetes. N Engl J Med 1976; 294: 241–245.
185. Heath H, Melton LJ, Chu CP. Diabetes mellitus and risk of skeletal fracture. N Engl J Med 1980; 303:567–570.
186. Aitken JM, Hart DM, Lindsay R. Oestrogen replacement therapy for prevention of osteoporosis after oophorectomy. Br Med J 1973; 3:515–518.
187. Lindsay R, Hart DM, Aitken JM, MacDonald EB, Anderson JB, Clarke AC. Long term prevention of postmenopausal osteoporosis by oestrogen: evidence for an increased bone mass after delayed onset of oestrogen treatment. Lancet 1976; 1:1038–1041.
188. Recker RR, Saville PD, Heaney RP. Effects of estrogens and calcium carbonate on bone loss in postmenopausal women. Ann Intern Med 1977; 87:649–655.
189. Weiss NS, Ure CL, Ballard JH, Williams AR, Daling JR. Decreased risk of fractures of the hip and lower forearm with postmenopausal use of estrogen. N Engl J Med 1980; 303:1195–1198.

190. Klibanski A, Neer RM, Beitins IZ, Ridgway EC, Zervas NT, McArthur JW. Decreased bone density in hyperprolactinemic women. N Engl J Med 1980; 303:1511–1514.
191. Austin LA, Heath H. Calcitonin: physiology and pathophysiology. N Engl J Med 1981; 304:269–278.
192. Nilsson BE, Westlin NE. Changes in bone mass in alcoholics. Clin Orthop 1973; 90:229–232.
193. Pennock JM, Kalu DN, Clark MB, Foster GV, Doyle FH. Hypoplasia of bone induced by immobilization. Br J Radiol 1972; 45:641–646.
194. Whedon GD, Lutwak L, Rambaut P, Whittle M, Leach C, Reid J, Smith M. Effect of weightlessness on mineral metabolism: metabolic studies on Skylab orbital space flights. Calcif Tissue Res 1976; (Suppl 21):423–430.
195. Kanis JA, Earnshaw M, Heynen G, Ledingham JGG, Oliver DO, Russell RG, Woods CG, Franchimont P, Gaspar S. Changes in histologic and biochemical indexes of bone turnover after bilateral nephrectomy in patients on hemodialysis: evidence for a possible role of endogenous calcitonin. N Engl J Med 1977; 296:1073–1079.
196. Schwartz KE, Wolfsen AR, Forster B, Odell WD. Calcitonin in nonthyroidal cancer. J Clin Endocrinol Metab 1979; 49:438–444.
197. Parthemore JG, Deftos LJ. Calcitonin secretion in primary hyperparathyroidism. J Clin Endocrinol Metab 1979; 49:223–226.
198. Deftos LJ, Parthemore JG. Scretion of parathyroid hormone in patients with medullary thyroid carcinoma. J Clin Invest 1974; 54: 416–420.
199. McElduff A, Clifton-Bligh P, Posen S. Metastatic medullary carcinoma of the thyroid complicated by Cushing's syndrome. Med J Aust 1979; 1: 186–188.
200. Trump DL, Mendelsohn G, Baylin SB. Discordance between plasma calcitonin and tumor-cell mass in medullary thyroid carcinoma. N Engl J Med 1979; 301:253–255.
201. Sizemore GW, Go VLW. Stimulation tests for diagnosis of medullary thyroid carcinoma. Mayo Clin Proc 1975; 50:53–56.
202. Wells SA, Baylin SB, Linehan WM, Farrell RE, Cox EB, Cooper CW. Provocative agents and the diagnosis of medullary carcinoma of the thyroid gland. Ann Surg 1978; 188:139–141.
203. Graze K, Spiler IJ, Tashjian AH, Melvin KEW, Cervi-Skinner S, Gagel RF, Miller HH, Wolfe JH, Delellis RA, Leape L, Feldman ZT, Reichlin S. Natural history of familial medullary carcinoma. Effect of a program for early diagnosis. N Engl J Med 1978; 299:980–985.
204. Goltzman D, Potts JT, Ridgeway EC, Maloof F. Calcitonin as a tumor marker. Use of the radioimmunoassay for calcitonin in the postoperative evaluation of patients with medullary thyroid carcinoma. N Engl J Med 1974; 290:1035–1039.
205. Silva OL, Wisneski LA, Cyrus J, Snider RH, Moore CF, Becker KL. Calcitonin in thyroidectomized patients. Am J Med Sci 1978; 275:159–164.

206. Silva OL, Snider RH, Moore CF, Becker KL. Urine calcitonin as a test for medullary thyroid cancer: a new screening procedure. Ann Surg 1979; 189:269–274.
207. Clifton-Bligh P, Robinson B, Poon T, Posen S. Calcitonin and the kidney. In *Hormones and the Kidney*, Stokes GS, Mahony JF (eds). Prog. Biochem. Pharmacol. (Karger, Basel) 1980; 17:204–211.
208. Becker KL, Nash DR, Silva OL, Snider RH, Moore CF. Urine calcitonin levels in patients with bronchogenic carcinoma. JAMA 1980; 243: 670–672.
209. Carey DE, Jones KL, Parthemore JG, Deftos LJ. Calcitonin secretion in congenital non-goitrous cretinism. J Clin Invest 1980; 65:892–895.
210. Heath H, Sizemore GW. Plasma calcitonin in normal man: differences between men and women. J Clin Invest 1977; 60:1135–1140.
211. Deftos LJ, Weisman MH, Williams GW, Karpf DB, Frumar AM, Davidson BJ, Parthemore JG, Judd HL. Influence of age and sex on plasma calcitonin in human beings. N Engl J Med 1980; 302:1351–1353.
212. Grunstein HS, Clifton-Bligh P, Posen S. Side effects of calcitonin therapy: a sex-related difference? N Engl J Med 1981; 305:286.
213. Watson CG, Steed DL, Robinson AG, Deftos LJ. The role of calcitonin and parathyroid hormone in the pathogenesis of post-thyroidectomy hypocalcemia. Metabolism 1981; 30:588–589.
214. Juan D. Hypocalcemia. Differential diagnosis and mechanisms. Arch Intern Med 1979; 139:1166–1171.
215. Fleischman AR, Rosen JF, Nathenson G. 25-Hydroxycholecalciferol for early neonatal hypocalcemia. Occurrence in premature newborns. Am J Dis Child 1978; 132:973–977.
216. Schedewie HK, Odell WD, Fisher DA, Krutzik SR, Dodge M, Cousins L, Fiser WP. Parathormone and perinatal calcium homeostasis. Pediatr Res 1979; 13:1–6.

PANCREATIC AND GASTROINTESTINAL DISORDERS

31
Diabetes Mellitus

Peter H. Sönksen
St. Thomas' Hospital Medical School, London, England

I. DIABETES MELLITUS: HISTORICAL BACKGROUND

Aretaeus, the Capadocian physician (A.D. 200), is generally credited with the introduction of the word *diabetes* (Greek, siphon). In his original description of the disease, he refers to the "siphoning off of flesh as urine" (1). He was referring to the wasting of flesh (proteolysis) with its conversion to glucose (gluconeogenesis) and the subsequent osmotic diuresis brought about by massive overproduction of glucose and consequent hyperglycemia. Thomas Willis (1621-1725) added the "mellitus" to "diabetes," following his description of sweet urine, and Mathew Dobson (?-1784) showed the sweetness to be due to sugar originating from the blood. Although in 1683 Brunner showed that pancreatectomy led to the diabetic syndrome in dogs (2), it was 200 years later that Von Mering and Minkowski repeated Brunner's experiments and extended them and concluded that the pancreas produced a substance that regulated glucose production by the liver. Baylis and Starling identified the first hormone (secretin) at the turn of the century, while Schäfer, a rival of Baylis and Starling, using remarkable powers of deduction concluded that the islets of Langerhans produced a hormone (or as he preferred to call it, an autacoid) that regulated hepatic glucose production. He named this substance "insuline" 8 years before it was isolated by Banting and Best. He also prophesied that it would be produced by activation of an inert precursor, "proinsuline," this time 54 years before its discovery in 1967 by Steiner. At the time Schäfer wrote his book *The Endocrine Organs* (3), he taught that insulin controlled blood glucose concentration by restraining hepatic glucose production, an effect that he described as the "chalonic" (or inhibitory) action of insulin (to distinguish it from any "stimulatory" or "autacoid" effect).

A. Action of Insulin

That insulin's major role was to inhibit hepatic glucose production in humans provided strong evolutionary arguments for the pancreatic endocrine products being drained into the portal circulation and a ready explanation of why, in the face of insulin deficiency (pancreatectomy or diabetes mellitus), the liver overproduced glucose. Thus much of the physiology of insulin as well as its pathophysiology had been worked out before it was isolated–initially by Paulescou (4) and subsequently by Banting and Best (5), who went on to use it effectively in the treatment of diabetes mellitus in January 1922. Banting was subsequently awarded a Nobel prize for his contribution to the discovery of insulin (6).

It remained standard teaching that insulin's major action in humans was the control of hepatic glucose production until the early 1950s, when insulin was shown to have a marked excitatory (autacoid) effect on glucose transport and metabolism in certain tissues–notably striated muscle and adipose tissue from the young rat–but to have no demonstrable effect on glucose transport and metabolism in the liver. With the documentation and characterization of the specific D-glucose transport system in the cell membrane, it became clear that although the transport process would work in the absence of insulin, it was under appropriate conditions exquisitely sensitive to the presence of insulin, which was capable of stimulating the rate of transport more than 10-fold. This resulted in the introduction of the first biological assay for insulin, which was sufficiently sensitive to measure circulating levels of insulin in normal humans and in the presence of diabetes mellitus. There then followed in the 1950s and 1960s a period of intensive research into the assay of insulin using a variety of different bioassays and the whole subject became very confused (largely as a result of the lack of specificity of the various assays). As a secondary effect of this intense activity on insulin-stimulated cellular pathways, the teaching emphasis changed. The emphasis was now on the excitatory (autacoid) actions of insulin in stimulating (1) glucose transport and oxidation, (2) lipid synthesis, (3) glycogen synthesis, (4) amino acid transport, and (5) protein synthesis. These in vitro actions of insulin documented in the rat were assumed to occur in humans, leading to the extrapolation that the hyperglycemia of diabetes mellitus was due primarily to a failure of glucose uptake and oxidation. (It is remarkable to see how quickly this became the accepted dogma.)

1. In Vivo Studies

It was the introduction of tracer methodology to the investigation of the pathophysiology of diabetes mellitus that showed this dogma to be wrong and the concepts put forward before the discovery of insulin to be correct! Initially in experimental diabetes in the dog (7) and subsequently in human diabetes (8) it was shown that the major hypoglycemic action of insulin in vivo is its inhibitory (chalonic) action on hepatic glucose production. At plasma insulin concentrations up to 50 mU/liter in the peripheral circulation (average value of peak insulin after 100 g oral glucose in normal subjects) the only demonstrable action of insulin is that of inhibition of hepatic glucose production. It is only at concentrations of insulin of 100 mU/liter and greater that stimulation of peripheral uptake of glucose is seen. These data were obtained with insulin infused into the peripheral circulation. Even more marked hepatic specificity is to be expected normally, with the liver receiving insulin concentrations in the portal vein approximately 10 times those in the peripheral circulation.

B. Hyperglycemia: Overproduction or Underutilization of Glucose?

Tracer methodology has again been helpful in confirming the hypotheses put forward by Schäfer and his contemporaries concerning the overproduction of glucose in the face of insulin deficiency. It has long been accepted (albeit intuitively) that the "severity" of diabetes is best measured by the concentration of fasting blood glucose. Figure 1 shows the relationship between fasting blood glucose and tracer-determined glucose production rate in a group of insulin-dependent diabetic patients from whom insulin has been withheld for 24 hr. Also shown is the fasting blood glucose and glucose production rate when the same patients have been maintained normoglycemic overnight with an intravenous infusion of insulin. Data for a group of normal subjects are shown for comparison. It can readily be seen that in the absence of insulin the increased concentration of fasting blood glucose is determined by the elevated hepatic glucose production rate and that insulin maintains a normal fasting blood glucose by inhibiting hepatic glucose production. Similar isotopic studies have shown that the elevated fasting concentrations of free fatty acids, ketone bodies, and branched-chain amino acids that are seen in insulin-withdrawn (or newly diagnosed) diabetic patients are also due to overproduction rather than underutilization.

1. Effects of Insulin Deficiency

It is possible to summarize the effects of insulin deficiency as in Figure 2. It should be noted that these four processes are all under the influence of the adenyl cyclase/cyclic AMP system and in each case insulin appears to be acting tonically to inhibit cyclic AMP generation while glucagon and catecholamines oppose this action. In vitro attempts to demonstrate such action of insulin have so far been unsuccessful. A knowledge of the pathophysiology of insulin deficiency makes it easy to understand why fasting measurements of the blood concentrations of glucose, amino acids, glycerol, free fatty acids, and ketone bodies give the best estimate of the severity of the disorder, since their concentration will in general be directly related to their production rate.

Although this is broadly true, there are several caveats. From the clinical management point of view, the most important indices of severity of the metabolic disturbance are: (1) degree of hyperglycemia, (2) degree of ketoacidemia, and (3) degree of dehydration and electrolyte disturbance. The extent of the dehydration and electrolyte disturbances in diabetic ketoacidosis (and hyperglycemic nonketotic coma/precoma) are to a great extent determined by the duration of the illness before diagnosis. The two basic features of the disrupted intermediary metabolism of diabetes–hyperglycemia and ketoacidemia–may together or independently kill the patient, the former by means of dehydration

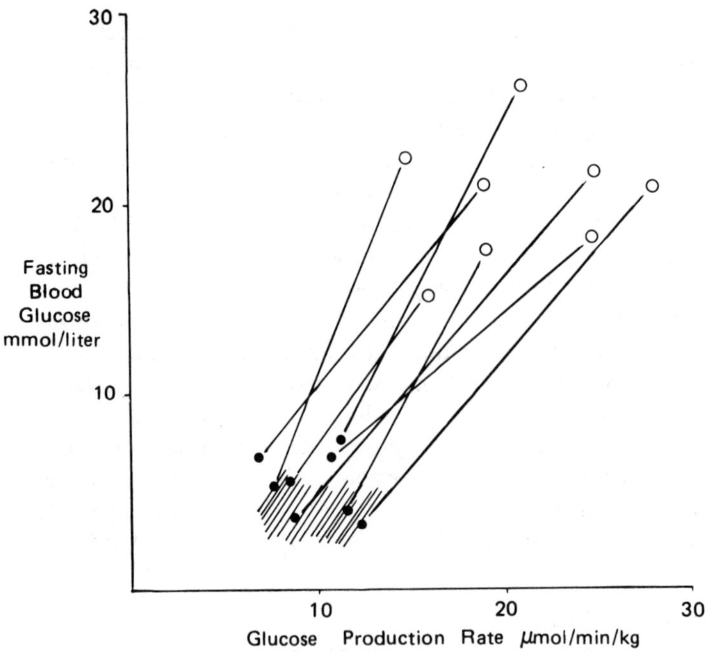

Figure 1 Relationship between fasting blood glucose and hepatic glucose production rate in diabetes and the effect of insulin. Open circles indicate results from diabetic patients 24 hr after their last injection of Actrapid insulin; closed circles indicate results from same patient on another occasion after overnight infusion of insulin. Shading indicates range of observations in 10 normal controls.

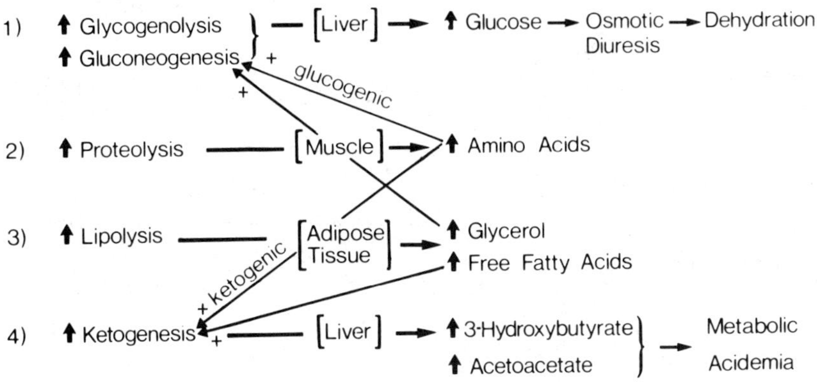

Figure 2 Summary of effects of insulin deficiency. (From Ref. 9.)

and electrolyte disturbance consequent on prolonged osmotic diuresis, the latter from acidemia (few patients survive in whom the pH has fallen below 6.8). The changes seen in the concentrations of the other intermediary metabolities do not pose a danger to life but do seem to give an accurate reflection of their rate of production. Not all amino acid levels and production rates are increased. It is notably the branched-chain amino acids leucine, isoleucine, and valine which are increased, while the concentration and production rate of what is normally the major glucogenic amino acid (alanine) are normal or reduced. No satisfactory explanation has yet been accepted for this but it is probably an indication of decreased rates of transamination of pyruvate (the major source of alanine in humans), almost certainly as a result of the elevated ketone body levels.

Thus, in summary, the liver in diabetes is working in an "unrestrained" fashion, processing all the substrates that are delivered to it in a very efficient manner. Since the provision of many substrates is still more than the liver can cope with, they accumulate in the plasma, despite the fact that the liver is producing a net increase in its export products, which in turn accumulate in the plasma because their production rates exceed the metabolic capacity of the tissues that rely on them for energy metabolism.

2. Oxygen Consumption and Respiratory Quotient

There is no evidence of a block in energy metabolism in diabetes–indeed, oxygen consumption is increased in severely ill patients in direct proportion to the degree of ketosis. This is an old observation from the classical studies of DuBois and Joslin at the beginning of the twentieth century. They observed

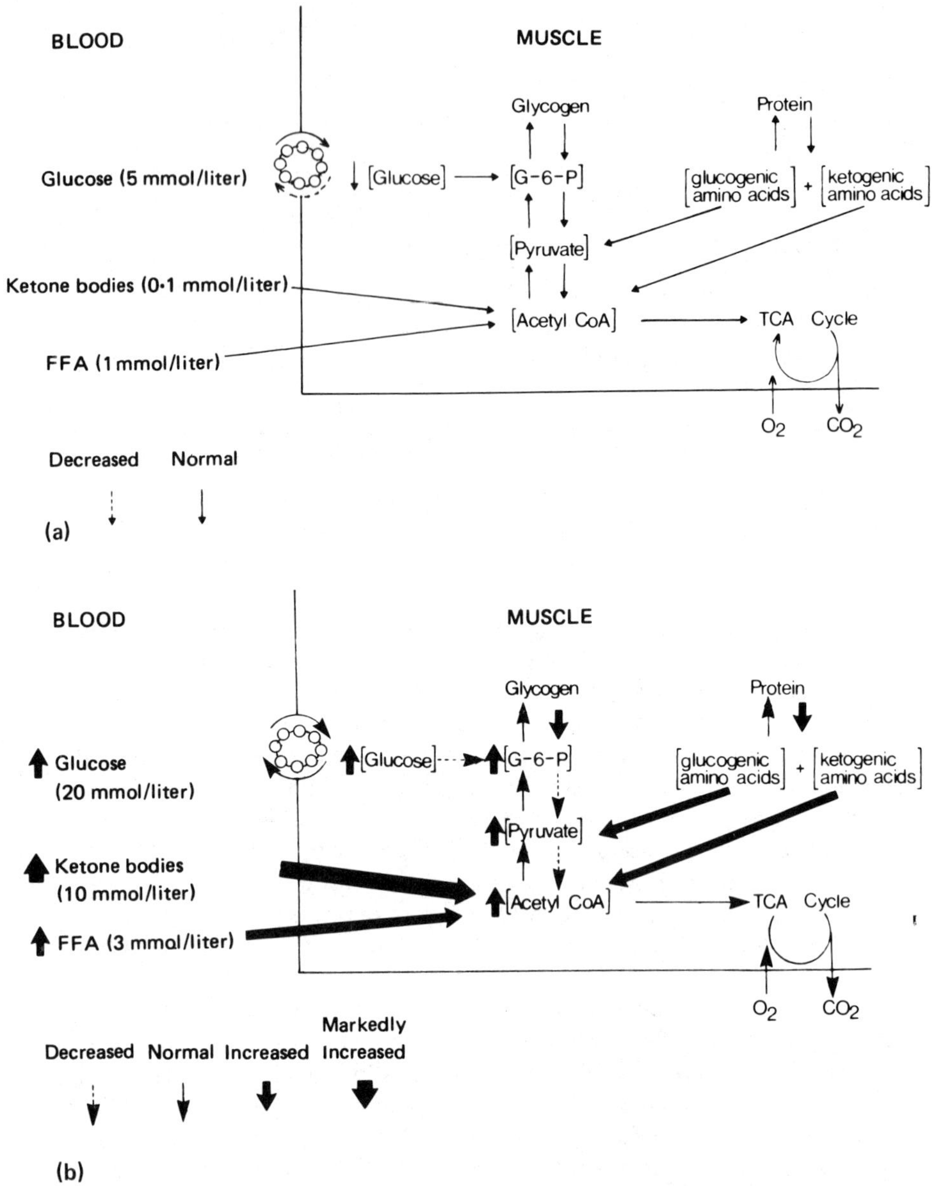

Figure 3 Glucose–fatty acid cycle. (a) Normal: note that the intracellular free [glucose] is very low and the substrate supply, regulated at the periphery by the insulin, balances energy requirements of tricarboxylic acid (TCA) cycle. (b) Uncontrolled diabetes: substrate availability exceeds the capacity of the TCA cycle with accumulation of extra and intracellular metabolites, including glucose-6-phosphate [G-6-P] and free [intracellular glucose], resulting in no net transport of glucose.

not only that oxygen consumption was normal but that the respiratory quotient could vary from less than 0.7 (the theoretical lower limit of normal when fat is the exclusive fuel) to 1.0, indicating rather surprisingly that even in the presence of severe diabetes, carbohydrate metabolism was accounting for all oxygen consumed.

3. Mechanisms Regulating Substrate Utilization in the Face of Insulin Deficiency

The mechanisms that determine the use of substrates in uncontrolled diabetes need further consideration. It has already been pointed out that glucose uptake by all cells is only by way of a highly specific transport protein which transports glucose into the cell, where in most tissues it is immediately phosphorylated and further metabolized so rapidly that the intracellular free glucose concentration is very low (Fig. 3a). In contrast to glucose, cell uptake of free fatty acid (FFA) and ketone bodies appears to be by simple diffusion since they, unlike glucose, are readily soluble in and pass through the lipid cell membrane. Cellular uptake is then obligatory and related to prevailing extracellular concentration, which in turn will be determined by the plasma concentrations of the various substrates. Thus in uncontrolled diabetes with high plasma FFA and ketonemia, the cells will be flooded with an excess of FFA and ketone bodies. Once in the cell they will enter into the metabolic pathways and their subsequent metabolism will be obligatory. Since both are metabolized to acetylcoenzyme A (acetyl-CoA) and thence into the Krebs cycle, it is possible that the capacity of Krebs cycle will not be adequate to oxidize all the available acetyl-CoA. The capacity of the basic oxidative pathway via the Krebs cycle is not readily increased in response to overprovision of substrate, and as a result intermediary metabolites must accumulate intracellularly (Fig. 3b). In the presence of significant ketonemia with high FFA turnover there is sufficient energy substrate available to satisfy all the requirements of the Krebs cycle and the resultant respiratory quotient (RQ) will be 0.7. If hepatic ketogenesis still continues and losses of ketone bodies occur in the urine and breath (which is the case), the RQ may fall below the theoretical lower limit of normal, and values of as low as 0.5 have been recorded (10, 11).

When fat is providing all the obligatory energy requirements for cellular metabolism, there is a process for inhibiting glucose metabolism which operates as a result of inhibition of the glycolytic pathway by accumulation of acetyl-CoA (because it is being produced faster than it is cleared via the Krebs cycle). Inhibition of the glycolytic pathway results in a rise in the concentration of glucose-6-phosphate intracellularly, with subsequent accumulation of intracellular free glucose and *no* further *net* entry of glucose into the cells. Thus there is a reciprocal relationship between glucose and FFA (and ketone body) metabolism in such a way that when all are present in excess (as in the case of the uncontrolled diabetic), FFA and ketone bodies are metabolized in preference to glucose (glucose-fatty acid cycle) (12).

4. Mechanisms Regulating Substrate Utilization in Normal Humans

In normal humans there is a reciprocal relationship between the metabolism of fat and carbohydrate, but in this case coordinated control is brought about by an entirely different mechanism—the supply of substrates—which in turn is governed by eating and insulin. After a high-carbohydrate meal, glucose is available as energy substrate and excess is available for storage as glycogen and, via hepatic lipoprotein synthesis, as triglyceride. Following a high-carbohydrate meal, insulin (the hormone of energy storage) is released and by way of its *chalonic* action inhibits lipolysis and cuts off the supply of FFA, which in turn facilitates the storage of available triglyceride and lowers the plasma FFA concentration, which by reducing FFA oxidation, in turn "opens up" the pathway of glucose, metabolism facilitating glucose entry into the cells. The rise in insulin concentration with feeding also inhibits hepatic glycogenolysis, gluconeogenesis, and ketogenesis; proteolysis is also inhibited, with net accumulation of structural protein and reduction in the supply of gluconeogenic (and ketogenic) substrates.

By these actions insulin has "prepared the way" for the ingested glucose (1) to replenish hepatic glycogen stores, and (2) to become the major substrate for cellular metabolism. This is brought about without a marked rise in the peripheral blood glucose concentration because hepatic glucose production is inhibited and the rate of glucose absorption from the gut is closely matched by the rates of conversion to glycogen and cellular metabolism. Any glucose absorbed that is in excess of these requirements is converted to lipoproteins by the liver under the influence of insulin and subsequently exported for storage in adipose tissue.

It should be noted that the use of glucose as the major substrate in the "fed" state, which is reflected by the rise in RQ to 1, is probably brought about as a result of "shutting off" the supply of alternative fuel (FFA) rather than "stimulating" glucose transport and cellular metabolism.

Once the readily available fuel from the meal has either been used up or stored, the continuing supply of glucose and alternative substrates is brought about primarily by a fall in insulin concentration (and also probably facilitated by a rise in glucagon and growth hormone). The inhibitory effect of insulin on glycogenolysis and gluconeogenis is reduced with a net increase in hepatic glucose production. Lipolysis is activated with provision of FFA as a substrate for cellular metabolism and ketogenesis. Proteolysis is activated and ensures the provision of substrates for gluconeogenesis.

Adaptation to Prolonged Fasting. The normal physiological response to fasting is a dynamic response which changes progressively with the continuation of the fast and is readily reversed on refeeding. Thus in the short-term fasting that occurs between meals, hepatic glycogen stores are adequate to maintain plasma glucose constant. If fasting is extended to 24 hr or longer, however, hepatic glycogen becomes depleted and the maintenance of a normal blood glucose concentration is entirely dependent on gluconeogenesis. Since the substrates for gluconeogenesis come mainly from structural protein and will thus be used up continuously during fasting, it has clearly been an evolutionary advantage to develop an adaptive mechanism to prolong survival in the face of famine. In humans this is reflected in a reduction in the obligatory requirement for glucose by the central nervous system and substitution of ketone bodies as an alternative substrate. Ketone body concentrations rise with prolonged withholding of food and after a week contribute about half of the obligatory energy requirements of the central nervous system (CNS). Breakdown of structural protein is consequently reduced, probably directly via the increased concentrations of plasma ketone bodies (3-hydroxybutyrate and acetoacetate), which in turn inhibit proteolysis.

Ketone bodies pass readily into the urine and during starvation losses may be as much as 10 g (100 mmol) per day. Although after an overnight fast, the ratio of 3-hydroxybutyrate/acetoacetate is approximately 1, the ratio increases with prolonged fasting to typical steady-state figures of 6 mmol/liter 3-hydroxybutyrate to aceto acetate, 1.5 mmol/liter a 4:1 ratio.

C. Ketosis in Diabetes

In the uncontrolled diabetic state, ketone body concentratioms may rise to as much as 25 mmol/liter in plasma, with appropriate increases in urinary excretion. The ratio of 3-hydroxybutyrate to acetoacetate may rise as high as 25:1, partly as a result of the mitochondrial redox changes consequent on insulin deficiency and partly as a result of accumulation of $[H^+]$. The extent of the metabolic acidemia will be reflected in the blood pH, values lower than 6.8 being seen only rarely and almost invariably being fatal. In uncomplicated ketoacidosis (minimal elevation of blood lactic acid) a blood pH of 6.8 usually reflects a total ketoacid concentration of approximately 25 mmol/liter but the 3-hydroxybutyrate/acetoacetate ratio can range from 5:1 to 25:1, this means that the acetoacetate concentration can vary from 5 to 1 mmol/liter. Since the conventional bedside tests for ketone bodies (Ketostix and Acetest) are sensitive only to acetoacetate, and require a concentration 1 mmol/liter or more to produce a positive response, it is occasionally possible to have life-threatening ketoacidemia with negative plasma Ketostix or Acetest, which may result in an (incorrect) assumed diagnosis of lactic acidosis.

D. Role of Other Hormones

The emphasis has so far been on the actions of insulin, since without doubt it is the most important regulatory hormone of energy storage and metabolism. In the presence of primary insulin deficiency (diabetes mellitus), however, there are secondary changes in the blood concentration of other hormones (in most but not all cases reflecting altered secretion rate). Insulin withdrawal leads to a rapid rise in circulating glucagon concentrations and the rate of rise in blood glucose is determined both by the degree of insulin deficiency and the magnitude of the rise in glucagon (13). Similarly, insulin withdrawal in most cases results in a rise in the concentration of adrenalin, noradrenalin, epinephrine, norepinephrine, growth hormone, and cortisol (14), all of which tend to compound the metabolic effects of insulin deficiency. It seems most likely that some of these hormonal changes are themselves a direct result of insulin deficiency. Thus glucagon levels rise rapidly following acute insulin deficiency and are rapidly suppressed by infusion of insulin (8), and it seems that insulin may itself have a direct inhibitory effect on glucagon secretion ("chalonic"), the implication of this being that an important part of insulin's action inhibiting hepatic glucose production is by inhibition of glucagon-stimulated glycogenolysis and glucogenolysis and gluconeogenesis. The available evidence suggests that these hormonal changes seen in diabetes mellitus are "epiphenomena" associated with insulin deficiency rather than primary events triggering the onset of the condition. There are changes in circulating thyroid hormone levels that seem to result from insulin deficiency or the metabolic disturbances secondary to insulin deficiency. Uncontrolled diabetes is associated with a low triiodothyronine (T_3) and high reverse T_3 concentration, almost certainly as a result of altered peripheral conversion of thyroxine (T_4) to T_3 (15). These changes are rapidly reversed by insulin therapy. T_4 concentrations are low-normal in untreated diabetes and rise to normal with insulin therapy.

II. INVESTIGATIONAL PROCEDURES

From the foregoing description of the background pathophysiology of diabetes mellitus it is clear that many biochemical disturbances are present as a consequence of insulin deficiency. By analogy with other endocrine conditions it might be anticipated that direct measurement of circulating insulin concentrations would be the most specific and accurate way of establishing the diagnosis and assessing its severity. In fact, this is not the case; because of the vital nature of the hormone, several clinical syndromes present before insulin deficiency becomes absolute, and in these cases the diagnosis and severity of the condition are best assessed by the clinical state of the patient combined with measurements of the biochemical disturbances. On the other hand, with milder degrees of insulin deficiency, dynamic testing may be required to demonstrate whether or not insulin secretion is normal.

A. Urine Glucose Measurements

Glycosuria has traditionally been the screening test for diabetes mellitus, mainly because of the widespread availability of simple specific tests for glucose in urine. When faced with a patient who has classic symptoms of diabetes mellitus, the finding of heavy glycosuria is to all intents and purposes diagnostic of the condition, although good clinical practice dictates that the inevitable accompanying hyperglycemia should be documented with at least one reliable blood glucose measurement. The majority of new cases of diabetes are diagnosed in this way and the accompanying hyperglycemia is unequivocal. This may not always be the case, however; because routine urinanalysis is an established feature of many medical examinations, the detection of glycosuria in a patient who has little or no history suggestive of diabetes is increasingly common. This raises the possible diagnosis of diabetes mellitus which needs to be distinguished from other causes of glycosuria. Since establishing a diagnosis of diabetes mellitus has quite profound social and medicolegal implications, care has to be taken to ensure that the diagnosis is, wherever possible, based on carefully executed diagnostic tests. Since most difficulty focuses on those patients in whom the biochemical defect is mildest, a provocative diagnostic test is indicated in all patients in whom glycosuria is not accompanied by unequivocally raised blood glucose concentrations (capillary blood glucose >11 mmol/liter, venous blood glucose >10 mmol/liter). Thus the finding of glycosuria can never in itself be diagnostic of diabetes mellitus but should just be one of several reasons why the diagnosis should be considered and further investigations instigated.

B. Blood Glucose Measurements

Despite continued efforts to find a better biochemical marker of diabetes mellitus, the concentration of glucose in the blood remains our best indication of the condition. One of the difficulties in obtaining international agreement on the diagnostic criteria for diabetes mellitus is the observation that in almost all epidemiological studies, blood glucose values appear to be unimodally distributed, albeit with a definite skew, the diabetic population appearing in this skew rather than forming a separate population. There is also a real tendency for average blood glucose to rise with age. It would seem that the only real epidemiological solution to this problem would be to construct a series of percentiles for population blood glucose by age (a universally agreed method used in determining normal growth and stature); it would then be a matter of mathematical precision as to what was within or without the 97th percentile range of normal for a given age. So far the epidemiologists have avoided this issue and have struggled to obtain international agreement as to what must be an arbitrary set of blood glucose values.* All the values used in this chapter are based on the WHO recommendations (16), and the classification of diabetes mellitus that they propose has also been adopted.

When considering glucose measurements in blood, care must be taken in distinguishing between plasma and whole blood glucose concentration and between capillary and venous blood. Whole blood glucose concentration is approximately 15% lower than plasma glucose, but the exact difference will vary with hematocrit; while capillary blood glucose is on average 7% higher than venous blood glucose in the fasting state (but much larger differences occur postprandially and during a glucose tolerance test). Wherever possible it is recommended that plasma glucose be measured. Methodological differences in glucose measurement do still exist but are less than in the past; glucose oxidase- and glucose dehydrogenase-based methods are the recommended techniques.

The use of "bedside" estimations of blood glucose has increased dramatically with the introduction of home blood glucose monitoring for diabetic patients and there are a number of enzyme-based reagent strips on the market which can be read by comparing the color against a color scale on the bottle or, more objectively, by reading the reflection from the strip in a special meter. With practice these methods are quick, cheap, and accurate, with a coefficient of variation of less than 12% (17). They are of considerable value in documenting an unequivocally raised blood glucose concentration, but undue reliance should not be placed on readings that are in the "gray area" between diabetes and normality. Even unequivocally raised values should be confirmed by an independent laboratory analysis before a firm diagnosis is made.

Random blood glucose is the most convenient since it can be done at any time and without any special preparation and can lead to an immediate and accurate diagnosis in a high proportion of cases in clinical practice, particularly if symptoms are present. *Fasting blood glucose* requires minimal preparation

---

*These were agreed to by a World Health Organization Expert Committee on Diabetes Mellitus and published in Technical Report 646 in 1980. They are in close agreement with the recommendations of the Diabetes Epidemiology Study Group of the European Association for the Study of Diabetes and to the National Institutes of Health Diabetes Data Group in the United States.

and is probably the most precise indication of the severity of the diabetic state because it is directly related to the degree of overproduction of glucose (see Sec. I.B). There is a gray area where it is difficult to distinguish normal from diabetic values, and in these cases an oral glucose tolerance test is recommended. Fasting blood glucose values are not necessary in patients who are symptomatic and who have a high random blood glucose measurement; in these cases, treatment should be started without delay. In noninsulin-treated cases, the fasting blood glucose will give the most accurate reflection of the success of treatment and is the most valuable reading for them to make at home.

C. Oral Glucose Tolerance Test

This dynamic test of glucose homeostasis has survived as the best (although by no means entirely satisfactory) stimulatory test of pancreatic endocrine function. It tests the body's ability to handle an unphysiological load of glucose and as such seems to be a remarkably effective measure of the secretory response of insulin-producing cells in the pancreas. Because the glucose response reflects whether or not the insulin response is adequate, it is rarely necessary to measure plasma insulin concentration during the test (just as measurement of cortisol during an insulin tolerance test in most instances eliminates the need to measure ACTH). The insulin response to oral glucose is always greater than that to the same dose given intravenously, despite much higher blood glucose concentration in the latter case. This is thought to be due to the concerted effects of the "enteroinsular axis," a term used to describe the secretion of other gastrointestinal hormones that are known to be able to modulate insulin secretion. Despite repeated claims to the contrary, diabetes mellitus remains a disease of insulin deficiency and the alterations in secretion of various components of the enteroinsular axis reflect this deficiency rather than cause it. In order to obtain valid and reproducible results from the oral glucose tolerance test, it is important to follow a standard protocol, which is dealt with in detail in Chapter 43.

The most important role of the oral glucose tolerance test in assessing pancreatic endocrine function occurs when the question of a diagnosis of diabetes mellitus has been raised but a random blood glucose or fasting blood glucose have failed to confirm or refute the diagnosis. It is essentially a diagnostic test that is more sensitive than the random or fasting blood glucose since it tests the maximal (or near-maximal) secretory capacity of the pancreas. It helps to resolve diagnostic difficulties that occur at the interface between normal and abnormal, but as one would expect from such a test, it is very susceptible to outside factors (such as previous nutrition; pyrexia; other illness, such as thyrotoxicosis; anxiety; etc.) and in patients in the borderline category is not highly reproducible. This lack of reproducibility is not a reflection of the inadequacy of the test but rather of the labile state of glucose metabolism under certain conditions (e.g., a normal person can have impaired glucose tolerance simply as a result of being 24 hr on a low-carbohydrate diet). Interpretation of slighly abnormal tests should be cautious and bear these points in mind. The WHO Expert Committee has recommended the use of the term "impaired glucose tolerance" for those with a mildly abnormal test, to avoid labeling these patients as "diabetic."

1. Classification of Diabetes Mellitus and Other Categories of Glucose Intolerance

The WHO Expert Committee has revised their recommended classification of diabetes mellitus in the light of long-term studies on the outcome of patients with mild degrees of glucose intolerance. In so doing they have incorporated the recommendations of the Diabetes Data Group of the National Institutes of Health in the United States.

The recommended simplified WHO classification is as follows:

1. *Clinical classes*
    - A. Diabetes mellitus
        1. Insulin-dependent, type 1
        2. Noninsulin-dependent, type 2
            - a. Nonobese
            - b. Obese
        3. Other types, including diabetes mellitus associated with certain conditions and syndromes: (1) pancreatic disease, (2) disease of hormonal etiology, (3) drug- or chemical-induced condition, (4) insulin receptor abnormalities, (5) certain genetic syndromes, (6) miscellaneous
    - B. Impaired glucose tolerance
        1. Nonobese
        2. Obese
        3. Associated with certain conditions and syndromes
    - C. Gestational diabetes
2. *Statistical risk classes* (subjects with normal glucose tolerance but substantially increased risk of developing diabetes)
    - A. Previous abnormality of glucose tolerance
    - B. Potential abnormality of glucose tolerance

D. Glucose Turnover Measurements

Although usually unnecessary for diagnostic purposes in clinical practice, the use of isotopically derived rates of glucose production and utilization have been available for many years but only recently have been widely accepted. There is no doubt about their technical ability to document the dynamic state of glucose in the body and they are to be recommended as investigative procedures when it is important to determine whether a high (or low) glucose concentration in the circulation is due to overproduction or underutilization (or vice versa) (18). They are also extremely helpful in the investigation of the mode of action of hormones (8, 11, 19) and newly introduced hormone analogs where the mode of action of the hormone may have been altered as a result of changes in structure (20). [^{3}H] 3-glucose seems to be the most widely accepted tracer for glucose, but if [^{14}C] glucose is used, its oxidation to $^{14}CO_2$ can readily be measured in the breath.

E. Ketone Bodies

The concentration of 3-hydroxybutyrate (3-OHB) and acetoacetate (AcAc) in plasma is primarily determined by, and gives an indirect measurement of, the rate of ketogenesis. Since 3-OHB and AcAc are in dynamic equilibrium,

$$\text{NAD} \quad \text{NADH}$$
$$\text{3-OHB} \rightleftharpoons \text{AcAc} + H^+$$

the equilibrium position of the reaction is dictated by the mitochondrial NADH/NAD ratio and the [H^+] concentration. In the blood of normal humans after an overnight fast the 3-OHB/AcAc ratio is approximately 1. The finding of an increased ratio indicates either an altered redox state or increased [H^+] or, most commonly, both. Ratios as high as 50:1 do occasionally occur.

Measurement of 3-hydroxybutyric and acetoacetate in blood is valuable in assessing the severity of metabolic disturbance in patients with diabetic ketoacidosis. Although the assays are technically quite straightforward, they are not widely available in routine laboratories, particularly on an emergency basis. Estimates of plasma acetoacetate can be made using Acetest tablets or Ketostix (plasma has to be diluted 1:1 with water before it will enter an Acetest tablet). The sensitivity of both techniques is approximately 1 mmol/liter acetoacetate. They do not react with the major ketone body 3-hydroxybutyrate and since on occasions, particularly in the presence of severe metabolic acidemia, the 3-hydroxybutyrate/acetoacetic ratio may be as high as 25:1, a negative plasma Acetest or Ketostix should not be taken as irrefutable evidence that any metabolic acidemia that is present must be something other than ketoacidosis. In the face of profound acidemia, even weak positive tests for acetoacetate indicate that it is almost certainly ketoacidosis. The important differential diagnosis is with lactic acidosis, and the diagnosis can only be made with certainty by direct measurement of ketone bodies and/or lactic acid concentrations.

F. Lactic Acid

The concentration of lactic acid in blood is determined by its production rate and disposal rate. A rise in blood lactic acid concentration may occur as a result of either overproduction of lactic acid (as associated with acute muscular exercise) and underutilization (phenformin-induced lactic acidosis), where conversion of lactate to pyruvate and hence either to glucose (gluconeogenesis) or $CO_2 + H_2O$ (oxidation) are inhibited. Lactate and pyruvate are in dynamic equilibrium, the position of the reaction being determined by the cytosolic redox state:

$$\text{Lactate} \overset{\text{NAD} \quad \text{NADH}}{\rightleftharpoons} \text{Pyruvate}$$

After an overnight fast, the lactate/pyruvate (L/P) ratio in normal humans is approximately 10:1 and the lactate concentration is approximately 1 mmol/liter. There are minor rises in lactate following meals, but in normal resting humans the concentration of lactate and the L/P ratio remain fairly constant. After exercise the lactate level may rise as high as 7 mmol/liter for a short time, the magnitude of the rise reflecting the extent of the exercise and the fitness of the individual. In lactic acidosis, lactate levels may rise as high as 25-30 mmol/liter and the L/P ratio to 50-100:1. Measurement of lactic acid is, like that of the ketoacids, quite straightforward but not widely available. There is as yet no "bedside test" for lactic acid, and if there are problems distinguishing the cause of a severe metabolic acidemia it is desirable to obtain an urgent analysis of lactic acid to distinguish lactic acidemia from ketoacidemia with a high 3-OHB/AcAc ratio. Lactate levels are often elevated in ketoacidosis (up to approximately 7 mmol/liter) but never to the values seen in lactic acidosis.

G. Free Fatty Acids

Free fatty acid concentrations in the plasma are determined primarily by rate of lipolysis of stored triglyceride in adipose tissue. These are transported bound to plasma albumin and rarely reach concentrations greater than 3 mmol/liter. They do not contribute significantly to the metabolic acidemia of uncontrolled diabetes. Free fatty acid uptake by tissues is determined by the plasma concentration; as with ketone bodies, uptake and production rate are closely related to plasma concentration.

H. Insulin

Insulin concentrations in plasma and other body fluids are measured by radioimmunoassay. Although there have been improvements over the 20 years that this assay has been available, it is still a difficult assay with poor reproducibility, particularly at the low levels seen in the fasting state. There have been difficulties due to the use of standards, but these have been ameliorated by adoption of an international standard. There is now general agreement that the average fasting insulin concentration in peripheral venous plasma from normal subject of ideal body weight is approximately 5 mU/liter (with a range of 1-12 mU/liter). Most radioimmunoassays do not distinguish proinsulin from insulin and in the fasting state much of this "apparent" insulin is in fact proinsulin. In healthy subjects given a 100-g oral glucose load, plasma insulin concentrations rise to an average peak figure of 50 mU/liter, but there is a very wide range of normal (20-250 mU/liter) (Fig. 4). The insulin responses between individuals show little if any correlation with the peak blood glucose concentrations reached. Thus in normal subjects the plasma glucose concentration is very tightly controlled by a very wide range of insulin responses. This represents different degrees of sensitivity to insulin between individuals, which is also reflected in their hypoglycemic response to exogenous insulin injection. Thus in Figure 4 the two extremes of the normal range are represented by two individuals, both of whom were able to keep their peak glucose below 8 mmol/liter, one with a rise in insulin from 4 to 20 mU/liter, the other with a rise from 4 to 250 mU/liter.

Fasting plasma insulin increases with obesity, as does the insulin response to oral glucose, only small differences in percentage ideal body weight accounting for considerable increases in insulin responses. For this reason it is always essential when examining insulin responses in any group of patients to ensure that the members of the control group are accurately matched for body weight and degree of obesity. Insulin concentrations also tend to increase with age in the nondiabetic population, so accurate age matching is important. Increased fasting plasma insulin is also seen in patients with acromegaly, Cushing's syndrome, hyperlipidemia, cirrhosis, and some exceedingly rare conditions with an insulin receptor defect.

In diabetes, fasting plasma insulin is usually within the range of normal, but the response to stimuli, particularly glucose, is impaired. There is a pattern of response that matches quite closely the severity of the disturbance in metabolism (see Table 1). These figures are all approximate and for nonobese patients with idiopathic diabetes mellitus and represent approximate responses to a 75-g oral glucose load.

It is sometimes stated that patients with noninsulin-dependent diabetes mellitus (NIDDM) have higher insulin values than do nondiabetic controls and

and the conclusion is drawn that NIDDM is therefore primarily a receptor or postreceptor disorder. These claims are usually found to be based on the comparison of an ill-defined population of NIDDM patients with variable degrees of obesity and unspecified prevalence of hyperlipidemia with a poorly matched group of younger, slimmer, and fitter controls (i.e., comparing apples with

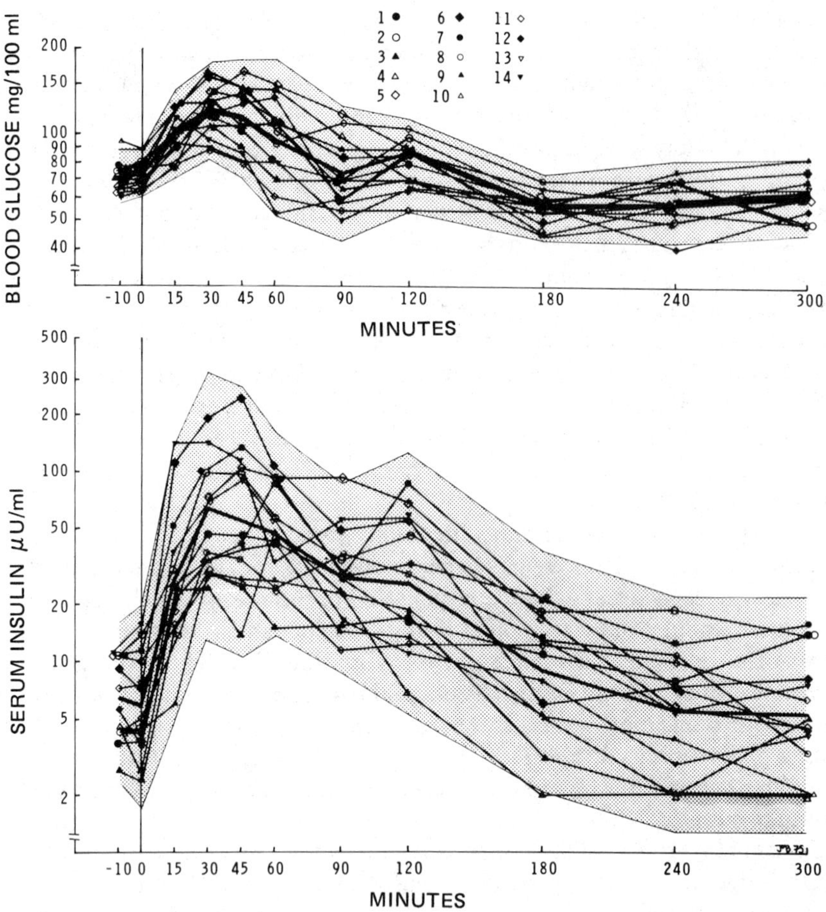

Figure 4 Blood glucose and serum insulin concentrations in 14 normal subjects during a 100-g oral glucose tolerance test. Data are presented on a logarithmic scale since all are log-normally distributed. Mean ±2 SD indicated by the heavy line and shading. (From Ref. 21.)

Table 1 Fasting Plasma Insulin and Glucose[a]

	Fasting		Peak		Time of peak (min)	
	G	I	G	I	G	I
Normal	4.5	5	6.5	50	30	45
↓						
Impaired glucose tolerance (IGT)	5	5	10	30	90	120
↓						
Diabetes mellitus (NIDDM)	10	5	30	10	120	150

[a]G, glucose, mmol/liter; I, insulin, mU/liter; NIDDM, noninsulin-dependent diabetes mellitus.

oranges). When controls are carefully matched and other possibly interfering diagnoses excluded (particularly hyperlipidemia), NIDDM is always associated with impaired insulin secretion.

The diminished insulin secretion in response to a glucose stimulus probably reflects two processes: (1) loss of β cells, and (2) loss of insulin storage in remaining β cells. Once there has been a rise in fasting blood glucose to 10 mmol/liter or greater, the β cells are near-maximally stimulated all the time and the fasting insulin concentration represents the near-maximal secretory capacity of the remaining β cells. It is not therefore surprising that there is little further rise with oral glucose. If this fasting plasma glucose is lowered with treatment, the remaining cells have the chance to regranulate and there is a return of an insulin response to oral glucose, albeit subnormal (Fig. 5).

In the case of secondary diabetes or impaired glucose tolerance (such as that seen with acromegaly) the insulin response is in proportion to the state of insulin resistance until glucose homeostasis is lost and there is a rise in fasting blood glucose. Once this occurs the insulin response to glucose disappears but can be restored by adequate treatment of the underlying condition (23, 24). If the condition is treated during the stage of impaired glucose tolerance, there is a fall in the insulin response as the glucose tolerance improves, indicating a reduction in the state of insulin resistance (25). In this way, the insulin response to glucose is a good index of the success of the therapy.

Assays of insulin in the plasma of insulin-treated patients is difficult because the majority of these patients have insulin-binding immunoglobulins in their plasma that: (1) interfere with radioimmunoassay, and (2) bind large amounts of insulin. It is possible to precipitate these immunoglobulins and their bound

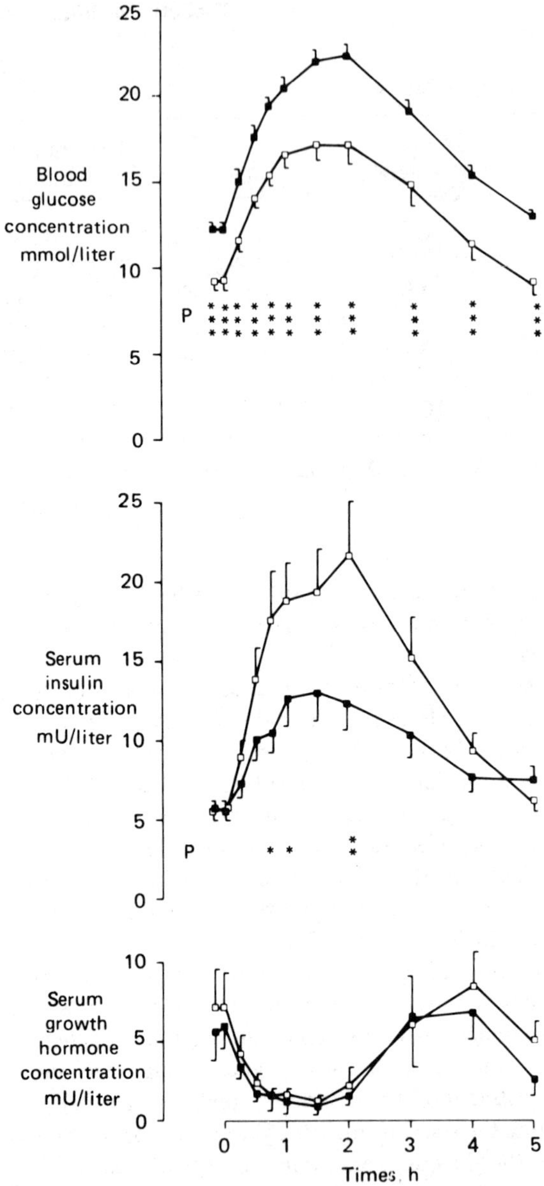

Figure 5 Oral glucose tolerance test showing glucose, insulin, and growth hormone concentrations in 35 diabetic patients before (closed box) and after (open box) a period of an average of 2 months dietary therapy. Results are given as mean ± standard error. The significance of the differences between tests is shown [*, $p < 0.05$; **$p < 0.01$; ***$p < 0.001$]. (From Ref. 22.)

insulin (with, e.g., polyethylene glycol) and measure "free" insulin in the immunoglobulin-free supernatant. Although in the right hands, these "free insulin" assays are valid, the uncertain nature and relevance of this measurement in terms of what is happening in the circulation limits its use to research procedures.

I. C Peptide

Since proinsulin is converted to insulin plus C-peptide during maturation of the β granule, one molecule of C peptide is always released at the time of insulin secretion. C peptide is immunologically quite distinct from insulin and in insulin-treated diabetic patients, who invariably have some antibodies to insulin in their circulation (which interfere with immunoassay of insulin), C-peptide measurements provide a valuable index of any residual β-cell secretory capacity.

C-peptide assays are essentially research procedures but have occasional clinical applications, such as in the diagnosis of iatrogenic hypoglycemia due to self-administration of insulin. In this case, plasma insulin concentration will be high (due to the injected insulin) but plasma C peptide undetectable (due to suppression of endogenous insulin secretion by hypoglycemia).

J. Islet Cell Antibodies

Using immunofluorescent techniques it is possible to demonstrate that a high proportion of newly diagnosed insulin-dependent diabetic patients have a circulating immunoglobulin that binds to islet cells in vitro (all cells). Recently, it has been shown that these antibodies may be present for some time before the onset of diabetes. The antibodies persist for a variable period after the onset of the clinical syndrome. Although largely a research procedure, it seems that it may in the future have limited prognostic value in assessing susceptibility to diabetes mellitus.

K. HLA Tissue Typing

Insulin-dependent diabetes mellitus occurs more (or less) frequently than would be expected by chance alone in patients with certain patterns of HLA antigens (e.g., DRW3 and DRW4 are found more commonly than expected in insulin-dependent diabetic patients).

In prospective studies it has been shown that siblings who inherit one of the susceptible haplotypes are more likely to develop diabetes and, as such, it has become an accepted "risk factor" when considering the likelihood of developing the disease (26).

Diagnostic Summary 1 Diabetes Mellitus

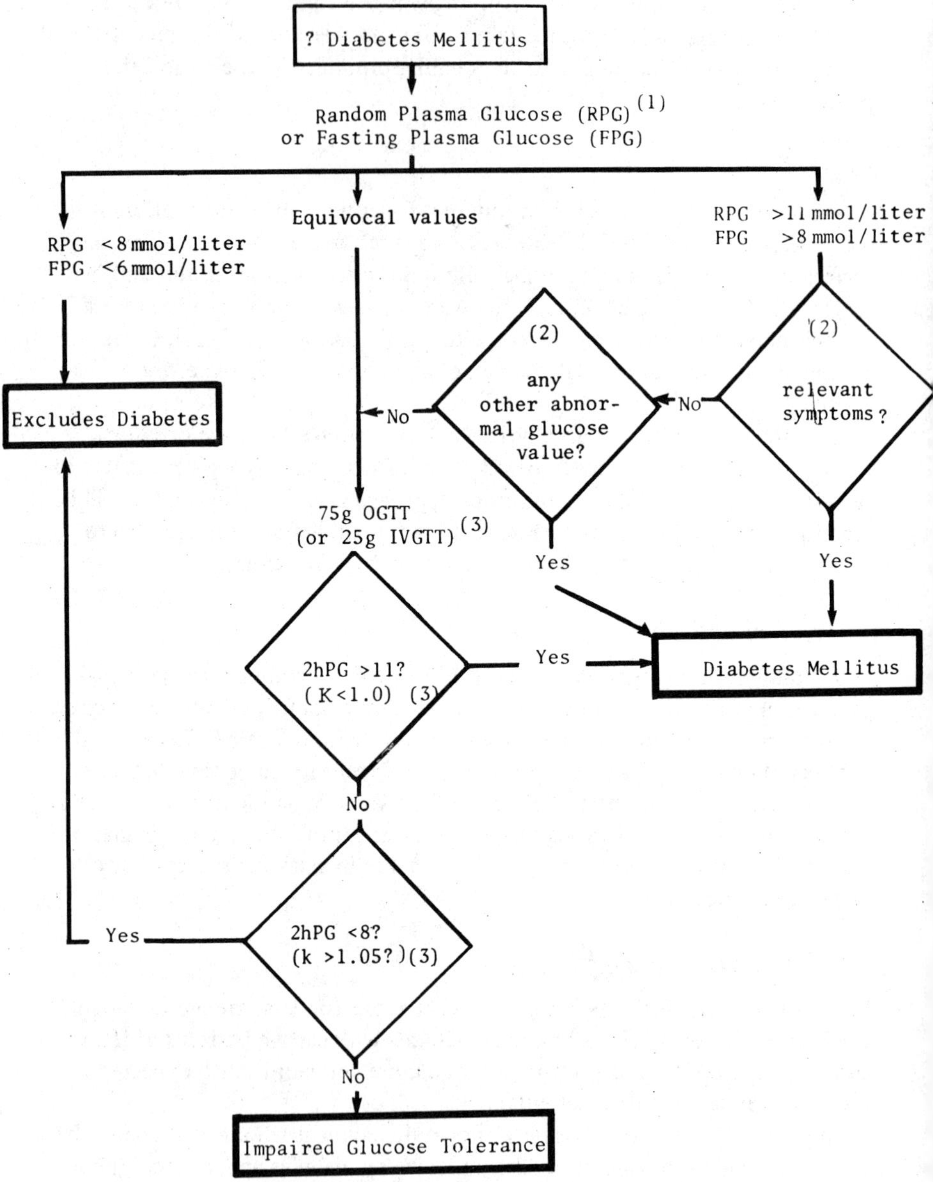

1. *Random plasma glucose* (RPG). All values in this table are given in terms of venous *plasma* glucose concentrations, based on the WHO recommendations. Criteria for whole blood glucose concentrations are 1 mmol/liter lower in all cases.
2. *Relevant symptoms.* The WHO recommends that even when unequivocally raised plasma glucose values are found on one occasion, a glucose tolerance test should be used to confirm the diagnosis unless other unequivocally abnormal values have been recorded on another occasion.
3. *Intravenous glucose tolerance test* (IVGTT). Although not included in the WHO recommendations, there are occasions where additional information might be obtained from intravenous rather than oral glucose tolerance tests. The criteria used here are based on a 25-g IVGTT and are those originally recommended by Lundbaek (27). More details are given in Chapter 43.

Note that urine tests are not referred to at all in establishing the diagnosis of diabetes mellitus. The finding of glycosuria on routine testing may be one of the (many) reasons why a possible diagnosis of diabetes mellitus may be considered.

REFERENCES

1. Major RH. *Classic Description of Disease*, 3rd ed. Blackwell, Oxford. 1948.
2. Brunner JC. In *Experimenta Nova Circa Pancreas*, Amstelaedami, 1683. (Available in the Library of the Royal Society of Medicine and Royal College of Physicians, London.)
3. Schäfer EA. *The Endocrine Organs.* Longmans, London, 1916; p. 128.
4. Paulescou NC. Recherches sur le rôle du pancréas dans l'assimilation nutrive. Arch Intern Physiol 1921; 17:85–109.
5. Banting FG, Best CH. The internal secretion of the pancreas. J Lab Clin Med 1922; 7:251–266.
6. Sönksen PH. The evolution of insulin treatment. J Clin Endocrinol Metab 1977; 6:481–497.
7. Issekutz B Jr, Issekutz TB, Elahi D, Borkow I. Effect of insulin infusions on the glucose kinetics in alloxan-streptozotocin dogs. Diabetologia 1974; 10:323–328.
8. Brown PM, Tompkins CV, Juul SM, Sönksen PH. Mechanism of action of insulin in diabetic patients: a dose-related effect on glucose production and utilisation. Br Med J 1978; 1:1239–1242.
9. Sönksen PH, Brown PM. Control of diabetic ketosis. In *Topics in Therapeutics*, Vere DW (ed). Pitman Medical, Marshfield, Mass, 1978; vol 4, pp 176–190.

10. Joslin EP. Diabetic Metabolism with high and low diets. Carnegie Institute, Washington, DC, 1923, Publ No 323.
11. Hall SEH, Saunders J, Sönksen PH. Glucose and free fatty acid turnover in normal subjects and in diabetic patients before and after insulin treatment. Diabetologia 1979; 16:297–306.
12. Randle PJ, Hales CN, Garland PB, Newsholme EA. The glucose-fatty acid cycle. Its role in insulin sensitivity and the metabolic disturbance of diabetes mellitus. Lancet 1963; 1:785–789.
13. Barnes AJ, Bloom SR, Alberti KGMM, Smythe P, Alford FP, Chisholm DJ. Ketoacidosis in pancreatectomized man. N Engl J Med 1977; 296: 1250–1253.
14. Schade DS, Eaton RP. The controversy concerning counter regulatory hormone secretion. An hypothesis for the prevention of diabetic ketoacidosis? Diabetes 1977; 26:596–601.
15. Saunders J, Hall SEH, Sönksen PH. Thyroid hormones in insulin requiring diabetes before and after treatment. Diabetologia 1978; 15:29–32.
16. WHO Expert Committee on Diabetes Mellitus (second report). Tech Rep Ser 646. World Health Organization, Geneva, 1980.
17. West TET, Judd SL, Sönksen PH. Evaluation in clinical practice of Dextrostix and Eyetone reflectance meter. Diabete Metab (Paris) 1977; 2:165–167.
18. Wilson NM, Brown PM, Juul SM, Prestwich SA, Sönksen PH. Glucose turnover and metabolic and hormonal changes in ethanol-induced hypoglycemia. Br Med J 1981; 282:849–853.
19. Gündogdu AS, Brown PM, Juul SM, Sachs L, Sönksen PH. Comparison of hormonal and metabolic effects of salbutamol infusion in normal subjects and insulin-requiring diabetics. Lancet 1979; 2:1317–1321.
20. Tompkins CV, Brandenburg D, Jones RH, Sönksen PH. Mechanism of action of insulin and insulin analogues: a comparison of the hepatic and peripheral effects on glucose turnover of insulin, proinsulin and three insulin analogues modified at positions A_1 and B_{29}. Diabetologia 1981; 20:94–101.
21. Sönksen PH. Double-antibody technique for the simultaneous assay of insulin and growth hormone. In *Hormones in Human Blood*, Antoniades HN (ed). Harvard University Press, Cambridge, Mass, 1976; pp 176–199.
22. Perkins JR, West TET, Sönksen PH, Lowy C, Iles C. The effects of energy and carbohydrate restriction in patients with chronic diabetes mellitus. Diabetologia 1977; 13:607–614.
23. Sönksen PH, Greenwood FC, Ellis JP, Lowy C, Rutherford A, Nabarro JDN. Changes of carbohydrate tolerance in acromegaly with progress of the disease and in response to treatment. J Clin Endocrinol Metab 1967; 27:1418–1430.
24. Sönksen PH. Aetiology and epidemiology of diabetes. Br J Hosp Med 1972; 7:151–156.

25. Sönksen PH. Clinical application of growth hormone assays. J R Coll Physicians Lond 1974; 8:220–236.
26. Cudworth AG. Type I diabetes mellitus. Diabetologia 1978; 14:281–291.
27. Lundbaek K. Intravenous glucose tolerance as a tool in definition and diagnosis of diabetes mellitus. Br Med J 1962; 1:1507–1513.

32

Pancreatic and Gastrointestinal Hormone-Secreting Tumors

Susan M. Wood and S. R. Bloom
Royal Postgraduate Medical School and Hammersmith Hospital, London, England

Since the discovery of secretin in 1902 an increasing number of gastrointestinal hormones have been identified. Many of these peptides have now been localized to both endocrine cells and to neurones, in the gastrointestinal tract, central nervous system, and other tissues (1). Their common neuroendocrine localization suggests that these peptides may act by endocrine, neurocrine, and paracrine mechanisms to regulate a wide variety of physiological processes.

The influence of disease on this peptide regulatory system and its derangement as the cause of disease are at present ill understood. Much information has come from hypersecretion of peptides from tumors (2), and these will be considered here because of their considerable clinical importance. Most recorded cases of gastrointestinal endocrine tumors have been documented during the last 20 years. This reflects the advent of sensitive radioimmunological techniques for measurement of peptides in plasma and tissue and the increasing awareness of tumor-related endocrine syndromes.

The endocrine tumors of the gut have been linked together, because of their common derivation from cells with APUD (amine precursor uptake and decarboxylation) characteristics. Such cells have similar ultrastructural and cytochemical features and possibly a common embryological origin (3). A glycolytic enzyme, neuron-specific enolase, has recently been found to be present in these cells, and is likely to be a further useful marker of neuroendocrine cells and their tumors.

These tumors (Table 1), apart from the carcinoids, are found most commonly in the pancreas. The peptides they secrete are the normal products of the cells of the islets of Langerhans—the A, B, D, and PP cells, which contain glucagon,

Table 1 Characteristics of Gut Endocrine Tumors

Name	Cell type	Hormone	Site	Benign (%)	Single (%)	MEA I[a] found in association (%)
Insulinoma	B	Insulin	Pancreas	95	90	5
Gastrinoma	G	Gastrin	Pancreas; occasionally in duodenum and stomach	40	30	25
Glucagonoma	A	Glucagon	Pancreas	40	70	5
Vipoma		Vasoactive intestinal peptide	(15–20% extra pancreatic ganglioneuroblastomas)	50	60	5
Somatostatinoma	D	Somatostatin	Pancrease, small intestine	10	60	5
PPoma	?	Pancreatic polypeptide	Pancreas	25	60	15
Neurotensinoma	NT	Neurotensin	Pancreas, sympathetic chain	50	85	10
Carcinoid	EC	5-Hydroxytriptamine Kallikrein Substance P	Large and small intestine, stomach, lung	>90	–	10

[a]Multiple endocrine adenoma, type I.

insulin, somatostatin, and pancreatic polypeptide, respectively. Tumors of each of these cell types have been described (5,6). It has been suggested, however, that these tumors originate not from islet cells but from multipotent stem cells (nesidioblasts) in the ductules, which differentiate into various types of peptide-producing cells (6). This would explain why many tumors contain more than one type of endocrine cell and often produce several peptides, and how the secretory product of a tumor can change with time, during treatment, or that metastases can contain only some of the original cells (7). It is therefore important to screen the plasma of patients for many peptides, as the biochemical marker for the primary tumor may vary and differ from that for the metastases.

I. RADIOIMMUNOASSAY

This technique allows accurate diagnosis of the tumor hypersecretory syndromes.

A. Collection of Samples

A number of precautions are necessary to obtain reliable results. Since plasma contains proteolytic enzymes, an enzyme inhibitor such as aprotonin (Trasylol) 200 μl per 10 ml whole blood should be used to reduce peptide degradation. The plasma should be separated within 15 min of venepuncture and stored frozen (−20°C) until assay. Thawing and freezing can cause significant loss of peptide activity, particularly of vasoactive intestinal peptide (VIP) and neurotensin, and must be avoided. Most gastrointestinal peptides are elevated by food; therefore fasting samples are necessary. Although uncommon among gut endocrine tumors, peptide release may be intermittent and therefore samples should be taken on several different occasions.

B. Assay Specificity

The specificity of the antibody used in radioimmunoassay is crucial. Antibodies with different regional specificities for a molecule can produce different results. There may be antibody cross-reaction between peptides of similar structure to the peptide to be measured, resulting in misleading high values for a peptide. Plasma constituents such as gamma globulins can also interfere. It is therefore important for samples to be measured by an experienced laboratory before important decisions regarding patient management are made on the basis of the result.

C. Normal Ranges of Fasting Plasma Peptides

Each laboratory has its own normal range for a particular peptide; any samples falling above this should be repeated, together with a further fresh sample. The normal upper limits of fasting plasma concentrations for our laboratory, which provides a screening assay service for tumors in the United Kingdom, are shown in Table 2. Positive diagnosis of a tumor, however, would require higher values and other criteria.

D. Nontumorous Causes of Elevation of Plasma Peptides

Certain conditions may give rise to high plasma peptide levels unrelated to tumors. For example, the achlorhydria of pernicious anemia or atrophic gastritis, both fairly common conditions, result in grossly elevated plasma gastrin levels, usually far exceeding those seen in the Zollinger-Ellison syndrome (8). Plasma gastrin is slightly elevated by gastric ulcer disease, after vagotomy, and during treatment with antacids and H_2 receptor antagonists (9). Serious illness is found nonspecifically to elevate peptides each as PP and glucagon, while acute tissue ischemia and systematic shock raises plasma VIP. Plasma levels of peptides excreted and metabolized by the kidney (e.g., PP) are increased by renal failure. Such factors may lead to an incorrect diagnosis and inappropriate investigation, with serious consequences for the patient.

E. Molecular Forms of Peptides

Many tumors synthesize two or more molecular forms of a given peptide (10), which can exhibit different biological activity compared to the naturally found peptide. These forms are best characterized by column chromatography. It is of interest that certain drugs, such as streptozotocin and metoclopramide, have been reported to alleviate symptoms in the watery diarrhea, hypokalemia achlorhydria (WDHA) syndrome by suppressing tumor production of the active peptide while leaving still elevated the plasma level of the inactive form (11).

Table 2 Normal Fasting Plasma Peptide Concentrations

Peptide	Fasting plasma concentrations (pmol/liter)
Glucagon	<30
Vasoactive intestinal peptide (VIP)	<30
Gastrin	<40
Pancreatic polypeptide (PP)	<200
Somatostatin	<100
Neurotensin	<50

II. SPECIFIC GUT TUMORS

This section describes the pathophysiology, clinical features, and diagnostic criteria for the main gut endocrine tumors. Early diagnosis is essential for surgical cure, but this requires a high index of suspicion often when the full clinical syndrome has not become manifest.

A. Glucagonoma

1. Pathophysiology

There are now some 90 cases of these pancreatic tumors reported in the literature (12,13). Although slow growing, 60% are malignant.

The clinical and biochemical features of the glucagonoma syndrome are due to the effects of glucagon released from the tumor. This readily explains the impaired glucose tolerance of these patients; it is of interest that their diabetes is mild with no complications of the disease, suggesting that glucagon plays little role in the etiology of these complications. The pathological basis for the necrolytic migratory rash is unknown. It is likely that the low plasma and tissue concentrations of amino acids and zinc secondary to hyperglucagonemia are in some way responsible (12).

2. Clinical Features

Most patients present in middle age and have mild diabetes and a characteristic skin rash, the necrolytic migratory erythema. Often both of these features have been present for months or years before the diagnosis is made. Less commonly, there is no specific clinical syndrome, the diagnosis being made during investigation of a patient with a pancreatic tumor or hepatic metastases, or with the pluriglandular syndrome.

The rash is the most useful diagnostic feature. It is characterized by bullous erythematous lesions, which form erosions and crusts, most commonly over the abdomen, groin, perineum, buttocks, and distal parts of the lower limbs. The edge of the lesions tend to migrate outward, while the center heals with pigmentation. Secondary infection may alter the picture and the rash can be confused with atypical psoriasis, pemphigus, and eczema. Most patients have angular stomatitis, glossitis, and a perioral rash. Abnormal glucose tolerance is common; the resultant diabetes is usually mild, controlled by diet or oral hypoglycemic agents. Other features of the disease include a normochromic, normocytic anemia present in most patients, and venous thrombosis in 30% of cases. There have been no reports of thrombophlebitis migrans. Weight loss, perhaps secondary to the catabolic effect of glucagon, is variable, but some patients become severely cachectic. Psychiatric disturbances, most frequently depression, are frequent. Much less common features include diarrhea and neurological deficit (12, 13).

3. Diagnostic Tests

The diagnosis is suspected on clinical grounds; an elevated fasting plasma glucagon (>30 pmol/liter) should lead to a search for a pancreatic tumor. The other biochemical abnormalities mentioned below support but are not essential for the diagnosis.

Glucose Tolerance. These patients have impaired or frankly diabetic glucose tolerance. Oral glucose results in an anomalous rise in plasma glucagon, in contrast to the suppression normally seen. Intravenous glucose, however, lowers or leaves plasma glucagon unchanged (13).

Amino Acids. Plasma levels of glucogenic and ketogenic amino acids are much reduced. Iatrogenic hyperglucagonemia is the only other situation in which such low levels are seen. Measurement of a single amino acid, such as alanine which is particularly low, can be helpful in patients with atypical dermatoses or marginally elevated glucagon levels (14).

Zinc. The plasma and tissue zinc concentrations are lower than normal. This has been suggested to be due to zinc uptake by the tumor for the synthesis of glucagon. Zinc deficiency impairs tissue healing and is likely to be one of the factors contributing to the necrolytic migratory erythema (12, 13). A similar rash is seen in acrodermatitis enteropathica and prolonged intravenous feeding, in both of which zinc deficiency occurs.

Skin Biopsy. Biopsy of the edge of a fresh lesion shows the diagnostic features of necrosis and lysis of the epidermis with a normal dermis. There is no suggestion of an immune basis for the rash; antiepithelial antibodies to cellular components or basement membrane are not seen on indirect immunofluorescence (12).

Arginine and Somatostatin. These have been used as research tools to investigate the secretory patterns of tumors. The responses of individual patients are variable, and as such we feel that these tests are not necessary or useful in diagnosis. We mention them for interest.

Arginine (0.5 g/kg infused intravenously over 30 min) results in a much greater release of glucagon, but less marked rise in insulin in patients with glucagon-secreting tumors compared to normal subjects (13,14).

Somatostatin, a peptide that suppresses the release of many hormones, in glucagonoma patients often reduces glucagon secretion more than insulin, and so produces hypoglycemia. A slowly increasing infusion of somatostatin (0.5, 2.0, 5.0, and 20.0 μg/min each for 1 hr) is used. Side effects include mild nausea, abdominal discomfort, and postural hypotension. In a number of patients with malignant tumors we have observed no suppression of glucagon release by somatostatin.

4. Differential Diagnosis (See Table 3)

Table 3 Differential Diagnosis of the Cutaneous Hyperglycemia Syndrome

Differential diagnosis	Distinguishing features
Pemphigus, infected eczema, psoriasis, candidiasis, epidermolysis, bullosa	No other features of glucagonoma syndrome; skin biopsy shows features of appropriate skin disease
Acrodermatitis enteropathica	Early onset in life; plasma glucagon not elevated
Glucagonoma	Elevated plasma glucagon, anemia, cachexia, etc.; pancreatic tumor

B. Insulinoma

1. Pathophysiology

The features of this islet cell tumor are a consequence of insulin-induced hypoglycemia. The presenting symptoms are commonly mistaken for other diseases, leading to delayed diagnosis. However, the tumors are usually benign and cure is limited only by resectability (15).

2. Clinical Features

Symptoms are extremely variable; they include those commonly associated with mild hypoglycemia—sweating, pallor, palpitations, and perioral paresthesiae—which then may progress to confusion, convulsions, and coma. Alternatively, patients present with features of other disorders, in particular those of neurological or cardiovascular disease (15).

Bizarre behavior as a consequence of acute or chronic neuroglycopenia has, not surprisingly, led to diagnoses of psychiatric illness.

3. Diagnostic Tests

The diagnosis depends on the demonstration of symptoms in the presence of hypoglycemia (glucose <2.2 mmol/liter) with an inappropriately high plasma insulin concentration (>15 mU/liter).

Fasting Insulin Concentration. The safest way of inducing hypoglycemia is by a 12- to 14-hr fast. More prolonged fasting may sometimes be required, and to further lower the glucose concentration the patient is encouraged to exercise under supervision, with free access to water. In children a ketogenic diet may provoke fasting hypoglycemia and is less traumatic than total starvation (16). An indwelling venous cannula is advisable to enable rapid intravenous glucose to be given once a sample for insulin has been taken.

Proinsulin and C Peptide. These are used as alternatives to plasma insulin, and also help in the diagnosis of factitious hypoglycemia. High levels of proinsulin and C peptide are strongly indicative of endogenous hyperinsulinism. Administration of exogenous insulin also raises proinsulin, but can be distinguished by a low C-peptide concentration. Sulfonylurea-induced hyperinsulinemia raises proinsulin, C-peptide, and insulin levels (17,18), and therefore drug levels are required if this is suspected.

Insulin Tolerance Tests. These are used to demonstrate failure of insulin suppression, diagnostic of these tumors, only when fasting has not done so (see Chap. 44). Other provocation tests, such as intravenous glucagon, tolbutamide, and oral leucine are no longer used; the results were difficult to interpret and the procedures often produce dangerous hypoglycemia.

4. Differential Diagnosis (See Table 4)

C. Gastrinoma (Zollinger-Ellison Syndrome)

1. Pathophysiology

In this condition high levels of circulating gastrin secreted from a pancreatic tumor result in gastric acid hypersecretion and consequently severe peptic ulceration poorly responsive to treatment (19). A similar clinical picture may rarely result from G-cell hyperplasia, which is diagnosed by antral biopsy (20). When the tumor occurs as part of the multiendocrine adenomatoses, hypercalcemia secondary to primary hyperparathyroidism exacerbates the hypergastrinemia. Parathyroidectomy results in only short-lived improvement in gastrin levels. Gastrinomas have a high incidence of malignancy and are seldom single tumors; surgical excision is therefore effective in less than 5% of cases.

2. Clinical Features

Primary jejunal and severe complicated recurrent duodenal ulceration are said to be characteristic of the Zollinger-Ellison syndrome (19). Tumors are often slow growing and some patients have mild symptoms for many years before requiring their first operation. The mean time for recurrence of ulcers reported by Stage and Stadil was 4.2 years; in the majority of patients the ulcer disease is therefore not classically fulminant (20). The diagnosis should always be suspected in patients with severe ulcer symptoms in their teens, or who develop initial ulcer symptoms late in life. Persistent diarrhea occurs in about one-third of patients; significant constipation may indicate the presence of an associated parathyroid adenoma, causing hypercalcemia.

3. Diagnostic Tests

Both hypergastrinemia and gastric acid hypersecretion are necessary for diagnosis of a gastrinoma in a patient presenting with recurrent peptic ulceration (20).

Table 4 Differential Diagnosis of Fasting Hypoglycemia

Differential diagnosis	Distinguishing features
Liver disease	Other features of liver disease
Adrenal disease	Other features of hypoadrenalism, low plasma cortisol, inadequate response to stimulation tests
Hypopituitarism	Features of hypopituitarism; abnormal pituitary function
Nonpancreatic tumors (retroperitoneal sarcoma, hepatocellular carcinoma)	Plasma insulin not usually elevated; tumor usually large and commonly retroperitoneal
Glycogen storage disease (von Gierke's disease)	Deficiency of glucose-6-phosphatase on liver biopsy
Factitious hypoglycemia due to insulin, oral hypoglycemic agents	High levels of insulin compared with C peptide; elevated plasma sulfonylurea levels
Insulinoma	Inappropriate levels of plasma insulin in the presence of hypoglycemia

Pentagastrin Stimulation Test (see Chap. 44 for details). In Zollinger-Ellison syndrome there is both hypersecretion of gastric juice and hyperacidity. The pentagastrin-stimulated secretion is often not much higher than the basal (20).

Plasma Calcium, Phosphate, and Parathormone. One-fourth of these patients have primary hyperparathyroidism (9); their hypercalcemia acts as a constant stimulus to gastrin secretion. Parathyroidectomy is often performed prior to pancreatic surgery but it tends only temporarily to relieve the hypergastrinemia.

Gastroscopy. Multiple ulcers may be present in unusual locations, such as the second or third portion of the duodenum and beyond the ligament of Treitz. The latter presentation occurs in about one-fifth of patients and has been regarded as pathognomonic of the Zollinger-Ellison syndrome (20). The gastric mucosa is thickened and folded; there is, however, no antral G-cell hyperplasia. The duodenum is often enlarged with a cobblestone appearance to the mucosa due to hyperplasia of Brunner's glands.

Secretion Test (see Chap. 44 for details). Patients with gastrinomas respond by a prompt rise in plasma gastrin of at least 50% of the basal value (20); normally, secretin lowers plasma gastrin. The criteria for interpretation of positive secretin test responses (9,21) vary in the literature, owing probably to lack of conformity in the procedure and dosage used. The test's diagnostic value has therefore not been adequately assessed.

Calcium Infusion (see Chap. 44 for details). In 80% of gastrinoma patients there is doubling of fasting gastrin levels by the fourth hour (20).

4. Differential Diagnosis (See Tables 5 and 6)

D. Vipoma [Synonyms: Watery Diarrhea, Hypokalemia, Achlorohydria (WDHA Syndrome); Pancreatic Cholera; Verner-Morrison Syndrome]

1. Pathophysiology

VIP-producing tumors are either pancreatic in origin or ganglioneuroblastomas, the latter occurring mainly in children. The majority of the pancreatic tumors are malignant and have metastasized to the liver by the time of diagnosis, while the childhood tumors are commonly benign. VIP, a 28-amino acid peptide, is widely found in the peripheral and central nervous system; its biological actions include stimulation of intestinal secretion, vasodilatation, stimulation of glycogenolysis, and production of hypercalcemia, which amply explains the clinical features found in the WDHA syndrome (22).

2. Clinical Features

Watery diarrhea of more than 1 liter per day is universally found at some stage in these patients. About half report intermittent diarrhea, but as the disease progresses the diarrhea tends to become continuous, although malabsorption and steatorrhea are rare. The diarrhea results in dehydration, which can be severe,

Table 5 Differential Diagnosis of Intractable Peptic Ulceration

Differential diagnosis	Distinguishing features
Recurrent duodenal ulceration	Mild or no elevation of plasma gastrin
Hyperparathyroidism	High plasma calcium and parathormone, low phosphate; cure by parathyroidectomy, but often gastrinoma associated
G-cell hyperplasia	Diagnosed on gastroscopic biopsy; no tumor found
Gastrinoma (Zollinger-Ellison syndrome)	Hyperacidity and inappropriately elevated plasma gastrin; pancreatic or rarely gastroduodenal tumor

Table 6 Differential Diagnosis of Persistent Severe Diarrhea

Differential diagnosis	Distinguishing features
Parasitic and infectious diseases	Positive blood and stool culture, ova, parasites
Inflammatory bowel disease	Characteristic barium follow-through, enema, and sigmoidoscopic biopsy
Coeliac disease	Malabsorption; characteristic villous atrophy
Villous adenoma	Seen on barium enema or sigmoidoscopic or colonoscopic biopsy
Purgative abuse	Psychological problems; elevated plasma or stool levels of purgatives
Zollinger-Ellison syndrome	Recurrent peptic ulcers; hyperacidity and hypergastrinemia
Carcinoid syndrome	Flushing, wheeze, etc.; elevated urinary 5-HIAA
Medullary carcinoma of thyroid	Thyroid tumor; elevated plasma calcitonin
Ganglioneuroblastoma	More common in children; elevated plasma VIP; tumor of neural origin found
Pancreatic vipoma	Elevated plasma VIP; pancreatic tumor

leading to acute tubular necrosis. Fecal loss of electrolytes results in hypokalemia, with the symptoms of lethargy, muscular weakness, nausea, vomiting, abdominal pain, and less commonly myocardial damage, leading to congestive cardiac failure. Loss of weight is common and this is not explained by dehydration alone. Facial flushing and impaired glucose tolerance are less common features of the syndrome. Tetany with hypercalcemia, perhaps due to hypomagnesemia, has been reported in four patients. Gallstones occur with increased frequency and this is perhaps related to the gallbladder dilatation and impaired bile concentration which VIP produces (22,23).

3. Diagnostic Tests

The diagnosis is made on the clinical features in the presence of an elevated plasma VIP concentration ($>$30 pmol/liter). The plasma VIP range reported for a series of VIP-producing tumors was 48-760 pmol/liter, with a mean of 203 ± 17 pmol/liter (22). Other features suggestive of the diagnosis are listed below.

Electrolyte Disturbance. Hypokalemic acidosis is frequent, due to potassium and bicarbonate loss in the stools. Plasma potassium and bicarbonate concentrations of <2.5 and <15 mmol/liter, respectively, have been reported in over 80% of patients (22). Raised plasma urea is usually indicative of dehydration. Both hypercalcemia and hypophosphatemia are common.

Achlorhydria. Although named as one of the major features of the WDHA syndrome, it probably occurs in less than half of the patients (22).

Abnormal Glucose Tolerance. This is sometimes seen, either secondary to pancreatic disease or due to VIP's stimulation of glycogenolysis.

Prednisolone Test. Prednisolone, 30–40 mg daily given orally, will suppress VIP-induced diarrhea. The mechanism is unknown, and escape from its effects occurs within a few weeks.

4. Differential Diagnosis (See Table 6)

E. PPoma

Pancreatic polypeptide hypersecretion has not been found to produce any specific clinical features. PP is produced in about half the pancreatic tumors where the other peptides are responsible for symptoms (24).

F. Somatostatinoma

Since 1979, when six somatostatinomas were reviewed by Krejs et al. (25), a further nine have appeared in the literature. All tumors were found in the pancreas; in most of these hepatic metastases were also present. The clinical symptoms common to all patients were weight loss, mild diabetes, and abdominal discomfort. Cholelithiasis, diarrhea, steatorrhea, and hypochlorhydria were seen in over 75% of patients, all of which can be explained by the pharmacological actions of somatostatin. The diagnosis is difficult with such a nonspecific presentation and will depend on a clinical suspicion and elevated plasma somatostatin concentration (26).

G. Other Peptide-Producing Tumors

Many tumors produce several peptides; neurotensin has recently been added to the list; in one series 11% of vipomas also secreted neurotensin (27). Other peptides frequently released by gut endocrine tumors include calcitonin, adrenocorticotropic hormone (ACTH) and thyroid releasing hormone (TRH) (7, 28).

H. Carcinoid

1. Pathophysiology

Carcinoids include a heterogenous group of tumors, producing a number of different active substances. Those in the midgut secrete 5-hydroxytryptamine

(5-HT), metastasize primarily to the liver, and produce the classic carcinoid syndrome. Those in the hindgut characteristically do not release biologically active substances, while those in the foregut secrete 5-hydroxytryptophan (5-HTP) because they lack the decarboxylase enzyme. These also produce a number of other neuroendocrine peptides; they tend to metastasize to skin and bone and result in an atypical carcinoid syndrome. Some features of the carcinoid syndrome can be explained by the actions of 5-HT; however, other substances, such as bradykinin and prostaglandins, are also likely to be involved (29).

2. Clinical Features

The features of the carcinoid syndrome include flushing, diarrhea, endocardial fibrosis, and bronchospasm, in order of frequency (29). There is usually no temporal relationship between symptoms such as flushing and diarrhea, suggesting that these have different humoral mediators. The duration, frequency, and color of the flush vary considerably depending on the site of the tumor. Lacrimation, facial swelling, and hypotension accompany severe episodes, especially in association with foregut tumors. Certain foods, excitement, or anxiety can precipitate attacks. In long-standing cases, reddening of the skin becomes permanent. In a few cases a pellagra-type syndrome develops because of diversion of tryptophan from nicotinamide to 5-HT synthesis (29).

The fibrotic lesions seen on the cardiac valves also occur on the pericardium pleura and peritoneum; these are often asymptomatic until a late stage in the disease.

3. Diagnostic Tests

Urinary 5-Hydroxyindoleacetic Acid (5-HIAA), 5-HT, and 5-HTP. The urinary excretion of 5-HIAA, the breakdown product of 5-HT, is greatly increased (>130 μmol per day is diagnostic). Tomatoes, pineapples, plums, walnuts, and bananas, which all contain 5-HT, should be excluded from the diet for 24 hr before a collection. If 5-HIAA excretion is normal in the presence of strong clinical evidence for the carcinoid syndrome, total 5-hydroxyindole excretion, which includes 5-HT, 5-HIAA, and 5-HTP, should be estimated. Plasma and whole blood 5-HT concentrations can be diagnostic when there is only a marginally raised 5-HIAA urinary excretion. Rauwolfia alkaloids, imipramine, and heparin lower blood 5-HT and should be discontinued prior to its measurement (29).

Provocation Tests. Oral alcohol, and infusions of calcium, glucagon, and epinephrine, have been used to provoke the carcinoid flush. All of these except epinephrine provoke similar responses in patients with medullary carcinoma of the thyroid.

4. Differential Diagnosis (See Table 6)

Diagnostic Summary 1 Insulinoma

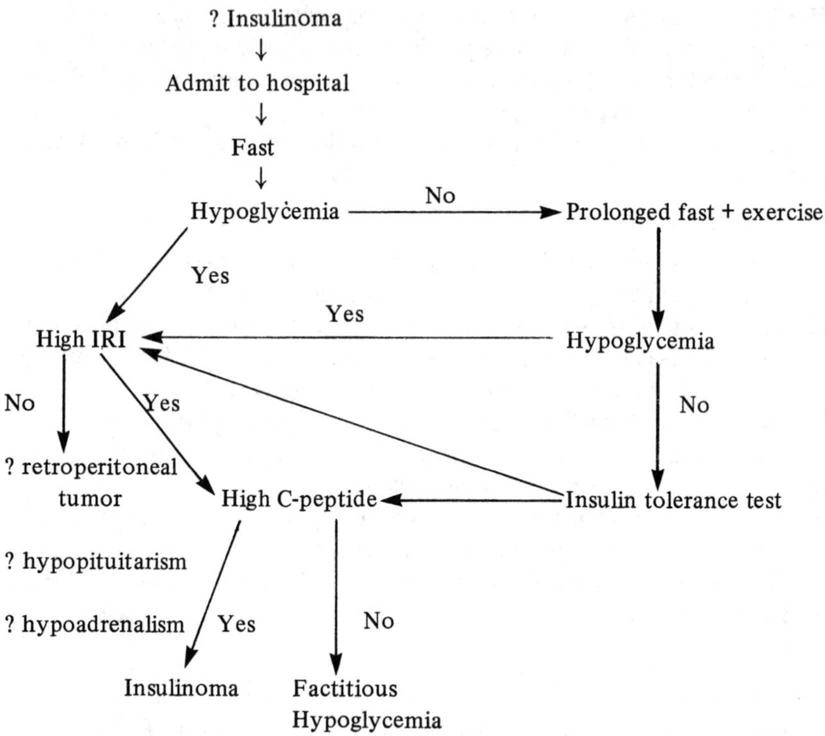

III. LOCALIZATION OF TUMORS

Identification of pancreatic and gut endocrine tumors at operation is often very difficult due to their small size and, in the case of gastrinomas, their multiple sites. A number of imaging techniques have therefore been used for preoperative localization.

A. Arteriography

Selective celiac and superior mesenteric arteriography using subtraction and magnification techniques has been reported to demonstrate between 50 and 90% of insulinomas (30), but many of these were also palpable at operation.

Diagnostic Summary 2 Zollinger–Ellison Syndrome

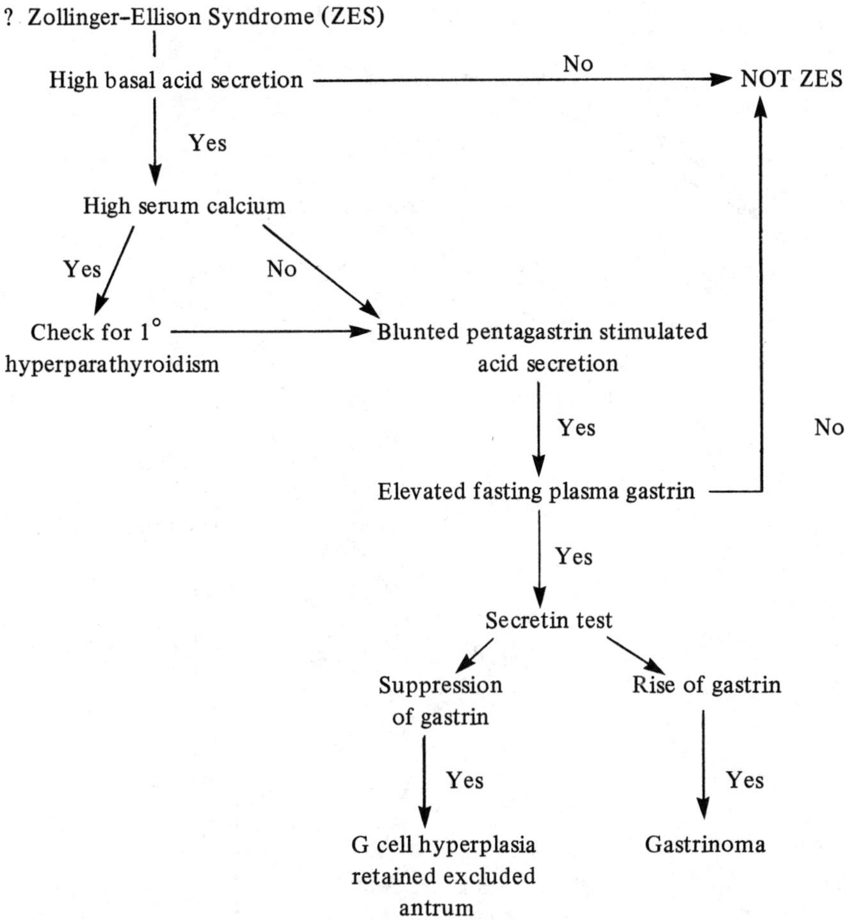

The accuracy of this technique in the localization of the other tumors has not been reported. Positive results can give valuable information not only on the site of the primary tumor, but also its size, vascularity, possible resectability, and presence of metastases. However, a negative arteriogram does not necessarily exclude a tumor.

Diagnostic Summary 3 Persistent Severe Diarrhea

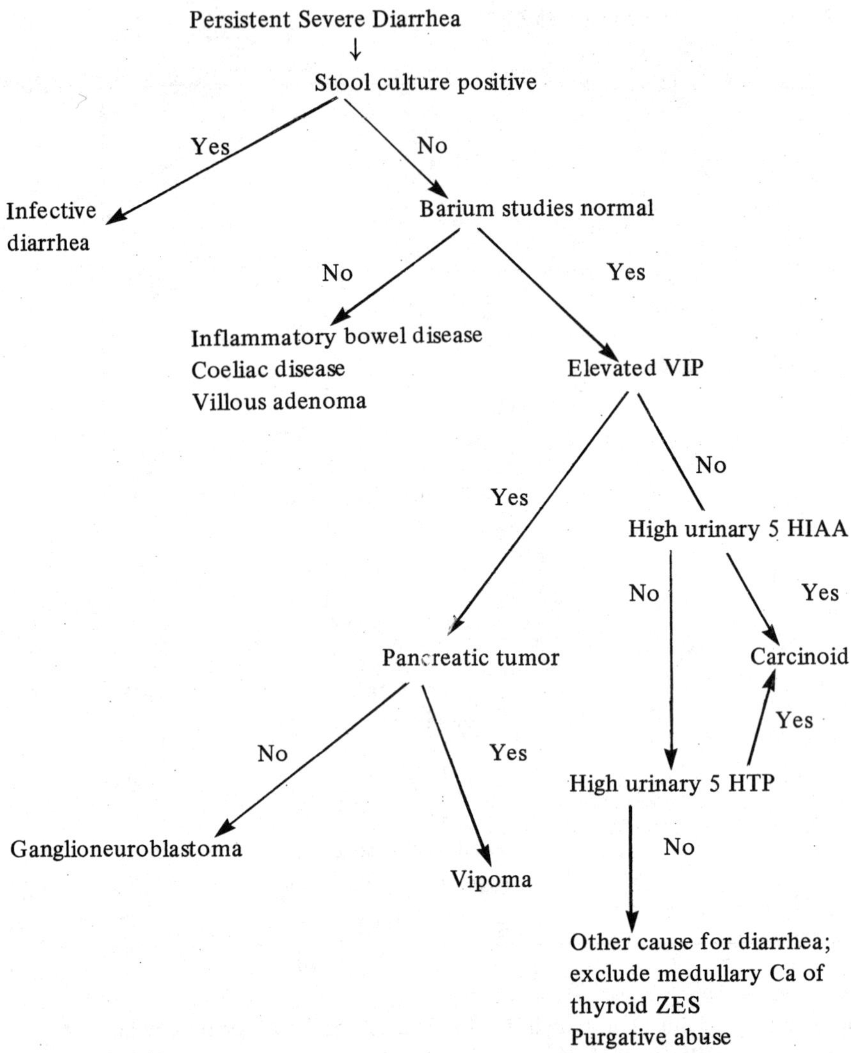

B. Percutaneous Transhepatic Portal Venous Sampling (THPVS)

This technique should be used if angiography fails to locate the primary tumor (30, 31). Use of the percutaneous transhepatic route to enter the portal circulation enables almost any vein in the splanchnic bed to be reached for sampling. Simultaneous sampling from arterial catheters allows arteriovenous peptide gradients to be measured. Despite the apparent advantages of this technique, it is not without complications and localization may be imprecise due to aberrant venous drainage. The reported success of THPVS is greater than 80% (30).

C. Other Techniques

Ultrasound, isotope scanning, and computerized axial tomography have inadequate power of resolution for localization of the primary tumor (31). However, they are noninvasive techniques and have proved useful for detecting hepatic metastases. Nuclear magnetic resonance techniques remain to be assessed.

REFERENCES

1. Bloom SR. Gut and brain. Endocrine connections. J R Coll Surg London 1980; 14:51–57.
2. Welbourn RB, Wood SM, Polak JM, Bloom SR. In *Gut Hormones*, 2nd ed., Bloom SR, Polak JM (eds). Churchill Livingstone, Edinburgh, 1980; ch. 83, pp. 547–554.
3. Pearse AGE. The cytochemistry and ultrastructure of polypeptide hormone producing cells of the APUD series and the embryologic, physiologic and pathologic implications of the concept. J Histochem Cytochem 1969; 17:303–313.
4. Tapia FJ, Barbosa AJA, Marangos PJ, Polak JM, Bloom SR, Dermody C, Pearse AGE. Neuron-specific-enolase is produced by neuroendocrine tumours. Lancet 1981; 1:808–811.
5. Kruseman ACN, Krugenburg G, de la Riviere GB, Bosman FT. Morphology and immunohistochemically defined endocrine function of pancreatic islet cell tumours. Histopathology 1978; 2:389–399.
6. Larsson LI. Endocrine pancreatic tumours. Hum Pathol 1978; 9:401–406.
7. Larsson LI, Grimelius L, Hakanson R, Rehfeld JF, Stadil F, Holst J, Angervall L, Sudler F. Mixed endocrine pancreatic tumours producing several peptide hormones. Am J Pathol 1975; 79:271–284.
8. Walsh J. Pathogenetic role of the gastrins. In *Gastrins and the Vagus*, Rehfeld JF, Amdrup E (eds). Academic, London, 1979.
9. Stadil F, Stage JG. The Zollinger-Ellison syndrome. Clin Endocrinol Metab 1979; 8:433–446.

10. Bloom SR, Bryant MG, Adrian TE. Multiple hormone forms in PPomas, VIPomas, and glucagonomas. Scand J Gastroenterol 1978; 13:24-25.
11. Long RG, Bryant MC, Polak JM, Bloom SR. Vipoma producing multiple molecular forms—studies with metoclopramide. Gastroenterology 1981; 80:1217.
12. Mallinson CN, Bloom SR, Warin AP, Salmon PR, Cox B. A glucagonoma syndrome. Lancet 1974; 2:1–5.
13. Leichter SB. Clinical and metabolic aspects of glucagonoma. Medicine 1980; 59:100–113.
14. Holst JJ, Helland S, Ingemannson, Pederson NB, von Schenck H. Functional studies in patients with the glucagonoma syndrome. Diabetologia 1979; 17:151–156.
15. Servide FJ, Dale AJD, Elveback LR, Jiang NS. Insulinoma: clinical and diagnostic features of 60 consecutive cases. Mayo Clin Proc 1976; 51: 417-429.
16. Marks V. The investigation of hypoglycaemia. Br J Hosp Med 1974; 11:731-734.
17. Fajans SS, Floyd JC. Diagnosis and medical management of insulinomas. Annu Rev Med 1979; 30:313–329.
18. Turner RC, Heding LG. Plasma proinsulin, C-peptide and insulin in diagnostic suppression tests for insulinomas. Diabetologia 1977; 13:571–577.
19. Zollinger RM, Ellison EH. Primary peptic ulceration of the jejunum associated with islet cell tumours of the pancreas. Ann Surg 1955; 142: 709–723.
20. Stage JG, Stadil F. The clinical diagnosis of the Zollinger-Ellison syndrome. Scand J Gastroenterol 1979; 14(suppl 53):79–91.
21. Feldman M, Walsh JH, Richardson CT. Serum gastrin response to secretin after vagotomy. Dig Dis Sci 1980; 25:921–923.
22. Long RG, Bryant MG, Mitchell SJ, Adrian TE, Polak JM, Bloom SR. Clinicopathological study of pancreatic and ganglioneuroblastoma tumours secreting vasoactive intestinal polypeptide (vipomas). Br J Med 1981; 282:1767-1771.
23. Verner JV, Morrison AB. Endocrine pancreatic islet disease with diarrhoea. Arch Intern Med 1974; 133:492–500.
24. Polak JM, Bloom SR, Adrian TE, Heitz PH, Bryant MG, Pearse AGE. Pancreatic polypeptide in insulinomas, gastrinomas, vipomas and glucagonomas. Lancet 1976; 1:328–330.
25. Krejs GJ, Orci L, Conlon M, Ravazzola M, Davis GR, Raskin PH, Collins SM, McCarthy DM, Baetens D, Rubenstein A, Aldor TAM, Unger RH. Somatostatinoma syndrome. Biochemical, morphological and clinical features. N Engl J Med 1979; 301:285–292.
26. Larsson LI, Hirsch MA, Holst JJ, Ingemansson S, Kuhl C, Jensen SL, Lundgvist G, Rehfeld JF, Schwartz TW. Pancreatic somatostatinoma, clinical features and physiological implications. Lancet 1977; 1:666–671.

27. Blackburn AM, Bryant MG, Adrian TE, Bloom SR. Pancreatic tumours produce neurotensin. J Clin Endocrinol Metab 1981; 52:820–822.
28. Belchetz PE, Brown CL, Makin HLJ, Trafford DJH, Stuart-Mason A, Bloom SR, Ratcliffe JG. ACTH, glucagon and gastrin production by a pancreatic islet cell carcinoma and its treatment. Clin Endocrinol 1973; 2:307–216.
29. Levine RJ. Serotonin and the carcinoid syndrome. In *Diseases of Metabolism*, Bondy PK, Rosenberg LE (eds). Saunders, Philadelphia, 1974; pp 1651–1684.
30. Reichardt W, Ingemansson S. Selective vein catheterisation for hormone assay in endocrine tumours of the pancreas. Acta Radiol Diagn 1980; 21:177–187.
31. Daggett PR, Goodburn EA, Kurtz AB, Le Quesne LP, Morris DV, Nabarro JDN. Is preoperative localisation of insulinomas necessary. Lancet 1980; 1:483–487.

OTHER ENDOCRINE DISORDERS

33

Placental Hormone Disorders

Tim Chard
St. Bartholomew's Hospital Medical College and the London Hospital Medical College, London, England

With the exception of a few extremely rare conditions, there are no placental hormone disorders in the sense that "hormone disorder" is normally understood, that is, as a defect in the gland of origin leading to abnormal hormone production and a clinical syndrome. Instead, measurement of placental hormones is used widely to provide diagnostic information on a series of primary fetoplacental disorders in which the purely endocrine aspects are of secondary significance. Hormones are employed as markers of fetoplacental function; they do not themselves play any known role in the conditions they are used to diagnose.

This concept differs very fundamentally from most traditional clinical endocrinology. In the present chapter the reasons for this difference are explored, together with aspects of physiology which reflect on the clinical use of placental hormone measurements, and selected examples of clinical application.

I. SPECIFIC HORMONES OF THE FETOPLACENTAL UNIT

The human fetoplacental unit produces a number of specific hormones and other products (Table 1). Some, such as the steroid hormones, are specific in the quantitative sense; thus the estriol of pregnancy is chemically identical to that of the nonpregnant adult but present in 10,000-fold greater concentration. Others, such as placental lactogen (hPL) and chorionic gonadotropin (hCG), are chemically different from their nonpregnancy analogs (growth hormone and luteinizing hormone) and are therefore specific in the qualitative sense. However, recent evidence for the occurrence of placental proteins in some normal tissues, especially seminal plasma, casts some doubt on the absolute "specificity" of these products (1, 2).

Table 1 Specific Hormones of the Human Fetoplacental Unit

Steroids:	Estrogens (includes estrone, estradiol, and estriol) Progesterone
Proteins and peptides:	Placental lactogen (hPL) Chorionic gonadotropin (hCG) Chorionic corticotropin (hCCT) Chorionic releasing hormones (includes hC-LHRH, hC-TRH)

II. CHEMISTRY OF PLACENTAL HORMONES

The chemistry of the estrogens is familiar and will not be considered further; aspects of their synthesis during pregnancy are described below.

Human placental lactogen is a polypeptide of 21,000 daltons with a single chain of 191 amino acides and two intrachain disulfide bonds (3). The amino acid composition is very similar to that of human growth hormone (hGH), the sole difference being in the number of methionine, histidine, and proline residues. The amino acid sequence of the two hormones is identical at 163 of the 191 residues (86% sequence homology), and the intrachain disulfide bonds are located in homologous portions of each molecule. The sequences of hPL and hGH are also somewhat similar to that of prolactin (13% sequence homology with hPL, 16% with hGH).

Human chorionic gonadotropin is a glycoprotein consisting of two subunits, termed α and β, which in the intact molecule are joined by noncovalent bonds. The α subunit has 92 amino acids and is very similar in all the glycoprotein hormones [luteinizing hormone (LH), follicle stimulating hormone (FSH), and thyroid stimulating hormone (TSH).] The β subunit, which is specific to the individual hormone, has 147 amino acids, of which the C terminus contains 32 residues which are unique to hCG.

III. BIOLOGICAL FUNCTIONS OF THE FETOPLACENTAL HORMONES

The biological functions of placental hormones (as opposed to biological effects in experimental systems) are very ill defined. It has even been suggested that placental products in general have no function but instead are waste products of the placenta as an independent organism (1,2).

The main functions proposed for the fetoplacental steroid hormones are the maintenance of early pregnancy (progesterone) and a role in the initiation of labor (estrogens/progesterone) (4). Several biological activities have been suggested for hPL, including lactogenesis and fetal growth promotion, stimulation of the corpus luteum, an effect on carbohydrate and lipid metabolism, erythropoiesis, inhibition of fibrinolysis, and immunosuppression (5). Chorionic gonadotropin has been proposed as the principal luteotropic factor of early pregnancy and as a possible stimulus to the gonad in the early male fetus (6).

The reality or otherwise of these functions is the subject of long and complex arguments. However, one definite conclusion can be reached here: *None* of the functions are reflected in any way in the clinical use of measurements of the hormones. They are used exclusively as diagnostic markers, a point further emphasized by the fact that *all* hormone parameters show virtually simultaneous alteration in pathological states.

IV. SYNTHESIS OF THE FETOPLACENTAL HORMONES

All specific placental hormones appear to be products of the syncytiotrophoblast. The main experimental evidence for this arises from immunohistochemical studies on protein hormones (7), although these have been criticized on both technical and theoretical grounds (8).

Studies on the localization of synthetic mechanisms within the trophoblast include the observations by Burgos and Rodriguez (9) of a clear differentiation between thick areas of the trophoblast cytoplasm which are rich in endoplasmic

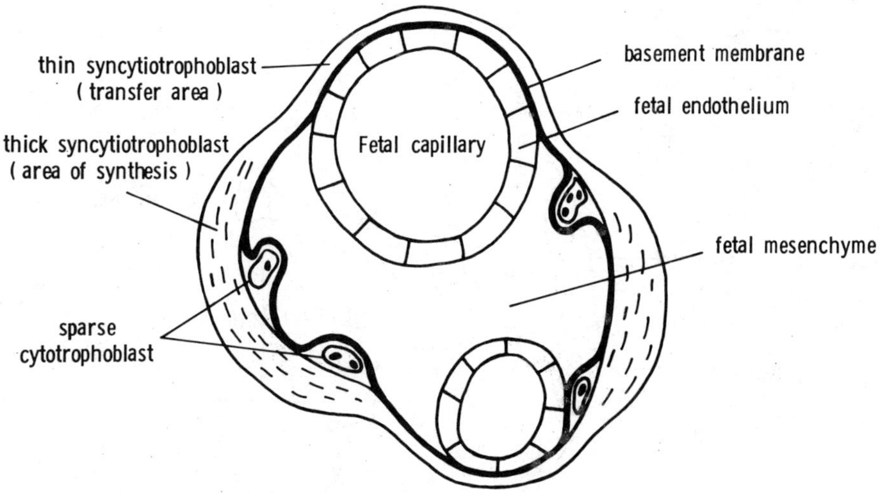

Figure 1 Structure of a chorionic villus of the human placenta. Note that separate areas of the trophoblast may be involved in synthesis and transfer.

reticulum and microvilli and therefore appear to be specialized for synthesis. together with thin areas without microvilli which lie in proximity to fetal capillaries and appear to be specialized for the transfer of nutrients and waste products (Fig. 1). The differentiation between these areas is of potential clinical significance because it is possible that a process which damages the critically important transfer areas could leave the synthetic areas intact. However, since the trophoblast pathology is usually secondary to factors such as blocking of maternal decidual arterioles or fetal capillaries in the chorionic villus, it seems likely in reality that all areas will be equally affected.

The synthesis of estrogens, in particular estriol (E_3), by the trophoblast is dependent on fetal androgenic precursors (Fig. 2). The clinical significance of this is that pathology which lies in the fetus would lead to falling levels of E_3, whereas exclusively placental products, such as hPL, would show no change. In practice, the vast majority of conditions which threaten fetal well-being have their origin in the placenta and the distinction between placental and fetoplacental products is clinically unimportant.

V. CONTROL MECHANISMS OF FETOPLACENTAL HORMONES

There is little evidence for the existence of control mechanisms for the fetoplacental hormones such as occur for comparable products of the normal adult. No releasing or inhibiting factors have been identified and where mechanisms have been suggested (e.g., the changes in hPL during experimental manipulation of carbohydrate metabolism), the evidence is often disputed and subject to

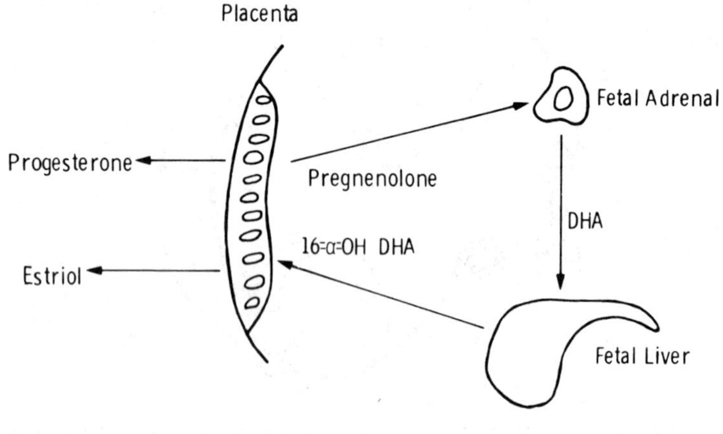

Figure 2 Simplified schema of the production of estriol from fetal androgenic precursors by the human fetoplacental unit. (From Ref. 10.)

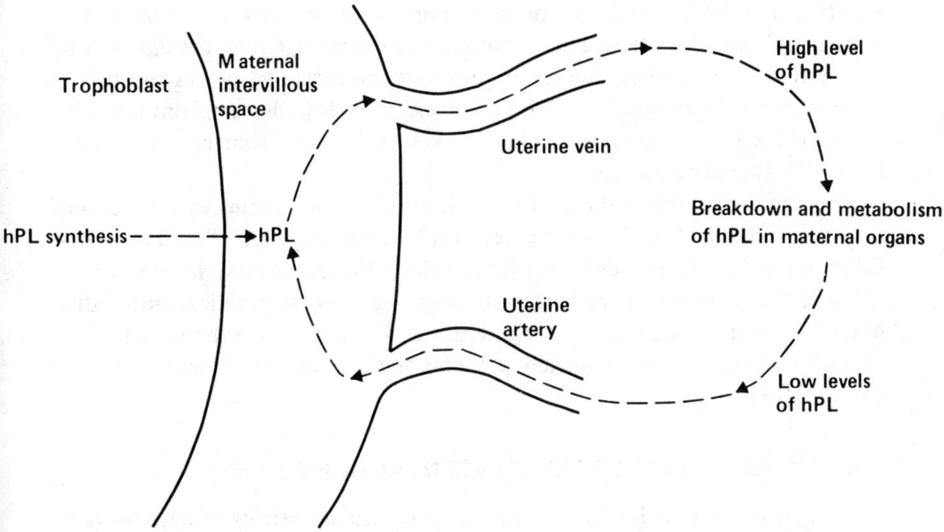

Figure 3 How uteroplacental blood flow may control the rate of production of hPL by the trophoblast. hPL is released into the intervillous space down a concentration gradient. The faster it is removed, the greater will be the gradient and the greater will be the rate of secretion, and secondarily, of synthesis. (From Ref. 2.)

alternative explanations (11). It has been proposed (Fig. 3) that the potential for placental synthesis is a function of the total mass of the trophoblast; that the rate of release depends on the concentration of the protein in the maternal blood in the intervillous space; and that this concentration, in turn, depends on the rate of blood flow in the intervillous space. Thus the hormone will diffuse from the trophoblast cell down a concentration gradient: the greater the rate of blood flow, the faster is the removal of the hormone and hence the steeper the gradient. This hypothesis has the implication that the rate of hormone production and its circulating levels in the mother will be closely related to the uteroplacental blood flow, and may further explain why products of the fetus and placenta, such as estriol, and the products of the placenta, such as hPL, usually show parallel changes in abnormal states.

VI. METABOLISM OF FETOPLACENTAL HORMONES

Maternal metabolism of the fetoplacental hormones takes place principally in the liver and the kidneys. Very little of the total hPL produced is excreted in urine, a rather larger proportion of hCG, and a very high proportion of E_3 (10). The latter explains the early popularity of urinary estrogens as a placental function test. The metabolism of the estrogens is complex, involving a series of conjugations and deconjugations and extensive cycling through the enterohepatic circulation (10). This complexity tends to detract from their clinical value because maternal physiology makes a substantial contribution to the levels in maternal compartments.

The half-life of hPL in the circulation is measured in minutes, of the steroids in hours, and of hCG in days. Theoretically, the clearance rate should be a useful criterion for clinical value: the shorter the half-life, the more rapidly will levels of the hormone reflect acute pathological events. In practice, most pathology in pregnancy is relatively long standing. The rare acute events, such as placental abruption, are clinically obvious and require no biochemical confirmation.

VII. MEASUREMENT OF FETOPLACENTAL HORMONES

The original methods for the measurement of urinary estrogens were by the classical techniques of colorimetry and fluorimetry. With the increasing trend toward measurement of estrogens in blood, the method of choice is radioimmunoassay (RIA), as it always has been for the quantitative measurement of hPL and hCG.

Two general points can be made about the measurement of fetoplacental hormones:

1. Because of the overlap between normal and abnormal populations (see below), precision of estimation is of the utmost importance—more so probably than in any other field of clinical endocrinology.
2. The very high circulating levels of the fetoplacental hormones make them ideal candidates for nonisotopic assays such as fluoroimmunoassay (FIA) (12). Such assays might also be suitable for emergency side-room use.

VIII. INTERPRETATION OF BIOCHEMICAL TEST OF PLACENTAL FUNCTION

Publications on the clinical use of biochemical tests of placental function are often confusing and contradictory. One group will show that a test is of great value, another will criticize the procedure. Furthermore, it can be asked whether any test is of value when set against the strict criterion of whether it contributes to a decrease in perinatal mortality and morbidity. However, certain generalizations can be made about the interpretation of these tests (see Ref. 13).

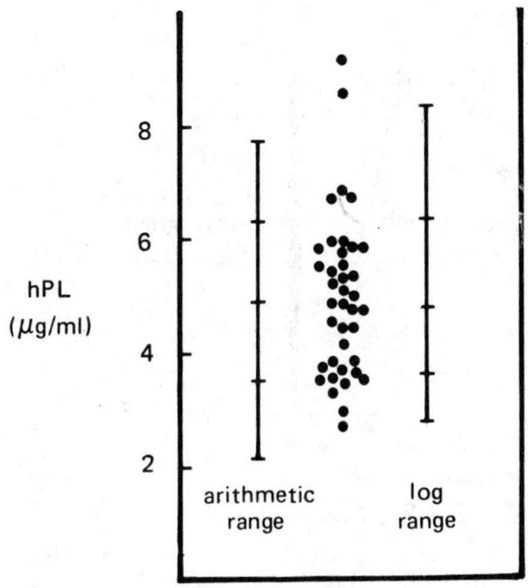

Figure 4 Skewed distribution; placental lactogen (hPL) values from a normal range for week 34 of pregnancy. When means and standard deviations are calculated in arithmetic form, the resulting statistical range is a poor fit to the observed spread of results. When the same calculation is made after logarithmic transformation, the resulting range is a much closer fit. It is likely that skewed distributions of this type will apply to the majority of biological parameters, including all hormonal tests of fetal well-being.

1. A test is valueless unless a carefully analyzed normal range is available. A normal range should usually be based on results from at least 50 subjects at each week of gestation, and a clear definition of "normality" should be stated.
2. The normal range should be analyzed by appropriate statistical procedures. A Gaussian distribution is unusual and results should usually be analyzed after logarithmic transformation or in nonparametric form (Fig. 4).
3. Every individual laboratory or group of laboratories should establish its own normal range. Because of differences in technique the use of a published normal range is often misleading.
4. Ranges should be established for clinical abnormalities according to whether or not they are associated with fetal risk. Thus there is little point in knowing that the levels of a given product are generally low in preeclampsia: the obstetrician needs to know which case of preeclampsia is at greatest risk.

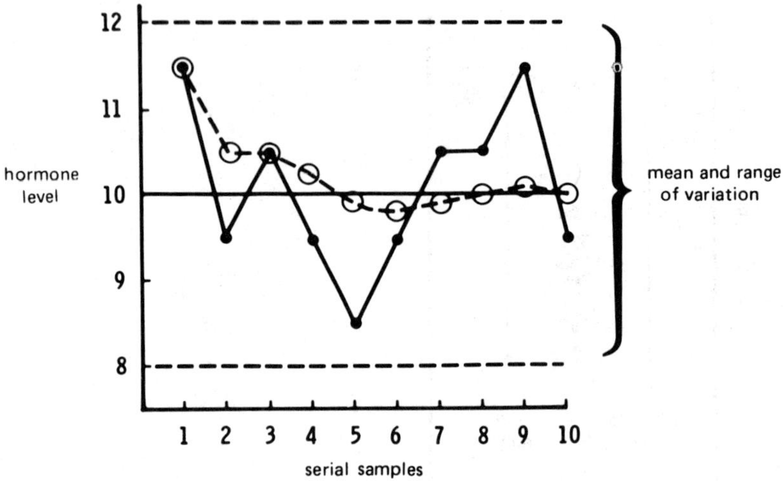

Figure 5 The value of serial samples. The hormone measured has an overall variation of ±20% and serial samples (●—●) show fluctuations within these limits. However, if the cumulative mean is calculated (o---o) the observed pattern stabilizes when five or more serial results are available, thus providing a much better estimate of the real situation in an individual subject. It should be noted that this analysis would not apply if the hormone levels show a progressive rise or fall over the period studied; for example, serial levels of plasma estriol at weekly intervals in late pregnancy.

5. There is no such thing as a perfect test. All show some overlap between normality and abnormality, with a "gray area" between. Results are better interpreted as risk and not certainty.
6. Serial levels are always more valuable than a single level. It is often thought that this is because a fall may be apparent in a high-risk case, but far more important is the fact that serial levels give greater confidence to the observed relation between an individual subject and the population of which that subject is part (Fig. 5).

IX. CLINICAL APPLICATION OF FETOPLACENTAL HORMONE MEASUREMENT

From the preceding sections it may already be apparent that the diagnostic significance of measurement of any one fetoplacental product is likely to be very similar to that of the others. There is little scientific evidence that this is not the case and the following discussion will therefore focus mainly on the protein hormones, especially hPL. The material presented is selected from an immense literature and is intended to be illustrative rather than encylopedic.

A. Threatened Abortion

About 15-20% of all pregnancies end in clinically obvious abortion and most of these patients require hospital admission. In addition, the outcome for the fetus is uncertain in many cases of vaginal bleeding in early pregnancy and these patients may require several days in hospital before the final diagnosis is apparent. It is generally agreed that low maternal levels of fetoplacental hormones after weeks 8-10 indicate that the outcome is likely to be unsatisfactory, and thus provide a guide to prognosis in this condition. This has been clearly shown for hPL (14-17) (Fig. 6). The biochemical tests seem to be complementary to sonography (18-19). Low levels, especially serially low levels after week 10 would be an indication for evacuation of the uterus in the absence of contradicting factors such as advanced maternal age or infertility.

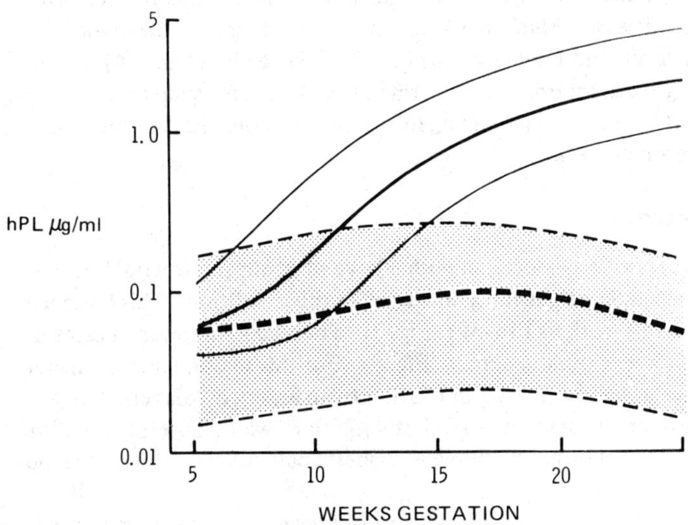

Figure 6 Circulating hPL levels in patients with vaginal bleeding who aborted on first admission to hospital (interrupted lines and shaded area). The mean and range for normal subjects are shown by the solid lines.

B. Low-Birthweight Infants

Maternal blood hPL levels correlate with the weight of the placenta (20, 21) and of the fetus (21-23). The latter relationship is presumably secondary to that between the weight of the fetus and placenta. Placental lactogen levels are a clinically efficient guide to the prediction of fetal weight in an individual patient. Low levels have been described in association with severe intrauterine growth retardation (IUGR) (24, 25), particularly in cases of maternal hypertension (26). The sensitivity of the test is around 40% (27), and the levels of hPL in IUGR become significantly lower than normal after 33 weeks of gestation (28). Low levels in midtrimester may also be predictive (29).

C. Hypertension and Preeclampsia

The confusion in the literature on hPL levels in preeclampsia can be attributed to two factors. First, the condition itself is very heterogeneous and often not clearly defined. Second, many authors fail to distinguish between preeclampsia per se and the fetal risk arising from the preeclampsia.

Spellacy and his colleagues (31) defined a "fetal danger zone" for subjects with hypertension: levels less than 4 μg/ml after week 30 indicated a fetal mortality of 24%. The levels are generally lower in multigravidae than in primigravidae (30, 31), and the lowest levels and greatest risk are associated with chronic vascular disease. Many workers have shown a similar association between low hPL levels and fetal outcome (24, 32, 33). Kelly et al. (34) showed a 75% fetal risk (growth retardation or perinatal asphyxia) for subjects developing hypertension after week 28 and having hPL concentrations that are lower than 2 SD below the normal mean.

D. Diabetes Mellitus

Diabetes mellitus is often associated with a large placenta and it would be expected that hPL would be generally increased in this condition. This has been shown by numerous workers (35-39) (Fig. 7). The levels are lower in cases in which fetal outcome is unsatisfactory (Fig. 8). For this reason levels in diabetic pregnancies have to be interpreted in relation to an elevated "diabetic range." Thus, under most circumstances, a level of 4 μg/ml provides a useful action line for the diagnosis of abnormality, while in diabetic patients the critical level becomes 5 μg/ml.

Conflicting results on the clinical value of hPL levels in diabetes can be attributed to a number of factors, including the definition of the severity of the condition, the failure to realize that abnormality should be judged in relation to the general elevation of levels, and the fact that perinatal death may occur due to

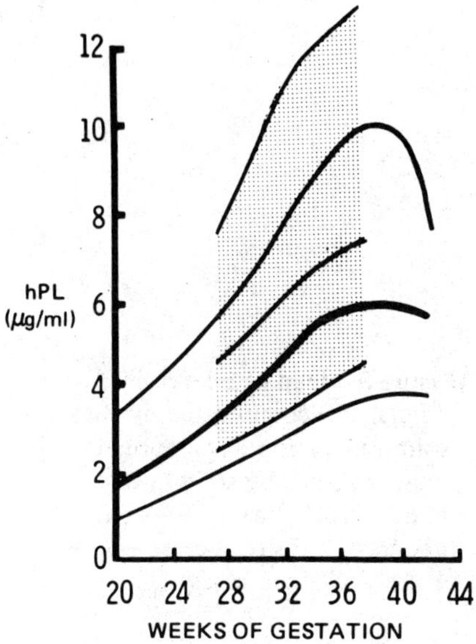

Figure 7 Circulating hPL levels in pregnancies complicated by diabetes mellitus in which there was no evidence of placental dysfunction (shaded area). The normal range is also shown.

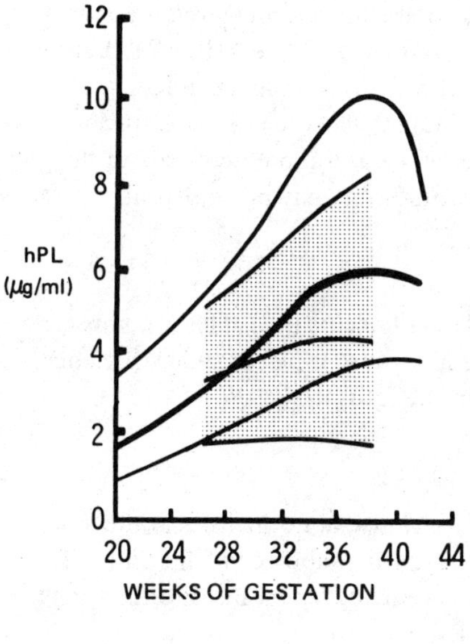

Figure 8 Circulating hPL levels in pregnancies complicated by diabetes millitus in which there was evidence of placental dysfunction (shaded area). The normal range is also shown.

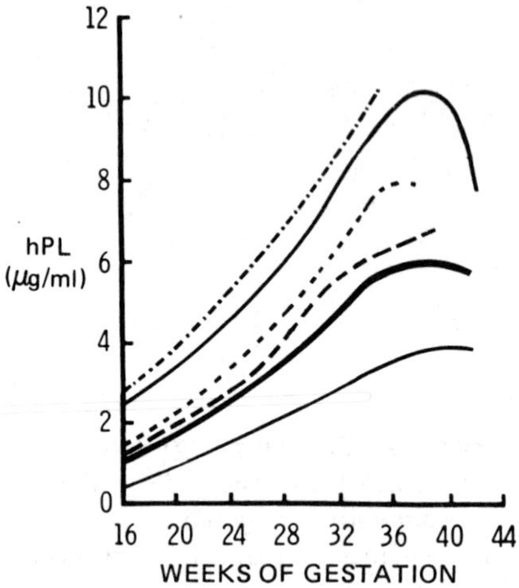

Figure 9 Mean hPL levels in pregnancies complicated by rhesus isoimmunization. The normal range is shown by solid lines; mildly affected cases; ————; moderately affected cases -----; severely affected cases —·—·—·—·.

metabolic dysfunction in the absence of obvious placental deficiencies. A new "problem" is the fact that the well-controlled diabetic pregnancy is effectively a normal pregnancy and should be treated as such.

E. Rhesus Isoimmunization

Maternal levels are generally elevated in this condition, and the levels are most elevated in cases in which the child is severely affected (24, 40) (Fig. 9). Before week 26, a value which is greater than 2 SD above the normal mean indicates a 90% likelihood that the case will be severe. Similar elevations are seen in amniotic fluid hPL (41). Thus the test may provide a useful predictive aid at the stage when other parameters, such as liquor bilirubin, may be equivocal.

F. Fetal Death

Maternal hPL levels usually fall before fetal death occurs (42). This is compatible with the fact that in most stillbirths the primary cause is placental insufficiency; only rarely does the primary cause lie within the fetus itself.

G. Fetal Distress and Neonatal Asphyxia

In approximately 12% of pregnancies with no clinical abnormalities in the antenatal period, fetal complications occur either during labor or at the time of delivery. A proportion of these cases can be predicted by means of estimations of hPL carried out as a routine screening procedure (30, 43); an apparently normal patient who has three or more levels below 4 μg/ml in the last 6 weeks of pregnancy has a 71% risk of fetal complications. Comparable observations have been reported in a mixed group of "risk" pregnancies, including patients with clinical evidence of fetal growth retardation, hypertension, preeclampsia, antepartum hemorrhage, and chronic renal disease (44) and very similar conclusions have been reached in studies on urinary estrogen excretion (45, 46). An association has been shown between abnormal hPL levels and an abnormal result of an oxytocin challenge test (47).

H. Prolonged Pregnancy

Maternal blood and amniotic fluid hPL decrease in prolonged pregnancy (43 weeks and more) (48). It is not clear whether they serve to define a special "at risk" group.

I. Miscellaneous Conditions

Several authors have described cases with an apparent absence of hPL in an otherwise uneventful pregnancy (49-51). Maternal hPL levels are generally lower in smokers than in nonsmokers (23, 31, 52.) The low levels in smokers seem to be related to the associated growth retardation rather than to the smoking itself (53). hPL levels are lower in mothers exposed to continuous aircraft noise (54).

X. ESTROGENS VERSUS PLACENTAL LACTOGEN

One of the principal reasons for selecting hPL to provide most of the clinical examples is the fact that the literature on this hormone, in terms of the criteria set out in Section VIII, is much superior to that on the estrogens. Furthermore, the switch from urinary estrogens to blood estrogens (stimulated by the fact that 24-hr urine collections are an obvious source of inaccuracy) requires that a new literature be generated on this topic. It is not intended to advocate one test over another; in the opinion of this author, measurement of either blood estrogens or hPL will provide very similar information, and the choice might well be dictated by factors such as cost and the technical preferences of a local laboratory.

XI. CONCLUSIONS

The very nonspecific nature of all parameters used in antenatal care (in turn, the result of the inaccessibility of the main patient–the fetus) generates frequent arguments for and against any one group of tests. The question may therefore be asked: Is placental function testing worthwhile? What value does an hPL or estrogen result have relative to other parameters recorded as part of antenatal care, and can the information lead to a significant reduction in mortality and morbidity? The first question has been answered in recent studies from Gordon and his colleagues (55) and Grudzinskas and his colleagues (56). Using a "relative risk factor" we have demonstrated that low hPL levels, observed as part of a routine screening program on an entire obstetric population, were as effective a predictor of poor fetal outcome as the occurrence of severe preeclampsia, low maternal weight at 32 weeks, and heavy smoking by the mother. All were superior to many other factors which are widely considered to be of great value in antenatal diagnosis. The second question has been addressed by a study from Spellacy et al. (57). Placental lactogen measurements were carried out on a large number of "at risk" subjects; the patients were divided into two randomized groups, one in which the results were reported to the clinician and the other in which they were not. In the first group the perinatal death rate was 3.5%, in the second 15%, a clear indication of the real practical value of these estimations. Since a substantial portion of perinatal mortality and morbidity cannot be identified by current clinical procedures, there is a good argument for the routine application of hPL or estrogen measurement in all pregnancies.

REFERENCES

1. Chard T, Klopper A. *Placental Function Tests.* Springer Verlag, Berlin, 1982.
2. Chard T. Proteins of the human placenta–some general concepts. In *Pregnancy Proteins*, Grudzinskas JG, Teisner B, Seppala M (eds). Academic, London, 1982, pp. 3-21.
3. Niall HD, Hogan ML, Tregear GW, Seagre GV, Hwang P, Friesen HG. The chemistry of growth hormone and the lactogenic hormones. Recent Prog Horm Res 1973; 29, 387-398.
4. Anderson ABM, Turnbull AC. Comparative aspects of factors involved in the onset of labour in ovine and human pregnancy. In *Endocrine Factors in Labour*, Klopper A, Gardner J (eds). Cambridge University Press, Cambridge 1973, pp 141-162.
5. Chard T. Human placental lactogen. In *Hormones in Blood*, Gray CH, James VHT (eds). Academic, London, 1979, pp 333-409.
6. Osathonondh R, Tulchinsky D. Placental polypeptide hormones. In *Maternal-Fetal Endocrinology*, Tulchinsky D, Ryan KJ (eds). Saunders, Philadelphia, 1980, pp 17–42.
7. de Ikonikoff LK, Cedard L. Localisation of human chorionic gonadotropin and somatomammotropic hormones by the peroxidase immunohistoenzymologic method in villi and amniotic epithelium of human placentas (from six weeks to term). Am J Obstet Gynecol 1973; 116:1124–1132.

8. Gau GS, Chard T. Location of the protein hormones of the placenta by the immunoperoxidase technique. Br J Obstet Gynaecol 1976; 83:876-878.
9. Burgos MH, Rodriguez EM. Specialised zones in the trophoblast of the human term placenta. Am J Obstet Gynecol 1966; 96:342–356.
10. Hull MGR, Chard T. Hormonal aspects of foetoplacental function. In *Fetal Physiology and Medicine*, Beard RW, Nathaneilsz PW (eds). Saunders, Philadelphia, 1976, pp 371–394.
11. Pavlou C, Chard T, Landon J, Letchworth AT. Circulating levels of placental lactogen in late pregnancy: the effect of glucose loading, smoking and exercise. Eur J Obstet gynaecol Rep Biol 1973; 3:45–49.
12. Chard T, Sykes A. Fluoroimmunoassay for human choriomammotropin. Clin Chem 1979; 25:979-975.
13. Chard T. Normality and abnormality. In *Plasma Hormone Assays in Evaluation of Fetal Well-Being*, Klopper A (ed). Churchill Livingstone, Edinburgh, 1976, pp 1-9.
14. Genazzani AR, Cocola R, Casoli M, Mello G, Scarselli EG, Neri P, Fioretti P. Use of human placental lactogen radioimmunoassay to predict outcome in cases of threatened abortion. Lancet 1969; 2:1385–1387.
15. Niven PAR, Landon J, Chard T. Placental lactogen levels as guide to outcome of threatened abortion. Br Med J 1972; iii:799–801.
16. Gartside MW, Tindall VR. The prognostic value of human placental lactogen (HPL) levels in threatened abortion. Br J Obstet Gynaecol 1974; 83:303–309.
17. Biswas S, Murrey M, Buffoe G, Graves L, Jelowitz J, Dewhurst J. Placental lactogen as a reliable index of fetal outcome in threatened abortion during early pregnancy. J Obstet Gynaecol 1980; 1:75–77.
18. Vorster CZ, Pannell PR, Slabber CF. The prognostic value of serum human placental lactogen determinations in early pregnancy. Am J Obstet Gynecol 1977; 128:879–880.
19. Jouppila P, Seppälä P, Chard T. Pregnancy-specific β_1-glycoprotein in complications of early pregnancy. Lancet 1980; i:667–668.
20. Sciarra JJ, Sherwood LM, Varma AA, Lundberg WD. Human placental lactogen (HPL) and placental weight. Am J Obstet Gynecol 1968; 1101: 413–421.
21. Lindberg BS, Nilsson BA (1973). Variations in maternal plasma levels of HPL in normal pregnancy and labour. J Obstet Gynaecol Br Common W. 1973; 80:619–6.
22. Letchworth AT, Boardman RJ, Bristow C, Landon J, Chard T. A rapid semi-automated method for the measurement of human chorionic somatomammotrophin. The normal range in the third trimester and its relation to fetal weight. J Obstet Gynaecol Br Common W. 1971; 78:542–548.
23. Boyce A, Schwartz D, Hubert C, Cedard L, Dreyfus J. Smoking, human placental lactogen and birthweight. Br J Obstet Gynaecol 1975; 82:964–967.
24. Lindberg, BS, Nilsson BA. Human placental lactogen (HPL) levels in abnormal pregnancies. J Obstet Gynaecol Br Common W. 1973; 80:1046–1053.

25. Hensleigh PA, Cheaton SG, Spellacy WN. Oxytocinase and human placental lactogen for prediction of intrauterine growth retardation. Am J Obstet Gynecol 1977; 129:675–678.
26. Granat M, Sharf M, Diengott D, Spindel A, Kahana L, Elrad H. Further investigation on the predictive value of human placental lactogen in high-risk pregnancies. Am J Obstet Gynecol 1977; 129:647–654.
27. Morrison I, Green P, Oomen B. The role of human placental lactogen assays in antepartum fetal assessment. Am J Obstet Gynecol 1980; 136: 1055–1060.
28. Daikoku NH, Tyson JE, Graf C, Scott R, Smith B, Johnson JWC, King TM. The relative significance of human placental lactogen in the diagnosis of retarded fetal growth. Am J Obstet Gynecol 1979; 135:615–520.
29. Salem HT, Lee JN, Sepälä M., Vaara L, Aula P, Al-Ani ATM, Chard T. Measurement of placental protein 5, placental lactogen and pregnancy specific β_1 glycoprotein in mid-trimester as a predictor of outcome of pregnancy. Br J Obstet Gynaecol 1981; 88:371–374.
30. Letchworth AT, Chard T. Placental lactogen levels as a screening test for fetal distress and neonatal asphyxia. Lancet 1972; 1:704–706.
31. Spellacy WN, Buhi WC, Birk SA, McCreary SA. Distribution of human placental lactogen in the last half of normal and complicated pregnancies. Am J Obstet Gynecol. 1974; 120:214–223.
32. Keller PJ, Baertschi U, Bader P, Gerber C, Schmid J, Solterman R, Kopper E. Biochemical detection of foetoplacental distress in risk pregnancies. Lancet 1971; 2:729–730.
33. Christensen A, Frayshov D, Fylling P. Hormone and enzyme assays in pregnancy. Acta Endocrinol 1974; 77:344–355.
34. Kelly AM, England P, Lorrimer JD, Fergusson JC, Govan ADT. An evaluation of human placental lactogen levels in hypertension of pregnancy. Br J Obstet Gynaecol 1974; 82:272–275.
35. Selenkow HA, Varma K, Younger D, White P, Emerson K. Patterns of serum immunoreactive human placental lactogen (IR-HPL) and chorionic gonadotropin (IR-HCG) in diabetic pregnancy. Diabetes 1969; 20:696–706.
36. Cohen M, Haour F, Dumont M, Bertrand J. Prognostic value of human chorionic somatomammotropin plasma levels in diabetic patients. Am J Obstet Gynecol. 1973; 115:202–210.
37. Ursell W, Brudenell M, Chard T. Placental lactogen levels in diabetic pregnancy. Br Med J 1973; 2:80–82.
38. Soler NG, Nicholson HO, Malins JM. Serial determinations of human placental lactogen in the management of diabetic pregnancy. Lancet 1975; 2:54–57.
39. Hertogh RD, Thomas K, Hoet JJ, Vanderheyden I. Plasma concentrations unconjugated estrone, estradiol-17β and estriol, and HCS throughout pregnancy in diabetics and gestational diabetics. Diabetologia 1976; 12:455–461.

40. Ward RHT, Letchworth AT, Niven PAR, Chard T. Placental lactogen levels in rhesus isoimmunization. Br Med J 1974; i:347–349.
41. Niven PAR, Ward RHT, Chard T. Human placental lactogen levels in amniotic fluid in rhesus isoimmunization. J Obstet Gynaecol Br Commonw. 1974; 81:988–990.
42. Ward H, Rochman H, Varnavides LA, Whyley GA. Hormone and enzyme levels in complicated pregnancy. Am J Obstet Gynecol 1973; 116:1105–1113.
43. England P, Lorrimer D, Fergusson JC, Moffatt AM, Kelly AM. Human placental lactogen: the watchdog of fetal distress. Lancet 1974; 1:5–7.
44. Edwards RP, Diver MJ, Davis JC, Hipkin LJ. Plasma oestriol and human placental lactogen measurements in patients with high risk pregnancies. Br J Obstet Gynaecol 1976; 83:229–237.
45. Beischer NA, Bhargava VL, Brown JB, Smith MA. The incidence and significance of low oestriol excretion in an obstetric population. J Obstet Gynaecol Br Commonw. 1968; 74:1024–1033.
46. Dickey RF, Grannis GF, Hanson FW, Schuster A, Ma S. Use of estrogen/creatinine ratio and the (estrogen) index for screening of normal and "high-risk" pregnancy. Am J Obstet Gynecol 1972; 113:880–886.
47. Spellacy WN, Cruz AC, Kalro PS, Kellner KR, Quinlan RW, Buhi WC, Birk SA. Oxytocin challenge test results compared with simultaneously studied serum human placental lactogen and free estriol levels in high-risk pregnant women. Am J. Obstet Gynecol 1979; 134:917-921.
48. Lolis D, Konstantinidis K, Papevangelou G, Kaskarelis D. Comparative study of amniotic fluid and maternal blood serum human placental lactogen in normal and prolonged pregnancies. Am J Obstet Gynecol 1977; 128:724-726.
49. Gaede P, Trolle D, Pedersen H. Extremely low placental lactogen hormone (hPL) values in an otherwise uneventful pregnancy preceding delivery of a normal baby. Acta Obstet Gynecol Scand 1978; 57:203–209.
50. Nielson PV, Pedersen H, Kampmann E-M. Absence of human placental lactogen in an otherwise uneventful pregnancy. Am J Obstet Gynecol 1979; 135:322–326.
51. Borody IB, Carlton MA. Isolated defect in human placental lactogen synthesis in a normal pregnancy. Br J Obstet Gynaecol 1981; 88:447-449.
52. Moser RJ, Hollingsworth DR, Carlson JW, Lamotte L. Human chorionic somatomammotropin in normal adolescent primiparous pregnancy. 1. Effect of smoking. Am J Obstet 1974; 120:1080–1086.
53. Lee JN, Grudzinskas JG, Chard T. Circulating placental lactogen levels in relation to smoking during pregnancy. J Obstet Gynaecol 1980; 1:87–89.
54. Ando Y, Hattori H. Effects of noise on human placental lactogen (HPL) levels in maternal plasma. Br J Obstet Gynaecol 1977; 84:115–118.
55. Gordon YB, Lewis JD, Pendlebury DJ. Is measurement of placental function and maternal weight worthwhile? Lancet 1978; i:1001-1003.

56. Grudzinskas JG, Gordon YB, Wadsworth J, Menabawey M, Chard T. Is placental function testing worthwhile? An update on placental lactogen. Aust NZ J Obstet Gynaecol 1981; 21:103–104.
57. Spellacy WN, Buhi WC, Birk SA, The effectiveness of human placental lactogen measurements as an adjunct in decreasing perinatal death. Am J Obstet Gynecol 1975; 212:835–843.

34
Ectopic Hormone Production

Lesley H. Rees
St. Bartholomew's Hospital Medical College, London, England

There is much unresolved controversy regarding the pathogenesis of ectopic hormone secretion, which although of great interest, is beyond the scope of this contribution and has been extensively reviewed fairly recently (1). Suffice it to say that caution should be exercised when applying this term to the description of a hormone within a nonendocrine tumor and it is better reserved for the few instances in which a well-defined clinical syndrome results from tumor hormone release. Both the APUD (amine precursor uptake and decarboxylation) concept (2) of tumor peptide production and the derepression theory (3) require reappraisal in the light of our better understanding of cellular differentiation. However, for the clinical endocrinologist these unresolved questions may not be strictly relevant and for them the impact of ectopic hormone production is twofold. Thus the metabolic abnormality caused by ectopic hormone secretion may be more malignant than the underlying histopathological nature of the neoplasm itself, which may be relatively benign. Furthermore, "silent" peptide production not associated with an overtly obvious clinical syndrome may occasionally provide a "marker" of tumor activity for use diagnostically or in following the progress of the disease.

I. THE "ECTOPIC" ADRENOCORTICOTROPIC HORMONE (ACTH) SYNDROME

A. Clinical Features

These are dominated by the sustained, high-circulating glucocorticoid levels, causing myopathy, diabetes mellitus, acne, hypertension, and edema. Severe pigmentation is unusual, but psychosis may be a prominent feature (4). If the underlying neoplasm is highly malignant, such as a small-cell carcinoma of the lung, the characteristic body habitus and Cushingoid facies may be absent, in which event survival can only be counted in weeks unless the hypercortisolemia is alleviated. In contrast, with a more benign lesion, the symptoms and clinical presentation may be indistinguishable from that observed in pituitary-dependent Cushing's disease. In my experience, hypokalemia is an invariable accompaniment of ectopic ACTH secretion, and is very unusual in pituitary-dependent disease and also unusual with adrenal tumors.

The reason for the almost invariable presence of hypokalemia is unclear. Thus, although an excellent correlation exists between plasma cortisol and serum potassium levels, suggesting that the low serum potassium reflects the severity of the hypercortisolemia, other factors may be involved. For example, it is possible that secretion of more potent mineralocorticoids, such as desoxycorticosterone (DOC), may occur or that the adrenocortical bioactivity of ACTH is potentiated by the secretion of other proopiocortin-derived peptides. Thus some novel peptides related to γ-melanocyte stimulating hormone (MSH) (5, 6) may be secreted only by the neoplastic tissue and not by the pituitary in Cushing's disease, although it must be stressed that this hypothesis remains highly speculative.

B. Diagnosis

Of 46 patients with Cushing's syndrome seen at St. Bartholomew's Hospital (G. M. Besser, personal communication, 1978) between 1968 and 1978, 20% were ultimately proven to have the ectopic ACTH syndrome. Any patient with a tumor and hypokalemia or with clinical Cushing's syndrome and either high ACTH levels, high cortisol levels, or hypokalemia should be considered to have the ectopic ACTH syndrome until proven otherwise. In some patients the tumor may be clinically occult due to its very small size, and thus may only become overt years after the initial presentation of the Cushing's syndrome. The tests used to try to prove ectopic ACTH production include:

1. Plasma ACTH levels. Although these may be higher than those seen in pituitary-dependent disease, this is not invariable, and in many patients levels may lie within the normal 9 am range and completely overlap with levels observed in patients with pituitary-dependent disease.
2. Metyrapone test (750 mg every 4 hr for 48 hrs). The majority of patients with the ectopic ACTH syndrome will not demonstrate a rise in urinary 17-OHCS or plasma ACTH when cortisol levels fall since tumor ACTH secretion is believed to be autonomous.
3. High-dose dexamethasone (2 mg every 6 hr for 48 hr). This will suppress ACTH and hence cortisol secretion by approximately 50% (as measured by

urinary 17 OHCS) in the majority of patients with Cushing's disease. However, some patients with ectopic production will show such supression, although this may of course reflect only coincident cyclical tumor production of ACTH.

C. Tumor Localization

This increasing recognition of encountered exceptions to the rules outlined above has led to the general acceptance that the differentiation between pituitary-dependent Cushing's disease and the ectopic ACTH syndrome may be very difficult or even impossible by these conventional means (7-9). Furthermore, the search for occult ectopic sources may not be possible using conventional radiological techniques (7, 8, 10). Thus, recently it has become clear that the judicious use of computerized axial tomography (CAT) scanning of organs known to harbor occult ACTH-secreting tumors or selective venous catheterization with ACTH measurements in an attempt at biochemical localization may both be useful adjuncts in investigation. In particular, the CAT scan may be invaluable for detecting occult thymic tumors (11-13), when conventional mediastinal x-ray tomography in untreated Cushing's syndrome may be misleading due to the presence of mediastinal adiposity (14), whereas a clear definition between fat and tumor is possible by CAT scanning (15). Other organs which may harbor occult ectopic ACTH-secreting tumors for which CAT scanning may be valuable include the adrenals (pheochromocytomas), pancreas, and lung (13).

The value of venous catheterization with selective blood sampling to locate other hormonally active tumors is well documented for adrenal tumors, both cortical and medullary and parathyroid adenomas, as is its use in the investigation of renovascular hypertension. Until recently, only single-case reports have been described of its use in Cushing's syndrome. Recently, however, Findling and colleagues (16) reported its used in 10 patients with Cushing's syndrome in which the inferior petrosal sinus was sampled. They found this of value in confirming the pituitary origin in five out of six patients, but failed to locate the ectopic sources in the others.

In a more extensive study, Drury and colleagues (17) studied 23 patients with ACTH-dependent Cushing's syndrome and confirmed high internal jugular vein ACTH levels in nine of ten patients with pituitary-dependent disease. Eight patients had 11 proven sites of ectopic ACTH production and six of these were correctly identified by the sampling techniques; furthermore, in four of them this was the only accurate method of localization. The results of one catheter were misleading, on 10 occasions were inconclusive, and five patients remained undiagnosed by any method. Overall, 15 of 28 catheterizations provided diagnostically valuable information.

In this latter study, multiple and simultaneous sampling to establish peripheral plasma concentrations as a "control" were used, since ACTH secretion from both pituitary and ectopic sources may be intermittent and pulsatile. Thus, unless the background variation can be established, the relevance of a single high value during the catheter cannot be correctly evaluated. In pituitary-dependent disease, high internal jugular vein sampling provided further evidence of the pituitary origin in 90% of patients. Since this is a safe procedure, well tolerated by the patient, it can be recommended as a useful diagnostic adjunct when other data, such as serum potassium or metyrapone testing, produce results which are atypical of pituitary-dependent disease.

In four of the six patients in whom an ectopic source was located, no other method, including CAT scanning, had shown any source of ACTH, and in four curative surgery was possible. However, 5 of the 23 patients remain undiagnosed and reasons for this high failure rate may include periodic hormone secretion (18), failure to cannulate the appropriate veins, or dilution and/or metabolism of ACTH from the bronchial or portal circulations.

In this regard it is of interest that the two bronchial carcinoids in the series were not located, and it may be that arterial sampling will prove superior for correctly locating small pulmonary tumors. Only one catheter provided misleading information, suggesting a definite pituitary source in a patient with a subsequently identified ectopic source. One may of course speculate that this tumor was producing a stimulus to pituitary ACTH secretion, such as corticotrophin releasing factor (19).

Finally, we must remember that tumors involved in ectopic ACTH secretion may elaborate an array of other peptides related to proopiocortin apart from ACTH itself. Thus concomitant β-lipotropin (β-LPH) secretion is usually the rule as well as secretion of the opiate-like peptide β-endorphin.

In particular, the secretion of β-endorphin and met-enkephalin (20) might have considerable clinical implications. Thus these opioid peptides can produce profound behavioral as well as analgesic effects in experimental animals and also in humans. It is interesting to speculate that their production might be responsible for suppressing the local clinical expression of the tumors as well as causing psychiatric disturbances observed in patients with malignant disease but without cerebral metastases. On a broader front we may surmise that elaboration of centrally active neuropeptides could combine to modify the clinical features of a wide spectrum of neoplasia.

II. MALIGNANT HYPERCALCEMIA

Hypercalcemia is a not uncommon accompaniment of cancer and is always associated with high morbidity and mortality. Cancer is the commonest cause of hypercalcemia; this occurs in approximately 10-20% of all patients suffering from cancer: in particular those with tumors of lung, breast, kidney, and patients with multiple myeloma. The accelerated bone resorption, which is usually the cause of the hypercalcemia, is believed to be mediated by hormonal and/or metabolic mechanisms.

The symptoms of hypercalcemia will not be elaborated, but their severity usually relates to the level of serum calcium. In most patients, regardless of the underlying pathology, the calcium is usually >3.0 mmol/liter and the serum phosphate low or normal. When secondary renal damage ensues, hypokalemic alkalosis may occur. The clinical features which help to distinguish this disorder from primary hyperparathyroidism include the rapidity of symptoms and absence of either periosteal bone resorption or nephrocalcinosis. Thus it is usually easy to diagnose malignant hypercalcemia and from most series of patients studied it is generally agreed that malignancy only rarely presents as a problem of hypercalcemia of unknown origin. Indeed, most surveys show that at least 75% of patients with hypercalcemia of malignancy have overt metastatic disease and probably another 15% will have metastases if a careful search is instituted (21). This leaves a residue of about 10% of patients who have hypercalcemia in association with localized neoplastic disease. Furthermore, these figures, which are generally accepted, are compatible with the poor prognosis of malignant hypercalcemia since most patients will have advanced disease, with 50% dying within 3 months and 80% within 1 year of the onset of hypercalcemia (21).

Cancer and primary hyperparathyroidism are common in the general population (cancer 1.4%; hyperparathyroidism approximately 0.7%), and in a review in 1976, Heath (22) noted 118 cases of the coexistence of these two diseases and Drezner and Lebovitz (23) proved primary hyperparathyroidism in 6 of 11 patients referred with hypercalcemia and cancer. However, in practice the differentiation between the diagnoses of primary hyperparathyroidism and malignant hypercalcemia is rarely a problem. However, if doubt exists, the hydrocortisone suppression test may be of value. If the test is performed as originally described (24) (120 mg hydrocortisone per day for 10 days, correcting the serum calcium for hemodilution), it provides excellent discrimination, since significant suppression of serum calcium does not occur in primary hyperparathyroidism, whereas malignant hypercalcemia is usually completely alleviated.

In patients with metastatic involvement of bone (mainly breast, bronchus, and kidney) factors such as prostaglandin release by the tumor tissue may cause local bone resorption, resulting in liberation of calcium. However, most interest has been shown not in the mechanisms by which bony metastases cause hypercalcemia (approximately 90% of patients), but in the mechanism by which hypercalcemia occurs in the other 10% with localized tumors.

Over 40 years ago Albright (25) suggested that the hypercalcemia he observed in a patient with a renal cell cancer could be due to elaboration by the tumor of a parathyroid hormone (PTH)-like substance. Initially, great credence was given to this hypothesis, although in recent years it has become clear that ectopic PTH secretion is a very uncommon event. Thus, if ectopic PTH production is indeed a rare occurrence, what is the etiology of nonmetastatic hypercalcemia? Various prostaglandins, especially those of the E series, are known to be potent stimulators of bone resorption in vitro and they may play a role in the excessive local bone destruction caused by metastatic tumors from kidney or breast (26) as well as facilitate the deposition of bony deposits. It is unlikely that circulating levels per se would ever be sufficient to cause bone resorption either as a physiological event or to be responsible for the production of hypercalcemia in the absence of metastases. However, although increased plasma prostaglandins and their urinary metabolites were shown in a small group of hypercalcemic patients without metastatic disease but with solid tumors (27), the response of such patients to treatment with prostaglandin synthetase inhibitors such as indomethacin has been uniformly disappointing.

A family of peptide substances, the osteoclast activating factors, have also been implicated in the pathogenesis of hypercalcemia associated with multiple myeloma and some lymphomas (28). These substances stimulate the number and activity of osteoclasts and their effects can be inhibited by glucocorticoids. Since steroids are often effective in reducing malignant hypercalcemia, this suggests their possible involvement in its pathogenesis (29).

More recently, studies by Stewart and colleagues (29) have suggested that hypercalcemia of malignancy might be explained by yet another mechanism. Thus, using measurements of nephrogenous cyclic AMP excretion as a marker of the biological activity of PTH, they conclude that some tumors might produce a non-PTH-like peptide which could mimic some of the hormonal activities usually associated with native PTH itself. Unfortunately, these observations remain highly controversial and as with so many other studies, the tumor tissues themselves were not examined for the presence of substances with such hormonal activity.

What then of true ectopic PTH secretion? Does it ever occur? A wide variety of different tumor types have been purported to secrete PTH, including a large number of squamous cell tumors originating in many different organs and tumors of breast and pancreas. Unfortunately, the strict criteria required for proof of ectopic hormone production are sorely lacking for PTH, whereas these criteria have been more than adequately fulfilled for some other hormones and in particular for ACTH. The few conclusive data compatible with true ectopic PTH secretion are contained within single-case reports which include the clear demonstration of an arteriovenous gradient of PTH across the tumor, in vitro PTH secretion by tumor cells, high levels of PTH-like material in extracts of tumor tissue, and high levels of PTH and increased urinary cyclic AMP in hypercalcemic patients. Furthermore, in one patient, hypercalcemia was maintained by ectopic PTH production in a parathyroidectomized patient whose requirements for calcium supplementation disappeared with he developed a lung tumor, PTH levels in his blood increased, and serum calcium fell on irradiation of the tumor (30). Thus, in the light of our poor understanding of the basic mechanisms underlying nonmetastatic hypercalcemia apart from conventional measurements of calcium, phosphate, and immunoreactive PTH, there is little point in the physician undertaking any other investigation as a routine during diagnosis, and attention should be directed at effective treatment when possible.

III. INAPPROPRIATE ANTIDIURESIS

The association of lung cancer and hyponatremia was first noted in 1938 by Winkler and Crankshaw (31), but it was not until 1957 that the cause was attributed to secretion of antidiuretic hormone. Elevated plasma and urinary vasopressin levels are reported and high tumor concentrations as well as in vitro synthesis by tumor tissue has been well documented. True ectopic vasopressin secretion is a feature only of small-cell lung cancer and its proven association with other cancers is rare. In contrast, inappropriate antidiuresis can occur in association with a wide variety of malignant and benign conditions, usually in association with either intrathoracic or intracerebral pathology.

Inappropriate antidiuresis is indeed a common accompaniment of small-cell lung cancer. In a series of 56 patients with this type of tumor proven histologically, 30% showed evidence of inappropriate antidiuresis when provocative water loading was employed, and levels of biologically active vasopressin (AVP) inappropriate for the plasma osmolality (>2.0 μU/ml) have been observed in such patients (32). In 10 patients studied after chemotherapy the syndrome resolved completely in three and partially in two. Furthermore, Odell and colleagues (33) detected elevated AVP levels of about 2.0 μU/ml in 41% and 43% of patients with lung and colonic cancer, respectively, compared with levels of 1.2 μU/ml in 46 normal subjects after dehydration.

Having said that the ectopic AVP secretion can occur, in many instances the cause of the water retention in patients with lung tumors may be due to other mechanisms. In a detailed study using hypertonic saline infusions, Robertson (34) looked at osmoreceptor responsiveness in these patients and defined several different response patterns. He concluded that about half of the patients with lung cancer and inappropriate antidiuresis had excess vasopressin secretion resulting from posterior pituitary stimulation due to abnormal signals received from an altered or defective osmoreceptor, and suggested different mechanisms to explain this defect. Thus carcinomatous involvement of the vagus nerve could interfere with baroregulatory input, which was one of the hypotheses postulated by Schwartz and his colleagues (35) in the original publication on this subject. Furthermore, neoplastic disease resulting in inferior vena cava obstruction may cause hypovolemia and/or hypotension, which can lower the threshold set point of the osmoregulatory system and stimulate vasopressin secretion. Finally, metastatic destruction of the hypothalamus could disturb posterior pituitary activity and, on a more speculative note, tumor production of substances capable of stimulating the posterior pituitary to secrete vasopressin remains a theoretical possibility.

In patients with true ectopic vasopressin secretion this is invariably accompanied by secretion of neurophysin I or II, although oxytocin production has also rarely been described. Recently, two studies have suggested that human neurophysin measurements may be of value, both in the differential diagnosis of inappropriate antidiuresis and as a tumor marker in patients without inappropriate antidiuresis but harboring small-cell lung tumors (36, 37). Pullan and colleagues (36) found that in a large number of patients with lung tumors ectopic vasopressin secretion was associated only with small-cell tumors and that raised neurophysin II levels were also observed, but not in patients with noncancerous causes of inappropriate antidiuresis. In another study North and colleagues (37) found raised levels of neurophysin I and II in 62% of 61 patients with small-cell cancer prior to treatment and a fairly good correlation between the levels and clinical response. Thus it seems that neurophysin measurements might be of value as a tumor marker for small-cell lung cancer, although, for obvious reasons their use in differential diagnosis will be of limited value since the tumor will usually be clinically overt. If neurophysin measurements are to be employed diagnostically, it must be remembered that drugs such as estrogens may cause neurophysin II levels to be raised, and hepatic and renal disease likewise. Finally, small-cell carcinoma is not the only tumor which can secrete ectopic vasopressin, and sporadic reports implicate carcinoma of pancreas, bladder, prostate, and deuodenum.

Minor degrees of hyponatremia are usually asymptomatic, but when the serum Na falls below 110 mEq/liter, water intoxication with fits and neurological disturbances leading to coma and death occur and urgent treatment may be required. The most effective and usually well tolerated treatment is water restriction alone (500–1000 ml per day), although there have been several vogues for the use of drugs such as demethylchlortetracycline, lithium, and more recently urea—all associated with their own particular problems (38).

Whenever possible, treatment, usually in the form of chemotherapy, should be directed at the underlying tumor, which if a small-cell tumor, will of course be unlikely to result in cure.

IV. ECTOPIC GONADOTROPIN AND PLACENTAL LACTOGEN (hPL) SECRETION

The early hopes that the secretion of human chorionic gonadotropin (hCG) or its subunits might be of great value as tumor markers have not been fulfilled. Thus the hypothesis that hCG should only be present in the circulation during pregnancy, in women with trophoblastic tumors, or in males with testicular neoplasia containing trophoblastic elements has clearly not been substantiated. Thus hCG is known to be synthesized by certain cells in normal adult tissues and hCG has been detected in normal human serum (39). Furthermore, hCG is present in adult human liver and throughout the gastrointestinal tract. However, there is some evidence that in these tissues the hCG may differ from normal placental hCG, and desialated forms of hCG with reduced biological activity may be present. Furthermore, hCG levels increase in rapidly regenerating tissues such as occurs in the hepatitic or cirrhotic liver.

From a diagnostic standpoint increased levels of hCG or its α or β subunits have been found in a high proportion of patients with islet cell pancreatic cancer, free α subunits being the commonest occurrence (40). Furthermore, Odell and colleagues (41) observed that in 186 patients with a variety of malignancies 41% have raised α-subunit levels compared with age-matched controls; intact hCG was detected in only 6% of the cancer group. Thus hCG or its subunits may be of value as a diagnostic marker for some tumors. Although the amounts of hCG secreted ectopically may equal that seen in the first trimester of pregnancy, no recognizable clinical syndrome may result. As mentioned earlier, this may be due to secretion of desialated hCG-like peptides with reduced half-life and little biological activity, since some tumors may lack the enzymes necessary for adding carbohydrate residues (42, 43).

However, two clear clinical syndromes are recognized in association with hCG production. Precocious puberty may occur in male children and interstitial cell hyperplasia with gynecomastia in adult males. In the male children the tumor is usually a hepatoma or hepatoblastoma and hCG measurement is of great value diagnostically, although the prognosis for these tumors is poor.

The reason for the production of gynecomastia in adult males is unclear. The underlying tumor is usually a large-cell lung tumor and it is possible either that hCG secretion results in increased testicular estrogen secretion, or that steroid interconversion occurs within the tumor mass, resulting in increased amounts of circulating estradiol. However, concomitant human placental lactogen (hPL) secretion often occurs and the incidence of hPL production in patients with nontrophoblastic neoplasia is approximately equal to that observed for intact-hCG production (5–6%), and gynecomastia also occurs in these patients.

In all cancer patients with detectable hPL levels, elevated plasma estrogens were observed. While the level of hPL alone might not be high enough to cause gynecomastia, the associated gonadotropin secretion causing increased amounts of testicular estrogen might, in combination, cause breast enlargement. Recently, the painful gynecomastia associated with ectopic hCG production by a lung cancer was successfully treated with antiestrogen tamoxifen (43).

While HCG and HPL measurements may have a limited diagnostic value, as discussed earlier, attempts to employ serial measurements as markers of therapeutic response have not been very useful since discordance between tumor growth and circulating hormone levels is often observed. This contrasts strongly with the serial use of hCG measurements in women with gestational trophoblastic tumors and men with germ cell tumors of the testes, where concordance is usually excellent between hormone level and tumor cell mass. hPL without hCG has been identified in a number of tumors, particularly pulmonary tumors, and has been studied extensively in carcinoma of the breast, where it can be identified in tumor tissue often in association with pregnancy specific β-glycoproteins (44). An improved prognosis was claimed when hPL was absent from the breast tissue, and in another study hPL was detected in serum of 10 of 72 women with breast cancer, with none detected in the control group (patients with mastitis, fibroadenosis, and in normal males and females) (45).

V. ECTOPIC GROWTH HORMONE (GH) AND PROLACTIN

Both of these events are rare, the literature consisting of a handful of case reports. Of greater importance is the possible secretion of substances with growth hormone releasing activity (GHRA). Thus the first reports of this phenomenon occurred in patients with clinical acromegaly in whom removal of bronchial carcinoids resulted in clinical and biochemical remission of the acromegaly (46-48). In a more recent study, Frohman and colleagues (49) described three patients with GH-secreting pituitary tumors and clinical acromegaly and three different tumors (one bronchial carcinoid, one abdominal carcinoid with hepatic metastases, and a pancreatic islet cell tumor) and attempted further biological and physicochemical characterization of the GHRA extracted from these tumors. They demonstrated dose-response relationships using GH release from dispersed rat anterior pituitary cells both in monolayer culture and in a perfusion system and also confirmed the peptide nature of the GHRA. While these observations are still of a preliminary nature, they are of great interest for two reasons: first, they suggest that prolonged stimulation of normal pituitary tissue by a releasing factor can result in tumor formation, and second, it reminds us to look carefully for the coexistence of nonpituitary tumors in every patient with acromegaly.*

---

*Since the preparation of this manuscript, the structure of growth hormone releasing factors isolated from human pancreatic tumors has been described (53, 54).

Ectopic prolactin secretion is a rare event, although raised prolactin levels have been observed in some patients with lung cancer, possibly due not to ectopic production, but to either "stress" or reflex neural stimulation of prolactin secretion associated with the presence of intrathoracic metastases. However, in a recent study of patients with testicular tumors, raised prolactin levels were observed in patients with nonseminomatous testicular tumors, those with seminomatous tumors having normal levels (50). The authors postulated that nonseminomatous testicular tumors may either elaborate factors such as estrogens which stimulate prolactin release, or that prolactin may be an ectopic tumor product. Again, no data on tumor tissue prolactin levels were provided.

A. Ectopic Calcitonin Secretion

Although the measurement of calcitonin is invaluable as a diagnostic marker for medullary carcinoma of the thyroid, its production by nonthyroidal cancers is less well known. Raised circulating immunoreactive calcitonin levels occur in approximately 50% of all patients with lung cancer (mean level 1250 pg/ml; normals <250 pg/ml); levels may also be raised in patients with nonmalignant lung disease as well as in patients with other tumors, such as carcinoma of the breast (51). In the study of patients with lung cancer, Silva et al. (51) undertook venous sampling in some patients and defined two groups: those in whom calcitonin appeared to originate from the thyroid, and those who appeared to have true ectopic calcitonin secretion. In 75% of patients the elevated calcitonin levels decreased when therapy was directed at the primary tumor, and the actual level correlated with clinical status in 67% of patients. Interestingly, the incidence of hypercalcemia was identical in the two groups, and therefore did not correlate with raised calcitonin levels. Furthermore, hypercalcitoninemia did not correlate with the presence of osseous metastases, which might be expected if thyroid calcitonin secretion was stimulated as a physiological response to the development of osseous metastases. Finally, these authors state that with the exception of CEA, no other substance is elevated so often in patients with lung cancer.

B. Multiple Ectopic Hormone Secretion

Multiple ectopic hormone synthesis and secretion is probably common and the reported pairing of ACTH with AVP and hPL with hCG may reflect only the special interests of the investigators. This supposition is probably true, since with the wider availability of the technically more exacting hormone measurements, it has become clear that many more single tumors may synthesize many more hormones. This, for example, is reflected in a recent report of a pancreatic islet cell tumor containing gastrin, ACTH, α-endorphin, somatostatin, and calcitonin in a patient with clinical Zollinger-Ellison syndrome and Cushing's syndrome (52). The pathogenesis of multiple ectopic hormone secretion by pancreatic islet cell tumors and other tumors remains unclear. However, such tumors could either be composed of mixed cell types or arise from undifferentiated pluripotential cells present in the pancreatic ductules.

From a diagnostic standpoint, multiple ectopic hormone secretion *is* important. Thus, in the difficult differential diagnosis of ACTH-dependent Cushing's syndrome, a tumor marker screen, using multiple hormone measurements as well as the measurement of nonhormonal proteins (such as AFP, CEA, and pancreatic polypeptide), may be of value in pointing more definitively toward the presence of an ectopic ACTH-secreting tumor.

REFERENCES

1. Baylin SB, Mendelsohn G. Ectopic (inappropriate) hormone production by tumors: mechanisms involved and the biological and clinical implications. Endocr Rev 1980; 1:45–77.
2. Pearse AGE. The cytochemistry and ultrastructure of polypeptide hormone-producing cells of the APUD series and the embryologic, physiologic and pathologic implications of the concept. J Histochem Cytochem 1969; 17: 307–313.
3. Gellhorn A. The unifying thread. Cancer Res 1963; 23: 961–970.
4. Jeffcoate WJ, Silverstone JT, Edwards CRW, Besser GM. Psychiatric manifestations of Cushing's syndrome: response to lowering of plasma cortisol. Br Med J 1979; 2:213–217.
5. Pedersen RC, Brownie AC. Adrenocortical response to corticotropin is potentiated by part of the amino-terminal region of pro-opiocortin/endorphin. Proc Natl Acad Sci USA 1980; 77:2239.
6. Al-Dujaili EAS, Hope J, Estivariz FE, Lowry PJ, Edwards CRW. Circulating pituitary pro-γ-melanotropin enhances the adrenal response to ACTH. Nature 1981; 291:156–159.
7. Aron DC, Tyrrell JB, Fitzgerald PA, Findling JW, Forsham PH. Cushing's syndrome: problems in diagnosis. Medicine 1981; 60:25–35.
8. Gold EM. The Cushing's syndrome: changing views of diagnosis and treatment. Ann Intern Med 1979; 90:829–844.
9. Crapo L. Cushing's syndrome: a review of diagnosis tests. Metabolism 1979; 28:955–977.
10. Flint LD, Jacobs EC. Belated recognition of adrenocorticotrophic producing hormone in post-adrenalectomized Cushing's syndrome. J Urol 1974; 112:688–688.
11. Thorner MO, Ragan G, Ortt B, Swgert N, Williamson BRJ, Macleod RM, Orth, DN. Thymic carcinoid tumor secreting ACTH intermittently and identified by CAT scan. Abstract 61st Annual Meeting of the Endocrine Society, 1979, p 155.
12. Drury PL, Pullan PJ, Wass J, Clement-Jones V, Edwards CRW, Rees LH, Besser GM. Variable weakness in a bar-maid. Paper presented to the Endocrine Section of the Royal Society of Medicine, 1979.

13. White FC, Drury PL, Kelsey Fry I, White P. The use of CT in the investigation of Cushing's syndrome. Proceedings of the 15th International Congress of Radiologists, 1982; in press.
14. Santini LC, Williams JL. Mediastinal widening (presumably lipomatosis) in Cushing's syndrome. N Engl J Med 1971; 284:1357–1359.
15. Bien ME, Mancuso AA, Mink MH, Hansen G. Computed tomography in the evaluation of mediastinal lipomatosis. J Comput Assist Tomogr 1978; 2:379–383.
16. Findling JW, Aron DC, Tyrrell JB, Shinsako JH, Fitzgerald PA, Norman D, Wilson CB, Forsham PH. Selective venous sampling for ACTH in Cushing's syndrome. Ann Intern Med 1981; 94:647–652.
17. Drury PL, Ratter SJ, Tomlin S, Williams J, Dacie JE, Rees LH, Besser GM. Experience with selective venous sampling in the diagnosis of ACTH-dependent Cushing's syndrome. Br Med J 1982;
18. Bailey RE. Periodic hormonogenesis–a new phenomenon. J Clin Endocrinol Metab 1971; 32:317–327.
19. Upton GV, Amatruda TT Jr. Evidence for the presence of tumour peptides with corticotrophin releasing factor-like activity in the ectopic ACTH syndrome. New Engl J Med 1971; 285:419–424.
20. Pullan PT, Clement-Jones V, Corder R, Lowry PJ, Rees GM, Rees LH, Besser GM, Macedo MM, Galvao-Teles A. Ectopic methionine enkephalin and β-endorphin. Br Med J 1980; 1:758–763.
21. Fisken RA, Heath DA, Bold AM. Hypercalcaemia–a hospital survey. QJ Med 1980; 196:405–418.
22. Heath DA, Hypercalcaemia and malignancy. Ann Clin Biochem 1976; 13: 555–560.
23. Drezner MK, Lebovitz HE. Primary hyperparathyroidism in paraneoplastic hypercalcaemia. Lancet 1978; 1:1004–1000.
24. Dent CE, Watson L. The hydrocortisone test in primary and tertiary hyperparathyroidism. Lancet 1968; 2:662–664.
25. Albright F. Case records of the Massachusetts General Hospital. Case 27461. N Engl J Med 1941; 225:789–794.
26. Greaves M, Ibbotson KF, Atkins D, Martin TJ. Prostaglandins as mediators of bone resorption in renal and breast tumors. Clin Sci 1980; 58:201–210.
27. Seyberth HW, Segre CV, Hamet P, Sweetman BJ, Potts TT, Oates JA. Characterisation of a group of patients with hypercalcaemia of cancer who respond to treatment with prostaglandin synthesis inhibitors. Trans Assoc Am Physicians 1976; 89:92–104.
28. Munday GR, Rick, ME, Turcotte R, Kowalski MA. Pathogenesis of hypercalcaemia in lymphosarcoma cell leukaemia. Role of an osteoclast activating activity factor-like substance and the mechanism of action for glucocorticoid therapy. Am J Med 1978; 65:600–606.
29. Stewart AF, Horst R, Deftos LT, Cadman EC, Lang R, Broadus AE. Biochemical evaluation of patients with cancer-associated hypercalcaemia. N Engl J Med 1980; 303:1377–1383.
30. Licata AA, Guccion JG, Glowitz RJ. Spontaneous return of normocalcaemia. JAMA 1938; 240:468–469.

31. Winkler WA, Crankshaw OF. Chloride depletion in conditions other than Addison's disease. J Clin Invest 1938; 17:1–6.
32. Gilby ED, Rees LH, Bondy P. Ectopic hormones as markers of response to therapy in cancer. Excerpta Medica Ser 1976; 375:132–138.
33. Odell W, Wolfsen A, Yoshimoto Y, Wertzinan R, Fisher D, Hirose F. Ectopic peptide synthesis: a universal concomitant of neoplasia. Trans Assoc Am Physicians 1977; 90:204–227.
34. Robertson GL. 1978. Cancer and inappropriate antidiuresis. In *Biological Markers of Neoplasia: Basic and Applied Aspects,* Ruddon, RW (ed). Elsevier, New York, p 277.
35. Schwartz WB, Bennett W, Curelop S, Bartter FC. A syndrome of renal sodium loss and hyponatraemia probably resulting from inappropriate secretion of antidiuretic hormone. Am J Med 1975; 23:529–542.
36. Pullan PT, Clappison BH, Johnston CI. Plasma vasopressin and human neurophysins in physiological and pathological states associated with changes in vasopressin secretion. J Clin Endocrinol Metab 1979; 49:580–587.
37. North WG, Maurer LH, Valtin H, O'Donnell JF. Human neurophysins as potential tumour markers for small cell carcinoma of the lung: application of specific radioimmunoassays. J Clin Endocrinol Metab 1980; 51: 892–896.
38. Decaus G, Genette F. Urea for long-term treatment of syndrome of inappropriate secretion of antidiuretic hormone. Br Med J 1981; 283: 1081–1083.
39. Borowski A, Muquardt C. Human chorionic gonadotrophin in the plasma of normal, non-pregnant subjects. N Engl J Med 1979; 301:298–302.
40. Kahn CR, Rosen SW, Weintraub BD, Fajans SS, Gordon P. Ectopic production of chorionic gonadotrophin and its subunits by islet cell tumours. N. Engl J Med 1977; 297:565–569.
41. Van-Hall EV, Vaitukaitis JL, Ross GT, Hickman JW, Ashwell G. Immunological and biological activity of HCG following progressive desialation. Endocrinology 1971; 88:450–464.
42. Yashimoto Y, Wolfsen AR, Odell WD. Glycosylation, a variable in the production of HCG by cancers. Ann J Med 1979; 67:414–420.
43. Jefferys, DB. Painful gynaecomastia treated with tamoxifen. Br Med J 1979; 1:1119–1120.
44. Horne CHW, Reid IN, Milne ED. Prognostic significance of inappropriate production of pregnancy protein by breast cancer. Lancet 1976; 2: 279–282.
45. Sheth NA, Suraiyz JN, Sheth AR, Randive KG, Jussawalla DJ. Ectopic production of human placental lactogen by breast tumours. Cancer 1977; 39:1093–1099.
46. Dabek JT. Bronchial carcinoid tumour with acromegaly in two patients. J Clin Endocrinol Metab 1974; 38:329–333.
47. Sonksen PH, Ayres AB, Braimbridge M, Corrin B, Davies DR, Jeremiah GM, Oaten SW, Lowy C, West TET. Acromegaly caused by pulmonary carcinoid tumours. Clin Endocrinol 1976; 5:503–513.

48. Gomez-Pan A, Scanlon ME, Thorner MO, Rees LH, Schally AV, Hall R, Besser GM. Effect of somatostatin on abnormal growth hormone and prolactin secretion in patients with the carcinoid syndrome. Clin Endocrinol 1979; 10:575-581.
49. Frohman LA, Szabo M, Berelowitz M, Stachura ME. Partial purification and characterisation of a peptide with growth hormone-releasing activity from extrapituitary tumours in patients with acromegaly. J Clin Invest 1980; 65:43-54.
50. Maclean GD, Holdaway IM. The serum prolactin level in testicular tumours: a new tumour marker. Aust NZ J Surg 1980; 50:384-386.
51. Silva OL, Broder LE, Doppman JL, Snider RH, Moore CF, Cohen MH, Becker KL. Calcitonin as a marker for bronchogenic cancer. 1979; 44: 680-684.
52. Asa SL, Kovacs K, Killinger DW, Marcon N, Platts M. Pancreatic islet cell carcinoma producing gastrin, ACTH, α-endorphin, somatostatin and calcitonin. Am J Gastrotenterol 1980; 74:30-35.
53. Rivier J, Spiess J, Thorner M, Vale W. Characterization of growth hormone-releasing factor from a human pancreatic islet tumor. Nature 1982; 300: 276-278.
54. Guillemia R, Brazeau P, Böhlen P, Esch F, Ling N, Wehrenberg WB. Growth hormone releasing factor from a human pancreatic tumor that caused acromegaly. Science 1982; 218:585-587.

35
Somatostatin

Lesley H. Rees
St. Bartholomew's Hospital Medical College, London, England

A number of somatostatin secreting tumors of the D cells of the pancreas have now been described (1-3). In the seven patients reported, the presenting symptom was hyperglycemia. Other symptoms included weight loss, anemia, hypochlorhydria, steatorrhea, and cholelithiasis. Many of these symptoms can be explained by the known inhibitory actions of somatostatin on the exocrine and endocrine functions of the pancreas and on gastric acid secretion. Most of the patients were women, five of the tumors were malignant, and three were also associated with the coincident secretion of adrenocorticotropic hormone (ACTH) and calcitonin (4). When measured, plasma immunoreactive somatostatin levels were found to be grossly elevated, and high tumor tissue concentrations have also been reported.

However, since many of the patients presented with mild symptoms and a long clinical history, despite the very high circulating plasma immunoreactive somatostatin levels, and since all the described biological effects of somatostatin were not observed in every patient, the in vivo bioactivity of the tumor somatostatin must be questioned. Indeed, since higher molecular weight forms of somatostatin have been observed in some plasmas and in tumor extracts (5) from these patients, the exact relationship of tumor somatostatin to authentic somatostatin-14 and its biological activity remains to be established.

Most pancreatic endocrine tumors are pleomorphic, containing mixed cell populations, and it is not surprising that somatostatin-containing cells have been identified in other tumors in which the chief secreted product is not somatostatin, but vasoactive intestinal polypeptide (VIP), insulin, glucagon, or gastrin (5, 6). In one patient, who presented in hypoglycemic coma with operative evidence of a metastatic pancreatic (7) malignancy immunohistochemical study of the biopsied tissue showed a major predominance of somatostatin-containing cells. Although the patient's symptoms were due to her inappropriate insulin levels, her circulating immunoreactive somatostatin levels ranged from 7500 to 16,800 pg/ml (NR 17-81 pg/ml). This patient's tumor has regressed dramatically on treatment with diazoxide, chlorthiazide, and 5-fluorouracil, and she remains very well 3½ years after initial diagnosis.

REFERENCES

1. Larsson L-I, Hirsch MA, Holst JJ, Ingemansson S, Kühl, C, Lindkaer-Jenson S, Lundquist G, Rehfeld JF, Schwartz TW. Pancreatic somatostatinoma. Clinical features and physiological implications. Lancet 1977; 1:666–668.
2. Ganda, OP, Weir GC, Soeldner JS, Legg MA, Chick WL, Patel WC, Ebeid AM, Gabbay KH, Reichlin S. Somatostatinoma–a somatostatin containing tumour of the endocrine pancreas. N Engl J Med 1977; 297:1352–1357.
3. Krejs GJ, Orci L, Conlon JM, Ravazzola M, Davis GR, Raskin P, Collins SM, McCarthy DM, Baetens D, Rubenstein A, Aldor JAM, Unger RH. Somatostatinoma syndrome: biochemical, morphological and clinical features. N Engl J Med 1977; 301:285–292.
4. Kovacs K, Horvath E, Ezrin C, Sepp H, Elkan I. Immunoreactive somatostatin in pancreatic islet cell carcinoma accompanied by ectopic ACTH syndrome. Lancet 1977; 1:1365.
5. Penman E, Lowry PJ, Wass JAH, Marks V, Dawson AM, Besser GM, Rees LH. Molecular forms of somatostatin in normal subjects and in patients with pancreatic somatostatinoma. Clin Endocrinol 1980; 12:611–620.
6. Bloom SR, Polak JM, West AM. Somatostatin content of pancreatic endocrine tumours. Metabolism 1978; 27 (suppl I): 1235–1238.
7. Wright J, Abolfathi A, Penman E, Marks V. Pancreatic somatostatinoma presenting with hypoglycaemia. Clin Endocrinol 1980; 12:603–609.

COMMONLY USED DYNAMIC TESTS

36

Hypothalamic Releasing Hormone Tests

Henry G. Burger and David M. Hurley
Prince Henry's Hospital, Melbourne, Australia

Two hypothalamic releasing hormone preparations are available for routine diagnostic use: thyrotropin releasing hormone (also called thyroliberin and TRH) and gonadotropin releasing hormone (also known as luteinizing hormone releasing hormone, luliberin, GnRH, or LHRH).* A third hypothalamic hormone, somatostatin, has not found a place in routine diagnosis.

I. THE TRH TEST

A. Preparations Available

Synthetic TRH (L-pyroglutamyl-L-histidyl-L-prolinamide) is marketed either as a lyophilized powder for dissolution in sterile saline or as a prepared solution for subcutaneous, intramuscular, or intravenous administration (e.g., 200 μg in 2 ml of sterile diluent), which is stable for at least 2 years if stored below 30°C. A tablet for oral use is rarely employed.

B. Dosage and Route of Administration

The conventional diagnostic test employs a single intravenous bolus of 200–500 μg, a dose giving a TSH response which is near-maximal (1).

---

*Corticotropin releasing hormone (CRF) and growth hormone releasing hormone (GHRH) are currently being evaluated for clinical use (see Grossman A, Nieuwenhuyzen Kruseman AC, Perry L et al. Lancet 1982; i:921–922. Wood SH, Ch'ng JLC, Adatis EF et al. Brit Med J 1983; 286: 1687–1691).

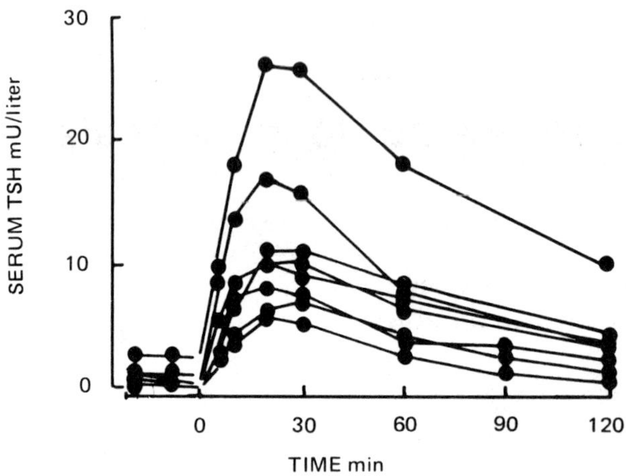

Figure 1 Serum Thyrotropin (TSH) response to the intravenous bolus administration of thyrotropin releasing hormone (TRH), 200 μg, to eight normal young men.

C. Hormonal Responses Measured

The TRH test is used most frequently to assess pituitary thyroid stimulating hormone (TSH) responsiveness; this requires measurement of TSH by radioimmunoassay prior to and following TRH administration. In normal subjects, serum prolactin (Prl) also increases and the test may therefore be used in the evaluation of prolactin secretion.

D. Protocol for the Routine TRH Test

No specific patient preparation is required; the patient need not be fasted. The following procedure is recommended:

1. Insert a scalp vein needle (21-23 gauge) into an antecubital vein, maintaining patency with heparinized saline.
2. Withdraw a blood sample for measurement of baseline serum TSH, and thyroid hormones [e.g., total thyroxine (T_4), T_3 resin uptake, total triiodothyronine (T_3) if indicated].
3. Inject TRH 200 μg rapidly. This may cause mild and transient nausea, flushing, and desire to micturate in 40–70% of subjects.
4. Collect further samples for TSH assay 20 and 60 min later. The latter sample terminates the test.
5. If Prl reserve is to be assessed, alone or simultaneously, samples for Prl assay are withdrawn before and 20 min after the TRH bolus (see Chapt 41).

E. The Normal TSH Response

In euthyroid subjects, serum TSH rises rapidly after the TRH bolus is given, reaching a maximum at 20 min, and falling significantly at 60 min (Fig. 1). The absolute quantitative response depends on the TSH assay procedure used, but representative mean responses in healthy adult males aged 20–40 years would be basal, 0-4 mU/liter; 20 min 9-14 mU/liter; 60 min, 7-10 mU/liter (2). Normal females have slightly greater responses and the response is blunted with increasing age in men but not in women. Responses in the evening may slightly exceed those in the morning.

II. THE GnRH (LHRH) TEST

A. Preparations Available

Synthetic GnRH (1-pyroglutamyl-L-histidyl-L-tryptophyl-L-seryl-L-tyrosyl-L-glycyl-L-leucyl-L-arginyl-L-prolyl-L-glycinamide) is marketed as a lyophilized powder for dissolution in sterile saline or as a prepared solution (e.g., 100 μg in 1 mL of sterile diluent), which is stable for at least 2 years if stored below 30°C.

B. Dosage and Route of Administration

The conventional diagnostic test employs a single intravenous bolus of 25–100 μg, the higher dose being necessary to elicit a significant follicle stimulating hormone (FSH) response in the normal adult male (3). A linear-log dose relationship has been demonstrated for the LH response in normal men over the range 1-3000 μg (4).

C. Hormonal Responses Measured

The GnRH test is used to assess pituitary gonadotropin reserve, and measurements are therefore made of both FSH and LH, by radioimmunoassay, prior to and following GnRH administration.

D. Protocol for Routine GnRH Test

No specific patient preparation is required; the patient need not be fasted. The following procedure is recommended:

1. Insert a scalp vein needle (21–23 gauge) into an antecubital vein, maintaining patency with heparinized saline.
2. Withdraw a blood sample for measurement of baseline serum FSH, and the appropriate gonadal steroid hormone (testosterone in the male, estradiol in the female).

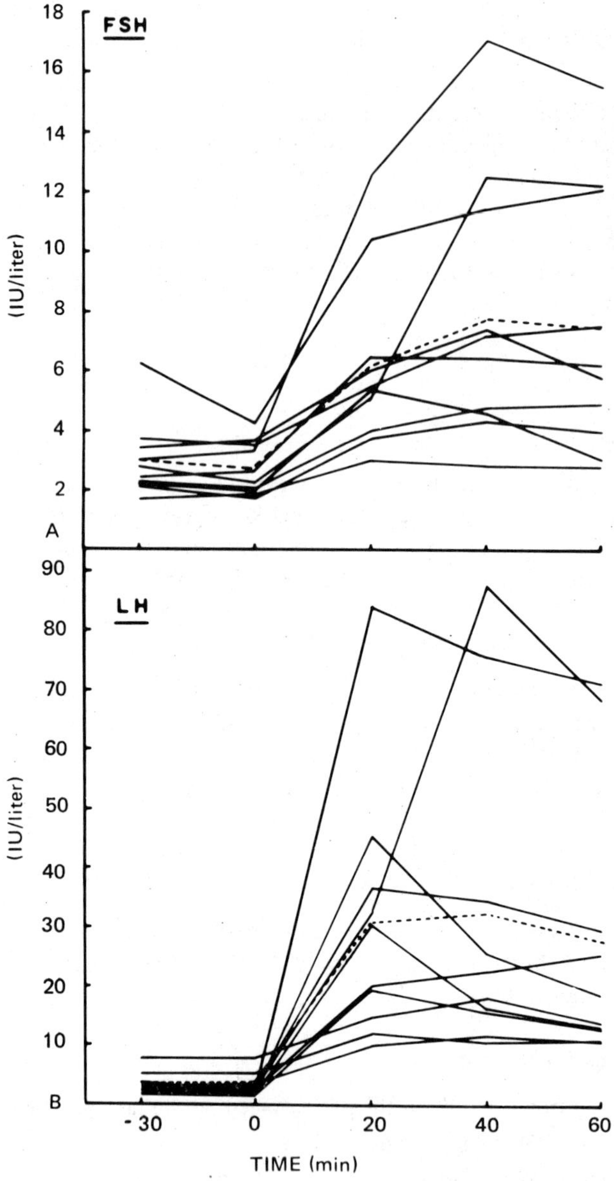

Figure 2 (A) Serum follicle stimulating hormone (FSH) and (B) luteinizing hormone (LH) responses to the injection of 100 μg of gonadotropin releasing hormone (GnRH) in 10 normal young adult men. The gonadotropins were measured using WHO matched reagents.

3. Wait 15 min, and obtain a further baseline sample for serum LH assay (the normal episodic secretion of LH makes it desirable to obtain two baseline samples).
4. Inject GnRH (25 μg in prepubertal subjects and females of reproductive age, 100 μg in adult males and postmenopausal females).
5. Collect further samples for FSH and LH assay at 15, 30, 45, and 60 min. The test is terminated at 60 min.

E. The Normal FSH and LH Response

In eugonadal subjects, serum LH rises rapidly after the GnRH bolus is given, reaching maximal levels at 20–30 min, and falling significantly by 60 min, while FSH rises more slowly and peaks between 20 and 60 min (Fig. 2). The absolute quantitative responses of FSH and LH vary with the sex and reproductive status of the subject, and depend also on the particular assay methods and standards used for measuring FSH and LH. In adult females, the responses vary with the stage of the menstrual cycle, being lowest in the early follicular phase; they rise in the middle to late follicular phase, reach a maximum at midcycle, and are generally higher during the luteal than the follicular phase. Representative values (using WHO reagents) in adult males challenged with 100 μg of LHRH would be as follows: for LH basal 2-8 (mean 3.8) IU/liter, peak 11-88 (mean 32) IU/liter; for FSH basal 2-6 (mean 3) IU/liter, peak 3–17 (mean 8) IU/liter.

In prepubertal children, baseline gonadotropin levels are lower, and the LH responses to GnRH are quantitatively less than those of adults. A clear-cut increase in the LH response is seen with pubertal development from stage I to Stage II (5) in boys and girls, with a further increase as puberty advances. FSH may rise little in prepubertal boys, and shows a relatively smaller enhancement of response than LH with the advent of puberty. In prepubertal girls, on the other hand, prepubertal FSH responses are greater than those seen in adults, and decline somewhat at the onset of puberty. Thus prepubertal girls show an increase in FSH which is relatively greater than that of LH, while in all other normal individuals, the LH response is relatively greater than that of FSH. It is important for individual laboratories to establish the range of normality with the particular gonadotropin assay being used.

III. COMBINED PITUITARY FUNCTION TESTS

The diagnostic indications for releasing hormone tests vary; in some circumstances, a comprehensive evaluation of anterior and posterior pituitary function is required, and under such circumstances, the TRH and GnRH stimuli may be applied simultaneously with insulin hypoglycemia, the latter being used to evaluate growth hormone, ACTH (and Prl) reserve. The concurrent administration of the three stimuli does not modify the responses to each given separately (6).

In performing the combined anterior and posterior pituitary function test, the following protocol is recommended:

1. The patient is asked to abstain from food and fluid following the previous evening meal (unless the patient has overt diabetes insipidus, when fluid restriction would be unsafe). The patient voids on rising and the urine is discarded. Patients undergoing assessment of ACTH reserve who are already taking cortisone acetate should discontinue this medication 36 hr before the test. If severe ACTH deficiency is suspected, admission to the hospital will be necessary.
2. At 8.00 A.M. the patient voids the second urine sample for the day, for measurement of urinary osmolality.
3. A scalp vein needle (21 gauge) is introduced into an antecubital vein, and attached to a three-way stopcock, to allow the maintenance of patency with heparinized saline, withdrawal of blood, and administration of the stimuli, and of glucose if necessary.
4. Blood is withdrawn for baseline measurements of serum osmolality, growth hormone (GH), cortisol (or ACTH), LH, and Prl.
5. Following a 30-min interval (to allow satisfactory basal conditions to be established following the venipuncture), blood is again withdrawn, for measurements of glucose, GH, cortisol, FSH, LH, Prl, TSH, total T_4 and T_3 resin uptake, and testosterone (or estradiol).
6. The three stimulatory substances are now injected intravenously:
   Insulin (Actrapid, glucagon-free insulin–0.1 U/kg in subjects without clinical evidence of obvious hypopituitarism; 0.05-0.08 U/kg in hypopituitary patients; 0.12-0.20 U/kg in patients with acromegaly or Cushing's disease).
   TRH: 200 μg
   GnRH: 25-100 μg, as discussed above.
7. Blood is withdrawn at the following times for glucose and hormone assay:
   +20 min: glucose, FSH, LH, TSH, Prl
   30 min: glucose, GH, cortisol, FSH, LH, Prl
   45 min: glucose, FSH, LH
   60 min: glucose, GH, cortisol, FSH, LH, TSH, Prl
   90 min: glucose, GH, cortisol
   120 min: glucose, GH, cortisol
8. If cortisol is being measured as an index of ACTH secretion, adrenal responsiveness should be checked: 0.25 mg synthetic α1-24 ACTH (Synacthen) is injected intravenously after 120-min blood sample, and a further sample for cortisol assay obtained 90 min later.

Precautions with respect to the insulin hypoglycemia test are considered in Chapters 40 and 37, the interpretations of GH and cortisol responses in Chapters 40 and 38 and the interpretation of tests of posterior pituitary function is discussed in Chapter 42. The test described above allows the comprehensive evaluation of pituitary and target organ function in a test of total duration 4 hr.

IV. THE DIAGNOSTIC VALUE AND INTERPRETATION OF HYPOTHALAMIC RELEASING HORMONE TESTS

A. General Considerations

Detailed critiques of the releasing hormone tests have been published (2, 7-10). Normal responsiveness to the hypothalamic releasing hormones depends on the presence of an intact hypothalamus and pituitary; lesions at either site may impair it. It depends further on the level of endogenous releasing hormone(s) present at the time of testing, and on the level of the physiological feedback substances, which may act at the hypothalamus, pituitary, or both. Other factors influencing the results of releasing hormone tests include drugs being taken by the patient, and the coexistence of stress, illness, depression, or dietary alteration.

It has become apparent (7) that it is a gross oversimplification to consider that hypothalamic lesions, resulting in defective releasing hormone secretion, would be characterized by preservation of normal pituitary responsiveness to exogenous releasing hormones, and that pituitary lesions causing hypopituitarism would be characterized by absent releasing hormone responsiveness, as was originally postulated. It has been demonstrated experimentally (11) that GnRH is itself important in regulating the number of GnRH receptors on the pituitary gonadotroph, thus providing a mechanism for loss of pituitary responsiveness in hypothalamic lesions. It is also to be noted that both hypothalamus and pituitary are affected in many patients with tumors or granulomatous lesions in the area.

The releasing hormone tests, particularly the TRH test, are, however, helpful in detecting subtle changes in the levels of the feedback signals affecting pituitary function, and in assessing whether endogenous releasing hormone secretion is intact.

B. The TRH Test: TSH Responsiveness

1. In Primary Thyroid Disease

The major practical application of the TRH test is in the diagnostic evaluation of patients with suspected hyperthyroidism. The experimental administration of even small quantities of thyroid hormones leads to blunting of the TSH response to TRH, while iodide-induced falls in circulating T_4 and T_3 cause hyperresponsiveness (7). Thus in patients with untreated hyperthyroidism, the TSH response to TRH is abolished; the extreme sensitivity of the thyrotroph to alterations in the levels of T_4 and T_3 causes difficulty in interpretation of this test, which may show an impaired TSH response in patients who are unequivocally euthyroid on standard clinical and biochemical criteria. Such situations have been documented in patients with autonomous thyroid nodules, and with orbital Graves' disease. The most valuable diagnostic information, serving to exclude the diagnosis, is obtained from the finding of a normal TSH response to TRH in a patient with suspected hyperthyroidism, in whom the results of standard tests of thyroid function have been equivocal. A diminished or absent response (interpreted in the light of the patient's age and sex, and in the absence of pituitary disease or other interfering factors) is suggestive but not diagnostic of hyperthyroidism. In previously treated thyrotoxicosis, the TRH response may remain subnormal for several months after clinical and biochemical remissions have occurred—again, a normal response is more helpful, as it can be used to exclude clinically significant recurrence.

The TRH test is of no practical value in hypothyroidism, where the baseline level of TSH, taken together with the free thyroxine index or an assay of free T_4 itself, serves to distinguish primary from secondary hypothyroidism in most instances (12).

2. In Disease of the Hypothalamus and Pituitary

The TRH test is of little diagnostic value in patients with suspected or known hypothalamic or pituitary disorders. Several reasons may be given:

1. The most useful diagnostic methods are history, physical examination, visual field examination, and neuroradiological investigations, particularly computerized tomographic (CT) scanning.
2. Baseline assessment of thyroid function (including TSH measurement) provides the endocrine information on which decisions regarding the need for thyroid hormone replacement will be based.
3. The results of standard TRH testing do not differentiate reliably between lesions of the hypothalamus and pituitary and provide little information of value for clinical decision making. Primary hypothalamic lesions are often associated with a TSH response which is somewhat exaggerated, and characterized by the fact that serum TSH at 60 min is greater than at 20 min. In contrast, extensive, destructive lesions of the pituitary are associated with an impaired or absent TSH response. Between these extremes, a variety of other responses may be observed: for example, normal or exaggerated TSH responses in hypothyroidism secondary to pituitary disease, or absent TSH responses, particularly in euthyroid patients with

Table 1 Basal TSH and TRH Responsiveness in Hypothalamic and Pituitary Lesions

Type of lesion	Basal TSH	Response to TRH
Hypothalamic	Low or normal or slightly elevated; often unstable	Normal or exaggerated; peak often delayed
Pituitary (other than acromegaly)	Low, normal, or slightly elevated	Absent, impaired, or normal; peak sometimes delayed
Acromegaly (euthyroid)	Low or normal	Absent, impaired, or normal

acromegaly. The difficulties in interpretation of the test have been discussed in detail (6); Table 1 summarizes the various possibilities.

From the practical aspect, an absent TSH response to TRH in a patient who does not have hyperthyroidism favors a pituitary lesion, and may be of most value in assessing the completeness of pituitary ablation. Patients with idiopathic hypopituitarism who show a normal or particularly a delayed TRH response may be presumed to have hypothalamic releasing hormone deficiency.

4. The preoperative assessment of TSH responsiveness does not serve a useful function, as the results cannot be expected to influence management decisions; even postoperative TRH testing provides little useful information. Thyroid hormone replacement should be based on clinical evidence of hypothyroidism, together with baseline thyroid function tests.

3. Prolactin Responses to TRH

It has been suggested that the assessment of Prl response to TRH may be of value in the differential diagnosis of idiopathic hyperprolactinemia and prolactin-secreting microadenoma (13). These authors claim that "a PRL-secreting adenoma in patients with galactorrhoea can be identified on the basis of the PRL response to TRH stimulation," with an absent or blunted Prl response indicating the presence of tumor, while a normal response is said to make a tumor unlikely. Such claims for the value of TRH testing remain controversial, however, as patients with normal pituitary radiology but absent Prl responses have not had surgical confirmation of the presence or absence of a microadenoma. Confirmed, clear-cut sustained hyperprolactinemia is almost invariably associated with absent Prl responsiveness to TRH (14), but in many patients the etiology remains uncertain.

4. Other Causes of Altered TRH Responsiveness

A number of disorders unrelated to previous disease of the hypothalamus, pituitary, or thyroid gland may affect TSH response to TRH. About 25% of patients with depression may show impaired responses, and prolonged fasting may blunt the response. TSH hypo- or unresponsiveness occurs in severe, life-threatening illness of any kind. Patients with Cushing's disease, or individuals treated with high doses of corticosteroids or dopamine, may show impaired responses. The influence of other agents have been described in detail (7).

5. Overall Conclusions Regarding the TRH Test

The most important practical indication to undertake a TRH test is in the evaluation of suspected hyperthyroidism when standard thyroid function tests have given equivocal results. The test has little practical value in the diagnosis and management of patients with disease of the hypothalamus and/or pituitary, despite its interest for the clinical research worker.

C. The GnRH Test

The value of GnRH as an elegant tool for the physiological and pathophysiological study of hypothalamic-pituitary function must be distinguished from its usefulness in endocrine diagnosis and management. From the latter viewpoint, the test is of very limited practical value. The situation has been complicated by the large variety of dosage schedules reported, by the lack of comparability of various gonadotropin radioimmunoassays, and by the difficulty of choosing the appropriate normal control group, particularly in the investigation of disorders of ovulation. A number of these problems have been reviewed (8, 10).

1. The GnRH Test in Delayed Puberty

In patients with delayed puberty not due to a primary gonadal disorder, the practical clinical question is whether the delay is functional, with a good prognosis for spontaneous development, or whether the patient has hypogonadotropic hypergonadism, requiring active therapy to bring about sexual maturation. In boys, this distinction can usually be made on the basis of family history (late onset of puberty is frequently familial) and of a careful evaluation of testicular volume, enlargement of the testes to 4 ml or more being the earliest clinical sign of puberty, and often long preceding other features. In girls, in whom the problem is less common, the clinical distinction may be much more difficult.

The GnRH test may be of some value in establishing prognosis where clinical evaluation has been unhelpful. Bourgignon et al. (15) reported that boys with simple pubertal delay showed LH and FSH responses similar to those of normal boys at stage II of puberty, while those with hypogonadotropic hypogonadism had prepubertal responses. Other authors have reported overlapping responses between the two groups. In girls with primary amenorrhea, it has been suggested that failure of gonadotropin response to GnRH is an indication for further investigation (10). Overall, the GnRH test appears to be of very limited value in practical patient management.

2. The GnRH Test in Hypothalamic and Pituitary Disease

As discussed earlier with respect to the TRH test, clinical and radiological assessment usually provides the practical basis for distinguishing hypothalamic from pituitary disorders. GnRH testing is unreliable, as absent, impaired, or normal responses can occur in both types of lesions (16). The test may be of some value in the assessment of women who have undergone surgical or radiotherapeutic pituitary ablation and in whom ovulation induction is to be undertaken. An absent GnRH response suggests that gonadotropin therapy should be the first choice, and that even if bromocriptine is used to lower elevated serum prolactin levels, reestablishment of ovulation is unlikely. In contrast, an intact gonadotropic response would be an indication for a trial of bromocriptine and/or clomiphene treatment before proceeding to gonadotropin therapy.

3. The GnRH Test in Menstrual Cycle Disorders

A large number of reports of the responses to GnRH in women with disorders of the menstrual cycle have been published. Interpretations of the results obtained are complicated by the difficulty of choosing an appropriate normal reference range, as the response in normal women is a function of the stage of the menstrual cycle at which testing is undertaken. From the clinician's viewpoint, there is usually no reason to undertake GnRH testing in patients with oligomenorrhea, or primary or secondary amenorrhea (8, 10). Since there is a good correlation between basal gonadotropin levels and the peak response to GnRH in the majority of patients, the GnRH test provides no useful information additional to the baseline measurements. The therapeutic uses of GnRH are beyond the scope of this chapter.

4. The GnRH Test in Male Infertility

GnRH testing may be of value in the assessment of men with infertility, where baseline gonadotropin levels, particularly those of FSH, are unexpectedly low for the degree of abnormality of the semen analysis (17). Thus an exaggerated response to GnRH in a patient with severe oligospermia and a normal baseline serum FSH concentration suggests the presence of a primary testicular lesion, while a diminished or absent response suggests the possibility of a disorder of the hypothalamus and/or pituitary.

REFERENCES

1. Snyder PJ, Utiger RD. Response to thyrotropin releasing hormone (TRH) in normal man. J Clin Endocrinol Metab 1972; 34:380-385.
2. Burger HG, Patel YC. Thyrotrophin releasing hormone–TSH. Clin Endocrinol Metab 1977; 6:83–100.
3. de Kretser DM, Burger HG, Hudson B, Keogh EJ. The pituitary-testicular response to luteinising hormone releasing hormone administration to normal men. Aust NZ J Med 1975; 5:227–230.
4. Woollesen F, Swerdloff RS, Odell WD. LH and FSH responses to luteinizing-releasing hormone in normal, adult, human males. Metabolism 1976; 25: 845–863.
5. Tanner JM. *Growth at Adolescence*. Blackwell, Oxford, 1962, pp 433–469.
6. Mortimer CH, Besser GM, McNeilly AS, Tunbridge MG, Gomez-Pan A, Hall R. Interaction between secretion of the gonadotrophins, prolactin, growth hormone, thyrotrophin and corticosteroids in man: the effects of LHRH, TRH and hypoglycaemia alone and in combination. Clin Endocrinol (Ox) 1973; 2:317-326.
7. Burger HG, Patel YC. TSH and TRH: their physiological regulation and the clinical applications of TRH. In *Clinical Neuroendocrinology*, Besser GM, Martini L (eds). Academic, New York, 1977, pp 67–130.
8. Burger HG. Clinical value of tests using hypothalamic releasing hormones. In Proceedings of the 6th Asia and Oceania Congress of Endocrinology, Singapore, 1978, vol 1, pp 24–30.
9. Snyder PJ, Jacobs LS, Rabello MM, Stirling FH, Shore RN, Utiger RD, Daughaday WH. Diagnostic values of thyrotropin-releasing hormone in pituitary and hypothalamic diseases. Ann Intern Med 1974; 81:751-757.
10. Wentz AC. Clinical applications of luteinizing hormone-releasing hormone. Fertil Steril 1977; 28:901-912.
11. Clayton RN, Catt KJ. Gonadotropin-releasing hormone receptors: Characterisation, physiological, regulation and relationship to reproductive function. Endocr Rev 1981; 2:186–209.
12. Burger HG, Patel YC. The values of serum thyrotrophin in the diagnosis and management of hypothyroidism. Med J Aus 1972; 2:293–297.
13. Marrs RP, Bertolli SJ, Kletsky DA. The use of thyrotropin-releasing hormone in distinguishing prolactin-secreting pituitary adenoma. Am J Obstet Gynecol 1980; 138:620–625.
14. Healy DL, Pepperell RJ, Stockdale J, Bremner WJ, Burger HG. Pituitary autonomy in hyperprolactinaemic secondary amenorrhoea–results of hypothalamic pituitary testing. J Clin Endocrinol Metab 1977; 44:809-819.
15. Bourgignon JP, Ernould CH, Brichant J, Franchimont, P. Diagnostic and prognostic interest of LH RH test in delayed puberty in males with a supportive longitudinal study. Convegno Internazionale di Endocrinologica Pediatrica, Bologna June 12-13, 1975; Pacini-Pisa 73-89.

16. Mortimer CH, Besser GM, McNeilly AS, Marshall JC, Harsoulis P, Tunbridge WMC, Gomez-Pan A, Hall R. Luteinising hormone and follicle stimulating hormone-releasing hormone test in patients with hypothalamic-pituitary-gonadal dysfunction. Br Med J 1973; 4:73–77.
17. de Kretser DM, Burger HG, Hudson B. The relationship between germ cells and serum FSH in males with infertility. J Clin Endocrinol Metab 1974; 38:449–455.

37
Hypothalamic-Pituitary-Gonadal Axis

Henry G. Burger and David M. Hurley
Prince Henry's Hospital, Melbourne, Australia

In this chapter, tests of hypothalamic, pituitary, and gonadal function, other than releasing hormone tests, are considered.

I. TESTS OF HYPOTHALAMIC-PITUITARY FUNCTION

As the measurement of luteinizing hormone releasing hormone (GnRH) in peripheral blood is not available as a practical diagnostic procedure, tests of hypothalamic function must rely on the assessment of gonadotropin or gonadal steroid responses. Absent responses can be due either to hypothalamic or to pituitary disease. However, it must be pointed out that the measurement of baseline gonadotropin and gonadal steroid levels is usually sufficient to localize lesions for clinical management purposes. Thus the finding of elevated gonadotropin levels [particularly follicle stimulating hormone (FSH)] with low normal or low levels of testosterone or estradiol is evidence in favor of a primary gonadal disorder, while normal or low gonadotropin levels with low steroid concentrations point to a hypothalamic or pituitary lesion—and in the absence of abnormal radiological findings, usually to a functional hypothalamic disturbance, particularly in ovulatory disorders.

A. Testing Negative Feedback: The Clomiphene Stimulation Test

The major clinical application of clomiphene is as a therapeutic agent for the induction of ovulation. It has also been used in the therapy of idiopathic oligospermia, although its efficacy remains unproven. However, it can be used to evaluate the integrity of the negative feedback relationship between the gonad and the hypothalamopituitary axis. Clomiphene is a weak estrogen, structurally related to trianisylchloroethylene (TACE), and may act as an estrogen agonist or more usually as an antagonist. It competes with estradiol for receptors in the hypothalamus and pituitary, and it is the hypothalamic blockade of estrogen action which leads to its effect in causing an elevation of both gonadotropins in normal subjects of both sexes. It has been used for clinical research purposes (reviewed in Ref. 1), but has not found a place for routine diagnosis.

The test is performed by the administration of 50–100 mg per day, usually for 5 days, to women, and 100-200 mg per day to men, for a variable time period of 7 days or more. Response is assessed by measurement of serum FSH and luteinizing hormone (LH), and/or the gonadal steroids, either in plasma or urine. A positive response consists of at least a twofold increase, usually seen on the third day of the test in women, while in men, gonadotropin levels increase after 2 days, with a peak in FSH occurring after about 7 days (average increase 64%), and in LH after 10 days (average increase 96%) (2). In anovulatory women who are fully responsive to clomiphene, the early rise in gonadotropin is followed by a rise in estrogens, and the subsequent development of changes typical of the ovulatory menstrual cycle (3), thus providing evidence of intact positive as well as negative feedback mechanisms. The clomiphene test is used most commonly as a combined diagnostic and therapeutic agent in anovulatory women. The failure to induce an ovulatory response with doses of clomiphene up to 150–200 mg per day is an indication to proceed to gonadotropin (or GnRH where appropriate) for ovulation induction. Such failure occurs most commonly in women with very low ovarian estrogen secretion.

B. Testing Positive Feedback: The Estrogen Provocation Test

The term "positive feedback" is conventionally used to describe the stimulating effect of estrogen on gonadotropin (particularly LH) release in the female, and there is now a large body of evidence in support of the concept that the normal midcycle preovulatory LH surge is triggered by the preceding increase in circulating levels of estradiol-17β.

The integrity of this positive feedback effect can be assessed following the administration of an appropriate estrogen in a way which will result in a sustained evaluation of circulating estrogen levels for 24–36 hr. The estrogen can be administered orally (e.g., ethinyl estradiol 200 μg per day for 3 days) or by intramuscular injection (e.g., estradiol benzoate 0.5-1 mg in two injections at an interval of 1 day, or a single injection of 2.5 mg). Midcycle-like LH peaks occur 36–72 hr later, after an initial suppression of both gonadotropins—the test thus evaluating negative as well as positive feedback. FSH responds inconsistently.

The test has been used to elucidate the pathophysiology of ovulatory disorders; thus many subjects with amenorrhea fail to show a surge of LH following estrogen administration, and only those subjects with a positive response were shown to ovulate following clomiphene administration (4). Women with hyperprolactinemia also fail to show a positive response (5). The response is blocked by progesterone, and cannot be elicited during the luteal phase of the menstrual cycle. It is noteworthy, however, that progesterone can itself induce a positive feedback release of gonadotropin, but only from an estrogen-primed hypothalamopituitary unit. The estrogen provocation test has not found a place in routine diagnosis and management.

II. TESTS OF GONADAL RESERVE CAPACITY

Although the gonads have the dual functions of gamete production and steroid secretion, only the latter is assessed in tests of gonadal reserve capacity. Human chorionic gonadotropin (hCG) is the standard stimulatory agent for assessing testosterone secretory capacity in the male, while mixed pituitary or urinary gonadotropin preparations, containing both FSH and LH, have been used to assess ovarian estrogen secretion.

A. The hCG Stimulation Test of Testicular Reserve

The assessment of testicular reserve capacity may be desirable in the following situations:

1. To establish the presence of absence of testicular tissue in patients without palpable testicular tissue (due either to bilateral cryptorchidism or to anorchia)
2. As a combined diagnostic and therapeutic test in boys with delayed puberty
3. To characterize fully the testicular function of patients with hypogonadotropic hypogonadism
4. To assess patients with oligospermic idiopathic infertility.

In most instances, careful clinical evaluation, together with baseline measurement of the gonadotropins and testosterone, will provide an adequate data base for clinical management.

Numerous regimens and doses of hCG have been described, and until recently, it has been customary to give multiple injections of hCG (e.g., 3000 IU per day intramuscularly for 4 days), with measurement of plasma testosterone before starting, at 48 hr after the first injection and 24 hr after the last (6). Results in normal men were reported by these authors: basal plasma testosterone 20.3 ± 4.1 (SD) nmol/liter day 2 32.8 ± 9.4 (64.7% increase); day 4 50.6 ± 13.8 (156% increase). Thus plasma testosterone showed a two- to threefold increase.

Recently, it has been demonstrated that the plasma testosterone response to single intramuscular injections of testosterone is dose related, biphasic, and prolonged (7, 8), with an initial peak at 2 hr, and a secondary rise, peaking 48–96 hr following the hCG. The maximal dose is approximately 3000 IU, and the peak response is again two to three times the basal level.

Although extensive studies of the single-dose test have not so far been recorded, it appears likely that it can be performed by taking a basal sample for testosterone measurement, giving a single intramuscular injection of 3000 IU and taking a further sample 72 hr later.

Normal responses to hCG have been published for prepubertal and pubertal boys (9). The finding of an absent response is strongly suggestive of a diagnosis of anorchia, while diminished responsiveness implies impaired Leydig cell reserve. An absent or markedly impaired response is found in some patients with hypogonadotropic hypogonadism but with repeated stimulation over weeks to months, particularly when FSH is added to therapy, normal testicular responsiveness together with spermatogenesis may occur, although some such patients have proved to be refractory to testicular stimulation (10).

B. The Combined Gonadotropin Stimulation Test of Ovarian Reserve

The assessment of ovarian responsiveness to exogenous gonadotropin in patients with hypogonadism has been reported infrequently, and is usually undertaken only as part of the evaluation of a patient who requires ovulation induction with gonadotropin. One suggested regimen, used in the Australian Ovulation Induction Program (11), consists of the collection of a baseline 24-hr urine sample for measurement of estrogen excretion, the administration of 150–200 IU FSH (the gonadotropin equivalent to a single pituitary) daily for 3 days, with further 24 hr urine collections on the third day of administration and again on the third day after the last dose (day 6). Estrogen excretion may be measured in terms of total urinary estrogen (by chemical assay) or as estrone-3-glucuronide (by radioimmunoassay). Failure to observe a significant increase in urinary estrogens on day 6 is an indication to repeat the test after a 1-week interval using twice the gonadotropin dose. Further failure of responsiveness leads to the use of a triple gonadotropin dose. A positive result is indicated by a threefold or greater increase in urinary estrogens on day 6: the dosage of FSH at which this is achieved provides a guide to the initial dose to be used in the ovulation induction program. For example, a response to 150 IU per day for 3 days might lead to the use of an initial dose of 100 IU per day in the actual treatment program. Failure to respond to a 3-day stimulation test with 600 IU per day indicates the absence of responsive ovarian follicles, and would ordinarily be an indication not to proceed with ovulation induction.

III. STIMULATION-SUPPRESSION TESTS OF GONADAL FUNCTION IN SUSPECTED ANDROGEN HYPERSECRETION

Various regimens of adrenocortical and gonadal steroid and tropic hormone administration have been described for the differential diagnosis of states of excessive androgen production in the hirsute or virilized female. There is a lack of agreement regarding the optimal schedules of steroid administration and the value of tropic hormonal stimulation, and there is, at least in some patients, lack of target organ specificity, with ovarian arrhenoblastomas having the ability to respond to adrenocorticotropic hormone (ACTH) and adrenal adenomas to hCG. Certain generalizations may be made:

(a) Dexamethasone is the synthetic glucocorticoid of choice to achieve ACTH suppression. When used in the differential diagnosis of a source of androgen overproduction, a suggested dosage is at least 2 mg daily for at least 3 days, to allow suppression of urinary metabolites. End points measured may include cortisol, testosterone, androstenedione, 17-hydroxyprogesterone, DHEA sulfate, and urinary 17-oxosteroids. Variable degrees of testosterone suppression have been reported in normal subjects; in idiopathic hirsutism, the polycystic ovary syndrome, and congenital adrenal hyperplasia, a greater than normal degree of suppression may occur. In virilizing ovarian tumors, there is usually failure of testosterone but not of 17-oxosteroid levels to suppress, but the test is not absolutely reliable (12). The other steroids show a variable degree of supression, but more prolonged dexamethasone administration (e.g., over 7 days) may allow evaluation of the other androgens (13).

(b) Gonadotropin suppression can be achieved by administering estrogen/progesterone combinations (e.g., ethinyl estradiol 50 μg plus medoxyprogesterone 10 mg daily) for at least 3 weeks. In normal subjects 50% suppression of plasma testosterone is expected.

(c) Theoretically, further information is obtained by administrating hCG to the dexamethasone-suppressed patient or ACTH to the gonadal-steroid-suppressed patient, but such tests have not been widely applied in routine endocrine diagnosis. References which may be consulted include papers by Osborn and Yannone (12), Abraham (14), and Abraham et al. (13).

(d) Overall, an adrenal source of androgen overproduction may be suspected in the presence of elevated 17-oxosteroids (and/or 17-hydroxycorticosteroids or urinary-free cortisol), hirsutism with normal menstrual function, early adrenarche with normal menarche, exaggerated diurnal rhythm of androstenedione, exaggerated androstenedione response to ACTH, elevated plasma pregnenolone, and gonadal steroid nonsuppressible elevated androstenedione and testosterone.

An ovarian cause may be suspected with normal 17-oxosteroids, bilaterally enlarged overaries, marked menstrual irregularity, a family history of polycystic ovarian disease, elevated LH relative to FSH, an exaggerated androstenedione or testosterone response to hCG, a blunted diurnal rhythm of androstenedione, and gonadal-steroid-suppressible elevated androstenedione and testosterone. Combined adrenal and ovarian overproduction is common.

The importance of establishing a source for the androgen overproduction is controversial, and unless the patient is clearly virilized or there is rapid progression of hirsutism, may be somewhat academic and depend on the treatment approach that is planned.

REFERENCES

1. Franchimont P, Burger HG. *Human Growth Hormone and Gonadotrophins in Health and Disease.* North Holland, Elsevier/Amsterdam, 1975, pp 246–250.
2. de Kretser DM, Burger HG, Hudson B, Keogh EJ. Effects of short term administration of clomiphene citrate on serum FSH and LH levels in men with idiopathic disorders of spermatogenesis. Andrologia 1974; 6:25–33.
3. Jacobson A, Marshall JR, Ross GT. Plasma gonadotropins during clomiphene induced ovulatory cycles. Am J Obstet Gynecol 1968; 102:284–290.
4. Shaw RW, Butt WR, London DR, Marshall JC. The estrogen provocation test: a method of assessing the hypothalamic-pituitary axis in amenorrhea. Clin Endocrinol (Oxf) 1975; 4:267–276.
5. Glass MR, Shaw RW, Butt WR, Logan-Edwards R, London DR. An abnormality of estrogen feedback in amenorrhea-galactorrhea. Br Med J 1975; 3:274–275.
6. de Kretser DM, Burger HG, Hudson B, Keogh EJ. The HCG stimulation test in men with testicular disorders. Clin Endocrinol (Oxf) 1975; 4:591–596.
7. Padron RS, Wischusen J, Hudson B, Burger HG, de Kretser DM. Prolonged biphasic response of plasma testosterone to single intramuscular injections of human chorionic gonadotrophin. J Clin Endocrinol Metab 1980; 50: 1100–1104.
8. Burger HG, Bremner WJ, de Kretser DM, Healy DL, Hudson B, Kovac G, Padron P, Wilson JD. Hypogonadotrophic hypogonadism in male and female. In *Endocrinology of Human Infertility–New Aspects*, Crosignani PG, Ruber BL (ed). Academic, London, 1981; pp. 185–205.
9. Winter JSD, Taraska S, Faiman C. The hormonal response to HCG stimulation in male children and adolescents. J Clin Endocrinol Metab 1972; 34:348–353.
10. Bardin CW, Ross GT, Rifkind, AB, Cargille CM, Lipsett MB. Studies of the pituitary Leydig cell axis in young men with hypogonadotrophic hypogonadism and hyposmia: comparison with normal men, prepubertal boys and hypopituitary patients. J Clin Invest 1969; 48:2046–2056.

11. The Human Pituitary Advisory Committee. Ovulation induction by human FSH—the results of the Australian programme. Aust NZ J Obstet Gynaecol 1976; 16:106-110.
12. Osborn RH, Yannone ME. Plasma androgens in the normal and androgenized female: a review. Obstet Gynecol Surv 1971; 25:195–228.
13. Abraham, GE, Chakmakjian ZH, Buster JE, Marshall JR, Ovarian and adrenal contributions to peripheral androgens in hirsute women. Obstet Gynecol 1975; 46:169–173.
14. Abraham GE. Ovarian and adrenal contributions to peripheral androgens during the menstrual cycle. J Clin Endocrinol Metab 1974; 39:340–346.

38
Hypothalamic-Pituitary-Adrenal Axis

A. Wayne Meikle and Don H. Nelson
University of Utah School of Medicine, Salt Lake City, Utah

Dynamic testing procedures employed in the estimation of adrenal hypo- or hyperfunction are of three types. Tests may stimulate secretion of the adrenal cortex by exogenous administration of adrenocorticotropic hormone (ACTH) or stimulate endogenous secretion of ACTH following the administration of insulin or metyrapone. Suppression tests employ the administration of dexamethasone, although in unusual circumstances, cortisol may be employed to suppress ACTH secretion. Finally, measurement of plasma cortisol and/or ACTH [or lipotropin (LPH)] may be performed using a multiple sampling technique.

I. STIMULATION TESTS

Stimulation tests are utilized chiefly for the demonstration of normal adrenal reserve, thus indicating that there is sufficient adrenal tissue present for increased cortisol secretion to occur following ACTH administration. These tests are thus most useful in the demonstration of adrenal insufficiency, but have also been found to have some application to the diagnosis of adrenal hyperfunction, particularly in the demonstration of partial enzyme deficiencies of congenital adrenal hyperplasia. A hyperactive response is characteristic of pituitary dependent Cushing's disease and lack of response is present in many but not all cortisol-secreting adrenal tumors.

A. Single-Dose ACTH Test

Synthetic $\alpha^{1\text{-}24}$-ACTH is generally employed for ACTH testing. Twenty-five units (0.25 mg) is given either intravenously or intramuscularly and plasma cortisol levels are measured 30 and 60 min later (1, 2). An increment of 7 μg/dl or greater above a baseline of greater than 5 μg/dl and a maximal poststimulation level exceeding 18 μg/dl are seen in normal subjects, while patients with adrenal insufficiency fail to respond. There is less regular absorption when the intramuscular test is employed and thus an increase in secretion indicates normal adrenal function but a lack of response cannot be taken as confirmatory of the presence of adrenal insufficiency. Patients who have partial deficiency of 21-hydroxylation may have a considerable increase in 17-hydroxyprogesterone when this test is employed, thus confirming the presence of a mild form of congenital adrenal hyperplasia (3). Patients with Cushing's syndrome of a pituitary-dependent type have increased secretion of 11-desoxycortisol when a modified form of this test is employed and 5 μg of $\alpha^{1\text{-}24}$-ACTH is given as a single intravenous injection (4).

B. ACTH Infusion Tests

ACTH infusion tests may consist of the administration of ACTH for periods of 2, 4, 8, or 24 hr. Multiple infusions, usually for 8 hr for a period of 2 or 3 days, also have been employed (5-7). These tests require demonstration of a significant increase in plasma cortisol or urinary corticosteroids to rule out primary adrenal insufficiency. A "normal" response consists of a doubling of the baseline value, although values slightly less than this are not necessarily abnormal. A longer rate of infusion results in a greater increase in plasma or urinary corticosteroids. Patients with primary adrenal insufficiency fail to have a significantly increased corticosteroid secretion when any of the modalities is employed. Patients with adrenal insufficiency secondary to pituitary disease and a deficiency of ACTH secretion fail to respond to short-term infusion, but with longer infusion and particularly ACTH infusion on successive days the atrophic gland present in these patients will begin to secrete cortisol.

When ACTH is administered for 24 hr in a constant infusion at the rate of 1-5 U/hr, urinary excretion of cortisol and its metabolic products may also be quantitated (7). The urinary tests commonly employed are free cortisol, 17-hydroxycorticosteroids (Porter-Silber chromogens), and 17-ketogenic corticosteroids. Each of these will usually double in a normal individual when a 24-hr constant infusion or two 8-hr infusions on successive days of ACTH is carried out (5, 6). There is a 24-30% variation in control levels when these types of determination are used and thus small increases should not be interpreted as a response to ACTH. 17-Ketosteroids may also be measured chiefly as an estimate of adrenal androgen secretion. These largely represent dehydroepiandrosterone sulfate and other androgens. Metabolic products of 21-OH steroids contribute in a small way to the total 17-ketosteroids excreted in the urine (8, 9). These urinary substances increase with a longer ACTH infusion period, and increase markedly in patients with hyperactive androgen secretion, such as those with congenital adrenal hyperplasia. Pregnanetriol is also increased considerably in the urine in the latter groups of patients, but measurement of the abnormal steroids produced in the various hydroxylase deficiencies can usually be carried out more easily in plasma than in urine using radioimmunoassay techniques (10).

C. ACTH Given Intramuscularly

Although the rapid screening test of 25 U of $\alpha^{1\text{-}24}$ ACTH intramuscularly with measurement of plasma cortisol levels 30 and 60 min later may rule out adrenal insufficiency (1, 2), if there is a deficient response it may be useful to give a larger dose (100 U intramuscularly) of a depot (zinc-complexed) preparation and have the patient return 24 or 48 hr later for a plasma cortisol determination. A doubling or greater in the cortisol level effectively rules out primary adrenal insufficiency if the control level is 7 μg or greater (5, 6). Occasionally, intramuscular ACTH is not absorbed well, however, and thus a negative response should not be taken as definitive for the diagnosis of primary adrenal insufficiency.

A 1-mg dose of depot ACTH, when injected intramuscularly, has a duration of action of 24 to 48 hr. A 1.0-mg dose of long-acting ACTH is administered intramuscularly on each of three consecutive mornings. A normal response, which may be observed in some patients with hypopituitarism as well as normal subjects, is indicated by a plasma cortisol value of over 25 μg/dl at 5-12 hr after the last dose. A lack of response documents primary adrenal cortical insufficiency.

D. Insulin Stimulation Test

This test should always be carried out under close supervision if adrenal insufficiency is suspected. An indwelling catheter is placed in an antecubital vein, a control plasma cortisol and blood glucose are drawn, and then insulin, 0.1-0.15 U/kg body weight, is administered intravenously and additional blood samples obtained at 30 and 60 min for estimation of glucose and cortisol (11). Normal subjects will have doubling or more of the plasma cortisol if significant hypoglycemia is produced (blood sugar less than 40 mg/dl). The lower insulin dose is preferred in patients who have a high liklihood of having adrenal insufficiency as patients with corticosteroid deficiency fail to mobilize glucose readily and may develop severe hypoglycemia and even convulsions. For this reason this test should be carried out with constant close observation and glucose should be administered orally or intravenously with the onset of symtomatology or at the conclusion of the test. An added difficulty in performing this test is that frequently the insulin dose given does not produce sufficient hypoglycemia to act as a stimulant to adrenal secretion. In this event, the test must be repeated using a larger insulin dose.

E. Metyrapone Test

Since the discovery that metyrapone blocks 11-hydroxylation, reduces cortisol secretion, and increases 11-desoxycortisol and ACTH secretion, it has been widely employed as a stimulator of ACTH secretion and for the determination of a normal adrenal-pituitary axis. It should be remembered that the metabolism of metyrapone may be increased by those substances which stimulate the mixed function oxidases, and increased drug metabolism by the liver may give a less than normal response (12, 15). In large doses, not just 11-hydroxylation but total secretion from the gland may be inhibited.

The administration of a single dose of metyrapone (approximately 30 mg/kg or approximately 3 g) at midnight with a small snack such as milk and crackers is followed by taking a blood sample for plasma cortisol, 11-desoxycortisol, and/or ACTH at 8 A.M. the next morning. This is a highly useful test in the diagnosis of primary or secondary adrenal insufficiency and in the differential diagnosis of Cushing's syndrome (12, 13). Normal subjects have an increase in 11-desoxycortisol of 7 μg or greater with some decrease but not total absence of plasma cortisol (12). Plasma ACTH usually more than doubles (12, 14) and exceeds 50 pg/ml. This type of response demonstrates the ability of both the pituitary gland and the adrenal cortex to respond to appropriate stimuli and can be considered a normal response. Patients with adrenal insufficiency of either the primary or the secondary type fail to respond and may develop symptoms of cortisol deficiency during the test. Plasma ACTH is already elevated in a patient with primary adrenal insufficiency but may increase further if there is suppression of some residual cortisol production. Similarly, if the adrenal cortex is capable of producing 7 μg/dl of cortisol, this may be converted to 11-desoxycortisol which will appear in the plasma, but due to the shorter half-life of the latter compound the level will be less than the previous cortisol level.

Patients with secondary adrenal insufficiency (ACTH deficiency) will have low to absent plasma ACTH which fails to increase, and also fail to have a significant increase in 11-desoxycortisol. Patients who have pituitary-dependent Cushing's syndrome generally have a hyperactive response to administration of metyrapone, while those with adrenal adenomas or ectopic ACTH-secreting tumors fail to respond (13). Patients in the latter group may have considerable

11-desoxycortisol in the plasma following metyrapone administration, but this is consistent with their initial high plasma cortisol and ACTH levels and usually does not result in misinterpretation of the test.

A multiple-dose metyrapone test is performed less commonly now, although it was the original approach used. This consists of the administration of usually 750 mg metyrapone every 4 hr for 48 hr or a total of 4.5 g per day for 2 days (13). This is the test generally employed when urinary 17-hydroxy or 17-ketogenic steroids are to be measured. There is a marked increased in urinary corticoids in the normal individual, lack of response in the patient with primary adrenal insufficiency or adrenal adenoma producing Cushing's syndrome, and usually a hyperactive response in the patient with pituitary-dependent Cushing's syndrome. It must be remembered that when 17-ketogenic steroids are measured in the patient with 21 hydroxylase deficiency, 17-hydroxyprogesterone and its metabolites are measured as 17-ketogenic steroids and thus are not a true reflection of cortisol secretion.

II. DEXAMETHASONE SUPPRESSION TESTS

Suppression tests are based on the physiological principle that administration of corticosteroids, usually dexamethasone, decreases secretion of ACTH by the anterior pituitary gland. This is largely secondary to a direct effect of the corticosteroids on the pituitary gland, but with large prolonged doses, action on both the hypothalamus and the adrenal cortex may occur. These tests were originally carried out with the potent corticosteroids 9α-fluorohydrocortisone but with the development of the even more potent compound dexamethasone, which has little sodium-retaining activity, this drug is now generally employed for carrying out these tests. It should be noted that a rare patient has been demonstrated to suppress ACTH secretion in response to cortisol and not dexamethasone, and other "abnormal" responses to dexamethasone have been described (see below). Suppression tests must take into account conditions which will modify the metabolism of the dexamethasone, including all of those drugs which increase drug metabolism by the liver (15-17). These compounds speed up the metabolism of the dexamethasone and suggest lack of suppression of ACTH and adrenal cortical secretion by the administered dose (false positive test).

A. Single-Dose Suppression Test

For this test 1 mg of dexamethasone is administered at midnight and a plasma cortisol is obtained at 8 A.M. the next morning. Almost all normal subjects will suppress plasma cortisol below 5 μg/dl when the test is performed in this manner (15-18). Patients with Cushing's syndrome usually fail to suppress, although a small percentage may demonstrate suppression, particularly if this is an abnormality of dexamethasone metabolism (17, 18). Patients with adrenal hyperactivity secondary to one of the enzymatic deficiencies of congenital adrenal hyperplasia are usually readily suppressible. In those patients who fail to show normal suppression, administration of 4 mg or rarely 8 mg of dexamethasone will usually differentiate between patients with pituitary-dependent Cushing's disease and those with Cushing's syndrome secondary to an adrenal tumor (17). ACTH produced by the pituitary gland in Cushing's disease is suppressed by the larger dose of dexamethasone, but is seldom suppressed in patients with adrenal adenomas or in those with ectopic ACTH-producing tumors (15). In the latter group, bronchial carcinoids often have been suppressible and a few other ectopic tumors or adrenal adenomas have been found to be suppressible with very large doses of dexamethasone (apparently due to a direct action of the drug on the tumor cell) (19-23). Fluorometric cortisol determination is often not satisfactory with this test due to the high blanks.

B. Multiple-Dose Test

Multiple-dose dexamethasone suppression tests were those originally described and usually consist of administration of the dexamethasone as 0.5 mg every 6 hr for 48 hr (low-dose test) or administration of 2 mg of dexamethasone every 6 hr for 48 hr [high-dose suppression test (13)]. Although this test may be performed with measurement of plasma cortisol, the test was originally described and is still usually employed when urinary corticosteroids are to be measured (24). Patients who have pituitary-dependent disease usually fail to suppress with the low dose, but these patients are then suppressed by the high-dose test. Patients with adrenal adenomas or ectopic-producing tumors fail to suppress with rare exceptions (15, 24).

Failure of suppression is not limited to patients with demonstrable adrenal or pituitary pathology. It is now recognized that patients with the familial form of endogenous depression fail to undergo normal suppression when single-dose or low-dose tests are carried out (25, 26). It has been found that a 4 P.M. cortisol after administration of 1 mg of dexamethasone the previous midnight is probably a better time for demonstrating lack of suppression in this group of patients than is the 8 A.M. value, although it is likely also to show a difference from normal (26). As depression may be associated with Cushing's syndrome, it is important to separate these patients who fail to suppress with dexamethasone from those who have true Cushing's syndrome. Patients with pseudo-Cushing's syndrome from alcoholism may also fail to suppress normally following dexamethasone administration (27). Using corticosterone measurements it is possible to adequately measure suppression in people receiving cortisol (33).

III. REPEATED SAMPLING FOR CORTISOL AND/OR ACTH.

Although not strictly a dynamic test, some mention of methods for the collection of cortisol and ACTH samples is indicated (28-32). The diurnal variation of both cortisol and ACTH with episodic spikes throughout this period is well known. Due to these types of variation, single samples drawn for either of these hormones may not be definitive. In the author's experience this is not generally a problem and thus a single sample demonstrating low cortisol and high plasma ACTH is very suggestive of primary adrenal insufficiency, and a high plasma cortisol with an absent ACTH value is suggestive of an adrenal tumor. A better way of establishing such levels, however, is to withdraw a number of samples at 30- to 60-min intervals over a period of 2 hr to as long as 24 hr, combine these samples quantitatively, and determine the mean cortisol or ACTH over a particular period of time. As 24 hr is too long for a routine measurement, collection over either a 2- or a 4-hr period is usually carried out.

REFERENCES

1. Lindholm J, Kehlet H, Blickert-Toft M, Dinesen B, Riishede J. Reliability of the 30 minute ACTH test in assessing hypothalamic-pituitary-adrenal function. J Clin Endocrinol Metab 1978; 47:272–274.
2. Dluhy RD, Himathongkam T, Greenfield M. Rapid ACTH test with plasma aldosterone levels improves diagnostic discrimination. Ann Intern Med 1974; 80:693–696.
3. Youssefnejadian E, David R. Diagnosis of congenital adrenal hyperplasia by measurement of 17α-OH-progesterone. Clin Endocrinol 1974; 4:451.
4. West CD. Unpublished results.
5. Besser GM, Butler PWP, Plumpton FS. Adrenocorticotrophic action of long-acting tetracosactrine compared with corticotropin gel. Br Med J 1967; 2:391–394.
6. Irvine WJ, Barnes EW. Adrenocortical insufficiency. Clin Endocrinol 1972; 1:549–594.
7. Nugent CA, MacDiarmid WD, Nelson AR. Rate of adrenal cortisol production in response to maximal stimulation with ACTH. J Clin Endocrinol Metab 1963; 23:684–693.
8. Sigrum-Schultz S, Levine LS, New MI. Dehydroepiandosterone sulfate (DS) levels, a rapid test of abnormal adrenal androgen secretion. J Clin Endocrinol Metab 1976; 42:1005–1013.
9. Culter GM Jr, Davis E, Johnsonbaugh RE, Loriax DL. Dissociation of cortisol and adrenal androgen secretion in patients with secondary adrenal insuffiency. J Clin Endocrinol Metab 1979; 49:604–609.
10. New MI, DuPont B, Pang S, Pollack M, Levine LS. An update on congenital adrenal hyperplasia. Recent Prog Horm Res 1981; 37:105–181.

11. Faglia G, Ambrosi B, Beck-Peccoz P, Travaglini P. Hypothalamic-pituitary-adrenal function in patients with pituitary tumours. Acta Endocrinol Copenh 1973; 73:223–232.
12. Spiger M. Jubiz W, Meikle AW, West CD, Tyler FH. Single dose metyrapone test. Review of four year experience. Arch Intern Med 1975; 135: 698–700.
13. Liddle GW, Island D, Meador CK. Normal and abnormal regulation of corticotropin secretion in man. Recent Prog Horm Res 1962; 18:125–164.
14. Meikle AW, Jubiz W, Matsukura S, West CD, Tyler FH. Effect of diphenylhydantoin on the metabolism of metyrapone and the release of ACTH in man. J Clin Endocrinol Metab 1969; 29:1553–1558.
15. West CD, Meikle AW. Laboratory tests for the diagnosis of Cushing's syndrome and adrenal insufficiency and factors affecting those tests. In *Endocrinology*. DeGroot LJ (ed). Grune & Stratton, New York, 1979, pp 1157–1177.
16. Jubiz W, Meikle AW, Levinson RA, West CD, Tyler FH. Effect of diphenylhydantoin in the metabolism of dexamethasone: mechanism of the abnormal dexamethasone suppression tests in humans. N Engl J Med 1970; 283:11–14.
17. Meikle AW. Dexamethasone suppression tests: usefulness of simultaneous measurement of plasma cortisol and dexamethasone. Clin Endocrinol 1982; 16:401–408.
18. Meikle AW, Lagerquist LG, Tyler FH. Apparently normal pituitary-adrenal suppressibility in Cushing's syndrome: dexamethasone metabolism and plasma levels. J Lab Clin Med 1975; 86:472–478.
19. Kendall JW, Sloop PR Jr. Dexamethasone-suppressible adrenocortical tumor. N Engl J Med 1968; 279:532–535.
20. Mathews JI, Pariss BL, Chertow B. Adrenal adenoma with variable response to dexamethasone suppression and metyrapone stimulation. J Clin Endocrinol Metab 1972; 34:902–905.
21. Kirschner MA, Powell RD Jr, Lippsett MB. Cushing's syndrome: nodular hyperplasia of adrenal glands with clinical and pathological features suggesting adrenocortical tumor. J Clin Endocrinol Metab 1964; 24:947–955.
22. Aron CD, Findling JW, Fitzgerald PA, Brooks RM, Fisher FE, Forsham PH, Tyrrell JB. Pituitary ACTH dependency of nodular adrenal hyperplasia in Cushing's syndrome. Am J Med 1981; 71:302–306.
23. Hidai H, Fujii H, Otsaku K, Abe K, Shimizu N. Cushing's syndrome due to huge adrenocortical multinodular hyperplasia. Endocrinol Jpn 1975; 22:555–560.
24. Liddle GW. Test of pituitary-adrenal suppressibility in the diagnosis of Cushing's syndrome. J Clin Endocrinol Metab 1960; 20:1539–1960.
25. Starkman MN, Schteingart DE, Schork MA. Depressed mood and other psychiatric manifestations of Cushing's syndrome: relationship to hormone levels. Psychosom Med 1981; 43:3–8.

26. Carroll BJ, Schroeder K, Mukhopadhyay S, Greden JR, Feinberg M, Ritchie J, Tarika J. Plasma dexamethasone concentrations and cortisol suppression response in patients with endogenous depression. J Clin Endocrinol Metab 1980;51:433-437.
27. Smals AG, Kloppenborg PW, Njo KT, Knoben JM, Ruland CM. Alcohol induced cushingoid syndrome. Br Med J 1976;2:1298.
28. Jeffcoate WJ, Rees LH, Lowry PJ, Besser GM. A specific radioimmunoassay for human β-lipotropin. J Clin Endocrinol Metab 1978;47:160–167.
29. Gilkes JJH, Rees LH, Besser GM. Relationship between plasma immunoreactive ACTH and LPH in Cushing's syndrome and Addison's disease. Br Med J 1977;1:966.
30. Kreiger DT. Plasma ACTH and corticosteroids. In *Endocrinology*, DeGroot LJ (ed). Grune & Stratton, New York 1979, Vol II, pp 1139–1156.
31. Krieger DT, Liotta AS, Suda T, Goodgold A, Condon E. Human plasma immunoreactive lipotropin and adrenocorticotropin in normal subjects and in patients with pituitary-adrenal disease. J Clin Endocrinol Metab 1979;48:566-571.
32. Berson SA, Yalow RS. Radioimmunoassay of ACTH in plasma. J Clin Invest 1968;47:2725-2751.
33. Meikle AW, Stanchfield JB, West CD, Tyler, FH. Hydrocortisone suppression test for Cushing's syndrome: therapy with anticonvulsants. Arch Intern Med 1974; 134: 1068–1071.

39
Hypothalamic-Pituitary-Thyroid Axis

H. K. Ibbertson
University of Auckland School of Medicine, Auckland, New Zealand

With the advent of the radioimmunoassay there has been a progressive simplification of thyroid function testing and many old "indirect" tests now have little place in routine diagnosis. In vivo radionuclide procedures have lost favor, although the thyroid uptake still retains an important secondary role. Only current first-line tests are described here.

I. SERUM TESTS

Routine assessment of thyroid function usually involves measurement of serum thyroid hormones (Chaps. 8 and 29) thyrotropin (TSH), and often thyroid antibodies. In special circumstances serum thyroglobulin (Tg) protein-bound ^{131}I and calcitonin (CT) (Chap. 29) have diagnostic value, and occasionally, chromatographic analysis of serum iodinated compounds may be needed to elucidate mechanisms of dyshormonogenesis (1).

A. Serum Thyrotropin (TSH)

The development of a radioimmunoassay for TSH (2) was made possible by the purification of human pituitary thyrotropin (3) and the production of specific antibodies in laboratory animals. Current TSH antibodies usually contain antigenic determinants directed against the common α subunit. Specific antisera have also been developed against both the α and β subunits, enabling measurement of these biologically inactive fragments even in the presence of elevated levels of (whole) TSH (4). To eliminate cross-reactivity, most assays employ antisera preabsorbed with HCG or with HCG added to the assay system. Falsely elevated TSH values have, however, been reported in mothers (and infants) with circulating heterophil antibodies from previous vaccination with serum containing rabbit IgG (5). Optimization of the assay by preincubation, use of TSH free serum, and a highly purified [^{125}I]TSH trace allows distinction between normal and low concentrations of TSH. Such modifications aim to allow evaluation of the borderline thyrotoxic in a single serum sample; suppression of TSH providing evidence of T_4, T_3 autonomy, thus obviating the need for a TRH test. In most reports TSH levels in Graves' sera lie below the lower limit of the normal range of the assay, which varies from 0.1 to 0.3μU/ml (6, 7), but low levels in about 10% of the normals make the distinction less than absolute. In practice, most TSH assays cannot distinguish normal from low levels and the TRH test still has an important role in borderline thyrotoxicosis.

Clear separation has in fact been achieved with the ultrasensitive cytochemical assay of Bitensky et al. (8). This technique which is 10 times more sensitive than current radioimmunoassays (RIAs), measures the increase in lysosomal permeability produced by TSH in guiea pig thyroid slices in vitro. This method can be regarded as the "gold standard" for TSH assay but is tedious and expensive and not suitable for routine diagnosis.

B. Serum Thyroglobulin (Tg)

Only small amounts of Tg reach the circulation (via intrathyroidal lymphatics) and in molar terms it is the least abundant iodine-containing compound in the blood. Serum levels are increased when there is distortion of destruction of thyroid architecture (multinodular goiter, subacute thyroiditis), extrinsic thyroid stimulation (iodine deficiency, Graves' disease), or autonomous overproduction from benign adenomata or differentiated carcinoma (9). Titers are higher in follicular than in papillary carcinoma and highest in the presence of metastases to bone or lung.

Many current radioimmunoassays are made invalid by the presence in the test sera of Tg antibodies (TgAb) which cause false elevation of normal levels and a decrease in high levels (10). Most studies exclude sera with positive TgHA titers measured by hemagglutination, but TgAb can be demonstrated by more sensitive methods in about 50% of "negative" sera. This difficulty can be overcome by a method which corrects for circulating TgAb by measuring the free (non-bound Tg) by double antibody RIA and derives total (F + B) by prior determination of the B/F ratio (11). This may not always be necessary and in one study neither the presence nor the titer of TgAb appeared to affect the Tg Assay (12).

Measurement of serum Tg provides a useful index of residual functioning thyroid tissue in patients with thyroid carcinoma who have received radioiodine ablation therapy (9, 13). Differences in assay sensitivity and interference by TgAb makes comparisons difficult, but most studies report good agreement with total body radioiodine scan data. In a review of 1323 cases of differentiated thyroid carcinoma (14) there were 284 patients with documented metastases. Total body scans were negative in 13% of these and all had either clinical or thyroglubulin abnormality. In only 4% was the serum Tg undetectable in the presence of a positive scan for metastases (9, 15) and this could relate to the insensitivity of the assays used. Although T_4 administration causes partial suppression of Tg in thyroid carcinoma (13), in two studies (12, 14) serum Tg allowed excellent discrimination between patients with and without disease even on T_4 therapy. Such data suggests that periodic withdrawal of T_4 and total body scanning can now be limited to patients in whom Tg levels remain elevated despite T_4 therapy.

C. Serum Thyroid Immunoglobulins

Knowledge of serum thyroid antibody levels can be important in the differential diagnosis of "simple" goiter, thyrotoxicosis, and unilateral exophthalmos as well as providing an autoimmune marker in patients with multisystem disease (16).

Five different antigen/antibody systems have been identified but only thyroglobulin (Tg) and microsomal (MC) are routinely measured. This has been simplified by the introduction of commercial hemagglutination (HA) kits which allow quantitation of TgHA and MCHA titers over a wide range. Although antibodies can still be detected by direct radioimmunoassay in HA negative sera (10), the sensitivity of the kits is adequate for routine clinical assessment. The assay is performed in plastic microtiter trays and with the Wellcome kit serial dilutions of the test serum are added to reconstituted (turkey) red cells coated with Tg or purified microsomal membranes. An even coating of cells on the bottom of the microtiter cups indicates positive hemagglutination. Titers are expressed in doubling dilutions of serum 1:10, 1:20, and so on, or in the case of MCHA, which is more sensitive, as fourfold dilutions: 10^2, 40^2, and so on.

In Hashimoto's thyroiditis titers are high and antibodies are present in almost 100% of patients. TgHA titers are high in the fibrous varient and low or absent in the oxyphil type (Chap. 29, Table 5). Moderate MCHA titers (40^2) are present in both, although they disappear in about 5% as thyroid tissue is progressively destroyed.

In Graves' disease serum thyroid antibodies are present in 70%. Low titers (TgHA less than 1:160, MCHA less than 1:40^2) are common and indicate nonprogressive multifocal thyroiditis. In 15% MCHA titers are high and these patients are liable to develop hypothyroidism. There is a fair correlation between the degree of thyroid destruction and the titer of microsomal antibodies which were formerly thought to be cytotoxic. High titers may, however, be observed without demonstrable loss of functional capacity and a specific cell membrane antigen has now been identified (17). In Graves' disease and in primary hypothyroidism MCHA alone is positive in about 30%, and in long-standing hypothyroidism both tests became negative in about 20%.

Thyroid stimulating immunoglobulins (TSI) are measured by a variety of techniques, which include the LATS protector (LATS-P) assay (18), human thyroid adenyl cyclase stimulation activity (HTACS) (19), and the receptor or thyrotropin binding inhibitor immunoglobulin assay (TBII), which measures inhibition of ^{125}ITSH binding to membrane receptors (20). The percentage of positive TSI in untreated Graves' disease ranges from 60 to 80% with the receptor assay to 70 to 90% with the HTACS assay. Neither LATS-P nor TBII assays measure thyroid stimulatory activity directly and there is little correlation between TBII, for example, and [^{99m}Tc] thyroid uptake in Graves' disease (21). These assay techniques have been invaluable in elucidating mechanisms of thyroid stimulation but have failed to provide data which can be used in a practical way in the day-to-day management of Graves' disease.

II. DYNAMIC TESTS

A. The TRH Test

The TSH response to TRH is dependent on thyrotrope nuclear T_3 occupancy and thus on the ambient levels of serum T_4 and T_3 (see Chap. 23). The sensitivity of the normal servomechanism is such that even within the normal range minimal deviations of serum thyroid hormones (particularly T_4) are accompanied by inverse changes in the serum TSH (22). The test is commonly performed with an intravenous bolus of 200 μg of synthetic TRH (23). Blood samples for TSH measurement are taken at 20 and 60 min and sometimes at 120 min. The response is dose related, but it is doubtful whether larger doses (400 μg, 500 μg) improve the discriminative value of the test. In normal subjects there is a prompt rise in serum TSH (and α and β subunits) with a peak level at 20–40 min and a slower decline to near normal between 60 and 120 min, the rate of fall being mainly dependent on feedback from the released T_3 and T_4. There is a linear correlation between the basal and peak serum TSH and the response is greater in the afternoon, when basal levels are higher (22). Response is greater in females and depressed by androgens (24). It is also blunted with age, although this may often reflect the presence of occult thyroid nodules (25). TRH also stimulates prolactin release and peak levels are achieved a little before TSH. Other trophic hormones are unaffected, but TRH suppresses the growth hormone response to insulin arginine stimulation (26) and growth hormone deficiency enhances the TSH response to TRH (27) actions, which must be re-

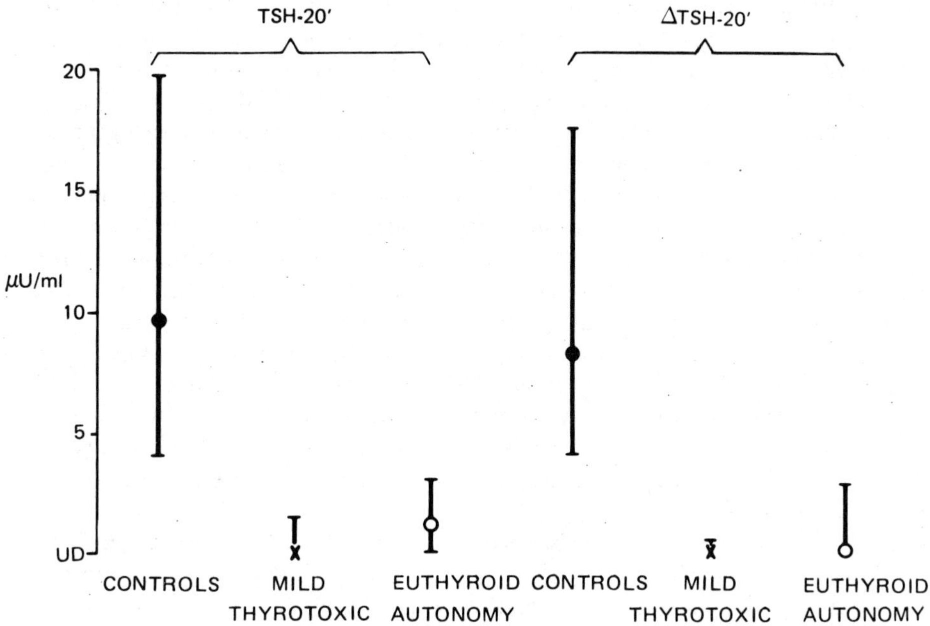

Figure 1 Short TRH test. Absolute and incremental (open triangle) TSH response at 20 min (20′) following an intravenous bolus of 200 μg (mean + 95% range). A normal or blunted response excludes thyrotoxicosis. When T_4 and T_3 are elevated, peak absolute and incremental responses of $\leqslant 1.5$ and $\leqslant 0.5$ μU/ml, respectively, confirm thyrotoxicosis. (Data from Ref. 25.)

membered when assessing children with growth defect. Side effects of TRH, which are immediate and usually transient, include mild nausea, a desire to micturate, dry mouth, and lightheadedness. By far the most important use of the TRH test is the detection of *thyroid autonomy* (Fig. 1). The response can be defined on the basis of the baseline and peak TSH value on serum samples at 0 and +20 min (25). An absent response with peak and increment values at 20 min which are equal to or less than 1.5 and 0.5 μU/ml, respectively, confirms thryotoxicosis when the serum T_4 or T_3 is elevated. A blunted TSH response (peak and increment values equal to or less than 2.9 and 2.7 μU/ml) indicates only partial thyroid autonomy and excludes thyrotoxicosis. The use of this test in borderline hyperthyroidism is discussed further in Chapter 29.

In *primary* (*thyroid*) *hypothyroidism* an exaggerated and prolonged TSH response is usual. This characteristic has been used to identify and grade borderline disease (28), but this adds little to a basal serum TSH measurement.

In *central hypothyroidism* a reduced or absent TSH response indicates an intrinsic pituitary defect, while a normal rise (peak and increment equal to or greater than 4 μU/ml) suggests a hypothalamic lesion. The distinction is often blurred, however, and the TSH response may be normal in the presence of a pituitary tumor despite unequivocal hypothyroidism. Failure of endogenous TRH delivery through distorted portal vessels could explain this finding. A prolonged TSH response is said to be characteristic of hypothalamic lesions and attributed to a sluggish release (and hence feedback of T_3 and T_4). A similar pattern can, however, be seen (for the same reason) when the TSH response is preserved in pituitary hypothyroidism. Thus the TSH test fails to diagnose the level of the lesion with any certainty and the distinction is usually made on other grounds. Measurement of serum T_3 during the TRH test allows assessment of the thyroid response to the released TSH, and peak levels occur at about 180 min. The integrity of the thyroid synthetic mechanism is not usually in question in central hypothyroidism but may be of occasional interest in patients with elevation of biologically inactive TSH when T_3 fails to rise despite an adequate TSH response.

The TSH response can be blunted by a variety of therapeutic agents, including glucocorticoids, growth hormone, somatostatin, L-dopa, bromocryptine, thiorodazine, phentolamine, cyproheptadine, acetylsalicylic acid, and many others (29). It may also be inappropriately low after withdrawal of carbimazole in Graves' disease or following longer-term administration of thyroxine for hypothyroidism.

B. In Vivo Radionuclide Studies

1. Thyroid Uptake Tests

Measurement of radionuclide thyroid uptake is no longer required to make the diagnosis of thyrotoxicosis, but it still has an important role in establishing its cause. It is particularly indicated in patients with suspected subacute thyroiditis, benign lymphocytic (painless) thyroiditis, iodide contamination, or factitious T_4 ingestion. ^{99m}Pertechnetate is the preferred isotope, with short half-life (6 hr) and minimal total body radiation dose (0.01 m rad/mCi). Uptake is maximal at about 20 min following intravenous injection of $[^{99m}Tc]0^-4$ and the "20-min uptake" exploits the rapid trapping pattern characteristic of thyrotoxicosis. The contribution to total uptake from increased gland vascularity can be assessed by continuous early phase recording (30). A progressive fall in the normal thyroid uptake values during the last decade has been attributed to increasing dietary iodide intake (31). This reduces the discriminative value of uptake tests but still allows detection of inappropriate suppression in the conditions mentioned above.

In vivo diagnostic ^{131}I has lost favor but is still useful for the calculation of dose retention in thyroid carcinoma and for the identification of functioning metastases by total body scintiscanning. Measurement of protein bound ^{131}I at 48 hr after the dose provides additional evidence of thyroid tissue ablation, levels of less than 0.006% dose per liter being confirmatory (32).

2. Perchlorate Discharge Test

This test is useful in identifying intrathyroidal defects in iodine binding. Iodide is normally trapped in the thyroid by an energy-dependent transport mechanism and immediately oxidized, organified, and bound to thyroglobulin. Perchlorate inhibits the thyroid trap and any unbound iodide is released into the circulation. A defect in iodine binding can be demonstrated in Pendred's syndrome, autoimmune thyroiditis, following radioiodine therapy and during treatment with carbimazole or propylthiouracil. The discharge test can also be used to check the adequacy of blockade by these drugs in acute severe thyrotoxicosis (33). The test usually involves the oral administration of 1 g of potassium perchlorate ($KClO_4$) 2 hr after a tracer dose of ^{131}I. Twenty-minute thyroid counts rise during the 2-hr period and show little change after that time. A reduction in counts of greater than 5% at 3 hr indicates an organification defect. The sensitivity of the test can be increased by a technique which measures neck ^{131}I uptake continuously for 20 min after the intravenous administration of ^{131}. A 200-mg dose of $KClO_4$ is given intravenously at 10 min and the test is positive if the 20-min neck count is reduced by more than 0.5% (34). With this technique the incidence of abnormality in Hashimoto's thyroiditis is increased from 40 to 80%, although the test is indicated only if serum thyroid antibody results are equivocal.

III. TESTS OF THYROID HORMONE ACTION

The poor sensitivity, specificity, and efficiency (35) of tests of thyroid hormone action limit their application in clinical practice. Such is the discriminative value of serum hormone measurements that "peripheral" tests now have a potential role only at the upper and lower limits of the normal serum ranges.

Serum values may be discrepant in nonthyroidal illness, but thyrotoxicosis can usually be excluded by the TRH test. It seems likely that the associated metabolic disturbance will preclude the future application of a specific test of peripheral hormone action. Such tests do have a potential role in patients with "compensated hypothyroidism." Older tests, such as the basal metabolic rate (BMR), serum cholesterol, and lipid levels (36), are too insensitive, and although the creatinine phosphokinase (CPK) and the cyclic AMP response to glucagon (37) both correlate with thyroid status in overt disease, they are of little value in borderline hypothyroidism. Assessment of cardiac ventricular performance by measurement of systolic time intervals (STI) (38) or by echocardiography (39) has been used to identify the myocardial disorder of hypothyroidism.

Systolic time intervals are measured by simultaneous recording of the electrocardiogram (ECG), phonocardiogram, and the carotid arterial pulse, and the preejection period (PEP) and left ventricular ejection time (LVET) are derived.

M-mode echocardiography which provides similar information more directly measures the left ventricular shortening fraction (LVSF) and derives left ventricular ejection time (LVET). Both STI and LVSF are prolonged in hypothyroidism, but only the latter has shown abnormality in borderline disease (39).

Achilles reflex half-relaxation time (ART) allows direct assessment of skelatal muscle function (40). Muscle contractility reflects thyroid status but is also altered by a number of nonspecific influences, including drugs such as epinephrine, β-adrenergic blockers, and glucocorticoids as well as pregnancy, hypoglycemia, and exercise. Following the latter the ART can remain shortened even after 60 min of rest (41). Using a carefully standardized technique and an automated photomotogram (42), the ART has been shown to be more discriminant than several other conventional tests of peripheral hormone action (43). In addition, the mean basal ART and the reduction with T_3 replacement was significantly different in patients with minor elevation of serum TSH compared with euthyroid controls (44). This was confirmed in a direct comparison in which ART but not STI was shown to discriminate between the two groups of patients (45). There is at present no specific yardstick against which to measure these indices of peripheral thyroid hormone action and the analysis of the "gray area" of TSH elevation remains an unresolved challenge. For the present, the simple visual assessment of ankle reflex relaxation remains a practical (though insensitive) test of thyroid hormone action and in this role is probably unique.

IV. TESTS OF THYROID MORPHOLOGY

A. Imaging Techniques

Thyroid imaging is indicated for the investigation of thyroid nodules, the qualitative assessment of the thyroid in thyrotoxicosis, the localization of ectopic thyroid tissue in congenital hypothyroidism, and for the management of thyroid carcinoma.

Thyroid scintiscanning is usually performed with ^{99m}Tc, although ^{131}I is still used for the detection of functioning metastases from thyroid carcinoma. Technetium may occasionally misclassify cold nodules as hot (46), and oblique views may be necessary to demonstrate a cold nodule obscured by functioning tissue (47). A repeat scan following TSH stimulation may demonstrate the presence of suppressed normal tissue in a patient with a hot nodule, and a repeat following T_3 administration can identify a warm nodule with more certainty. A number of other radionuclides, including ^{67}Ga, ^{74}selenomethionine, and ^{32}phosphate, have been used to delineate autonomous thyroid tissue, and *positive* uptake can be demonstrated despite failure of iodide concentration. None of these techniques have proved consistently helpful in the differential diagnosis of thyroid carcinoma. The fluorescent scan is a novel technique which involves focal irradiation of the thyroid gland by gamma rays derived from a ^{124}Am source. Interaction with intrathyroidal iodine (^{127}I) causes a characteristic fluorescent x-ray emission which can be picked up by lithium-silicone detector (48). This gives a semiquantitative estimate of the thyroidal content of stable iodine and can be used in the same way as the scintiscan and also to measure thyroid iodine content during antithyroid drug treatment or in the evaluation of Hashimoto's thyroiditis. This refinement can hardly be justified for routine use.

Thyroid ultrasonography is a valuable adjunct to the evaluation of the cold nodule and can distinguish between solid and cystic lesions larger than 1 cm. It also gives a relatively accurate measurement of thyroid size and can be used to follow the effects of T_4 replacement in autoimmune thyroiditis and simple goiter (49). The conventional B-mode ultrasonogram is simply performed without risk or discomfort in children, adults, and also during pregnancy. Its main use is for the selection of nodules for diagnostic and therapeutic needle aspiration (50).

B. Thyroid Biopsy

Fine needle biopsy (FNB) and core needle biopsy (CNB) have both become reestablished as important diagnostic aids (51) and previous fears of dissemination of malignant cells have proved unfounded. The biopsy is performed with the patient lying, and the neck is hyperextended by placing a small pillow beneath the shoulders.

For *FNB*, local anesthetic is preferable although not essential, since this allows several aspirations without discomfort. The procedure is performed with a 25-gauge needle and moderate suction. The orange pink aspirate from a solid lesion is smeared on a microscope slide fixed and stained using the Papanicolaou technique. Standard cytological criteria are used for microscopic assessment. If the initial aspiration yields fluid a larger needle (18-20 gauge) is substituted and the cyst aspirated. The aspirate varies in color and is yellow from simple cysts, brownish from degenerate cysts, and red from recent haemorrhage. A clear opalescent fluid is characteristic of a parathyroid cyst and measurement of parathyroid hormone (PTH) by radioimmunoassay (RIA) in the cyst fluid will confirm its origin.

For *CNB*, local anesthetic is usual. A small nick is made in the skin on the inferomedial side of the nodule to allow introduction of the needle, which is directed in the long axis of the neck. The Trucut needle with 11.4-cm cannula and 20-mm specimen notch has proved very satisfactory in practice. The tissue sample is fixed immediately in formalin. Complications are very uncommon but can include local bleeding, puncture of the trachea, and transient damage to the laryngeal nerve.

FNB and CNB can be used together or separately in the investigation of the cold nodule. FNB is possible in nodules as small as 0.5 cm in diameter but CNB is restricted to nodules greater than 2 cm. In practice, FNB can be employed for nodules up to 4 cm. If the diagnosis is thyroiditis, anaplastic, papillary or metastatic carcinoma, no additional diagnostic procedure is necessary. If the specimen is unsatisfactory or follicular grade I or II, CNB can give additional information, although more often surgical excision is advised. In nodules larger than 3-4 cm, degenerative changes are common and FNB may be unsuccessful. For these nodules CNB is preferable. Both FNB and CNB can be undertaken at the same session and this may be helpful when sampling difficulty is anticipated. If the core sample proves satisfactory, it may not be necessary to process the FNB. By a judicious use of these techniques it may be possible to avoid surgery altogether or to temporize in an older patient with an apparently benign neoplasm. In younger patients neither technique can be relied on to exclude carcinoma with 100% certainty, and surgical excision with frozen section is the logical management.

REFERENCES

1. Barsano CP, De Groot LJ. Dyshormogenetic goitre. J Clin Endocrinol Metab 1979; 8:145–165.
2. Odell WD, Wilber JF, Utiger RD. Studies on thyrotropin physiology by means of radioimmunoassay. Recent Prog Horm Res 1967; 23:47–85.
3. Condliffe PG, Purification of human thyrotropin. Endocrinology 1963; 72: 993–96.
4. Kourides IA, Ridgeway EC, Weintraub BD, Bigos ST, Gershengern MC, Maloof F. Thyrotropin-induced hyperthyroidism: use of alpha and beta subunit levels to identify patients with pituitary tumours. J Clin Endocrinol Metab 1977; 45:534–543.
5. Czernichow P, Vandalem JL, Hennen G. Transient neonatal hyperthyrotropinemia: a factitious syndrome due to the presence of heterophil antibodies in the plasma of infants and their mothers. J Clin Endocrinol Metab 1981; 53:387–393.
6. Spencer CA, Nicoloff JT. Improved radioimmunoassay for human TSH. Clin Chim Acta 1980; 108(3):415–424.

7. Smith SR, Burton DW, Izenstark MD. Levels of serum thyroid-stimulating hormone in hyperthyroidism. Arch Intern Med 1979; 139:756–760.
8. Petersen V, Rees Smith B, Hall R. A study of thyroid stimulating activity in human serum with the highly sensitive cytochemical bioassay. J Clin Endocrinol Metab 1975; 41:199-204.
9. Schlossberg AH, Jacobson JC, Ibbertson HK. Serum Thyroglobulin in the diagnosis and management of thyroid carcinoma. Clin Endocrinol 1979; 10:17–27.
10. Ratcliff JG, Ayoub LAW. Determination of total serum thyroglobulin in the presence of thyroglobulin antibodies. In *Thyroid Research VIII*, Stockigt JR, Nagataki S (eds), Proceedings of the VIIIth International Thyroid Congress, Sydney. Australian Academy of Science, Canberra 1980; 493–498.
11. Ratcliffe JG, Ayoub LAW, Pearson D. The measurement of serum thyroglobulin in the presence of thyroglobulin antibodies. Clin Endocrinol 1981; 15:507–578.
12. Black EG, Cassoni A, Gimlette TM, Harmer CL, Maisey MN, Oates GD, Hoffenberg R. Serum thyroglobulin in thyroid cancer. Lancet 1981; 2: 443–445.
13. Pacini F, Pinchlhera Giani C, Grasso L, Doveni F, Baschieri L. Serum thyroglobulin in thyroid carcinoma and other thyroid disorders. J Endocrinol Invest 1980; 3:283-292.
14. Ashcraft MW, VanHerle AJV. The comparative value of serum thyroglobulin measurements and iodine 131 total body scans in the follow up study of patients with treated differentiated thyroid carcinoma. Am J Med 1981; 71:806–814.
15. Bridgman MC, Cooper RA, Luttrell BM, Reeve TS, Stiel JN, Wilmshurst EG, Hales B. Evaluation of serum thyroglobulin levels in the follow up of thyroid cancer following ablative therapy. In *Thyroid Research VIII*, Stockigt JR, Nagataki S (eds), Proceedings of the VIIIth International Thyroid Congress, Sydney. Australian Academy of Science, Canberra 1980; pp 483–485.
16. Doniach D, Bottazzo GF, Russell RCG. Goitrous autoimmune thyroiditis (Hashimoto's disease). J. Clin Endocrinol Metab 1979; 8:63–80.
17. Khoury EL, Hammond L, Botazzo GF, Doniach D. Presence of the organ-specific "microsomal" autoantigen on the surface of human thyroid cells in culture: its involvement in complement-medicated cytotoxicity. Clin Exp Immunol 1981; 45:316-328.
18. Hardisty CA, Hanford CA, Munro DS. The prediction of relapse after drug treatment of Graves' disease by assay of long acting thyroid stimulator-protector (LATS-P). Clin Endocrinol 1981; 14:509–517.
19. McKenzie JM, Zakarija M, Sato A. Humoral immunity in Graves' disease. J Clin Endocrinol Metab 1978; 7:31–45.
20. Smith BR, Hall R. Thyroid stimulating immunoglobulins in Graves' disease. Lancet 1974; 2:427–431.

21. Croxson MS, Lim TMT, Graham FM, Ibbertson HK. Thyrotropin displacement activity of serum ummunoglobulins in health and disease. Aust NZ J Med 1980; 10:151–156.
22. Weeke J. The influence of the circadian thyrotrophin rhythm on the thyrotropin response to thyrotropin-releasing hormone in normal subjects. Scand J Clin Lab Invest 1974; 33:17–20.
23. Ormston BJ, Garry R, Cryer RJ, Besser GM, Hall R. Thyrotropin-releasing hormone as a thyroid function test. Lancet 1971; 2:10–14.
24. Morley JE, Sawin CT, Carlson HE, Longscope C, Hershman JM. The relationships of androgen to the thyrotropin and prolactin responses to the thyrotropin-releasing hormone in hypogonadal and normal men. J Clin Endocrinol Metab 1981; 52:173–176.
25. Croxson MS, Wilson TM, Ballantyne GH. TRH testing, T4 thyrotoxicosis and the aging thyroid gland. NZ Med J 1981; 93:417–420.
26. Maeda K, Kato Y, Chihara K, et al. Suppression by thyrotropin-releasing hormone (TRH) of human growth hormone release induced by arginine and insulin-induced hypoglycemia in man. J Clin Endocrinol Metab 1976; 43:453–456.
27. Cobb W, Reichlin S, Jackson I. Growth hormone secretory status is a determinant of the thyrotropin response to thyrotropin-releasing hormone in euthyroid patients with hypothalamic-pituitary disease. J Clin Endocrinol Metab 1981; 52:324–329.
28. Basterin PA, Bonnyns M, VanHaelst L. Grades of subclinical hypothyroidism in asymptomatic autoimmune thyroiditis revealed by the thyrotropin releasing hormone test. J Clin Endocrinol Metab 1980; 51:163–166.
29. Wensel KW. Pharmacological interference with in vitro tests of thyroid function. Metabolism 1981; 30:717–732.
30. Armstrong DI, Rogers TGH, Brownlie BEW, Turner JG. Thyroid vascularity and trapping function: analysis of very early thyroid technetium "uptake." Int J Nucl Med Biol 1970; 3:65–70.
31. Park YK, Hortand BF, Vanderween JE, Shank FR, Prosky L. Estimation of dietary iodine intake of Americans in recent years. Research 1981; 79: 17–23.
32. Pochin EE. Radioiodine therapy of thyroid cancer. Semin Nucl Med 1971; 1:503–515.
33. Barnes HV, Bledsoe T. A simple test for selecting the thionamide schedule in thyrotoxicosis. J Clin Endocrinol Metab 1972; 35:250–255.
34. Gray HW, Greig WR, Thomson JA. Intravenous perchlorate test in the diagnosis of Hashimoto's disease. Lancet 1974; 1:335–338.
35. Galen RS, Gambino SR. *The Predictive Value and Efficacy of Medical Diagnoses*. Wiley, New York, 1975.
36. Kulty KM, Bryant DG, Farid NR. Serum lipids in hypothyroidism: a reevaluation. J Clin Endocrinol Metab 1978; 46(1):55–56.

37. Lazarus JH, Shelty KJ, Siddle K. The value of glucogen induced rise in plasma adenosine 3′,5′-cyclic monophosphate in assessing thyroid status. In *Thyroid Research*, Robbins J, Braverman IE (eds). Exerpta Medica, Amsterdam, 1975, 378:606-609.
38. Plotnick GD, Vassar DL, Parisi AF, Hamilton BP, Carliner NH, Fisher ML. Systolic time intervals in hypothyroidism: end organ functions as a reflection of clinical status. Am J Med Sci 1979; 277:263–268.
39. Davies HA, Dawdle RJ, Lazarus JH, Davies CJ. Do peripheral thyroid indicators reflect response to treatment in latent hypothyroidism. In *Thyroid Research VIII*, Stockigt JR, Nagataki S (eds), Proceedings of the VIIIth International Thyroid Congress, Sydney. Australian Academy of Science, Canberra, 1980, pp 529-532.
40. Gilson WE. Achilles-reflex recording with a simple photomotograph. N. Engl J Med 1959; 260:1027-1028.
41. Ballantyne GH, Croxson MS. The effect of exercise, thyroid status and insulin induced hypoglycaemia on the Achilles tendon reflex time in man. Eur J Appl Physiol 1981; 46:77-83.
42. Tuck DL. Improved measurement of the achilles tendon reflex. Med Biol Eng 1974; 12:170-174.
43. Croxson MS, Naden RP, Ibbertson HK. Diagnostic efficiency in primary hypothyroidism. Aust NZ Med 1974; 4:98.
44. Croxson MS, Ibbertson HK. Subclinical hypothyroidism. NZ Med J 1980; 91:89-91.
45. Ooi JL, Whitlock MG, Frengley PA, Ibbertson HK. Systolic time intervals and ankle reflex time in patients with minimal serum TSH elevation: response to triiodothyronine therapy. Clin Endocrinol 1980; 13:621-627.
46. Steinberg M, Cavalieri RR, Choy SH. Uptake of technetium 99-pertechnetate in a primary thyroid carcinoma: need for caution in evaluating nodules. J Clin Endocrinol Metab 1970; 31:81-85.
47. Karelitz JR, Richards JB. Necessity of oblique views in evaluating the functional status of a thyroid nodule. J Nucl Med 1974; 154:782-785.
48. Jonckleer MH, Vanhaelst L, Deconinck F, Michotte Y. Atrophic autoimmune thyroiditis: relationship between the clinical state and intrathyroidal iodine as measured in vivo in man. J Clin Endocrinol Metab 1981; 53:476-479.
49. Hansen JM, Kampmann J, Madsen SN, Skovsted L, Solgaard S, Grytier C, Grontvedt T, Norry Ragaussen S. L-Thyroxine treatment of diffuse nontoxic goitre evaluated by ultrasonic determination of thyroid volume. Clin Endocrinol (Oxf) 1979; 10:1-6.
50. Walfish PG, Hazani E, Strawbridge HTG, Misken M. Combined ultrasound and needle aspiration cytology in the assessment and management of hypofunctioning thyroid nodule. Ann Intern Med 1977; 87:270-274.
51. Gershengorn ML, McClung MR, Chee EW, Weintraub BD, Robbins J. Fineneedle aspiration cytology in the preoperative diagnosis of thyroid nodules. Ann Intern Med 1977; 87:265-269.

40
Growth Hormone Secretion

Leslie Lazarus
St. Vincent's Hospital, Sydney, Australia

I. EXERCISE

Background. Physical exercise is a profound stimulus to growth hormone (GH) release. The use of exercise as a screening procedure is well established and has the advantage of being an outpatient procedure requiring little preparation. The manner in which exercise stimulates GH release is not known, although it has been observed that for a reliable response the subject should be exercised to exhaustion. In physically fit subjects this may require a large work load. Some clinicians have reported a high failure rate of 25-30% with this test in normal subjects, but this can be reduced to 10% with careful attention to the mode of exercise and the work load used.

Contraindications. Should not be used in subjects with exercise-induced asthma or coronary artery insufficiency.

Procedure. The test may be performed at any time of day and no special preparations are necessary. The exercise is best done using a bicycle ergometer with adjustable loads. An indwelling needle is inserted in a forearm vein. Following two basal samples for human growth hormone (hGH) the subject exercises for 20 min and then rests for a further 20 min. Blood samples for hGH are taken at the end of the 20-min exercise period and at the completion of the 20-min rest period. The work load should be sufficient to achieve a pulse rate of 180 beats per minute in the child or 150 beats per minute in an adult.

Side Effects. In the unfit subject a feeling of exhaustion may last for some time following the exercise.

Interpretation. As a screening procedure a normal response of 20 mU/liter or greater eliminates the need for further investigation of hGH status.

II. SLEEP

Background. A surge of GH release occurs during the onset of slow-wave sleep [electroencephalogram (EEG) stages 3 and 4] and sampling of this GH peak is well established as a physiological test of GH secretion.

Preparation. Ideally, the subject should be admitted to the hospital and the study performed on the second night after an initial night's sleep in the same surroundings for the purpose of acclimatization. However, a number of workers have reported that the test may be performed without EEG monitoring and by the taking of a single blood sample at 60-90 min after the onset of sleep, at the anticipated time for the onset of slow-wave sleep. No sedatives or soporifics should be used and the subject should be allowed to sleep in quiet, comfortable surroundings.

Contraindication. None.

Procedure. An indwelling venous catheter should be inserted for blood sampling and maintained patent with a slow saline infusion. EEG monitoring should be undertaken using long leads. Blood samples should be taken prior to the onset of sleep and at 30-min intervals until the completion of the sleep cycle.

When this test is performed without monitoring the subject should be observed for the onset of sleep and blood samples taken via the catheter at intervals over the period of from 60 to 120 min after the observed onset of sleep.

Side Effects. None.

Interpretation. By consensus it has been agreed that a growth hormone-deficient child will fail to achieve a peak hGH level of 10 mU/liter and a child with partial GH deficiency will fail to achieve a peak hGH level of either 15 mU/liter or 20 mU/liter depending on the criteria used.

It should be noted that while a peak hGH of greater than the criterion indicates normal GH secretion and eliminates the diagnosis of GH deficiency, a failure to achieve the criterion does not establish a diagnosis of GH deficiency. The sleep GH test is usually accepted as a physiological screening procedure and a failure to achieve the criterion indicates that a further diagnostic procedure should be undertaken (e.g., insulin-induced hypoglycemia).

III. ARGININE

The administration of amino acids results in a release of GH. The amino acids may be given complexed in a protein meal, as a beef extract (Bovril), or as an amino acid infusion. L-Arginine infusion has been the most widely used either as a single test or as a sequential test with insulin-induced hypoglycemia.

Preparation. The test should be performed in the morning after an overnight fast.

Contraindication. None.

Procedure. The arginine is given in an intravenous infusion of a 10% solution of L-arginine monochloride in saline at a dose of 0.5 g/kg body weight (to a maximum of 30 g) over a period of 30 min. The subject should be at rest throughout the procedure. An indwelling venous catheter or needle should be inserted into an antecubital vein for blood sampling and for the infusion. At least two blood samples should be taken at 15-min intervals for basal hGH measurements prior to commencement of the infusion. Then the arginine infusion is given over a period of 30 min and blood samples are taken at the completion of the infusion and at 15-min intervals until 90 min following commencement of the infusion. When combined with insulin as a sequential test a dose of intravenous insulin (as described for the insulin hypoglycemia test) is given at 90 min.

Side Effects. None.

Interpretation. Women and children respond more consistently and have a greater rise than do adult men. The response of men can be augmented by the prior administration of estrogens. A normal response is the achievement of a serum hGH level of 20 mU/liter or greater at some time during the test.

IV. INSULIN-INDUCED HYPOGLYCEMIA

Background. Hypoglycemia is a profound stimulus to the release of hGH and acts via the hypothalamus. The induction of hypoglycemia by the intravenous administration of insulin has become established as a standard stimulus for hGH release. The insulin-induced hypoglycemia (IIH) test is based on the older insulin tolerance test, with which it should not be confused. The insulin tolerance test which was used to demonstrate hypoglycemia unresponsiveness in pituitary or adrenal hypofunction used as a criterion the inability of the hypopituitary subject to recover euglycemia rather than the measurement of hormonal responses.

As the aim of the IIH is to use hypoglycemia as an hypothalamic-pituitary stimulus, it is mandatory that an adequate degree of hypoglycemia be achieved. By consensus, hypoglycemia is defined as a blood glucose of 2.2 mmol/liter or less or a level 50% or less of the basal level. As hypoglycemia is also a stimulus to adrenocorticotrophic hormone (ACTH) release, the simultaneous measurement of cortisol allows for another parameter of hypothalamic-pituitary function.

The IIH may be performed either as a solitary test, as part of a sequential study following arginine infusion, or as a combined test together with TRH and GnRH.

A. Solitary Test

Preparation. The test is best performed in the morning after an overnight fast with the subject comfortably at rest on a bed. The test may be performed as an outpatient procedure. The subject should be counseled regarding the symptoms of hypoglycemia.

Contraindication. The test is potentially dangerous and should not be performed in subjects with coronary artery disease or epilepsy, both of which may be activated by the hypoglycemia. A medical officer should always be in attendance, with adequate facilities for resuscitation and the administration of hydrocortisone or intravenous glucose.

Procedure. An indwelling cannula or needle should be inserted into an antecubital vein for the taking of serial venous blood samples and as an avenue for the rapid administration of glucose should this be necessary. The needle should be kept patent with a slow saline infusion. A bedside glucose monitor should be available for the immediate measurement of blood glucose levels to assess whether an adequate degree of hypoglycemia has been achieved.

After a suitable rest period basal blood samples should be taken for the measurement of glucose, hGH, and cortisol. Two basal samples at an interval of 15 min should be taken before the administration of the insulin.

Neutral purified insulin should be used by intravenous bolus injection. The standard dose used is 0.1 U/kg body weight for children or 0.15 U/kg for adults, and this may be diluted in normal saline to make a larger volume for administration. A smaller dose of 0.05 U/kg may be used in insulin-sensitive patients with profound hypopituitarism and a larger dose of up to 0.3 U/kg may be required in patients with acromegaly and insulin resistance.

An adequate degree of hypoglycemia must be achieved and should be verified by immediate blood glucose measurement using a bedside glucose monitor. If hypoglycemia has not been achieved within 45 min after the injection of insulin, a further dose should be administered.

Blood samples for the measurement of glucose, hGH, and cortisol should be taken at 30-min intervals until 120 min after the insulin administration.

If normoglycemia is not achieved by 120 min intravenous glucose may be administered. Following the procedure the subject should be given a light meal before leaving the clinic to return home or to a ward. Steroid-deficient subjects should be given a dose of hydrocortisone intramuscularly at the completion of the test.

Side Effects. Apart from the changes of profound hypoglycemia mentioned above there are no significant side effects of the procedure.

Interpretation. By consensus, severe growth hormone deficiency is present if the hGH fails to rise above 10 mU/liter following the induction of an adequate degree of hypoglycemia. Partial growth hormone deficiency is defined by some workers as a failure to achieve a peak level of 15 mU/liter and by others as failure to achieve a peak level of 20 mU/liter. A number of factors may influence the hGH response to IIH, as detailed in Chap. 21, Tables 2 and 7.

B. Sequential Test (Arginine Infusion/Insulin-Induced Hypoglycemia)

The IIH test may be performed in sequence with an arginine infusion test as a single outpatient procedure. The arginine infusion is performed first and then at 75 min following the commencement of the arginine infusion, an intravenous dose of insulin is given following the same protocol as for the solitary test. The same criteria for performance, safety, and interpretation apply when the test is performed in this manner. The sequential test has the advantage of providing two tests of GH secretion at a single attendance for the patient.

C. Combined Test [Insulin-Induced Hypoglycemia/Thyroid Releasing Hormone (TRH)/Gonadotropin Releasing Hormone (GnRH)]

The IIH test may be combined with the simultaneous intravenous administration of TRH (200 μg) and GnRH (100 μg) to provide a combined test of anterior pituitary function to assess the responses of GH, thyroid stimulating hormone (TSH), prolactin, luteinizing hormone (LH), follicle stimulating hormone (FSH), and ACTH.

The same criteria and precautions apply to this combined test as for the solitary IIH test. In order to assess the response of all hormones it is common practice to extend the observation period to 180 min following the combined stimuli.

V. L-DOPA (1-DIHYDROXYPHENYLALANINE)

Background. The oral administration of L-dopa stimulates the release of hGH in the normal subject and a paradoxical fall in serum hGH levels in the acromegalic patient. L-Dopa is thought to act via its conversion to dopamine and the subsequent perturbation of hypothalamic biogenic amines. The test is used to stimulate hGH release in children with possible hGH deficiency and in adults with hypopituitarism. A failure of response may occur in 25-40% of normal subjects, but this failure rate may be reduced to 5-10% by the prior administration of propranolol, which potentiates the GH response to L-dopa. While the test is well suited for use as an outpatient screening procedure, it induces vomiting and nausea in up to 40% of subjects.

Preparation. The test is best performed in the morning after an overnight fast.

Contrainidications. None.

Procedure. The subject should be at rest for 30 min prior to the test and throughout the test. Venous blood samples for the measurement of serum hGH should be taken via an indwelling needle or catheter. At least two samples should be taken at 15-min intervals prior to the oral administration of the L-dopa. In the adult a dose of 500 mg is used and in children a dose of 10 mg/kg body weight up to a maximum of 500 mg is recommended. When used as a combined propranolol/L-dopa test a dose of 0.75 mg/kg (up to a maximum of 40 mg) of propranolol is given orally 20 min prior to the L-dopa. Blood samples are taken at 30-min intervals until 2 hr after the L-dopa dose.

Side Effects. Vomiting and nausea may occur in up to 40% of subjects.

Interpretation. In the possible GH-deficient subject a normal response is the achievement of a serum hGH level of 20 mU/liter or greater at any time during the test. A peak serum hGH of between 10 and 20 mU/liter may indicate partial GH deficiency and a level of less than 10 mU/liter indicates severe GH deficiency. As 25-40% of normal subjects fail to respond to L-dopa, the test alone is not diagnostic unless a normal response occurs. This latter observation excludes GH deficiency.

VI. CLONIDINE

Clonidine is an α-adrenergic drug used as an hypotensive agent. It has been observed to stimulate GH release and proposed as an alternative to insulin-induced hypoglycemia.

Preparation. The test should be performed in the morning after an overnight fast.

Contraindications. None.

Procedure. Clonidine is given as an oral dose of 0.15 mg/m^2 or as an intravenous dose of 0.2 μg/kg body weight over a period of 10 min. The subject should be at rest and two basal samples at least 15 min apart should be taken prior to the dose. A peak of hGH occurs at 60-90 min following ingestion and at 60 min following the intravenous dose. Blood samples should be taken at 30-min intervals until 120 min following the oral dose or 90 min following the intravenous dose.

Side Effects. In all subjects there is a fall in blood pressure of 20–25 mmHg and drowsiness which may persist for 1–3 hr. The blood pressure should be checked before allowing the subject to leave the clinic.

Interpretation. A normal response is the achievement of a peak serum hGH level of 20 mU/liter or greater. Similar to other tests, some 25% of normal subjects fail to respond to this test.

VII. GLUCAGON

Glucagon stimulates the release of insulin and subsequently GH in normal subjects. The peak of hGH response occurs at 120–180 min postinjection and there is some evidence to suggest that the GH response follows the rapid drop in blood glucose. The incidence of failed GH responses in normal subjects may be as high as 40%, but this can be reduced to 10–15% by the prior administration of propranolol.

Contraindications. Should not be used in diabetic subjects.

Procedure. The test is performed after an overnight fast and the subject should be at rest throughout. Blood samples are taken via an indwelling needle or catheter. After two basal samples for hGH and glucose a dose of 1.0 mg of glucagon is given subcutaneously. The dose used is 0.5 mg for children, 1.0 mg for nonobese adults and 1.5 mg for adults of weight greater than 90 kg. Blood samples for hGH and glucose are taken at 30-min intervals from 60 to 180 min. The peak hGH response usually occurs around 150 min following injection.

Side Effects. In some subjects nausea, vomiting, and a feeling of apprehension may occur. Delayed hypoglycemia, especially if given together with propranolol.

Interpretation. A normal response is the achievement of a hGH level of 20 mU/liter or greater at any time during the test.

VIII. PROPRANOLOL

Propranolol is a β-adrenergic blocker which has been noted to enhance the hGH responses to stimuli. When given together with L-dopa or glucagon it may reduce the incidence of failed GH responses in normal subjects from 40 to 10%.

Contraindications. Should not be used in subjects with bronchial asthma.

Procedure. The dose used is 0.75 mg/kg body weight up to a maximum of 40 mg. It is given orally and most workers suggest that it be given 20 min prior to the stimulus. Some workers give propranolol and L-dopa or glucagon simultaneously.

Side Effects. Prolonged hypoglycemia has been noted in some subjects following propranolol-augmented tests.

Interpretation. The same criteria apply as for the test procedure using L-dopa or glucagon alone.

IX. ANDROGEN/ESTROGEN-PRIMED TESTS

Background. The GH responses of pubertal children are greater than those of prepubertal children, and it has been demonstrated that spontaneous puberty as well as androgen/estrogen administration enhances the GH response to stimuli in an individual child. The use of sex hormone priming has been advocated by some workers to differentiate the partial GH deficiency associated with delayed puberty from organic disease.

Procedure. A stimulation test (exercise, insulin-induced hypoglycemia) is repeated after 3 days of sex hormone administration. For boys androgens are administered using testosterone propionate 25 mg intramuscularly daily or methyltestosterone 10 mg orally thrice daily or fluoxymestrone 10 mg orally twice daily. For girls, ethinyl estradiol 50 μg orally per day is given.

Side Effects. Nausea may be induced in some girls by the estrogen administration.

Interpretation. In the child with simple delayed puberty the previously subnormal hGH response to stimulation should be converted to a normal response by sex hormone priming.

X. TRH TEST OF GH RELEASE

Background. Thyrotrophin releasing hormone (TRH, protirelin) stimulates the release of TSH and prolactin but not growth hormone in normal subjects. It causes the release of GH in 50% of acromegalics, and this rise can be used both for diagnosis and for the prediction of responses to therapy. A positive correlation has been reported between the GH response to TRH and the outcome of surgery or bromocriptine therapy. The paradoxical GH response to TRH is not unique to acromegaly and may be seen in a number of other conditions (Chap. 21, Table 4). While the TSH response to TRH is suppressed in acromegaly, there is no correlation between the paradoxical rise in GH and the TSH response, and thyroid hormone administration does not block the GH response to TRH.

Preparation. Due to possible blood pressure changes and episodes of smooth muscle spasm which may occur, the subject should be supine when the intravenous TRH is given.

Contraindication. The TRH test should be avoided in patients with bronchial asthma, other forms of obstructive airway disease, or coronary artery insufficiency.

Procedure. The subject should be at rest and supine. An indwelling cannula or needle should be inserted into an antecubital vein for the taking of serial venous blood samples. After a suitable rest period two basal blood samples at an interval of 15 min should be taken for the measurement of hGH. A bolus dose of 200 μg of TRH should be given intraveneously and blood samples taken for hGH measurement at 30-min intervals until 120 min, when the test may be terminated.

Side Effects. Following an intravenous bolus of TRH, a number of transient reactions are common. These include nausea, a desire to micturate, a feeling of flushing, dizziness, a metallic taste, and abdominal discomfort. These side effects have been attributed to a local action of the TRH on smooth muscle of the gastrointestinal-genitourinary tracts.

Interpretation. No significant change in hGH is noted in normal subjects. A paradoxical rise in hGH indicates an abnormality of hypothalamic-pituitary control of GH secretion and may be seen in a number of conditions (Chap. 21, Table 4), including 50% of acromegalics.

XI. ORAL GLUCOSE LOAD

Background. In the normal subject the serum hGH level is suppressed following an oral glucose load. In patients with acromegaly the serum hGH level is not suppressed to normal levels by 2 hr after an oral glucose load of 50-100 g, and this has been considered a criterion of diagnosis. In some acromegalic patients a paradoxical rise of serum hGH may occur following an oral glucose load and this response is considered by some to be diagnostic of acromegaly. It should be noted, however, that the failure of suppression and the paradoxical response of serum hGH may occur in a number of other conditions (Chap. 21, Table 3.) and is thus not diagnostic of acromegaly but is a sign of abnormal hypothalamic-pituitary control of GH release.

Preparation. The test is best performed as part of an oral glucose tolerance test.

Contraindications. The test should not be performed if the subject has uncontrolled diabetes mellitus with hyperglycemia.

Procedure. Using the criteria suggested by the WHO, the test should be performed in the morning after a fast of at least 8 hr and not more than 16 hr.

Table 1 Dynamic Tests of Growth Hormone Secretion

1. Stimulation tests
   a. Physiological
      Exercise
      Sleep
   b. Nutrient challenge
      Arginine infusion
      Insulin-induced hypoglycemia
         Solitary test
         Sequential test with arginine infusion
         Combined with TRH and GnRH
   c. Pharmacological
      L-dopa
      Clonidine
      Glucagon
      Propranolol
         Propranolol/L-dopa
         Propranolol/glucagon
      Androgen/estrogen-primed tests
      TRH
2. Suppression test
   Oral glucose

The patient should rest for at least 30 min prior to the glucose load and during the course of the procedure.

Venous blood samples are best taken via an indwelling needle or catheter and should be taken 15 min prior to the glucose, immediately prior to the glucose, and at 60 min and 120 min following the glucose load. A glucose load of 75 g (416 mmol) should be dissolved in 250–350 ml of water and drunk within 5 min. The blood samples should be assayed for glucose and serum hGH. Some workers also advocate the measurement of insulin in the same samples.

Side Effects. None.

Interpretation. While the majority of references suggest that the 2-hr serum hGH should be suppressed to 10 mU/liter or less, others advocate suppression to below 5 mU/liter. There are no statistical data to support either figure, which are based on anecdotal data and clinical consensus only. A paradoxical rise is considered to have occurred if at any stage during the procedure the serum hGH rises to a level significantly greater than the basal.

The blood glucose measurements may also be used to assess whether the subject has diabetes mellitus.

Tables 1 and 2 summarize the tests described above.

Table 2 Dynamic Tests of Growth Hormone Release

Test	Dose	Time of maximum response (min)	Side effects	Limitations
Exercise		20	None in otherwise healthy subjects	Contraindicated in bronchial asthma, coronary insufficiency, and elderly
Sleep		60–120	None	Should have EEG monitoring for stage of sleep
Arginine	0.5 g/kg body weight i.v. over 30 min	30–60	None	None
Insulin-induced hypoglycemia	0.05–0.30 U/kg	30–90 postinjection	Hypoglycemia	Medical attendant must be present throughout test with glucose and cortisol available; contraindicated in epilepsy, ischemic heart disease, and elderly
L-Dopa	10 mg/kg body weight orally in children; 500 mg orally in adults	30–120	Nausea and vomiting in 40%	None
Clonidine	0.15 mg/m^2 orally	60–120	Hypotension and drowsiness	None
Glucagon	1.0 mg subcutaneous	120–180	Nausea, Vomiting, apprehension, hypoglycemia	Risk of hypoglycemia unreliable in diabetes

Table 2 (Continued)

Test	Dose	Time of maximum response (min)	Side effects	Limitations
Propranolol	0.75 mg/kg body weight orally (but not exceeding 40 mg) is given 2 hr prior to L-dopa or glucagon		Hypoglycemia	Prolonged hypoglycemia; avoid in subjects with bronchial asthma
TRH	200 μg i.v.	30–60	Nausea, desire to micturate, feeling of flushing, dizziness, abdominal discomfort	Should not be used in subjects with bronchial asthma, chronic obstructive airways disease, or ischemic heart disease
Oral glucose	75 g orally	120	Nil	Nil

41

Prolactin Secretion

Stephen Franks
St. Mary's Hospital Medical School, University of London, London, England

A large number of dynamic tests of prolactin secretion have been devised, making use of the wide range of drugs which have been shown to cause rapid stimulation or suppression of prolactin. These tests have provided useful information on the dynamics of prolactin secretion in normal subjects and, in particular, have confirmed the importance of tonic inhibitory control of prolactin by dopamine. However, dynamic function tests have proved of very limited value in assessment of hyperprolactinemic states (as discussed below and in Chap. 22). Details of the more commonly used tests are given and the less common testing procedures are briefly summarized.

I. PROLACTIN STIMULATION TESTS

A. Insulin Hypoglycemia

Stimulation of prolactin by insulin hypoglycemia was described in the initial clinical studies which followed the development of a specific radioimmunoassay for prolactin some 10 years ago (1). A standard insulin tolerance test is performed as described in Chapter 38. The peak prolactin response to insulin hypoglycemia is, however, very variable, ranging from 2 to 19 times basal levels (1). Because of this and of the problems associated with hypoglycemia, this test is rarely used as a primary test of prolactin reserve, but it is convenient to measure prolactin levels in patients with pituitary disease who are undergoing insulin hypoglycemia for assessment of human growth hormone (hGH) or adrenocorticotropic hormone (ACTH) secretion (2).

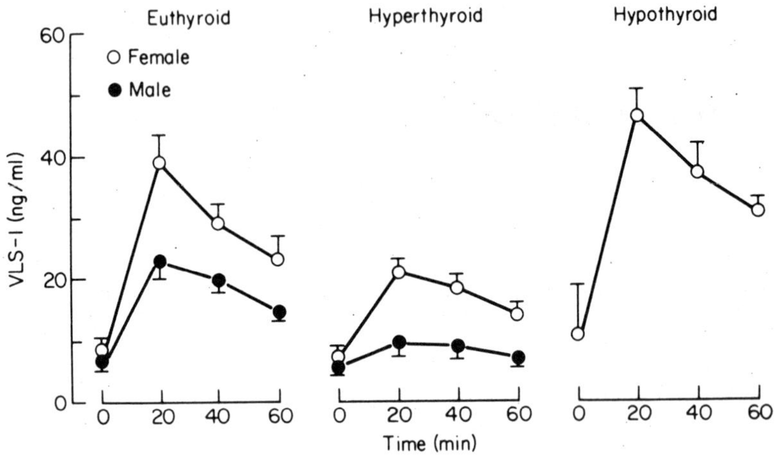

Figure 1 Prolactin response to TRH. Mean ± SE prolactin concentration before and after 200 μg of TRH are shown in normal subjects and in those with thyroid disease. (From Ref. 13.)

B. Thyrotropin Releasing Hormone (TRH)

An intravenous injection of synthetic TRH causes a rapid rise in serum prolactin levels with a peak at 15-30 min (3). The prolactin response to TRH is influenced by similar factors to that of TRH-induced TSH secretion; it is greater in women than in men and is affected by the thyroid status of the subject (Fig. 1). Since basal prolactin levels are usually within the normal range in hypopituitarism, the response to TRH may be a useful index of the functional capacity of the lactotrope in such patients. However, impaired prolactin secretion is rarely of clinical importance and routine testing of the prolactin response to TRH in patients with suspected hypopituitarism (e.g., following pituitary surgery) is not advocated. It may, however, provide useful information in patients who fail to lactate following pregnancy (i.e., in the diagnosis of Sheehan's syndrome). The TRH test is of limited value in evaluation of hyperprolactinemic states. The prolactin response to TRH is usually impaired when basal prolactin concentrations are elevated, irrespective of whether the patient has a pituitary tumor (4). The exception to this is hyperprolactinemia due to primary hypothyroidism; in this case the prolactin response to TRH is exaggerated and predicts that treatment with thyroxine will result in lowering of prolactin levels to normal.

The procedure for the TRH test is as follows. No preparation of the patient is required and the test can easily be performed on an outpatient visit. A baseline blood sample is taken and is followed by an intravenous injection of 200 μg of TRH. Blood samples are usually taken at 20-min intervals for 1 hr, but two samples at 30 and 60 min are in fact sufficient.

C. Dopamine Receptor Antagonists

The phenothiazine chlorpromazine was used to stimulate prolactin secretion in early studies (5). An intramuscular injection of chlorpromazine (25 or 50 mg) causes a rise in prolactin levels which reach a maximum 1-2 hr after the dose. Pimozide and the benzamide sulpiride are more potent stimulators of prolactin secretion and have been used as provocation tests (6, 7). Another drug of the benzamide group, the antiemetic metoclopramide, has enjoyed wide use in dynamic testing of prolactin secretion (8, 9). The peak response of prolactin occurs about 30 min after intravenous injection of metoclopramide (Fig. 2). As with TRH the responsiveness is greater in women than in men but does not appear to be affected by the thyroid status of the subject (10). The increment in prolactin concentrations which follows an intravenous dose of 2.5 mg of metoclopramide is almost twofold greater than that observed after 400 μg of TRH. Thus many investigators favor this test over the TRH test as an index of prolactin reserve. Since the response of prolactin to metoclopramide (or other dopamine receptor antagonists) depends on endogenous dopaminergic control by the hypothalamus, it may be impaired in hypothalamic hyperprolactinemia while the response to TRH may be preserved (9). Unfortunately, the response of prolactin to TRH may also be impaired in some patients with hypothalamic disease, so this combination of tests is not a reliable way of differentiating pituitary from hypothalamic causes of hyperprolactinemia. Thus, like the TRH test, the metoclopramide test is perhaps most valuable as a research tool rather than as a routine test of clinical value. Recent studies with a new dopamine receptor antagonist, domperidone (which is thought not to cross the blood-brain barrier), have provided an interesting insight into dopaminergic control of other anterior pituitary hormones in hyperprolactinemia (11), but it is too early to assess its clinical usefulness in the differential diagnosis of hyperprolactinemia. A suggested protocol for the metoclopramide test (Fig. 2) is as follows. No preparation of the patient is required. Following a baseline blood sample metoclopramide 2.5 mg is given intravenously and blood is collected at 30 and at 60 min.

D. Cimetidine

During the course of clinical trials of the histamine H_2 receptor antagonist cimetidine in patients with peptic ulceration it was found that this drug was a

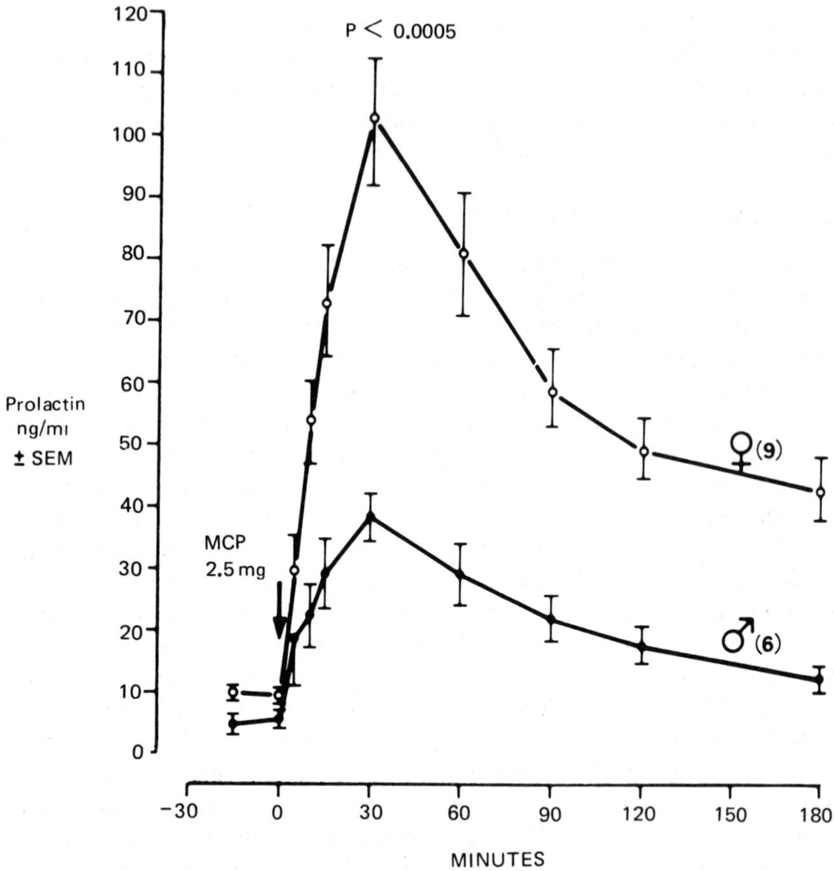

Figure 2 Stimulation of prolactin by intravenous metoclopramide (MCP) in six men and nine women. The peak response of prolactin was significantly higher in women than in men. (From Ref. 9.)

potent stimulator of prolactin. A recent study has made an extensive evaluation of its use in normo- and hyperprolactinemic patients (12), and although it confirms the prolactin-stimulating action of cimetidine, it does not claim that the test has any significant advantage over the TRH or metoclopramide stimulation tests.

III. PROLACTIN SUPPRESSION TESTS

Dopamine receptor agonists such as L-dopa and bromocriptine lower prolactin levels and it was thought that the prolactin response to a single dose of L-dopa

(250 or 500 mg) or bromocriptine (2.5 mg) might help differentiate between hyperprolactinemia of hypothalamic and pitutitary origin. However, it has become clear that these drugs act directly on the pituitary and suppress prolactin secretion in normal subjects and in hyperprolactinemic patients whether or not the patient has a pituitary tumor. These tests have no place in the routine investigation of disorders of prolactin secretion.

REFERENCES

1. Frantz AG, Kleinberg DL, Noel GL. Studies on prolactin in man. Recent Prog Horm Res 1972; 28:527–590.
2. Franks S, Brook CGD. Basal and stimulated prolactin levels in childhood. Horm Res 1976; 7:65–76.
3. Jacobs LS, Snyder PJ, Utiger RD, Daughaday WH. Prolactin response to thyrotrophin releasing hormone in normal subjects. J Clin Endocrinol Metab 1973; 36:1069–1073.
4. Jacobs HS, Franks S, Murray MAF, Hull MGR, Steele SJ, Nabarro JDN. Clinical and endocrine features of hyperprolactinaemic amenorrhoea. Clin Endocrinol 1976; 5:439–454.
5. Turkington RW. Phenothiazine stimulation test for prolactin reserve: the syndrome of isolated prolactin deficiency. J Clin Endocrinol Metab 1972; 34:247-249.
6. L'Hermite M, Vekemans M, Delvoye P, Nokin J, Robyn C. Prolactin studies in normal subjects. Proc R Soc Med 1973; 66:865–865.
7. Thorner MO, Besser GM, Hagen C, McNeilly AS. Introduction of a new stimulation test for prolactin: the sulpiride test: a comparison with other dynamic function tests. J Endocrinol 1974; 61:xxxii.
8. McNeilly AS, Thorner MO, Volans G, Besser GM. Metoclopramide and prolactin. Br Med J 1974; 2:729.
9. Judd SJ, Lazarus L, Smythe G. Prolactin secretion by metoclopramide in man. J Clin Endocrinol Metab 1976; 43:313–317.
10. Eskildson PC. Effect of metoclopramide and TRH on the release of prolactin in hypo- and hyper-thyroidism. Proceedings of the XIII Acta Endocrinologica Congress, Cambridge, England. Acta Endocrinol (Copenh) 1981; 97(Suppl 243), Abstract 415.
11. Scanlon MF, Rodriguez-Arnao MD, McGregor AM, Weightman D, Lewis M, Cook DB, Gomez-Pan A, Hull R. Altered dopaminergic regulation of thyrotrophin release in patients with prolactinomas: comparison with other tests of hypothalamic-pituitary function. Clin Endocrinol 1981; 14:133–143.
12. Gonzales-Villapando C, Szabo M, Frohman LA. Central nervous system-mediated stimulation of prolactin secretion by cimetidine, a histamine H_2-receptor antagonist: impaired responsiveness in patients with prolactin-secreting tumors and idiopathic hyperprolactinemia. J Clin Endocrinol Metab 1980; 51:1417–1424.
13. Franks S Prolactin. In *Hormones in Blood*, 3rd Ed, Academic, London, 1979, vol I. pp 280–332.

42
Posterior Pituitary Function

Peter H. Baylis
Royal Victoria Infirmary, Newcastle-Upon-Tyne, England

Three commonly used tests of vasopressin (AVP) secretion are described. Preparation of the patient is the same for all tests. They should be fasted from midnight but encouraged to drink water only. Tea, coffee, alcohol, and smoking are not allowed during this period. There are no common tests of oxytocin (OXT) secretion.

I. DEHYDRATION TEST (MODIFIED DASHE TEST)

A. Protocol

1. Prepare patient as above.
2. Patient to empty bladder and weigh.
3. Insert intravenous cannula in antecubital vein.
4. No fluids for 8 hr. Patient must be supervised. Dry food snacks are permitted.
5. Consider stopping test if there is weight loss of more than 5% of initial body weight.
6. Take blood and urine samples at time zero and intervals of 2 hr.
7. Urine–record volume and osmolality. Plasma–record osmolality.
8. After 8 hr, give desmopressin 40 μg intranasally or 2 μg intramuscularly.
9. Patient may drink.
10. Take urine and blood samples at intervals of 2 hr for further 4 hr.

B. Interpretation

1. Maximal urine osmolality after 8-hr dehydration greater than 700 mmol/kg—normal; less than 500 mmol/kg (hypotonic)—abnormal. 500-700 mmol/kg—borderline. Maximal plasma osmolality greater than 300 mmol/kg suggestive of cranial diabetes insipidus (CDI) or nephrogenic diabetes insipidus (NDI).
2. Patients with hypotonic urine
   a. Maximal urine osmolality after desmopressin greater than 650 mmol/kg—CDI.
   b. No increase in urine osmolality after desmopressin—NDI or primary polydipsia (PP).
   c. Other responses—borderline.

II. WATER LOAD

A. Protocol

1. Prepare patient as above.
2. Patient to empty bladder and weigh.
3. Insert intravenous cannula in antecubital vein.
4. Give water (20 ml/kg) to drink over 15 min.
5. Take blood and urine samples at time zero and at ½-hr intervals for 4 hr.
6. Urine—record volume and osmolality. Plasma—record osmolality.

B. Interpretation

1. Plasma osmolality should fall 8-12 mmol/kg to check absorption of water.
2. Minimum urine osmolality (usually at 2 hr after ingestion) less than 150 mmol/kg—normal.
3. Percentage of water load excreted by 4 hr is 80-120%—normal.

III. HYPERTONIC SALINE INFUSION

A. Protocol

1. Prepare patient as above.
2. Patient to empty bladder and weigh.
3. Insert two intravenous cannulae into each antecubital vein.
4. Infuse 5% saline at 0.06 ml/kg per minute for 2 hr.
5. Take blood samples at time zero and at ½ hr intervals.
6. Blood sample taken into ice-chilled tubes and plasma separated immediately in cold centrifuge. One aliquot for osmolality, another for AVP deep frozen at −30°C.

7. Note the time of thirst onset.

B. Interpretation

1. Normal response falls within shaded area of Figure 3a in Chapter 24.
2. NDI and PP patients fall in normal range (Chapter 24, Fig. 3a).
3. CDI patients fall to right of normal range.
4. Most patients with the syndrome of inappropriate antidiuresis (SIAD) have values to left of normal range.

43
Pancreatic Function

Peter H. Sönksen
St. Thomas' Hospital Medical School, London, England

The oral glucose tolerance test remains the most satisfactory dynamic test of endocrine pancreatic function and should be used wherever possible to establish or refute the diagnosis of diabetes mellitus. The WHO Expert Committee have put forward some recommendations for standardization of this procedure which are likely to be accepted worldwide.

The main indication for doing a dynamic test of endocrine pancreatic function (usually the oral glucose tolerance test) is when there is need to establish whether or not a patient has diabetes mellitus and the random and/or fasting blood glucose values leave this diagnosis in doubt. The recommended procedure for investigation of such patients is summarized in Chap. 31, p. 519.

An oral glucose tolerance test is indicated if the possible diagnosis of diabetes mellitus has been raised and is in doubt:

1. Random plasma glucose $\geqslant 8$ and < 11 mmol/liter
2. Fasting plasma glucose $\geqslant 6$ and < 8 mmol/liter
3. Random plasma glucose $\geqslant 11$ mmol/liter or fasting plasma glucose $\geqslant 8$ mmol/liter when the patient has *no* symptoms suggestive of diabetes mellitus *and no* other abnormal blood glucose concentrations documented

A standard 75-g glucose load is recommended for adults and 1.75 g/kg body weight (to a maximum of 75 g) for children. The glucose should be dissolved in 250–350 ml of water.

Formal dietary preparation is not recommended unless the diet consists of less than 125 g of carbohydrate per day. In such subjects at least 3 days of

Table 1 Glucose Concentration

	Venous whole blood	Capillary whole blood	Venous plasma
Diabetes mellitus (DM)			
Fasting	≥7.0 mmol/liter (≥1.2 g/liter)	≥7.0 mmol/liter (≥1.2 g/liter)	≥8.0 mmol/liter (≥1.4 g/liter)
and/or			
2 hr after glucose load	≥10.0 mmol/liter (≥1.8 g/liter)	≥11.0 mmol/liter (≥2.0 g/liter)	≥11.0 mmol/liter (≥2.0 g/liter)
Impaired glucose tolerance (IGT)			
Fasting	<7.0 mmol/liter (<1.2 g/liter)	<7.0 mmol/liter (<1.2 g/liter)	<8.0 mmol/liter (<1.4 g/liter)
and			
2 hr after glucose load	≥7.0–<10.0 mmol/liter (≥1.2–<1.8 g/liter)	≥8.0–<11.0 mmol/liter (≥1.4–<2.0 g/liter)	≥8.0–<11.0 mmol/liter (≥1.4–<2.0 g/liter)

preparation is advisable, during which the intake of carbohydrate is limited to 150 g per day.

The test should be performed after an overnight fast of 10–14 hr, although water is permitted. The first step is to take a fasting blood sample, after which the patient is given 75 g of glucose in water to be consumed in between 5 and 15 min. Special testing solutions are available for use instead of glucose. They consist of partial hydrolysates of cornstarch and are less likely to cause nausea but they are more expensive than glucose. Further blood samples are taken after glucose, at least a sample at 1 and 2 hr after the glucose load. Smoking must not be allowed during the test; the patient should be resting quietly throughout in either a chair or a couch. It is sensible to collect a urine sample before and 2 hr after the glucose load and to test these for glucose.

It must be borne in mind that many factors, including drugs, can affect the glucose tolerance test (1). Plasma or whole blood glucose must then be measured using a reliable and preferably specific glucose method (see Chap. 31).

It is recommended that in the absence of symptoms, at least one additonal abnormal blood glucose value is needed to confirm the diagnosis of diabetes mellitus [e.g., a 1-hr postglucose value of 11 mmol/liter (2.0 g/liter) or more during the first test or an elevated 2-hr or fasting glucose value on a subsequent occasion].

The criteria described in Table 1 may be used for pregnant women as well as for all patients with suspected diabetes, although different clinical action is necessary. It should be noted that the National Institutes of Health Diabetes Data Group has suggested that a separate set of criteria be used for pregnant women.

The WHO Committee note that even though the new criteria are more soundly based than earlier values, the cutoff levels remain somewhat arbitrary. Action to be taken in the case of individuals with values near the limits may be influenced by individual circumstances. They also emphasize that it is essential that patients with impaired glucose tolerance not be labeled as "normal" and returned to the comminity by default. They have an increased risk of worsening to diabetes and of developing atherosclerosis. Different courses of action will be necessary depending on age, obesity, and the presence of other diseases. During pregnancy, the treatment for impaired glucose tolerance should be the same as for diabetes.

I. INSULIN RESPONSES

Much of this has been covered in Chapter 31. Insulin responses must always be judged in relationship to (1) the prevailing glucose concentrations; (2) the age, weight, sex, and degree of obesity; and (3) other underlying conditions or treatment. The characteristic pattern of idiopathic (primary) diabetes is an inappropriately low insulin concentration in relation to the prevailing blood glucose, particularly in the early part of the test (0-30 min). A high fasting insulin and/or an exaggerated response to the glucose load always suggests secondary diabetes mellitus (acromegaly, hyperlipidemia, etc.).

II. THE STANDARDIZED MEAL

The glucose tolerance test has been justly criticized as being unphysiological. Insulin and glucose responses to mixed meals may be quite different from those of oral glucose. Although there is a strong case for using standardized meals in research studies examining the effect of treatment, their use as a diagnostic procedure cannot be recommended because of the lack of agreement on what should be used.

III. THE INTRAVENOUS GLUCOSE TOLERANCE TEST

Although less commonly used than the oral glucose tolerance test, the intravenous glucose tolerance test has at least two advantages:

1. The glucose load is administered intravenously and the result is thus independent of the rate of absorption from the gut (which can vary

considerably between individuals as well as from time to time in the same individual).
2. The result can be represented by a single number, the K value, which is directly related to the rate of fall of blood glucose after the glucose load. Having a single number as an index of glucose tolerance facilitates epidemiological studies both in terms of pooling results from a given group of patients as well as in assessing changes in glucose tolerance with time.

These advantages have to be compared with the disadvantages before deciding whether the intravenous or oral glucose tolerance test is appropriate for the circumstances under consideration. The disadvantages of the intravenous tolerance tests are:

1. More complex to execute; requires frequent blood samples and involves intravenous injection of 50% dextrose solution.
2. Bypasses gut and therefore independent of enteroinsular axis (less of a stimulus to insulin secretion).

The problem of repeated blood samples can easily be overcome by the use of an indwelling plastic cannula with a three-way tap. Great care must be exercised over the intravenous injection of 50% dextrose; any leakage from the vein into subcutaneous tissues is intensely painful, leads to much local swelling and often thrombophlebitis, and completely invalidates the test.

With these provisos the intravenous glucose tolerance test can be recommended. There are several variants described, but the simplest remains that described by Lundbaek (2) and the others offer little if any advantage. Preparation for the test is identical to that for the oral glucose tolerance test—at least 3 days on a diet containing at least 150 g/day of carbohydrate and an overnight fast of 10-14 hr during which intake of water is not restricted.

The patient is best rested on a couch or bed and the intravenous cannula inserted using local anesthetic. The cannula with three-way tap is flushed and kept filled with isotonic saline after insertion and after each blood sample. When the cannula is inserted and the patient is warm, rested, and relaxed, the fasting blood sample is taken and 50 ml of 50% dextrose for intraveous use is injected via a vein on the opposite arm. The injection is best carried out with a fairly wide bore needle; since dextrose is quite viscous, it is essential that the needle be well placed intravenously. The injection should take between 1 and 3 min and the timing of the test (with a stopwatch) should be started from the end of the injection. The patient should be asked what he or she feels when the injection is started. If the dextrose is going smoothly into the vein there is *no* pain and the only thing the patient will notice is a cool feeling at the site of injection. *Any local pain* or discomfort indicates extravasation of the dextrose and the injection should be stopped immediately and the test abandoned. After the injection has been accomplished, the arm should be placed behind the head or raised in the air, to reduce the risk of subsequent thrombosis.

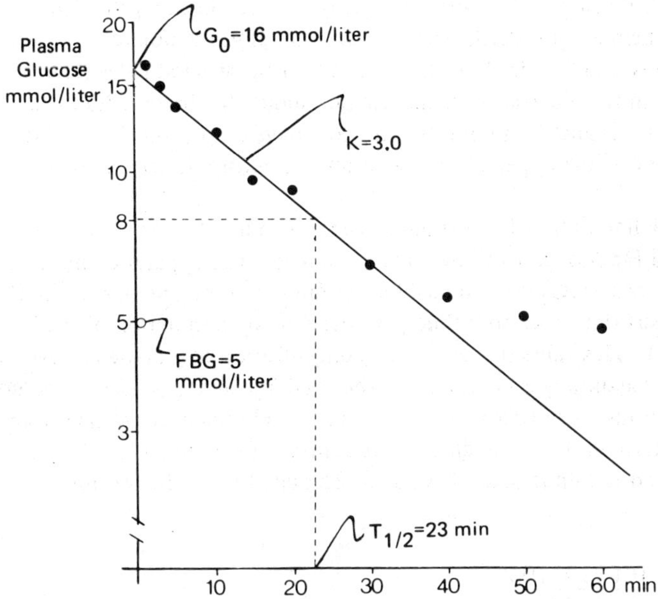

Figure 1 Intravenous glucose tolerance test in a 70 kg normal male: method of plotting data and calculating results (D.S. = 12.6 liters; 186 ml/kg).

The majority of patients feel a flush during or after the injection, which is greatest when the injection is rapid. It is not usually unpleasant, but the patient should be warned in advance that this may happen and be reassured that it is harmless and will only last a few seconds if it does happen. Blood samples are taken through the cannula at 1, 3, 5, 10, 15, 20, 25, 30, 40, 50, and 60 min for measurement of glucose (and if indicated, insulin).

IV. INTERPRETATION OF RESULTS

Blood or plasma glucose values are plotted against time on two-cycle semilog graph paper. When plotted in this manner, the data points tend to fall on a straight line and the "line of best fit" is drawn using a transparent ruler, ensuring that the ruler is placed such that it passes through the points with equal scatter on either side of the line (Fig. 1).

In normal subjects, where blood glucose concentration falls rapidly and may be back to the fasting value within 30 min, the linear portion of the data may only extend from 1-30 min (occasionally 1-20 min), in which case data points beyond the time when glucose has nearly reached "fasting" value should be ignored. On the other hand, in patients with diabetes, where blood glucose declines only slowly, all the points 1–60 min usually fall on a line and the line of best fit can take them all into consideration. Occasionally, the points at the very early part of the test tend to lie above the line of best fit; this indicates slow mixing of glucose in the glucose pool, and the line should be drawn with little consideration of the 1- and 3-min points. (It often pays to plot the data points in ink but to draw the line in pencil, so that if unsatisfactory, it can be erased and replaced.)

Having drawn a line of best fit, it should extend through the vertical axis at time 0 and extend far enough to allow $T_{1/2}$ to be read. The apparent concentration of glucose at time 0 (G_0) is obtained by extrapolating the line of best fit of blood glucose versus time back to 0 time (i.e., the time of completion of the injection of glucose). This value represents the concentration of glucose achieved in the glucose pool assuming even mixing of the total injected dose (25 g) and no loss through metabolism or urinary excretion. $T_{1/2}$ is obtained by reading from the graph the time when the blood glucose concentration had fallen to 50% of the G_0 value; if read in minutes, the K value is calculated from the formula.

$$K\ (\%/\text{min}) = \frac{0.693 \times 100}{T_{1/2}\ (\text{min})}$$

and represents the rate of fall of blood glucose, the units being percent per minute.

From the data can also be calculated the "apparent distribution space" (DS)–the volume of body fluid in which the 25 g (138.9 mmol) glucose dose is distributed, assuming the concentration of glucose to be uniform throughout.

$$DS\ (\text{liter}^{-1}) = \frac{138.9}{G_0 - \text{fasting blood glucose (mmol/liter)}}$$

For example, in a normal subject weighting 70 kg, the intravenous injection of glucose (25 g) resulted in a G_0 value of 16 mmol/liter, fasting blood glucose was 5 mmol/liter and $T_{1/2}$ was 23 min.

$$DS = \frac{138.9}{16 - 5} = \frac{138.9}{11} = 12.6 \text{ liters} = 180.4 \text{ ml/kg body weight}$$

$$K = \frac{0.693 \times 100}{23} = 3.0\%/\text{minute}$$

V. INTERPRETATION

The apparent distribution space is a good index of extracellular fluid volume. In normal subjects the K value is greater than 1.05, while in diabetic patients it is 1.0 or less. Values in the range 1.0–1.05 are considered borderline. Patients with diabetes mellitus and an elevated fasting blood glucose value have unequivocally low K values, generally in the range of 0.3–0.5% per minute. The test is of little or no value in this group since the low K value is as much a reflection of the elevated fasting blood glucose as any disturbance in glucose metabolism. Its use should for this reason be confined to those with normal or only marginal elevated fasting blood glucose values. The insulin response to an intravenous glucose load is normally very brisk, with peak insulin occurring at either the 1- or 3-min point, the insulin levels running closely parallel to the glucose values. With detailed analysis it is possible to demonstrate that the insulin response normally consists of two phases: an immediate response that occurs in the interval 0–10 min and a later response occurring between 10 and 60 min (3). In early diabetes the immediate peak is severely impaired or absent, while the second peak may be relatively preserved. The amount of insulin secreted in the interval 0–10 min is the major determinant of the subsequent rate of fall of blood glucose.

REFERENCES

1. National Diabetes Data Group. Classification and diagnosis of diabetes mellitus and other categories of glucose intolerance. Diabetes 1979; 28:1039–1057.
2. Lundbaek K. Intravenous glucose tolerance as a tool in definition and diagnosis of diabetes mellitus. Br Med J 1962; 1:1057–1513.
3. Turner RC, Schneelock B, Nabarro JDN. Biphasic insulin secretory response to intravenous Xylitol and glucose in normal, diabetic and obese subjects. J Clin Endocrinol Metab 1971; 33:301–307.

44
Pancreatic Tumors

Susan M. Wood and S. R. Bloom
Royal Postgraduate Medical School, Hammersmith Hospital, London, England

I. INSULIN TOLERANCE TEST FOR INSULINOMA

Insulin tolerance tests are used to demonstrate failure of insulin suppression diagnostic of these tumors only when fasting has not done so. Hypoglycemia is induced either by fish insulin, which is biologically active but does not cross-react with the human insulin assay, or by porcine insulin when C peptide is measured; in either case allowing endogenous β-cell activity to be tested. Insulin (0.1 U/kg body weight) is given as a bolus intravenous injection. Samples for glucose, insulin, and C peptide are taken at −30, −15, 0, 10, 20, 30, 60, 120, and 180 min. Other provocation tests, such as intravenous glucagon, tolbutamide, and oral leucine, are no longer used; the results were difficult to interpret and the procedures often produced dangerous hypoglycemia.

II. TESTS FOR GASTRINOMA

Both hypergastrinemia and gastric acid hypersecretion are necessary for the diagnosis of gastrinoma in a patient presenting with recurrent peptic ulceration.

(a) *Pentagastrin stimulation test–procedures.* After an overnight fast a naso-gastric tube is passed under x-ray control, and all gastric juice aspirated for a "resting secretion sample." Over the next hour aspiration continues to obtain a "basal secretion sample." Pentagastrin 6 μg/kg is then injected intramuscularly and 15-min samples aspirated over 1 hr. In Z–E–S (Zollinger-Ellison Syndrome) there is both hypersecretion of gastric juice ($>$100 ml/hr) and hyperacidity: basal acid output is $>$15 mEq/hr. The pentagastrin-stimulated secretion is often not much higher than the basal; the ratio of basal to maximal acid secretion usually exceeds 0.6.

(b) *Secretin test procedures.* Synthetic Squibb or pure natural porcine secretin 0.44 μg/kg (approximately 2 clinical units/kg) is given by rapid intravenous bolus. Venous samples for gastrin are taken before and at 2, 5, 7, 10, 15, 20, and 30 min after injection of secretin. Patients with gastrinomas respond by a prompt rise in plasma gastrin of at least 50% of the basal value; normally secretion lowers plasma gastrin. The test has been used to help differentiate patients with Zollinger-Ellison Syndrome from those with ulceration after vagotomy and primary hyperparathyroidism, both of which result in elevated basal gastrin. The rise after secretin is usually much less than in the tumor patients. The criteria for interpretation of positive secretin test responses vary in the literature owing probably to lack of conformity in the procedure and dosage used. The test's diagnostic value has therefore not been adequately assessed.

(c) *Calcium infusion procedure.* Calcium gluconate (15 mg/kg) is infused intravenously over 4 hr. Venous samples are taken before and hourly during infusion. In 80% of gastrinoma patients there is doubling of fasting gastrin levels by the fourth hour.

45
Calcium Homeostasis

Solomon Posen
University of Sydney, Sydney, Australia

I. THE ASSAY OF NEPHROGENOUS CYCLIC AMP (1)

Protocol. After an overnight fast (water may be taken ad libitum) the patient drinks 200 ml of water at 7 A.M. and a further 200 ml at 7.30 A.M. At 8 A.M. the patient empties his bladder and discards the urine. The patient then collects all urine voided during the next 2 hr. During this period the patient drinks as much water as possible to ensure an adequate urinary volume (some protocols call for 200 ml every 30 min). Blood (15 ml) is taken into an ethylenediaminetetraacetic acid (EDTA) tube in ice at 9 A.M. A final urine specimen is voided at 10 A.M. The 2-hr urine volume is noted and an aliquot is kept for cyclic AMP and creatinine assays. The blood is centrifuged as soon as possible after collection and the plasma kept at −20°C until assay.

Assay and Calculation of Results. Creatinine and cyclic AMP are measured in plasma and urine. Nephrogenous cyclic AMP is calculated according to the formula

$$\text{NcAMP} = \frac{(\text{UcAMP} \times \text{V}) - (\text{PcAMP} \times \text{C}_{\text{cr}})}{\text{C}_{\text{cr}}} \times 100$$

where NcAMP is the nephrogenous cyclic AMP (in nmol per 100 ml glomerular filtrate), UcAMP the concentration of urinary cyclic AMP (in nmol/ml), V the urine volume (in ml/min), PcAMP the plasma cyclic AMP (in nmol/ml), and C_{cr} the creatinine clearance (in ml/min).

Interpretation. The normal range of NcAMP is 0.29–2.81 nmol/100 ml GFR. The large majority of hyperparathyroid patients (primary or secondary) have values above the upper limit of the normai range.

Warning. This measurement becomes imprecise when the glomerular filtration rate is low (as in secondary hyperparathyroidism due to advanced renal failure).

II. STEROID SUPPRESSION TEST (2, 3)

Protocol. Cortisone acetate (50 mg three times a day) is given to the patient for 10 days. Blood is taken for serum calcium on days 0, 5, 8, and 10.

Interpretation. A fall in serum calcium to normal values with a rise into the abnormal range after steroid withdrawal constitutes strong evidence in favor of the presence of some disorder other than (or in addition to) hyperparathyroidism.

Warning. A course of corticosteroids administered in this fashion results in adrenal suppression. This is particularly important in patients about to be subjected to surgery. False positive tests occur (4, 5).

III. PARATHYROID HORMONE INFUSION (7, 8)

Protocol. Medications including supplemental calcium and vitamin D are withheld for 8 hr before and during the actual test. Food is withheld from midnight before each collection day until the end of the collection period. The patient is encouraged to drink water throughout the test (the original protocol recomments 250 ml of water by mouth each hour from 6 A.M. until noon, but many patients cannot drink these amounts).

Infusions are performed on two successive days. On day 1, 50 ml of 0.9% NaCl containing 0.5% human serum albumin are given between 9 and 9.15 A.M. Urine is collected hourly from 8 A.M. until noon. On day 2, 300 USP units parathyroid hormone (Lilly) are given in 50 ml of 0.9% NaCl containing 0.5% human serum albumin. Urine is again collected each hour from 8 A.M. until noon. Urinary creatinine, cyclic AMP, and inorganic phosphate are estimated in each specimen. (Several other injection schedules exist, but each involves urine collection on a "control" day as well as on a "test" day.)

Interpretation. In normal subjects and in patients with all forms of hypoparathyroidism (other than "classical" pseudohypoparathyroidism) the first two urine specimens after the infusion of bovine parathyroid hormone (PTH) show at least a 10-fold rise in urine cyclic AMP (expressed in nmol/mmol creatinine). The mean rise in normal subjects is 15-fold, with even greater rises in hypoparathyroidism of non-"pseudo" origin. In pseudohypoparathyroidism there is either no response or at most a twofold rise.

During the same infusion procedure, urinary phosphate rises by a mean of 230% in normal subjects (PTH day versus control day), whereas little or no rise is seen in pseudohypoparathyroid individuals. Urinary phosphate is more inconsistant even under control conditions than urinary cyclic AMP and there is much overlap between "pseudo" and other forms of hypoparathyroidism.

Warning. Lilly PTH is no longer being manufactured. New infusion techniques based on human PTH are currently being evaluated (6).

IV. PENTAGASTRIN STIMULATION TEST FOR MEDULLARY CARCINOMA OF THE THYROID (9, 10)

Protocol. No particular patient preparation is necessary, although the test is usually performed in the fasting state. Pentagastrin (Peptavlon, Ayerst) is given intravenously in 5 ml of normal saline at a dose of 0.5 μg/kg over a period of 5 sec. Blood is taken through an indwelling cannula from the opposite arm before the intravenous injection and at 1, 2, 3, 5, and 10 min afterwards. Plasma or serum may be used for calcitonin assay.

Interpretation. In normal subjects the calcitonin concentration does not exceed 200 pg/ml in any specimen. In patients suspected of suffering from medullary carcinoma a rise above this level is usually seen in the 1- to 5-min specimens. Occasionally, only one value is elevated.

Warning. Some subjects develop transient chest or upper abdominal pain immediately after pentagastrin injection. This usually subsides within 2 min.

REFERENCES

1. Broadus AE, Mahaffey JE, Bartter FC, Neer RM. Nephrogenous cyclic adenosine monophosphate as a parathyroid function test. J Clin Invest 1977; 60:771–783.
2. Dent CE. Cortisone test for hyperparathyroidism. Br Med J 1956; 1:230.
3. Dent CE. Some problems of hyperparathyroidism. Br Med J 1962; 2: 1419–1425.
4. Posen S, Kleerekoper M, Ingham JP, Hirshorn JE. Parathyroid hormone assay in clinical decision making. Br Med J 1976; 1:16–19.
5. Watson L, Moxham J, Fraser P. Hydrocortisone suppression test and discriminant analysis in differential diagnosis of hypercalcaemia. Lancet 1980; 1:1320–1325.
6. Slovik DM, Adams JS, Neer RM, Holick MF, Potts JT Jr. Deficient production of 1,25-dihydroxyvitamin D in elderly osteoporotic patients. N Engl J Med 1981; 305:372–374.
7. Chase LR, Melson GL, Aurbach GD. Pseudo-hypoparathyroidism: defective excretion of 3′,5′-AMP in response to parathyroid hormone. J Clin Invest 1969; 48:1832–1844.

8. Aurbach GD, Marcus R, Winickoff RN. Urinary excretion of 3′,5′-AMP in syndromes considered refractory to parathyroid hormone. Metabolism 1970; 19:799–808.
9. Rude RK, Singer FR. Comparison of serum calcitonin levels after a 1-minute calcium injection and after pentagastrin injection in the diagnosis of medullary carcinoma. J Clin Endocrinol Metab 1977; 44:980–983.
10. Wells SA Jr, Baylin SB, Lineham WM, Farrell RE, Cox EB, Cooper CW. Provocative agents and the diagnosis of medullary carcinoma of the thyroid gland. Ann Surg 1978; 188:139–141.

46
Sodium and Potassium Homeostasis

Eric A. Espiner
Christchurch Clinical School of Medicine, and Princess Margaret Hospital, Christchurch, New Zealand

It is essential that tests be adequately planned and executed if faulty interpretation is to be avoided. Laboratory requirements for sample collection should be ascertained in advance. Readers are referred to Chapter 26 for information on drugs and other factors affecting the renin-angiotensin-aldosterone axis in clinical practice.

I. PLASMA RENIN ACTIVITY (PRA)

Indications. In the diagnosis of hypertension (mineralocorticoid excess states such as primary aldosteronism, renal ischemia, renin-producing tumors). Also in the diagnosis of adrenocortical insufficiency, in assessing the adequacy of mineralocorticoid replacement treatment, and in the diagnosis of Bartter's syndrome and hyporeninemic syndromes. Most useful if done in conjunction with plasma aldosterone.

Patient Preparation. The patient's posture, salt intake, and drug treatment may profoundly alter PRA. Except in urgent situations, time of blood sampling should be standardized (e.g., 8-10 A.M.) because of the prominent diurnal rhythm in PRA. The following preparation should apply.

1. Nonessential drugs should be stopped at least 2 weeks before the test. If hypotensive drugs cannot be stopped, consider changing to prazosin and/or methyldopa treatment, since these drugs have less effect on the renin-angiotensin-aldosterone axis.

2. Patient reports to the laboratory between 8 and 10 A.M. with a 24-hr urine collection for Na and K excretion, collected over the previous 24 hr. This provides data on the subject's sodium intake. Urine aldosterone excretion may also be measured.
3. As well as blood for PRA, samples should be drawn for plasma aldosterone and plasma Na and K. In some cases, samples for plasma adrenocorticotropic hormone (ACTH) and cortisol may be necessary if adrenocorticortical insufficiency is suspected.
4. N.B. *Inpatients* should be made to walk for at least 30 min before sampling. Overnight supine (8 A.M.) and 10 A.M. erect (2 hr upright posture) conditions for PRA sampling may give additional information.

Interpretation. *Low* PRA is seen in mineralocorticoid excess syndromes, in many patients with essential hypertension, and in the elderly. *High* PRA is seen in adrenocortical insufficiency, fluid and salt-wasting syndromes, Bartter's syndrome, severe renal ischemia, malignant hypertension, and reninomas. High PRA values occur in neonates and in normal infants, particularly in the first year of life.

II. PLASMA ALDOSTERONE

Indications. In the diagnosis of primary aldosteronism and other forms of hypokalemic hypertension. For diagnosis of adrenocortical insufficiency, particularly where hypoaldosteronism is suspected. Most useful in conjunction with PRA.

Patient Preparation. As for PRA.

Interpretation. *High* plasma aldosterone is seen in primary aldosteronism. Elevated values also occur in secondary hyperaldosteronism, in stressed subjects, and sometimes in patients taking estrogen preparations. Potassium depletion may attenuate aldosterone secretion. *Low* plasma aldosterone is seen in adrenal insufficiency and hyporeninemic syndromes. Low values may also occur in normal subjects ingesting liberal salt or licorice.

III. RENIN STIMULATION TESTS

Indications. In the diagnosis of primary aldosteronism and other forms of hypokalemic hypertension. In the differential diagnosis of "low-renin" forms of hypertension. For the diagnosis of hyporeninemic hypoaldosteronism.

Sodium Deprivation

The patient is placed on a diet containing 10 mmol Na, 60–100 mmol of K daily. Drug therapy should be stopped 2 weeks previously and it is usually necessary to admit the patient to hospital.

If it is hazardous to stop hypotensive therapy, the treatment should be changed to either prazosin and/or methyldopa at least 2 weeks before testing. On the morning of the fifth day of salt restriction, blood for PRA is drawn at 8 A.M. after the patient has been supine overnight, and the test is repeated after 2 hr of ambulation at 10 A.M.

Urinary electrolyte excretion should be monitored to ensure that Na excretion is less than 20 mmol/per day on the day of renin sampling. Interpretation of results is helped by simultaneous assessment of plasma aldosterone, plasma Na, K, and creatinine, and urinary excretion of aldosterone.

Risks. Include postural hypotension and/or severe volume depletion, and hyperkalemia, particularly if *hypo*aldosteronism or other disorder of sodium wasting is suspected.

Interpretations. Depending on the PRA method, normal subjects show a three- to fivefold rise in PRA using the combined stimulation of salt restriction and upright posture. In primary aldosteronism the renin increment is small and does not rise above the normal range for ambulant normal subjects on normal diets, except when long-term diuretic (or spironalactone) therapy has been used. The renin response is less in the elderly (over 60 yr), in subjects habituated to a high-salt (>250 mmol) diet, in automatic insufficiency, and in hyporeninemic hypoaldosteronism.

Aldosterone. Plasma aldosterone should be double the upper limit of normal (normal 8 A.M. range 150–550 pmol/liter, 5–18 ng/per 100 ml; 40–100 ng/per 100 ml) after salt restriction. Urine aldosterone (acid labile metabolite) should be greater than 60 μg/per day (normal 5-20 μg/per day, 15–60 nmol/per day) on normal salt intake. The response is reduced in primary adrenal insufficiency, in subjects habituated to a high-salt diet, in autonomic insufficiency, and in hyporeninemic hypoaldosteronism.

Diuretic-Induced Volume Depletion

A variety of tests have been used. One convenient test is listed below:

The patient attends fasting between 8 and 9 A.M.

Blood is drawn for PRA, electrolytes, and aldosterone.

An intravenous injection of frusemide 40 mg is then given and the subject is asked to stand for 30 min when the tests are repeated.

Risks. The test should not be done in patients with marked potassium depletion.

Interpretation. PRA should rise to 1 ng/ml/per hour or more.

IV. SALT LOADING TESTS

Indications. To assess autonomy of aldosterone (or other mineralocorticoid) secretion and responsiveness of the renin-angiotensin-aldosterone axis to volume expansion.

Oral Salt

The subject is given a diet containing 200 mmol of Na daily for 4-5 days. NaCl capsules (1 g = 17 mmol Na) can be used to augment dietary sodium intake. The 8 A.M. plasma Na and K and aldosterone are measured before and on the morning of the fifth day of high salt intake. Interpretation is assisted by assessing 24-hr urinary electrolyte and aldosterone excretion before and on the last day of high salt.

Lesser sodium loads (e.g., 120 mmol Na) may be advisable if the patient has marked hypokalemia (plasma K < 2.8 mmol/liter) or if cardiac complications such as left ventricular failure are likely.

Interpretations. Plasma K should not fall below 3.5 mmol/liter. Urine aldosterone should be less than 8 μg per day, plasma aldosterone $<$5-7 ng per 100 ml.

Intravenous Saline: 4-hr Infusion of 2 Liters (Outpatient Test)

The patient attends at 8-8:30 A.M. An intravenous needle is inserted and blood is drawn for plasma aldosterone and electrolytes at 9 A.M. Two liters of 0.9 g% saline is then given over 4 hr (9 A.M.–1 P.M.) with the patient supine throughout. Plasma aldosterone and electroytes are repeated at 1 P.M.

Risks. Plasma K should be $>$2.8 mmol/liter prior to testing. The test should be done cautiously in those with cardiac or renal pathology.

Interpretation. Plasma aldosterone should fall to less than 5-7 ng/per 100 ml after saline.

Two-Day Infusion Test After Salt Restriction

This test combines a stimulatory test for PRA (low-salt diet for 5 days) and a suppressive test to assess aldosterone autonomy. An additional advantage is the ability to measure potassium clearance during the second day of salt infusion.

Patient Preparation. The patient is hospitalized and placed on a fixed metabolic balance diet containing 10 mmol of Na and 100 mmol of K daily. Dietary K (e.g., 40-80 mmol/per day) may need to be supplemented by K supplements. This diet is maintained throughout the 6-day period of assessment.

On the fifth day of the diet, blood samples are drawn for PRA (see Sec I.C., sodium deprivation). Two liters of 0.9 g% saline is then given intravenously from 10 A.M. to 2 P.M. on day 5 and repeated on day 6. The test is concluded after completion of the 24-hr urine at 8 A.M. on day 7.

Blood for aldosterone and electrolytes is drawn at 8 A.M. (overnight supine) on days 5, 6, and 7. Urinary electrolytes and aldosterone excretion are measured on days 5, 6, and 7.

Risks. Plasma K should be >2.8 by the morning of day 5 and >2.5 on the morning of day 6. Patients with cardiac or renal disease should be more closely monitored.

Interpretation. Plasma aldosterone should fall to <5-7 ng/100 ml on day 7 and urine aldosterone to <8 μg/day on day 6. The urine potassium discriminant $[(\Delta K/U_{Na}V)/(K^+)]$ should be <0.035 (1).

Fludrocortisone Suppression

The test can be done as an outpatient with the subject taking a normal diet. After a 24-hr collection is complete and blood has been drawn at 8-10 A.M. for electrolytes and plasma aldosterone, the subject takes 9α-fluorohydrocortisone 0.2 mg twice daily (0.4 mg/per day) for three successive days. Urine is again collected on the third day and the patient attends on the following day for repeated (8-10 A.M.) measurement of electrolytes and plasma aldosterone.

Risks. As for intravenous saline tests.

Interpretation. Plasma aldosterone should fall to less than 5 ng/per 100 ml: urinary aldosterone excretion should be less than 8 μg/per day on the third day of fluorocortisone.

V. MISCELLANEOUS

Plasma Aldosterone Response to 4-hr Erect Posture

Indications. In the differential diagnosis of primary aldosteronism.

Procedure. With the patient taking a normal Na diet (>100 mmol/per day) and off all drug therapy for at least 2 weeks, blood is drawn at 8 A.M. (overnight supine) for plasma aldosterone and cortisol. The patient is then asked to remain in the erect position until 12 noon, when a further blood sample for aldosterone and cortisol is drawn.

Interpretation. Plasma aldosterone either falls or shows no change in patients with adenoma, whereas a distinct rise occurs in patients with hyperplasia. Plasma cortisol may help to interpret stress effects, which may invalidate the test. Note that PRA response to 4-hr posture, while small or negligible in both categories, does not discriminate between the two pathologies.

Plasma Aldosterone Response to ACTH.

Indications. To assess glomerulosa function (e.g., in adrenocortical insufficiency and/or hypoaldosteronism). To distinguish patients with ACTH deficiency from those with primary adrenocortical insufficiency.

Procedure. Blood for cortisol and aldosterone is drawn at 10 A.M. just before an injection of ACTH (0.25 mg α1-24-ACTH or 25 U of ACTH) intramuscularly. Repeat samples are taken 1 hr later.

Interpretation. In normal subjects and most patients with ACTH deficiency, there is a distinct rise in plasma aldosterone (increment $>$10 ng/per 100 ml). No significant rise occurs in patients with primary adrenocortical insufficiency. The plasma cortisol response is likely to be reduced in both categories of adrenal insufficiency, although it may be normal in ACTH deficiency, particularly if partial or only recently acquired.

Similar results can be obtained using an intravenous ACTH stimulation test (e.g., 25 U of ACTH given over 8 hr, or alternatively 1.25 μg over 1 hr) if samples for steroids are drawn before and after the first hour of this stimulation.

Adrenal Vein Sampling for Aldosterone

Indications. To distinguish patients with primary aldosteronism due to adenomas from those with bilateral hyperplasia. To lateralize the disorder of primary aldosteronism prior to surgical intervention.

Procedure. This investigation should only be done if tests have conclusively proven that the patient has primary aldosteronism. The test requires a radiologist with experience in adrenal vein catheterization. Patients should be on normal sodium intake and preferably off drug therapy. Comparison of the sample's cortisol concentration with a simultaneously drawn peripheral blood sample is essential for interpretation of the catheter's position. We have also found that rapid fluctuations in aldosterone and cortisol secretion may seriously affect results. We now routinely perform the study under conditions of low-dose ACTH stimulation (1.25 μg of α1-24-ACTH per hour commencing 30 min before the femoral vein cannulation).

An ACTH infusion is commenced 30 min before the procedure is started and is maintained throughout the test at a constant rate (1.25 μg/hr). When the catheter is thought to be correctly placed in the adrenal vein, blood is allowed to drip (or is gently aspirated) into a collection tube for steroid analysis. At the same time blood is drawn from an arm vein and the time of sampling recorded. The procedure is repeated for the second adrenal vein. The patient should be carefully monitored in the next 24 hr (see below).

Risks. (1) Acute: the patient may experience sudden pain during injection of contrast into adrenal veins; (2) Adrenal hemorrhage or infarction: Continued pain and/or fever in the next 24 hr suggests adrenal infarction. If this is suspected, the patient should be confined to bed, and assessment made of blood pressure, and hormonal status.

Interpretation. Cortisol measurements are essential to confirm placement of the catheter. If the cortisol gradient (catheter sample/peripheral sample) is less than 1.5, interpretation is unreliable. Adrenal vein aldosterone/peripheral aldosterone ration >30 suggests ipsilateral adenoma. Adrenal vein aldosterone/peripheral aldosterone ratio <2-3 suggests contralateral adenoma, *provided* that the cortisol ratio on the sample is high (preferably >10).

Aldosterone/cortisol ratios, calculated from their concentrations in adrenal venous blood, are also useful in determining the site of adenoma. If an adenoma is present, the ratio should be at least five times greater than that for the contralateral gland. Again interpretation depends on the demonstration of a gradient for cortisol (adrenal vein cortisol/peripheral cortisol >1.5) in the catheter samples.

Renal Vein Renin Sampling

Indications. In the diagnosis of unilateral renal ischemia and renin secreting tumors and to predict blood pressure response to surgery in patients with renal ischemia.

Procedure. Patients are usually hospitalized and drugs stopped if possible. Renin suppressants (particularly beta-blocker drugs, clonidine, etc.) should be avoided and stopped at least 1 week before the test.

1. *Without stimulation.* Catheters are passed into each renal vein and their position confirmed by venography. Samples are then drawn from both right and left renal veins, as well as from a peripheral vein, for PRA.
2. *With stimulation.* Frusemide 80 mg is given orally the night before and again on the morning of the test.

Other stimulation tests include salt restriction (see Sec. I.A) and tilt-table stimulation. The procedure is otherwise the same as described in (1) above.

Interpretation. Renal vein renin ratios >1.5 (affected/unaffected) are consistent with unilateral ischemia. This is strengthened by the finding of suppressed renin secretion on the contralateral side. A very high renal vein ratio on one side with contralateral suppression is consistent with reninoma.

REFERENCE

1. Christlieb AR, Espiner EA, Amsterdam EA. The pattern of electrolyte excretion in normal and hypertensive subjects before and after saline infusions. Am J Cardiol 1971; 27:595-601.

47
Pheochromocytoma Testing

M. Gary Nicholls
Princess Margaret Hospital, Christchurch, New Zealand

I. SPECIFIC BIOCHEMICAL DIAGNOSIS

(a) *Urine collection* over 24 hr in 15 ml of 6 N HCl for the measurement of metanephrines, vanillylmandellic acid (VMA), and catecholamines. Avoid vigorous exercise and all medications (especially those containing catecholamines). Alternatively, collect urine after a symptomatic episode (express result per gram of urine creatinine) or over the nocturnal 12 hr. Make a note of all current medications to facilitate interpretation of the results.

(b) *Plasma catecholamines* (radioenzymatic assay). The patient must be resting supine for 30 min prior to withdrawal of blood through an indwelling venous catheter. Caffeine-containing drinks, smoking, and vigorous exercise, and all medications noted, should be avoided for 12 hr before the blood is drawn to allow accurate interpretation of the results. Blood drawn during a symptomatic episode or with a rise in arterial pressure should secure the diagnosis if initial results are equivocal.

(c) *Pharmacologic testing.* Provocative tests, using histamine, tyramine, or glucagon, are potentially dangerous, must not be used when the blood pressure is greater than about 170/100 mmHg, and are negative in 20% of patients with a pheochromocytoma. A positive response requires a rise in arterial pressure of at least 20/15 mmHg above that obtained during a standard cold-pressor test. A supranormal increase in plama catecholamines during glucagon stimulation may improve diagnostic accuracy. For the patient with arterial pressure readings above 170/110 mmHg, a decline of 35/25 mmHg or more with phentolamine (1-5 mg, i.v.) is suggestive of pheochromocytoma. A lack of specificity limits its usefulness, however, and the decline in arterial pressure can be fatal.

Where the usual biochemical indices are borderline, a catecholamine suppression test using either clonidine (1) or pentolinium (2) may be helpful—although widespread experience with these tests is lacking. For the former test, a single dose of oral clonidine 300 μg is given. In pheochromocytoma, plasma norepinephrine levels are not reduced at 3 hr, whereas a distinct fall is observed in non-pheochromocytoma subjects (1, 3). In that catecholamine production from a tumor may be variable with time, and since clonidine might reduce norepinephrine release from sympathetic nerve endings which are loaded with excess catecholamines, it would be no great surprise if circulating norepinephrine levels declined after clonidine in a few patients with pheochromocytoma (4). The pentolinium test uses an intravenous injection of 2.5 mg pentolinium. Pheochromocytoma patients show little or no fall in plasma catecholamine levels at 10 min, whereas a major decline (approximately 50% below baseline) is observed in those without a pheochromocytoma (2). Blood pressure measurements must be carried out after clonidine or pentolinium administration as hypotension has been reported, especially in patients already taking antihypertensive medications.

(d) *Platelet catecholamine content.* The possibility that platelet catecholamine content is a helpful aid to the diagnosis of pheochromocytoma has been raised (5, 6). These authors found markedly elevated platelet catecholamines in the pheochromocytoma patients compared to controls—using radioenzymatic techniques to measure catecholamine content. If confirmatory results are forthcoming from other laboratories, this could provide a relatively simple method of biochemical diagnosis.

REFERENCES

1. Bravo EL, Tarazi RC, Fouad FM, et al. Clonidine-suppression test. A useful aid in the diagnosis of pheochromocytoma. N Engl J Med 1981; 305: 623–626.
2. Brown MJ, Allison DJ, Jenner DA, et al. Increased sensitivity and accuracy of phaeochromocytoma diagnosis achieved by use of plasma-adrenaline estimations and a pentolinium-suppression test. Lancet 1981; 1:174–177.
3. Levinson PD, Lance BK, Kowarski AA, et al. Catecholamine suppression testing in patient with phaeochromocytoma and normal plasma catecholamine levels. Lancet 1983; 1:1216–1217.
4. Halter JB, Beard JC, Pfeifer MA, et al. Clonidine-suppression test for diagnosis of pheochromocytoma. N Engl J Med 1982; 306:49–50.
5. Feldman JM, Klatt C. Elevated platelet norepinephrine concentration in patients with pheochromocytoma. Clin Chim Acta 1981; 117:279–288.
6. Zweifler AJ, Julius S. Increased platelet catecholamine content in pheochromocytoma. A diagnostic test in patients with elevated plasma catecholamines. N Engl J Med 1982; 306:890–894.

Appendix: Practical Details and Reference Ranges for Hormone Assays

Richard A. Donald
Christchurch Clinical School of Medicine and Princess Margaret Hospital, Christchurch, New Zealand

EXPLANATORY NOTE

It is emphasized that the following ranges are intended only as a guide and to help the reader interpret both gravimetric and molar (International System or SI) units. Reference ranges, detection limits, assay precision and bias, standardization, and reporting times may vary considerably between different laboratories, as do sampling, storage, and transport requirements. It is important that all the relevant details be obtained from the local laboratory. In some countries (e.g., the United Kingdom, New Zealand) a nationwide hormone assay service with detailed instruction booklets is available.

Assay results may be meaningless or misleading if various factors affecting hormone secretion, the stability of the hormone in the sample, or drug effects are ignored. These factors have been discussed in detail in previous chapters and are briefly summarized in the following table, together with the major clinical indications for using hormone assays. Many protein and steroid hormone assays have an interassay coefficient of variation of 10-20%. For best results serial samples should be assayed together. It is most unwise to compare results from different laboratories, as assay standardization, procedure, and performance often vary considerably. Your local laboratory will generally provide error limits if requested and in return will expect correctly processed and labeled samples and requisition forms (see Chap. 11). Good liaison between the clinic and the laboratory benefits all concerned, including the patient.

Hormone	Adult reference range	Sampling precautions	Clinical indications
ACTH (corticotropin) Plasma	0–85 ng/liter (0–19 pmol/liter) >150 ng/liter follow-insulin hypoglycemia or metyrapone	Avoid stress; note time of sampling and details of steroid therapy; keep plasma frozen	Differentiation of primary and secondary adrenal insufficiency, differential diagnosis of Cushing's syndrome and monitoring response to treatment ACTH deficiency; cortisol assay cheaper
ADH: *see* Vasopressin			
Aldosterone Plasma	50–200 ng/liter (140–500 pmol/liter)	Stop all drugs 2 weeks if possible; take 10 A.M. ambulant sample with plasma electrolytes and urine electrolytes over previous 24 hr; keep plasma frozen; state blood pressure and plasma renin if known	Differential diagnosis of hypokalemic hypertension; localization of aldosterone adenoma; salt-wasting and hyporeninemic syndromes
Urine	3–20 μg/day (9–60 nmol/day)	Precautions as for plasma; request Na^+ K^+, creatinine on the 24-hr collection; acidify to pH 5 with HCl and take 20-ml aliquot	Also for plasma (except localization of adenoma) Urine assay easier and cheaper than plasma

Androstenedione Plasma	*Male*: 0.05–0.29 μg/100 ml (2–11 nmol/liter) *Female*: 0.05–0.35 μg/100 ml (2–13 nmol/liter)	Give therapy details and timing of sample	Differential diagnosis of hirsutism, virilization, androgenic adrenal or ovarian tumors
Angiotensin II Plasma	20–75 pg/ml (20–70 pmol/liter)	*See* Renin activity; keep plasma frozen	Renin assay generally an adequate substitute
Calcitonin Plasma	<0.1 μg/liter (<27 pmol/liter) or <1.0 μg/liter following provocative tests	Keep plasma frozen; consider taking samples from other family members and provocative tests (e.g., calcium infusion or whiskey)	Diagnosis of medullary carcinoma of the thyroid and monitoring response to treatment
Catecholamines Urine	<0.6 mol/day	Acidified urine essential; correct pH to 2 with HCl	Diagnosis of pheochromocytoma
VMA ratio	1.58–2.26 (0.41–1.16 in (pheochromocytoma)	As for urine	As for urine
Chorionic gonadotropin (hCG, βhCG) Plasma or serum	<2 IU hCG/liter	State clinical details drug or surgical therapy; store serum frozen	Detection and management of molar pregnancy, choriocarcinoma, testicular tumors; diagnosis of early and ectopic pregnancy and implantation disorders
Urine	<30 IU/day	First morning specimen; send 20-ml aliquot at ambient temperature	As for serum; commonly used in diagnosis of pregnancy

Hormone	Adult reference range	Sampling precautions	Clinical indications
Cortisol Plasma	80–300 μg/liter (8 A.M.) (210–830 nmol/liter) After dexamethasone 1 mg at midnight <100 nmol/liter After synacthen or insulin hypoglycemia; increment >300 nmol/liter (normal), <220 nmol/liter (subnormal)	Sample at 8 A.M. for deficiency states; 12 midnight for Cushing's syndrome; use manipulative tests, e.g., dexamethasone (Cushing's), Synacthen test (Addison's) insulin tolerance test (hypopituitrism); avoid stress, state drugs (especially steroids, contraceptives, phenytoin)	Diagnosis of Cushing's syndrome, Addison's disease, hypopituitrism, congenital adrenal hyperplasia, adrenal atrophy; check on therapeutic levels
Urine	30–170 μg/day (100–500 nmol/day)	Stop drugs if possible 2 days before; used with ACTH stimulation and dexamethasone suppression (see above)	Good screening test for Cushing's syndrome; adrenal insufficiency following ACTH stimulation
C Peptide Plasma	0.9–1.5 μg/liter (300–500 pmol/liter)	Give therapy details; store plasma deep frozen	Diagnosis of residual pancreatic function in insulin-treated diabetics, insulinoma, and factitious hypoglycemia
Dehydroepiandrosterone (DHA) Urine	<100 μmol/day in basal state <5 μmol/day after 3 days dexamethasone suppression	Acidify to pH 2–3 with HCl; store at 4°C or below	Diagnosis of DHA secreting adrenal or ovarian tumors

Dihydrotestosterone (DHT) Plasma	Contact local laboratory	Take baseline and sample 48 hr post-1500 IU hCG	Differential diagnosis of ambiguous genitalia and 5α-reductase deficiency
Epinephrine (adrenaline) Plasma	25–150 ng/liter (140–820 pmol/liter)	Avoid smoking, caffeine 12 hr beforehand; fast overnight and resting; take sample 30 min after inserting i.v. line and again 10 min later, (standing); note drug therapy; special collection tubes required	Diagnosis of pheochromocytoma (urine catechols and VMA preferable as routine screening tests
Estradiol-17β Plasma	*Male*: <82 ng/liter (<300 pmol/liter) *Female*: follicular 4.9–41 ng/100 ml; luteal 12–22 ng/100 ml; menopausal <5.4 ng/100 ml	Menstrual and oral contraceptive details essential	Assessment of ovarian function, ovarian response in infertile women treated with gonadotropins, and diagnosis of precocious puberty and estrogen secreting tumors
Estrogens	*Male*: 5–40 nmol/day *Female*: premenopausal 20–300 nmol/day; postmenopausal 10–55 nmol/day; children <10 years: 0–59 nmol/day		
Urine Nonpregnancy	Risk of ovarian hyperstimulation of estrogen output more than doubles or is >500 nmol in 24 hr after hPG	As for plasma; correct pH to 2–3 with HCl; store at 4°C or less	As for plasma estradiol

Hormone	Adult reference range	Sampling precautions	Clinical indications
Pregnancy	Refer to reference chart from local laboratory	5-ml aliquot of a 24-hr specimen; no preservatives required; corticosteroids and ampicillin interfere; repeated sampling necessary	To monitor fetoplacental function during the third trimester of pregnancy
Follicle stimulating hormone (FSH) Plasma	*Male*: 1–6 IU/liter *Female*: Premenopausal 1–10 IU/liter, postmenopausal >15 IU/liter	Must state age, sex, last menstrual period, contraceptive or sex steroids; plasma stable at ambient temperature 3–4 days	Investigation of hypogonadism, delayed puberty, infertility, amenorrhea, assessment of hypothalamic-pituitary function (LHRH stimulation generally unnecessary)
Gastrin	30–120 ng/liter (15–60 pmol/liter)	Fast overnight; details of acid secretion test assist interpretation; keep plasma frozen	Diagnosis of the Zollinger-Ellison syndrome
Glucagon Plasma	0–120 ng/liter (0–34 pmol/liter)	Store plasma at –20°C; if anticoagulated with EDTA, trasylol or benzamidine probably unnecessary; do simultaneous blood glucose and state drugs	Diagnosis of glucagon secreting tumors
Growth hormone (hGH somatotropin) Plasma	0–5 μg liter (0–10 mU or 0–238 pmol/liter) Response to stimulation tests >20 μg/liter (adults); >7 μg/liter (prepubertal children) (Chaps. 21–40)	Patient resting and unstressed; multiple sampling and glucose suppression test useful (acromegaly); stimulation tests (e.g., hypoglycemia, sleep) essential if hGH deficiency suspected)	Diagnosis acromegaly, gigantism, and response to therapy; differential diagnosis of short stature and assessment of pituitary function

17α-Hydroxyprogesterone Plasma	<3 μg/liter (<10 nmol/liter)	State details of glucocorticoid therapy; some laboratories offer blood spot assays for neonatal screening; sample should be taken >48 hr after birth; keep plasma frozen	Diagnosis congenital adrenal hyperplasia and monitoring response to treatment
Insulin Plasma	0–20 μU/ml 0–20 mU/liter (0–150 pmol/liter)	Plasma glucose must be taken simultaneously; refer to Chaps. 32 and 44 manipulative procedures; state drug therapy; antibodies following insulin therapy interfere; keep plasma frozen	Diagnosis of insulinoma, or nesidioblastosis; occasionally used in the early diagnosis of diabetes (during IVGTT)
Luteinizing hormone (LH, ICSH) Plasma	*Male and female*: 1–8 IU/liter *Female* (midcycle): 8–50 IU/liter; postmenopausal >10 IU/liter	*See* FSH; note that hCG crossreacts in assay and very high results in pregnancy; high values at midcycle, hence date of last period important	*See* FSH; can be substituted for CG assay if this is not available for diagnosis of trophoblastic tumors
Norepinephrine (noradrenaline) Plasma	100–850 ng/liter 590–5000 pmol/liter	*See* Epinephrine	*See* Epinephrine
Normetanephrine and metanephrine Urine	<1.0 mg/day	Correct pH of urine to 2 with HCl	*See* Epinephrine

Hormone	Adult reference range	Sampling precautions	Clinical indications
17-Oxogenic steroids (17-OGS) Urine	*Male*: 11–26 mg/day (30–85 μmol/day) *Female*: 3–20 mg/day (20–50 μmol/day expressed as cortisol)	Acidify to pH 2 with HCl; 200-ml aliquot desirable if KS and AGS also required; state steroid and drug therapy (penicillins may interfere)	Assessment of adrenocortical function; diagnosis of congenital adrenal hyperplasia; differential diagnosis of Cushing's syndrome and ACTH deficiency (response to metyrapone)
17-Oxosteroids (17-OS) Urine	*Male*: 11–30 mg/day (38–104 μmol/day) *Female*: 3–20 mg/day (10–70 μmol/day expressed as DHA)	As for 17-OGS	Differential diagnosis hirsutism and virilization; an obsolescent test (*see* Androstenedione, DHA, Testosterone)
Oxygenation index (11-desoxy/11-oxy ratio)	<0.5	As for 17-OGS; unreliable in first week of life	Diagnosis of 11-hydroxylase deficiency; assessing adequacy of metyrapone blockade
Pancreatic polypeptide (PP) Plasma	<415 ng/liter (<100 pmol/liter) >300 pmol/liter abnormal	Patient must be fasting; keep plasma frozen	Diagnosis of pancreatic endocrine tumors

Parathyroid hormone Plasma	Very antiserum dependent; check with local laboratory	Simultaneous serum calcium, albumin, phosphate, and renal function results necessary for interpretation; keep plasma frozen	Investigation of primary hyperparathyroidism; differential diagnosis of hypercalcemia or hypocalcemia
Placental lactogen Plasma	Refer to reference chart (see Chap. 33)	Pregnancy details essential; serial sampling is important	Monitoring placental function during the third trimester of pregnancy
Pregnanediol Urine	Anovulatory and follicular 0.1–1 mg/day (0.3–3 μmol/day) Luteal phase (postovulatory) 2.0–12.2 mg/day (8–38 μmol/day)	50 ml urine (random sample); correct pH to 2–3 with HCl; store at 4°C; sample on day 21 of cycle or 17–20 days after clomiphene dose; state last menstrual period and drugs; correct for creatinine	Assessment of ovulation and corpus luteum function in infertility
Pregnanetriol Urine	*Male*: 1.9–4.1 mg/day (5.6–12.2 μmol/day) *Female*: 0.8–2.9 mg/day (2.4–8.6 μmol/day)	State details of steroid therapy; send 50-ml aliquot of a 24-hr collection	Diagnosis of congenital adrenal hyperplasia and assessing response to treatment

Hormone	Adult reference range	Sampling precautions	Clinical indications
Progesterone Plasma	Anovulatory and follicular 0.16 μg/100 ml (<5 nmol/liter) Luteal phase (postovulatory) >25 nmol/liter	Time of sampling and menstrual and drug history as for pregnanediol; some laboratories will measure salivary progesterone	As for pregnanediol
Progesterone-17-α-hydroxy: *see* 17α-hydroxyprogesterone			
Prolactin Plasma	Normal *Male*: 0–15 μg/liter *Female*: 0–20 μg/liter (0–950 pmol/liter) *Male*: 50–250 mIU/liter *Female*: 50–400 mIU/liter Borderline *Male*: 250–400 mIU/liter *Female*: 400–500 mIU/liter	Avoid stress; clinical and drug details vital; phenothiazine derivatives, butyrophenones, rauwiloid, methyldopa, metoclopramide, oral contraceptives, opiates, TRH, etc. cause hyperprolactinemia, also hypothyroidism and renal failure; repeat sample if result borderline	Investigation of galactorrhea, amenorrhea, hypogonadism, infertility; differential diagnosis of pituitary tumors; assessment of hypothalamic-pituitary function and response to treatment of prolactinomas

Renin activity (PRA) Plasma	10 A.M. standing 500–3500 ng/liter/hr (0.38–2.69 nmol/liter/hr)	Stop nonessential drug therapy 2 weeks before; collect 24-hr urine for Na and K; sample at 10 A.M. (patient ambulant); keep plasma deep frozen	Etiology of hypertension (especially primary aldosteronism), localizing renal ischemic disease, diagnosis and treatment of adrenocortical insufficiency, diagnosis Bartter's syndrome
Sex hormone binding globulin (SHBG) Plasma	*Male*: 10–48 nmol/liter *Female*: 48–100 nmol/liter	State time, menstrual and pregnancy status; mention drugs, particularly oral contraceptives	Hirsutism and virilization; monitoring estrogen therapy in males with cancer; indirect assessment of "free testosterone"
Testosterone Plasma	*Male*: 2.56–10.84 μg/liter (9–38 nmol/liter) *Female*: 0.14–0.90 μg/liter (0.5–3 nmol/liter)	Mention drugs; may be helpful to use with hCG stimulation, dexamethasone suppression and SHBG assessment	Diagnosis of hypogonadism and delayed puberty in males, hirsutism or virilization in females, precocious puberty, testicular feminization
Thyroglobulin	Check with local laboratory	Clinical details regarding extent of residual normal and neoplastic thyroid tissue are essential	To test for the adequacy of ablation of thyroid carcinoma and differential diagnosis of thyroid and other carcinomas

Hormone	Adult reference range	Sampling precautions	Clinical indications
Thyroid stimulating hormone (TSH) Plasma	0–5 mU/liter	State therapy: thyroid surgery, irradiation, and drugs; also available as a blood spot test in neonates; plasma stable at ambient temperature 3–4 days	Diagnosis of hypothyroidism; differential diagnosis of hypothyroidism and hypopituitrism; in association with TSH releasing hormone stimulation, diagnosis of borderline thyrotoxicosis and hypopituitrism
Thyroxine (T_4) Plasma	35–100 μg/liter (55–140 nmol/liter)	Markedly affected by estrogens (oral contraceptives, pregnancy) and drugs (phenytoin) which influence thyroxine binding; can be corrected by assessing "TBG binding ratio" or "T_3 resin uptake"; also available as a blood spot test in neonates	Diagnosis of hyperthyroidism or hypothyroidism (most useful screening test); monitoring response to T_4 (but not T_3) therapy
Triiodothyronine (T_3) Plasma	0–78–1.76 μg/liter (1.2–2.7 nmol/liter)	State age, whether there is acute severe nonthyroidal illness or malnutrition (above factors lower T_3)	A confirmatory test for hyperthyroidism if T_4 result borderline; differential diagnosis of exophthalmos
Vasoactive intestinal peptide (VIP)	$<$60 ng/liter ($<$20 pmol/liter) $>$60 pmol/liter abnormal	Patient fasting	Pancreatic tumors or ganglioneuroma secreting VIP

Vasopressin (AVP, antidiuretic hormone)	1–5 ng/liter (0.9–4.6 pmol/liter)	Stop all drugs if possible; plasma and urine osmolality should be recorded at same time; keep plasma frozen	Diagnosis of diabetes insipidus and inappropriate ADH syndrome; plasma/urine osmolalities cheaper and generally as informative
Vitamin D (25 OH D_3)	4–32 μg/liter (10–80 nmol/liter)	State calcium and phosphate albumin values and give therapy details	Diagnosis of vitamin D deficiency or toxicity

Note: Some rounding of numbers has occurred in the conversion of gravimetric to SI units. The implied conversion factors are therefore not exact.

Sources: *Specialised Assay Services for Hospital Laboratories* (provided by the British Supraregional Assay Service), 3rd ed, Stitch SR, Hobbs J (eds). University Printing Service, Leeds, 1980. *Handbook and Protocols for Hormone Assays*, National Hormone Assay Service (New Zealand). Issued by the National Hormone Committee (Medical Research Council) and the Department of Health, New Zealand, 1980. Ratcliffe JG. Hormone assays. Medicine: Endocrine Disorders 1982; 6:348–357.

Author Index

Numbers in parentheses are reference numbers and indicate that an author's work is referred to although the name is not cited in the text. Italic numbers give the page on which the complete reference is listed.

C

D

E

F

H

I

J

K

L

N

O

Q

R

U

V

W

Y

Z

Subject Index

A

D

H

J

K

L

M

P

R

T

X

Y

Z

ABOUT THE BOOK

Comprehensive, authoritative, and completely up to date, this timely work provides a practical guide to the diagnosis of *Endocrine Disorders*, examining the applications, interpretation, and limitations of the tests currently in use. With this unique resource, it is now possible to develop more effective diagnostic strategies, allowing improved treatment and saving valuable time and money.

In concise papers by experts from around the world, *Endocrine Disorders* stimulates cooperation between clinical and laboratory personnel with an informative overview of methodology . . . illustrates the background to the various investigative procedures through a discussion of pathophysiology . . . and provides how-to-do-it details of commonly used dynamic testing procedures—all presented with a variety of helpful features for enhanced clarity and simplicity.

Endocrine Disorders serves equally well in the office, laboratory, research library, and classroom, providing an unmatched resource for endocrinologists, pediatricians, gynecologists, internists, laboratory personnel involved in endocrine testing and organ imaging, and medical students.

ABOUT THE EDITOR

RICHARD A. DONALD is Endocrinologist, and Professor of Medicine at the Christchurch Clinical School of Medicine, Christchurch, New Zealand. He received the M.D. degree (1966) from the University of Otago, New Zealand and the Ph.D. degree (1969) from the University of London, England. His research interests include the radioimmunoassay of peptide hormones and in vivo and in vitro studies with hypothalamic releasing hormones, and he has published over 100 papers in the professional literature. In addition to his other duties, Dr. Donald serves as Chairman of the New Zealand Medical Research Council subcommittees responsible for the National Hormone Assay Service and the distribution of growth hormone and gonadotrophins. Dr. Donald is a Fellow of the Royal Australasian College of Physicians and is a member of the New Zealand Endocrine Society, the Endocrine Society of Australia, and the Fertility Society of Australia.